MANUAL OF
VASCULAR DISEASES
Second Edition

MANUAL OF
VASCULAR DISEASES
Second Edition

Editors

Sanjay Rajagopalan, MD, FACC, FAHA
John W. Wolfe Professor of Cardiovascular Medicine
Co-Director, Cardiovascular MR/CT Imaging Program
Section Director, Vascular Medicine
Department of Cardiovascular Medicine
The Ohio State University Medical Center
Columbus, Ohio

Steven M. Dean, DO, FACP, RPVI
Associate Professor of Medicine
Clinical Associate Professor
Program Director Vascular Medicine, Department of Cardiovascular Medicine
The Ohio State University Medical Center
Columbus, Ohio

Emile R. Mohler III, MD
Associate Professor of Medicine
University of Pennsylvania School of Medicine
Director, Vascular Medicine
University of Pennsylvania Health System
Philadelphia, Pennsylvania

Debabrata Mukherjee, MD, MS, FACC
Professor
Department of Internal Medicine/Cardiology
Texas Tech University
Chief, Cardiovascular Medicine
Department of Internal Medicine/Cardiology
Texas Tech University Hospital
El Paso, Texas

Wolters Kluwer | Lippincott Williams & Wilkins
Health
Philadelphia · Baltimore · New York · London
Buenos Aires · Hong Kong · Sydney · Tokyo

Acquisitions Editor: Frances DeStefano
Product Manager: Leanne McMillan
Production Manager: Alicia Jackson
Senior Manufacturing Manager: Benjamin Rivera
Marketing Manager: Kimberly Schonberger
Design Coordinator: Holly McLaughlin
Production Service: SPi Global

Printed in China

Library of Congress Cataloging-in-Publication Data
Manual of vascular diseases / editors, Sanjay Rajagopalan ... [et al.]. —2nd ed.
     p.; cm.
  Includes bibliographical references and index.
  ISBN 978-1-60913-422-8
  1. Blood-vessels—Diseases—Handbooks, manuals, etc. I. Rajagopalan, Sanjay.
  [DNLM: 1. Vascular Diseases—diagnosis. 2. Vascular Diseases—therapy. WG 500]

  RC691.M17   2011
  616.1'3—dc22

                                                                                          2011007850

Care has been taken to confirm the accuracy of the information presented and to describe generally accepted practices. However, the authors, editors, and publisher are not responsible for errors or omissions or for any consequences from application of the information in this book and make no warranty, expressed or implied, with respect to the currency, completeness, or accuracy of the contents of the publication. Application of the information in a particular situation remains the professional responsibility of the practitioner.

The authors, editors, and publisher have exerted every effort to ensure that drug selection and dosage set forth in this text are in accordance with current recommendations and practice at the time of publication. However, in view of ongoing research, changes in government regulations, and the constant flow of information relating to drug therapy and drug reactions, the reader is urged to check the package insert for each drug for any change in indications and dosage and for added warnings and precautions. This is particularly important when the recommended agent is a new or infrequently employed drug.

Some drugs and medical devices presented in the publication have Food and Drug Administration (FDA) clearance for limited use in restricted research settings. It is the responsibility of the health care provider to ascertain the FDA status of each drug or device planned for use in their clinical practice.

To purchase additional copies of this book, call our customer service department at (800) 638-3030 or fax orders to (301) 223-2320. International customers should call (301) 223-2300.

Visit Lippincott Williams & Wilkins on the Internet: at LWW.com. Lippincott Williams & Wilkins customer service representatives are available from 8:30 am to 6 pm, EST.

I would like to dedicate this edition to my wife Kyle and my wonderful children Tejas and Shreyas. All three of them are intimately familiar with this edition as I have had to take time that I would have ordinarily spent with them to writing and editing chapters for this book. I would also like to thank my parents (Narasimhan and Shanthi Rajagopalan) and my uncle and aunt (Narasimhan and Saroja Ranganathan) who continue to inspire me and find the balance between work and play.

Sanjay Rajagopalan

To my wife and daughter, Jennifer and Annie Dean, as well as my parents, Merrell and Sherma Dean, for their unyielding support, tolerance, and love.

Steven Dean

To my family for their patience, understanding, and support throughout this writing and many other endeavors.

Emile R. Mohler

To all the outstanding faculty, fellows, residents, and students I have worked with throughout the years. I am grateful to them for sharing their insight, thoughts, and talents.
To Suchandra with love.

Debabrata Mukherjee

Aamer Abbas, MD, FACC
Assistant Professor
Interventional Cardiologist
Department of Internal Medicine/
   Cardiovascular Diseases
Texas Tech University
Paul L. Foster School of Medicine
Director
Cardiac Cath Lab
Department of Cardiology/Vascular
   Medicine
University Medical Center
El Paso, Texas

Shadi Abu-Halimah, MD
Senior Fellow
Department of Surgery
Division of Vascular Surgery
University of North Carolina
   at Chapel Hill
Chapel Hill, North Carolina

Anil K. Agarwal, MD
Professor of Internal Medicine
Division of Nephrology
The Ohio State University
Director of Interventional Nephrology
Division of Nephrology
The Ohio State University Medical
   Center
Columbus, Ohio

Robert Bahnson, MD, FACS
Dave Longa-berger Chair in Urology
Department of Urology
Ohio State University
Columbus, Ohio

Siddharth Bhende, MD
Vascular Surgery Fellow
Department of Vascular Surgery
Ohio State University Medical Center
Columbus, Ohio

Quinn Capers IV, MD, FACC, FSCAI
Associate Dean, Admissions
College of Medicine
Associate Professor and Director
Peripheral Vascular Interventions
Department of Cardiovascular Medicine
Richard Ross Heart Hospital
The Ohio State University
Columbus, Ohio

Teresa L. Carman, MD
Assistant Professor
Department of Medicine
Case Western Reserve University
   School of Medicine
Director, Vascular Medicine
Harrington-McLaughlin Heart &
   Vascular Institute
University Hospitals Case Medical
   Center
Cleveland, Ohio

Leslie Cho, MD
Director, Women's Cardiovascular
   Center
Section Head, Preventive Cardiology
   and Rehabilitation
Robert and Suzanne Tomsich
   Department of Cardiovascular
   Medicine
Cleveland Clinic
Cleveland, Ohio

Vineet Chopra, MD
Assistant Professor
Department of General Internal
   Medicine
University of Michigan
Ann Arbor, Michigan

Mark A. Crowther, MD, MSc, FRCPC
Professor
Department of Medicine
McMaster University
Chief
Department of Laboratory Medicine
St. Joseph's Healthcare and Hamilton
   Health Sciences
Hamilton, Ontario, Canada

Steven M. Dean, DO
Clinical Associate Professor
Department of Cardiovascular Medicine
The Ohio State University Medical
   Center
Columbus, Ohio

Rekha Durairaj, MD
Postdoctoral Research Fellow
Davis Heart and Lung Research
   Institute
The Ohio State University
Columbus, Ohio

Jonathan L. Eliason, MD
Assistant Professor of Surgery
Section of Vascular Surgery
University of Michigan-Cardiovascular
    Center
University of Michigan
Ann Arbor, Michigan

Sean J. English, MD
Research Fellow
Department of Surgery
University of Michigan Health System
Ann Arbor, Michigan

Mark A. Farber, MD
Associate Professor
Departments of Surgery and Radiology
University of North Carolina
Director
Center for Heart and Vascular Care
Chapel Hill, North Carolina

James B. Froehlich, MD, MPH
Associate Professor
Department of Internal Medicine
University of Michigan
Clinical Associate Professor
Department of Internal Medicine
University of Michigan Medical
    Center
Ann Arbor, Michigan

Michael R. Go, MD
Assistant Professor
Department of Surgery
Division of Vascular Diseases
    and Surgery
The Ohio State University
Columbus, Ohio

Justin B. Hurie, MD
Fellow
Section of Vascular Surgery
University of Michigan
Ann Arbor, Michigan

Michael R. Jaff, DO
Associate Professor
Department of Medicine
Harvard University
Medical Director
Vascular Center
Massachusetts General Hospital
Boston, Massachusetts

Wael Jarjour, MD, FACP
Associate Professor
Department of Internal Medicine
The Ohio State University
Division Director of Immunology/
    Rheumatology
Department of Internal Medicine
The Ohio State University Medical
    Center
Columbus, Ohio

Joshua Joseph, MD
Internal Medicine Resident
Department of Internal Medicine
Yale University
Yale-New Haven Hospital
New Haven, Connecticut

Maria Litzendorf, MD
Vascular Surgery Fellow
Department of Vascular Diseases
    and Surgery
Ohio State University
Columbus, Ohio

Gregory Lowe, MD
Chief Resident
Department of Urology
Ohio State University Medical Center
Columbus, Ohio

Matthew A. Mauro, MD, FACR, FSIR, FAHA
Ernest H. Wood Distinguished
    Professor of Radiology and Surgery
Chairman, Department of
    Radiology
University of North Carolina School
    of Medicine at Chapel Hill
Chapel Hill, North Carolina

Georgeta Mihai, PhD
Research Assistant Professor
Department of Cardiovascular
    Medicine
The Ohio State University
Columbus, Ohio

Marc E. Mitchell, MD
James B. Hardy Professor
    and Chairman
Department of Surgery
University of Mississippi Medical
    Center
Jackson, Mississippi

Emile R. Mohler III, MD
Associate Professor of Medicine
University of Pennsylvania School
  of Medicine
Director, Vascular Medicine
University of Pennsylvania Health
  System
Philadelphia, Pennsylvania

Debabrata Mukherjee, MD, MS
Professor
Department of Internal Medicine/
  Cardiology
Texas Tech University
Chief
Cardiovascular Medicine
Department of Internal Medicine/
  Cardiology
Texas Tech University Hospital
El Paso, Texas

Shane Parmer, MD
Director of Vascular Services
Department of Vascular Surgery
Marietta Memorial Hospital
Marietta, Ohio

Sanjay Rajagopalan, MD
Wolfe Professor of Medicine
  and Radiology
Co-Director, Cardiovascular MR/CT
  Imaging Program
Director, Vascular Medicine
  Program
Department of Cardiovascular
  Medicine
The Ohio State University Medical
  Center
Columbus, Ohio

Stanley Rockson, MD
Allan and Tina Neill Professor of
  Lymphatic Research and
  Medicine
Department of Medicine
Division of Cardiovascular
  Medicine
Stanford School of Medicine
Stanford, California

Bhagwan Satiani, MD, MBA, FACS
Professor of Clinical Surgery
Department of Surgery
Division of Vascular Diseases and
  Surgery
The Ohio State University
Medical Director, Vascular Labs
Ohio State University Heart and
  Vascular Center
Ross Heart Hospital
The Ohio State University
Columbus, Ohio

Jeffrey A. Skiles, MD, FACC
Cardiologist
Department of Cardiology
Selma Medical Associates, Inc.
Winchester, Virginia

David Paul Slovut, MD, PhD
Lecturer in Medicine
Departments of Cardiology and
  Vascular Medicine
Massachusetts General Hospital
Boston
Department of Cardiology and
  Vascular Medicine
North Shore Medical Center
Salem, Massachusetts

Timothy M. Sullivan, MD
Chairman
Departments of Vascular/Endovascular
  Surgery
Minneapolis Heart Institute
Abbott Northwestern Hospital
Minneapolis, Minnesotav

Walter A. Tan, MD
East Carolina Heart Institute at Pitt
  County Memorial Hospital
East Carolina University
Greenville, North Carolina

Paaladinesh Thavendiranathan
Clinical Instructor
Cardiovascular Medicine
Davis Heart and Lung Research Institute
The Ohio State University
Columbus, Ohio

Gilbert R. Upchurch Jr, MD
William H. Muller Jr. Professor
Chief of Vascular and Endovascular
    Surgery
Department of Thoracic and
    Cardiovascular Surgery
University of Virginia
Charlottesville, Virginia

Patrick S. Vaccaro, MD
Chief
Division of Vascular Diseases and
    Surgery
The Ohio State University
Columbus, Ohio

Thomas W. Wakefield, MD
S. Martin Lindenauer Professor of
    Surgery
Head, Section of Vascular Surgery
Staff Surgeon
Department of Surgery
University of Michigan
Ann Arbor, Michigan

Michael C. Walls, MD
Fellow in Advanced Cardiovascular
    Imaging
Division of Cardiovascular Medicine
Ohio State University Medical Center
Columbus, Ohio

Cynthia Wu
Department of Clinical Hematology
University of Alberta
Edmonton, Alberta, Canada

A decade has passed since the first inception of an idea for a book in Vascular Medicine—an eternity in the field of medicine where changes occur nearly every week. When the original idea for this book was conceived, there were very few books in Vascular Medicine that allowed the reader to acquire a quick update on common vascular disorders from the vantage of a coat pocket. Since the last edition, there have been many other textbooks that have come and gone. Furthermore, the field has seen many changes including advances in endovascular therapy, imaging-based diagnostics, new discoveries in the genetic underpinnings of vascular disease, and even a newly consecrated board to certify practitioners of the field.

A new edition that incorporated these changes was a necessity, as many of our notions and beliefs in the field continue to evolve. Another objective, which was never planned when the first edition of the book was conceived, was the utility of the book in preparing for boards in cardiology, vascular medicine, and vascular surgery. In keeping with this function, we have provided questions following each chapter to prepare individuals who may be taking these exams.

This edition is made possible by excellent contributions from leaders in the practice of vascular medicine and my co-editors who continue to amaze me with their understanding and insights into the field I would like to acknowledge Debabrata Mukherjee for his knowledge in the field of endovascular therapy and the alacrity of his responses during the review of this book, Emile Mohler for his knowledge of peripheral arterial disease and vasospastic diseases, and finally, my good friend Steven Dean for his incredible breadth of experience in venous and lymphatic disorders. This edition would not have happened without the tireless efforts of Rebecca Abbott who kept us organized throughout the yearlong process. Finally this edition would not be possible without the efforts of Leanne McMillan who steered us towards the finish line. Thanks Leanne!

We hope that this edition continues to inspire all of you toward providing outstanding care to our patients.

Sanjay Rajagopalan, MD

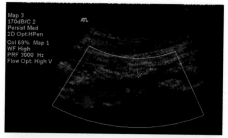

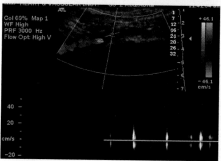

FIGURE 2-3. Duplex ultrasound of the abdominal aorta in the same patient as in Figure 2.2. **Top panel:** Color image demonstrating occluded infra-renal aorta. **Bottom panel:** Doppler analysis demonstrating preocclusive "thump" characteristic of occlusion.

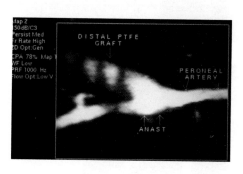

FIGURE 2-5. Duplex ultrasound demonstrating color power angiography technique of the distal anastomosis of a synthetic external iliac artery to peroneal artery bypass graft.

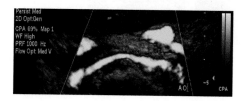

FIGURE 2-7. Color power angiography technique demonstrating the right renal artery from the aorta (*AO*) to the hilum of the kidney.

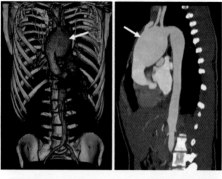

FIGURE 5-4. Volume rendered (**right**) and MIP (**left**) display of a large ascending thoracic aortic aneurysm.

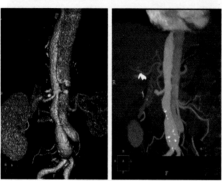

FIGURE 5-7. An aortic dissection with extension into the abdomen. **A:** Three-dimensional volume reconstruction (*upper left*). **B:** A maximum intensity projection with a 60-mm thickness (slab-MIP) demonstrates calcium in the abdominal aorta and reveals segments of the celiac, superior mesenteric, and lumbar arteries in relation to the hepatic parenchyma (*bottom left*).

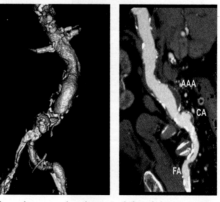

FIGURE 5-8. The volume-rendered image (**left**) of this aorta does not adequately reveal diffuse aneurysmal involvement. A curved multiplanar reconstruction (**right**) of this tortuous area enables electronic linearization of the aorta perpendicular to the flow of blood and provides a more reliable assessment of abdominal aneurysm length. (Reprinted from Goldman C, Sanz J. CT Angiography of the abdominal aorta and its branches with protocols. In: Mukerjee D, Rajagopalan S, eds. *CT and MRI angiography of the peripheral circulation: practical approach with clinical protocols*. London, UK: Informa Health Care, 2007:117, with permission.)

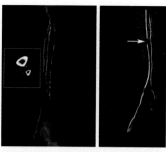

FIGURE 5-10. A volume-rendered display of lower extremity atherosclerotic disease (**left**). Axial CTA image (**inset**) illustrates calcification within the walls of the anterior tibial, posterior tibial, and peroneal arteries with poor luminal visualization. Occlusive disease (**right**). Three-dimensional CTA volume-rendered image (*left anterior oblique view*) shows a segmental occlusions of the anterior tibial artery (*arrow*) with small bridging collateral arteries. (Reprinted from Cohen E, Doshi A, Lookstein, R. CT angiography of the lower extremity circulation with protocols. In: Mukerjee D, Rajagopalan S, eds. *CT and MRI angiography of the peripheral circulation: practical approach with clinical protocols.* London, UK: Informa Health Care, 2007:139, with permission.)

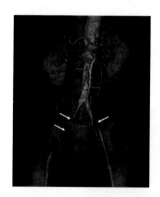

FIGURE 5-11. Volume-rendered image illustrating occlusion of bilateral common iliac arteries and the proximal portion of the right external iliac artery secondary to giant cell arteritis. (Reprinted from Cohen E, Doshi A, Lookstein R. CT angiography of the lower extremity circulation with protocols. In: Mukerjee D, Rajagopalan S, eds. *CT and MRI angiography of the peripheral circulation: practical approach with clinical protocols.* London, UK: Informa Health Care, 2007:141, with permission.)

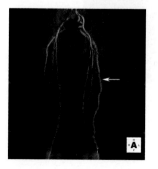

FIGURE 5-12. Persistent sciatic artery. Three-dimensional CTA volume-rendered image (*anteroposterior view*) shows occlusion of the distal left superficial femoral artery. The left popliteal artery is supplied by a persistent left sciatic artery fed by the internal iliac artery (*arrow*). (Reprinted from Cohen E, Doshi A, Lookstein R. CT angiography of the lower extremity circulation with protocols. In: Mukerjee D, Rajagopalan S, eds. *CT and MRI angiography of the peripheral circulation: practical approach with clinical protocols.* London, UK: Informa Health Care, 2007:143, with permission.)

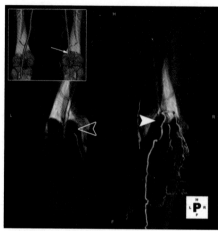

FIGURE 5-13. Popliteal artery entrapment. Three-dimensional CTA volume-rendered image (*posteroanterior view*) of a young patient with right calf pain on exertion. The medial head of the right gastrocnemius muscle demonstrates an abnormal origin lateral to the popliteal artery (*closed arrowhead*). *Inset* image shows complete occlusion of the right popliteal artery (*arrow*) with multiple superficial collateral arteries originating just proximal to this level. The normal origin of the medial head of the left gastrocnemius medial to the popliteal artery (*open arrowhead*) is shown for comparison. (Reprinted from Cohen E, Doshi A. Lookstein R. CT angiography of the lower extremity circulation with protocols. In: Mukerjee D, Rajagopalan S, eds. *CT and MRI angiography of the peripheral circulation: practical approach with clinical protocols*. London, UK: Informa Health Care, 2007:143, with permission.)

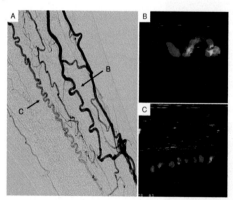

FIGURE 9-1. A: Digital subtraction angiography shows corkscrew collaterals around the area of occlusions in the right lower leg. Continuous-wave Doppler ultrasound shows corkscrew collaterals as color Doppler flows of a snake sign [**A** (*arrow B*), and **B**] and a dot sign [**A** (*arrow C*) and **C**]. (From Fujii Y, Nishioka K, Yoshizumi M, et al. Corkscrew collaterals in thromboangiitis obliterans (Buerger disease). *Circulation* 2007;116:e539–e540, with permission.)

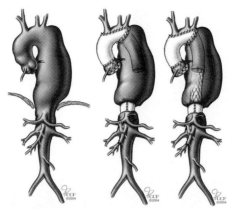

FIGURE 14-4. Elephant trunk procedure. **Left:** Preoperative disease. **Middle:** Stage I with replacement of the ascending aorta and arch with a Dacron graft with the distal graft sutured circumferentially to the aorta distal to the left subclavian artery and the free end of the graft ("elephant trunk") within the descending aneurysm. **Right:** Completion of the procedure using an endovascular stent graft attached proximally to the "elephant trunk" and the distal end secured to a Dacron graft cuff. (Adapted from 2010 ACCF/AHA/AATS/ACR/ASA/SCA/SCAI/SIR/STS/SVM guidelines for the diagnosis and management of patients with thoracic aortic disease. *Circulation* 2010;121;1544–1579.)

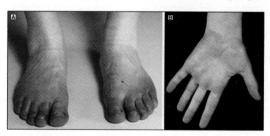

FIGURE 18-3. Erythermalgia affecting the feet and the hand. (Reprinted from Sandroni P, et al. *Arch Dermatol* 2006;142:283–286, with permission.)

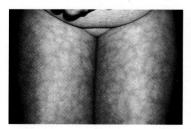

FIGURE 18-4. Livedo reticularis. Note the symmetric, regular, "unbroken" rings.

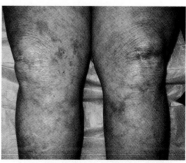

FIGURE 18-5. Livedo racemosa. Note the asymmetric and irregular appearance of the cones.

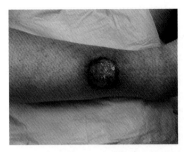

FIGURE 18-6. Pyoderma gangrenosum.

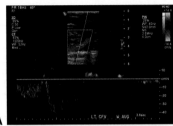

A

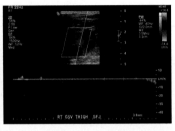

B

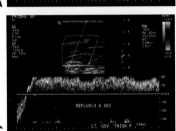

C

FIGURE 19-4. Demonstration of competency of the SFJ by duplex ultrasound. During quiet respiration (A, B), blood flows cephalad in the greater saphenous and the common femoral veins as indicated by the arrows. With performance of the Valsalva, there is complete cessation of flow (B) with a competent SFJ. In contrast, in (C), there is blood flow in the opposite direction with the Valsalva suggesting reflux of the SFJ. From Zwiebel WJ. *Introduction to vascular ultrasonography*, 4th ed. Philadelphia: W. B. Saunders, 2000:356–357.

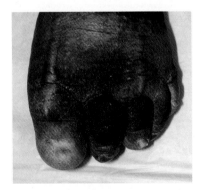

FIGURE 26-4. Hyperkeratotic, papillomatous skin along the dorsum of the second toe prohibits the ability to pinch or "tent" the affected area, thus fulfilling the definition of a *positive Stemmer's sign*.

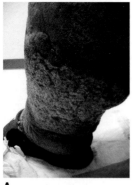 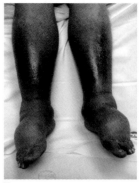

A　　　　　　　　**B**

FIGURE 26-5. Chronic venous insufficiency is an increasingly recognized secondary cause of lymphedema. Note the constellation of marked venous stasis hyperpigmentation and profound lymphedematous dorsal foot swelling.

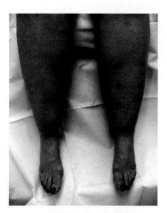

FIGURE 26-6. Classic lipedema of the lower extremities. Observe the symmetric calf involvement and "ankle cutoff sign" with sparing of the feet and toes. These clinical features delineate lipedema from lymphedema.

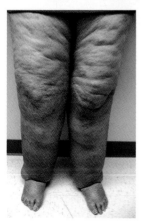

FIGURE 26-7. Lipolymphedema. Rarely, long-standing lipedema can eventuate in secondary lymphedema. Although this female patient experienced a 40-year history of familial symmetric thigh and calf swelling without foot involvement, for the last several years, dorsal pedal edema evolved.

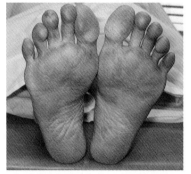

FIGURE 30-1.

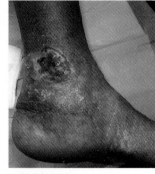

FIGURE 30-2A.

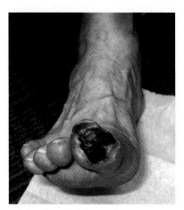

FIGURE 30-2B.

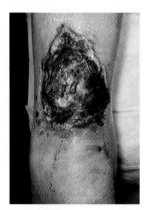

FIGURE 30-2C.

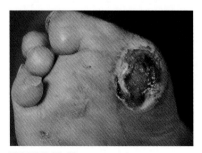

FIGURE 30-2D.

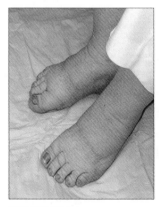

FIGURE 30-3.

CONTENTS

CHAPTER 1 ■ History and Examination of the Arterial System

Sanjay Rajagopalan and Rekha Durairaj

The goal of a vascular history and examination is to arrive at a diagnosis and to structure appropriate investigations. This may often involve a detailed evaluation of the patient to look for systemic manifestation of vascular disease. A superficial approach devoid of detail and accuracy may often result in therapeutic decisions being delayed.

VASCULAR HISTORY

Patients with arterial disease often present with characteristic symptoms and signs that may enable one to arrive at a diagnosis even prior to the physical examination. This section will deal with elements of a vascular history that may facilitate this process.

Demographics

Atherosclerotic peripheral arterial disease typically presents after the age of 40, whereas Buerger's disease and certain forms of large vessel vasculitis (Takayasu's arteritis) often presents between 20 and 40 years. Temporal arteritis and atherosclerotic aneurysms present typically after the age of 65 years. A strong female predilection may be seen in some vasculitic disorders such as primary Raynaud's syndrome, lupus vasculitis, and Takayasu's arteritis.

History of Presenting Illness

The type of symptoms and duration, mode of onset, aggravating and relieving factors (effects of elevation, exercise, rest, dependency, temperature, pressure, etc.) should be noted.

Type and Duration of Symptoms

The nature of symptoms may provide a clue to the diagnosis. Historical differentiation of large-vessel from small-vessel disease is possible in both the upper and lower extremities. The most common problems suggesting upper extremity large arterial insufficiency are pain, coldness, ulcers, and gangrene. Small-vessel vasospastic diseases such as Raynaud's syndrome present as characteristic cold sensitivity, with or without a classic triphasic response (sequential development of digital pallor, cyanosis, and rubor following cold exposure and warming). Although the symptom of Raynaud's suggests vasospasm of the small arteries of the hand, it may sometimes represent a manifestation of a more proximal etiology (e.g., emboli from the axillary or subclavian artery) that exaggerates the physiologic cold responsiveness of the digital vascular bed. The presence of tissue necrosis in the upper extremity almost always suggests fixed obstructive disease, even if the patient has Raynaud's symptoms. A critical historical clue in differentiating upper extremity vasospasm from fixed arterial obstruction is whether the symptoms are constant or intermittent. Thus, fixed cyanosis and ulceration in the finger(s) in a patient with otherwise typical worsening of symptoms on cold exposure is almost always because of fixed disease. Symptoms caused by vasospasm alone are intermittent, and the extremity is asymptomatic and normal in appearance between attacks. Upper extremity large artery involvement is frequently asymptomatic with chronic stenosis of presenting as muscle fatigue or arm claudication, only after physiologic compensatory mechanisms including collateral support have been exhausted. Thoracic outlet syndrome may present as recurrent bouts of pain or numbness with activity, typically involving a dermatomal pattern.

Chronic arterial stenoses of the lower extremity is most often asymptomatic (see claudication) with atypical symptoms being relatively common. As lower extremity arterial disease progresses, the patient may experience pain at rest or may present with tissue necrosis and/or gangrene (chronic critical limb ischemia). With atherosclerotic peripheral arterial disease, disease progression is gradual occurring slowly over several years, with many patients reporting no change in their symptoms for years. Abrupt deterioration of symptoms should raise the question of superimposed thrombosis or embolism.

Intermittent claudication (derived from "claudicatio," Latin for limp) is classically described as cramping pain or weakness occurring with exercise and relieved by rest. Atypical manifestations are more common than classic claudication and may include a variety of symptoms including weakness. Symptoms in claudication are caused by inadequacy of the blood supply to contracting muscles and are therefore localized to muscle groups, including those of the buttocks, thigh, and the calf. Calf symptoms typically predominate in most patients irrespective of the level of disease, perhaps because the calf is metabolically more active than other muscle groups when walking. Aortoiliac disease may present as aching discomfort in the hips and thighs along with a sensation of weakness that may mimic spinal stenosis.

The amount of exercise producing pain is generally reproducible, and patients can typically quantify their exercise capacity in terms of walking distance or time. Factors such as time of day, meals, medications, and a host of other factors may influence symptoms in a number of patients. The pain of intermittent claudication is typically relieved by rest, usually within 5 minutes, and may be relieved by slowing the pace of walking. The amount of exercise required to precipitate pain is roughly inversely related to the severity of the narrowing of the vessel, and pain is usually manifested one segment below the area of stenosis (assuming a single focal lesion at these levels). One may approximately deduce the level of involvement by considering the location of symptoms although this is frequently not predictive. Thus in some patients, aortic disease is manifested by buttock pain, iliac disease by thigh muscle pain, and superficial femoral arterial disease (the most commonly affected artery) by calf claudication. However, since multilevel disease is usually the norm in atherosclerosis, the symptoms typically reflect the most distal significant disease or the area with the poorest collateral support.

Upper Extremity Claudication. This is seen in individuals with subclavian artery stenosis. Radiologic subclavian steal may be seen if the stenosis is proximal to the origin of the vertebral artery (Chapter 16).

Differential Diagnosis of Claudication. Table 1.1 lists conditions that may mimic lower extremity claudication (pseudoclaudication) and their characteristics. Nocturnal cramps are by far the commonest nonvascular cause of cramping and are thought to represent an exaggerated neuromuscular response to stretch. Table 1.2 lists causes of true claudication that are nonatherosclerotic.

Rest Pain. Rest pain becomes a prominent feature as blood flow becomes insufficient to supply the basal needs of extremity and its sensory nerve supply. Rest pain is classically defined as severe nocturnal pain or burning that begins in the feet especially over the metatarsal heads, is relieved by dependency, and is aggravated by elevation of the legs above the level of the heart. Rest pain is a sign of very severe ischemia that may be limb threatening if no intervention is undertaken. Metatarsalgia is an occasional differential diagnosis for rest pain. This is usually seen with DJD or rheumatoid arthritis, is aggravated by dependency, and may be relieved on standing.

Neuropathic Pain and Causalgia. Neuropathic pain and causalgia (see Chapter 18, complex regional pain syndrome) are both often described as burning discomfort involving the extremities. The former is commonly seen in conditions such as diabetes that have a propensity to involve the nerves and is often associated with additional deficits in a typical glove-and-stocking distribution typically in the lower extremity. Complex regional pain syndrome (previously referred to as reflex sympathetic dystrophy) is a distinct pain syndrome that is an important differential diagnosis for upper extremity pain. It usually occurs in response to an inciting trauma (which may be trivial and may not be recalled by the patient), including medical conditions such as myocardial infarction, deep venous thrombosis, and hip fracture. It is additionally characterized by hyperalgesia, allodynia, and abnormal sudomotor activity that is disproportionate to the inciting injury and occurring beyond the territory of a single nerve.

    Erythermalgia (erythromelalgia) is a characteristic condition associated with burning pain discomfort and redness of the extremities (lower more common than upper) that is typically worsened by heat. This may be primary or secondary to conditions such as myeloproliferative disorders, lymphoma, diabetes, hypertension, and drugs such as calcium channel blockers and bromocriptine (Chapter 18).

Mode of Onset of Illness

Acute arterial insufficiency is typified by the five Ps (pain, pallor, paresthesias, paralysis, poikilothermia) (Chapter 7). Abrupt onset of pain with pallor often suggests an embolic phenomenon. Acute arterial thrombosis superimposed on a preexisting atherosclerotic plaque or stenosis is the other major cause of acute limb ischemia. With arterial thrombosis the clinical presentation is not as dramatic as embolism. The patient is, however, aware

TABLE 1.1

DIFFERENTIAL DIAGNOSIS OF INTERMITTENT CLAUDICATION

Condition	Description	Effect of Exercise and Cessation Activity	Other Special Features
PSEUDOCLAUDICATION OF THE CALF			
Nocturnal cramps	Cramping pain in calves; nocturnal predilection; spontaneously relieved in a few minutes	Occurs at rest	May be relieved by postural adjustment
Chronic compartment syndrome	Bursting pain, typically in muscled athletes or cyclists	Provoked by strenuous exercise (e.g., jogging or cycling). Subsides gradually	Relief speeded by elevation
Venous claudication	Tight or bursting calf pain in patients with extensive proximal DVT (iliofemoral)	Walking exacerbates; subsides gradually	Relief speeded by elevation; signs of chronic venous insufficiency present
Radiculopathy (e.g., herniated disc)	Sharp lancinating pain in patient with prior back problems that radiates down the posterior aspect of the leg	Provoked by change in posture and minimal activity. Not relieved by resting	May be relieved by changes in posture
Symptomatic Baker's cyst	Tenderness and swelling behind the knee	Worsens with activity and not relieved by rest	Signs of inflammation at the back of the knee
PSEUDOCLAUDICATION OF THE HIP/BUTTOCK			
Hip arthritis	Aching discomfort, symptoms relate to level of activity	Worse with activity. Not relieved by rest	More relief in non-weight-bearing situations. Weather-sensitive symptoms
Neurogenic claudication (spinal cord compression)	Weakness rather than pain	Symptoms start shortly after standing up. Immediate relief on sitting or change of posture	May or may not have a history of back problems. Relieved by stopping only if position changed (lumbar spine flexion)
PSEUDOCLAUDICATION OF THE FOOT			
Arthritic/inflammatory processes	Aching pain that may be continuous and relate to activity	Aggravated by weight bearing. Not quickly relieved and may be present at rest	

TABLE 1.2

NONATHEROSCLEROTIC CAUSES OF ARTERIAL STENOSIS AND RESULTANT SYMPTOMS

Collagen vascular diseases
Giant-cell arteritis (Takayasu's and temporal)
Buerger's disease
Embolism (proximal sources)
    Heart (LV thrombus, paradoxic embolus)
    Aneurysm
Dissection
    Traumatic
    Inherited disorder of collagen metabolism (PXE, Ehlers-Danlos)
Adventitial cystic disease
Popliteal artery entrapment
Retroperitoneal fibrosis
Drugs
    Ergot derivatives
    Sympathomimetics
    5HT1A/D agonists

of a change in clinical status. Table 1.3 enumerates the differences between an embolic and an *in situ* thrombotic episode. The symptoms may then worsen or may abate depending on the patient's ability to recruit collateral pathways. A common site of thrombosis in the lower extremity is the superficial femoral artery, although it may occur anywhere from the aorta to the

TABLE 1.3

DIFFERENTIATING EMBOLISM FROM THROMBOSIS AS THE ETIOLOGY OF LIMB ISCHEMIA

	Embolism	Thrombosis *in Situ*
History	Abrupt-onset pain	Onset may not be abrupt; change in
	Prior cardiac event	symptoms acute but not abrupt
Physical exam	Cold, mottled, paralyzed	Cool, bluish, limb (slower progression);
	(rapid progression)	abnormal contralateral pulse exam
	Normal contralateral limb	No distinct demarcation
	Clear demarcation	
Etiology	Cardiac thrombus (75–85%)	Native artery plaque rupture
	Aortic atheroma	Graft occlusion
	Proximal aneurysm	
Prior vascular intervention	Usually no	Often yes

digital arteries. Occasionally thrombosis may be precipitated by a decrease in blood flow velocity because of a low cardiac output state, as may occur with congestive cardiac failure or after myocardial infarction.

The site of affliction may offer a clue to the diagnosis. Atherosclerosis and Buerger's disease typically affect the lower extremities and present with claudication generally in a bilaterally symmetric manner. Foot claudication is generally seen in disorders that cause medium-vessel and small-vessel involvement such as Buerger's disease and thromboembolization. Bilateral involvement of the upper extremity should suggest a systemic process such as a vasculitic disorder. A patient who presents with gangrene or an ulcer in the fingers unilaterally of fairly acute onset should raise the suspicion of an embolic episode (intracardiac sources, embolization from a proximal vessel/aneurysm, etc).

Past Medical History

The patient should be asked about concurrent diseases and atherosclerotic risk factors (hypertension, diabetes, tobacco abuse, dyslipidemias, strokes, blood clots, or amputations). A prior history of peripheral vascular intervention (percutaneous or surgical graft) in the extremity is helpful in suspecting relevant complications (restenosis vs. graft failure).

Personal History

(a) Occupation: Usage of vibratory tools may place one at risk for Raynaud's phenomenon, whereas occupations that involve repetitive trauma to the hand should raise suspicion of the hypothenar-hammer syndrome. Exposure to vinyl chloride should raise suspicion for acroosteolysis. (b) Smoking: Smoking has a strong association with Buerger's disease, and the absence of smoking may cause one to reconsider the diagnosis. (c) Iliac artery compression should be recognized as an important differential diagnosis of lower extremity symptoms in competitive cyclists. (d) The presence of sexual dysfunction is common in patients with atherosclerotic peripheral arterial disease.

Medication Usage

A careful list of all the medications that the patient is currently on or has previously used should be determined. Migraine medications such as 5-HT(1B/1D) receptor agonists and ergot derivatives may potentiate vasospasm; β blockers may precipitate Raynaud's symptoms; and medications such as sulfonamides, allopurinol, phenytoin, carbamazepine, cholorthalidone, methylthiouracil, spironolactone, and tetracycline have all been associated with toxic vasculitis.

Family History

A history of premature arterial disease suggests inherited disorders of thrombosis, lipoprotein metabolism, or hyperhomocystenemia. A family history of aneurysmal disease, sudden death, or skin or joint laxity should raise the threshold for suspecting inherited disorders of collagen metabolism including Ehlers-Danlos and Marfan's syndromes.

PHYSICAL EXAMINATION OF THE ARTERIAL SYSTEM

General Examination

An examination of the patient's general appearance can often provide clues in a patient with a suspected arterial disorder. The distinctive appearance of a patient with Marfan's syndrome (arm span greater than height, longer pubis-to-head distance than pubis-to-foot, arachnodactyly, and chest deformities), pseudoxanthoma elasticum (characteristic yellowish orange papules over the neck and flexural areas and angioid streaks in the retina), neurofibromatosis, and/or café au lait spots (association with coarctation of the pararenal aorta and proximal stenosis of the renal arteries) is often apparent. Tendinous xanthomas (seen subcutaneously or over extensor tendons in patients with type II hyperlipoproteinemia) and tuberoeruptive xanthomas seen over the extremities and over the palms (xanthoma striatum palmare) are often manifestations of systemic atherosclerosis. Cutaneous telangiectasias may be seen and may often be associated with arteriovenous malformations. [Nevus vinosus (port wine stain) shows no tendency to regress (unlike nevus flammeus or the ordinary birthmark) and is associated with three syndromes (Sturge-Weber: port wine stain in distribution of trigeminal in association with seizures and vascular malformations of the retina and leptomeninges; Klippel-Trenaunay: port wine stain involving an extremity with associated venous varicosities and absent deep venous system; Parke-Weber syndrome: a subset of Klippel-Trenaunay with direct arteriovenous malformations/communication with a tendency for high-output congestive heart failure).]

Examination of the Head, Neck, and Chest

Inspection

HEENT. The mucous membranes of the oral cavity and eyes should be examined for evidence of clues that may suggest systemic vascular disease. The presence of sub-conjunctival hemorrhages and petechiae may suggest a diagnosis of infective endocarditis. Blue sclerae may suggest osteogenesis imperfecta and its association with aneurysmal disease. Hollenhorst's plaques may be seen in the retina in individuals who present with monocular symptoms and transient ischemic attacks.

Neck and Chest. Pulsatile masses in the neck may represent aneurysms, kinking or coiling of the vessels, or masses overlying a vessel (lymph node or carotid body tumor). The commonest location for a carotid artery aneurysm is in the common carotid artery; it presents as a pulsatile mass at or below the level of the angle of the mandible. Aneurysms of the internal carotid artery may often not be visible externally, because the overlying fascia prevents expansion in this direction. Pulsations in the supraclavicular fossa are usually secondary to involvement of the subclavian artery or its thyrocervical branch. The most common expansile lesion in the neck that needs to be distinguished from an aneurysm is "kinking" or "coiling" of the carotid artery. The pulsations with a "kinked" common carotid artery is typically along the long axis of the vessel, as opposed to a true aneurysm that pulsates in an expansile manner at right angles to the long axis of the vessel.

Palpation

Palpation of the pulses is perhaps the important part of examination of the arterial system. When examining the arterial pulse, the following points are to be noted: (a) The volume of the pulse (an expansile pulsation may indicate aneurysmal expansion, while a diminished pulse may indicate a proximal occlusion), (b) The condition of the arterial wall, whether atheromatous or not. When reporting pulses it is best to follow a systematic approach and report pulse volume on a scale of 0 to 4 (0, absent; 1, trace; 2, moderately decreased; 3, mildly decreased; 4, bounding). The *common carotid artery* is felt in the carotid triangle just in front of the sternomastoid muscle against the carotid tubercle of the 6th cervical vertebra. It is often difficult to separate the internal carotid artery from the common carotid artery pulsations. Contrary to what one may expect, carotid artery pulsations are often felt well in total occlusions of the internal carotid artery. The *superficial temporal artery* is felt just in front of the tragus of the ear. The presence of prominent superficial temporal artery pulsations almost certainly excludes significant stenosis of the common or external carotid artery. A carotid body tumor is typically a painless mass at the angle of the mandible, often called into attention because of unrelated reasons. Although cranial nerve lesions may occur owing to the invasive nature of this tumor, these are typically absent. The mass is laterally mobile but vertically fixed owing to its adherence to the carotid sheath. A bruit may sometimes be heard either due to extrinsic compression of the vessel or concomitant atheromatous involvement. The vertebral artery cannot be palpated along its course.

Auscultation

Auscultation for bruits should be performed over all superficial arteries including swellings. Bruits over the carotid artery could originate from the chest as in aortic stenosis. These transmitted murmurs are loudest at the base of the chest or at the apex and have a characteristic "crescendo–decrescendo" quality. The presence of a carotid bruit does not translate into a stenosis and neither does it provide any clues as to the severity. Noninvasive vascular studies are indispensable to assess the lesion. Bruits may be heard over the subclavian artery and suggest a stenosis.

Examination of the Lower Extremity

Inspection

Change in color may be a noticeable feature of an acutely ischemic limb. Placing the limb side-by-side with the contralateral limb may highlight minor differences. An acutely ischemic limb is characterized by the five Ps as outlined previously. Not all of these symptoms and signs may necessarily be present concurrently. Most often, the patient presents with abrupt onset of pain below the level of the occlusion, with the color and temperature changes distal to the level of occlusion. With severe ischemia, the patient complains of paresthesias and has impaired sensation to light touch and position that may progress to complete anesthesia. With more prolonged ischemia, paralysis and gangrene develop. Signs of chronic ischemia include diminished hair growth, loss of subcutaneous fat, shininess, trophic changes in the nails (brittleness and the development of transverse ridges), and ulcerations. The foot may often appear purple—"dependent rubor." This phenomenon is due to filling of the dilated skin capillaries with deoxygenated blood. In cases of lower extremity distal embolization, the clinical picture is characterized by cyanotic discoloration of the toes, often in the presence of palpable pulses ("blue toe syndrome").

Capillary Refill Time on Inspection. The patient is asked to sit up and hang his legs by the side of a table. A normal leg will remain pink in the elevated and the dependent position. An ischemic limb, however, becomes pale in the elevated position and gradually becomes pink in the dependent posture. The time for the change in color is called the capillary refill time. In severely ischemic limbs it takes 20 to 30 seconds to improve pallor. Subsequently, the ischemic limb changes color and become purple-red quickly. This is referred to as dependent rubor refill.

Examination of Gangrenous Area. The location and extent of gangrene may provide clues regarding the level and severity of arterial occlusion. The type of gangrene also should be noted. In other words is the area "dry" or "wet" and putrefying (as seen in diabetic gangrene). The line of demarcation between the gangrenous area and normal tissue should be noted.

Livedo Reticularis. This is a mottled discoloration of the skin ("fishnet" or reticular pattern) typically seen in the lower extremities and the trunk with atheroembolism (Chapter 18). The webs of the "fishnet" are usually pink or a violaceous hue that may worsen with cold exposure. This may occur as a primary disorder in young women (20 to 40 years) but may occur secondary to a number of processes including embolic disease, collagen vascular disease (SLE, PAN, dermatomyositis), hyperviscosity syndromes, malignancies (lymphoma), infections (lyme disease, tuberculosis, syphilis), intra-arterial injection in drug addicts, and drugs such as amantidine.

Pernio. This is a disorder typically seen in women in the lower extremity, in which raised red and blue lesions are seen in the toes and shins (may need to be distinguished from atheroembolism). These are typically described as burning and are intensely pruritic. These lesions typically last less than 10 days. Chronic pernio is referred to as chilblains and is seen in areas, such as the toes, repeatedly exposed to cold (also see Chapter 18).

Palpation

Skin Temperature. This is best felt with the back of one's hand. The apparent line of demarcation between ischemic tissue and normally perfused tissue (at rest) may be made this way.

Acrocyanosis. This is a persistent bluish discoloration of the hands (less commonly the feet). This disorder is not associated with changes in the skin such as ulcerations, sclerodactyly, or alterations in digital waveforms/pressures and may additionally be distinguished from Raynaud's symptoms in being persistent rather than episodic.

Capillary Refill Time with Palpation. Applying firm pressure on the foot or the pulp of the lower extremity and determining the time it takes for the pallor to improve can assess this. Alternatively, one can elevate the legs (to empty the capillaries). Normally the capillaries fill rapidly in less than 5 seconds. In cases of ischemia it may take longer than 20 seconds for the pallor to disappear.

Pulse Evaluation. The disappearance of arterial pulsations below the level of occlusion in the extremity is generally the rule. The only exception is the presence of good proximal collateral circulation when the pulse may be diminished but does not disappear. The *dorsalis pedis artery* is felt lateral to the tendon of the extensor hallucis longus in the foot and is congenitally absent in 10% of individuals. The anterior tibial artery is typically felt anteriorly, midway between the two malleoli against the lower end of the tibia just above the ankle joint and just lateral to the tendon of the extensor hallucis. The posterior tibial artery is felt behind the medial malleolus midway between the latter and the Achilles tendon. Palpation of the *popliteal artery* may be difficult as it lies deep behind the knee. The artery can be located by turning the patient to the prone position and by feeling the artery with the fingertips after flexing the knee passively with the other hand. Alternatively, with the patient in the supine position, the knee is flexed to 40 degrees with the heel resting on the bed, so that the muscles around the popliteal fossa are relaxed. The clinician places his fingers over the lower part of the popliteal fossa and the fingers are moved sideways to feel the pulsation of the popliteal artery against the posterior aspect of the tibial condyles. The *femoral artery* is felt just below the inguinal ligament midway between the anterior superior iliac spine and the pubis.

Neurologic Evaluation

Early sensory deficits in cases of advanced limb ischemia may be subtle, and it should be noted that light touch, two-point discrimination, vibratory perception, and proprioception are usually lost well before deep pain and pressure. Motor deficits are indications of advanced, limb-threatening ischemia (Table 1.4; see Table 7.1). Patients with diabetes may have preexisting sensory deficits, which may lead to confusion.

TABLE 1.4

CATEGORIES OF ACUTE LIMB ISCHEMIA

Category	Description	Motor and Sensory Findings	Arterial Doppler Signals
I Viable	Not immediately threatened	None	Audible
IIa (Marginally threatened)	Salvageable if promptly treated	Minimal sensory defect (toes) or none	Often inaudible
IIb (Immediately threatened)[a]	Salvageable with immediate revascularization	Mild, moderate weakness; sensory deficit extends to beyond toes, associated with rest pain	Usually inaudible
III	Major tissue loss or permanent nerve damage inevitable	Profound motor paralysis with extensive sensory deficits	Inaudible; venous sounds also absent

When presenting early, the differentiation between class IIb and III acute limb ischemia may be difficult.

[a]In level IIa patients there is time for angiography before embarking on revascularization; In level IIb, immediate revascularization is required.

(Adapted from Rutherford RB, Baker JD, Ernst C, et al. Recommended standards for reports dealing with lower extremity ischemia: revised version. *J Vasc Surg* 1997;26:517–538.)

Evaluation of the Upper Extremity

Inspection

Severe pallor may be noted in acute ischemia but may also be seen during an attack of Raynaud's syndrome. Note should be made of nail-bed changes (such as pitting and hemorrhages), cyanosis, ulcerations, and gangrene. The presence of abnormally dilated capillaries visualized through capillary microscopy (Chapter 16) may suggest a diagnosis of PSS/CREST, whereas abnormal capillary rarefaction may suggest collagen vascular disease such as SLE or rheumatoid arthritis in a patient presenting with secondary Raynaud's syndrome.

Palpation

Temperature. The skin temperature is assessed as before using the back of the examining hand, with the level of the skin temperature providing the demarcation zone between ischemic and normal tissue.

Capillary Refill Time. This can be determined by applying firm pressure on the finger pulp region and determining the time for the pallor to disappear.

Pulse Evaluation. The *subclavian artery* is felt just above the middle of the clavicle. The *brachial artery* is felt in the medial upper arm between the bellies of the biceps and triceps. In the antecubital fossa the *brachial artery* is felt in front of the elbow just medial to the tendon of the biceps. The *radial and ulnar arteries* are felt at the wrist on the lateral and medial volar aspects respectively. The ulnar artery is congenitally absent in 2 to 3% of individuals. Absence of radial and brachial pulses in a young individual should raise the question of Takayasu's arteritis. Aneurysms of the upper extremities are located most commonly in the subclavian artery, and can be palpated in the supraclavicular fossa.

Auscultation

Blood pressure should always be procured in both upper extremities. A discrepancy of greater than 10 mm Hg is abnormal. Abnormally low brachial pressures in both upper extremities should prompt blood pressure assessment in the lower extremity to avoid missing conditions such as coarctation and Takayasu's arteritis.

Thoracic outlet syndrome maneuvers (also see Chapter 17): These tests are performed to rule out vascular thoracic outlet syndrome. These maneuvers may often be positive in normal individuals and are of limited value by themselves. However, when used in conjunction with the appropriate history, the tests can be helpful. In each of the maneuvers the radial artery pulse is felt digitally or with the aid of a Doppler at rest and after the provocative maneuver. With a positive test, there is a diminution of the pulse amplitude with the maneuvers.

Adson's test: The patient while sitting upright is asked to take a deep breath, look upward, and turn his face to the affected side.

Hyperabduction maneuver: The patient is asked to hyperabduct the symptomatic extremity (typically to 180 degrees). This will cause the disappearance of the pulse due to compression of the artery in the event of a compression syndrome and the reappearance with restoration of normal position.

Costoclavicular maneuver: The patient is asked to thrust both his shoulders backward and downward maximally.

EAST maneuver (external rotation–abduction stress test): This may be the most reliable. The patient is asked to adopt the "stick-up posture" with arms extended, externally rotated, and behind the head. The patient then repeatedly makes fists repetitively for 3 minutes, and pulses are felt at the end of this period.

Branham's sign: This is performed when an arteriovenous fistula is suspected. A pressure on an artery proximal to the fistula will cause reduction in size of the swelling, and disappearance of bruit, as well as a fall in pulse rate.

Examination of the Abdomen

No examination of the arterial system is complete without examination of the abdomen.

Inspection

The inspection of the abdomen should focus on evaluation of pulsations. Although pulsations of the aorta are not seen normally in the vast majority of patients, they may be visualized in thin subjects.

Palpation

Normal aortic pulsations are roughly the width of the patient's thumb. An aortic aneurysm may be suspected when the aortic pulse is expansile and larger than a full centimeter. Extension of the pulsations to the xiphoid or costal margins should also raise suspicions for a thoracoabdominal or suprarenal aneurysm. Presence of tenderness over a known aneurysm is an ominous sign and may indicate impending rupture.

Auscultation

Asymptomatic abdominal bruits are common findings on abdominal examination of older adults. These may arise as a consequence of atherosclerotic involvement of the abdominal aorta or may signify a stenosis in the aorta, renal or mesenteric arteries. Renal artery bruits that are hemodynamically significant are often systolic–diastolic (Chapter 10). The presence of a diastolic component indicates that the degree of narrowing of the artery is severe since there is continued flow during diastole. Aortoiliac disease causes bruits in the middle of the lower abdomen and femoral areas.

ASSESSING OUTCOMES AND IMPROVEMENTS IN ARTERIAL DISEASE

Classification of arterial disease allows standardization of reporting practices and allows for assessment of outcomes. Table 1.4 (Table 7.1) lists the SVS-ISCVS joint classification of acute limb ischemia. Patients with

TABLE 1.5

CATEGORIES OF CHRONIC LIMB ISCHEMIA: FONTAINE AND RUTHERFORD CLASSIFICATION OF PERIPHERAL ARTERIAL DISEASE

Fontaine			Rutherford	
Stage	Clinical	Grade	Category	Clinical
I	Asymptomatic	0	0	Asymptomatic
IIa	Mild claudication	I	1	Mild claudication
IIb	Moderate to severe claudication	I	3	Moderate claudication
III	Ischemic rest pain	II	4	Ischemic rest pain
IV	Ulceration or gangrene	III	5	Minor tissue loss
		III	6	Major tissue loss

(Adapted from the Norgen L, Hiatt WR, Dormandy JA, et al. Inter-Society Consensus for the Management of Peripheral Arterial Disease (TASC II). *J Vasc Surg* 2007;45(Suppl):S5–S67.)

evidence of advanced irreversible ischemia (class III) need to be treated with an emergent amputation rather than revascularization, as a washout of the large quantity of muscle metabolites will often lead to rapid multiorgan failure and death. Patients who present with severe limb ischemia (class IIB) progress to class III in 6 hours or less, when irreversible changes occur and amputation may be necessary. This time frame may not allow diagnostic workup such as angiography. Table 1.5 lists the SVS/ISCVS classification of chronic limb ischemia. This classification is principally meant for clinical research and as such does not provide gradations in

TABLE 1.6

PARAMETERS TO ASSESS IMPROVEMENT WITH THERAPY IN EXTREMITY ISCHEMIA

Clinical Parameters

Patient-based parameters

   Mortality

   Limb salvage

   Ankle-brachial indices

   Absolute and initial claudication distance

Procedure-based parameters

   Technical success

   Primary and secondary patency rates (percutaneous or graft)

   Procedural morbidity and mortality

Surrogate markers

  Perfusion-related end points

    Doppler blood flow

    $TcPO_2$

    Skin perfusion by laser doppler perfusion

    MRI based perfusion assessment

    Reactive hyperemia perfusion by various modalities

Metabolic end-points

   NMR spectroscopy of phosphocreatine and ATP (^{31}P) at rest and exercise

Vessel-related end points

   Contrast arteriography

   Intravascular ultrasound

   Magnetic resonance and CT angiography

Biomarkers

   Numerous

Quality-of-life Instruments

General Health (SF-36v2)

PAD Specific Questionnaires

   Walking Impairment Questionnaire

   PAD-Physical activity recall (PAD-PAR)

severity of claudication pain, which is relevant in clinical practice. Thus, follow-up of patients based on absolute or initial claudication distance is preferable. Table 1.6 lists parameters that may be used to assess improvement in PAD patients.

CONCLUSIONS

A careful history and systematic evaluation of the arterial system is indispensable to accurate diagnosis, diagnostic planning, and therapy. Differential diagnostic considerations in the upper extremity tend to be more numerous and complex than in the lower extremity. Atherosclerosis still tends to be the most common form of arterial disease in the lower extremity and presents as intermittent claudication.

PRACTICAL POINTS

- Symptoms caused by vasospasm alone are intermittent and the extremity is asymptomatic and normal in appearance between attacks.

- The presence of tissue necrosis in the upper extremity almost always suggests fixed obstructive disease, even if the patient has Raynaud's symptoms.

- Acrocyanosis and pernio may mimic critical limb ischemia and should be differentiated.

- Aortoiliac disease may also produce aching discomfort in the hips and thighs along with a sensation of weakness in the lower extremity.

- Renal artery bruits that are hemodynamically significant are often systolic–diastolic.

- Thoracic outlet syndrome maneuvers such as Adson's tests are positive in normal individuals.

- The most common expansile lesion in the neck that needs to be distinguished from an aneurysm is "kinking" or "coiling" of the carotid artery.

CHAPTER 2 ■ Noninvasive Vascular Testing for the Diagnosis of Lower Extremity, Carotid, Renal Artery, and Abdominal Aortic Diseases

Michael R. Jaff

A thorough clinical evaluation and accurate noninvasive testing remain the cornerstones of successful patient stratification in vascular medicine. Given the myriad of therapeutic options in these complex patients, and the systemic nature of atherosclerosis, diagnostic methods must be accurate, safe, painless, and reproducible. Comprehensive methodical testing promotes improved outcomes through appropriate patient selection. Ultrasound-based testing in the four major peripheral arterial beds are reviewed in this chapter: lower extremity, extracranial carotid, abdominal aortic, and renal. Magnetic resonance imaging and CT angiographic techniques for the diagnosis of arterial disease are discussed in later chapters (see Chapters 4 and 5, respectively).

BASICS OF VASCULAR ULTRASOUND

An understanding of the principles of ultrasonography is an essential prerequisite for successful vascular testing as this modality is used in the diagnostic evaluation of most vascular beds. Vascular ultrasound is based on the principle of Christian Doppler, who described a "frequency shift" of an emitted sound wave beam. This "shift" is the difference between the frequency of transmission and the frequency of reflection. The frequency of the sound waves used in diagnostic ultrasound, measured in megahertz (MHz), is above the frequency heard by the human ear. As the ultrasound beam is emitted into the body, it hits flowing blood, among other targets (bone, soft tissue structures, etc.) and is reflected back to the ultrasound transducer crystal. This information is then converted into a gray-scale image on a monitor. The addition of the Doppler waveform to the gray-scale B-mode ("brightness" mode) image is known as *duplex ultrasonography (DUS)*. Modern, commercially available ultrasound machines add color to the gray-scale image. This provides more rapid identification of vascular structures and shortens the examination time significantly. Estimation of peak velocities requires the ultrasound beam to be parallel to the flow in the vessel. This can be adjusted on the machine (Fig. 2.1).

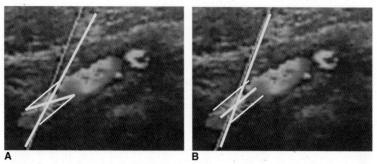

FIGURE 2-1. **A:** Incorrect Doppler angle. **B:** Correct Doppler angle where the angle of insonation is parallel to the direction of arterial flow.

DIAGNOSTIC EVALUATION OF LOWER EXTREMITY ARTERIAL DISEASE

Lower Extremity Arterial Testing

The evaluation of patients with peripheral artery disease (PAD) includes a historical review of patient symptoms and atherosclerotic risk factors, physical examination, and the use of noninvasive vascular tests. The equipment and training required to perform these examinations are minimal; therefore, these may be performed readily in the office in the initial diagnostic evaluation, immediately after or concomitant with physical examination.

Overall Approach to Lower Extremity Diagnostic Testing

Although many vascular practices, in conjunction with their vascular laboratories, use different algorithms for the diagnosis of PAD, there are some consistent patterns. Ankle-brachial indices (ABIs) are performed in every patient suspected of having PAD. If general information regarding the anatomic location of PAD is required, physiologic testing with segmental limb pressures (SLPs) and pulse volume recordings (PVRs) is sufficient. The addition of an exercise treadmill test to assess response of the ABI may be extremely helpful in confirming or excluding an arterial basis to lower extremity pain of a "claudication" nature. In addition, exercise testing provides an objective documentation of the true functional limitation of PAD and can be used to demonstrate physiologic improvement after intervention (Table 2.1). If specific information regarding the precise location of arterial stenoses or occlusion is required, DUS may be performed from the infrarenal abdominal aorta through the distal tibial arteries. In a number of vascular labs, ABIs, SLPs, and PVRs are obtained simultaneously as initial diagnostic tests in patients with suspected PAD, or limb discomfort without an obvious cause prior to or at the time of the initial visit.

TABLE 2.1

NONINVASIVE DIAGNOSTIC TESTING FOR PERIPHERAL ARTERIAL DISEASE

Vascular Laboratory Examination	Information Obtained	Clinical Indication	Limitations
Segmental limb pressures	Localizes disease to specific segments of the lower extremity arteries; may aid in predicting wound healing potential	Moderate to severe claudication or limb ischemia with consideration to revascularization	Inaccurate in patients with noncompressible arteries; requires special cuffs; proximal thigh cuff occasionally uncomfortable for the patient
Pulse volume recordings	Localizes disease to specific segments of the lower extremity arteries; may aid in predicting wound healing potential	Moderate to severe claudication or limb ischemia with consideration to revascularization; useful in calcified arteries	Requires a skilled and meticulous technologist; mainly qualitative information
Segmental Doppler waveforms	Localizes disease to specific segments of the lower extremity arteries; easy to perform and interpret	Moderate to severe claudication or limb ischemia with consideration to revascularization	Not accurate in calcified arteries; less accurate in selected centers than PVRs
Exercise ABI	Confirms diagnosis of peripheral arterial disease when resting ABI is >0.90	Atypical symptoms of exertional limb discomfort; Serial examinations to demonstrate clinical effects of intervention	Requires calibrated treadmill and close observation; many patients may not be able to complete exercise study; technologist must be competent to rapidly perform postexercise arterial pressures
Arterial duplex ultrasonography	Specific identification of sites of atherosclerotic disease: stenosis, occlusion; can accurately clarify options for invasive therapy	Advanced intermittent claudication, critical limb ischemia with need for revascularization; postcatheterization access site complication (i.e., pseudoaneurysm, hematoma, arteriovenous fistula)	Requires expensive equipment; requires skilled technologist; prolonged examination time; calcified arteries cause acoustic shadowing and inability to obtain Doppler velocities; provides only anatomic information and does not describe functional limitation

(Reprinted from Hiatt WR, Hirsch AT, Regensteiner J. *Peripheral arterial disease handbook.* Philadelphia: Lippincott, Williams & Wilkins, 2001:88–89, Table 5.1, with permission.)

Ankle-Brachial Index

The first objective test in the evaluation of PAD is the ABI. The test is inexpensive, painless, reproducible, quick, and relatively easily performed during an office visit. This test compares the blood pressure obtained with a handheld Doppler in the dorsalis pedis or posterior tibial artery (whichever is higher) to the blood pressure in the higher of the two brachial pressures. Oscillometric determination of the ABI may also provide an accurate determination of the ABI in an outpatient population and may be used in the absence of a Doppler. Generally, an ABI of 0.9 is considered normal, greater than 0.4 to less than 0.9 reflects mild to moderate PAD, and 0.4 or less suggests severe PAD. These categories do not always reflect the clinical status of the patient and are rough indices of disease severity. The latter is altered by a number of factors including lifestyle, concomitant disease modifiers, and collateralization to name a few factors. Limitations of the ABI include artifactually high ABI in patients with medial calcification, especially of the tibial vessels, resulting in high ankle pressures that sometimes may exceed 250 mm Hg and incorrect ABIs (≥ 1.3). In this case, the ABI is unreliable, and other objective tests must be utilized. Since digital vessels are usually not affected by medial calcification, a toe-brachial index (TBI) may be performed when ABIs are elevated. A TBI of less than 0.7 is considered abnormal. A high ABI is also associated with greater cardiovascular risk and thus may have prognostic implications. Recently, an alternate definition of PAD using the lower pressure in the involved lower extremity (rather than higher) has been proposed. Patients diagnosed with PAD by the alternate definition (up to 10% of the overall population) but not according to the current definition were found to be at higher risk on follow-up (median of 6.6 years).

Another limitation of the ABI, particularly in patients with moderate stenosis of the infrarenal abdominal aorta or common iliac arteries, is the finding of normal resting ABI. These patients may undergo exercise treadmill testing, particularly if the index of suspicion for PAD is high.

Exercise Ankle-Brachial Indices

Exercise ABIs are extremely helpful in making the diagnosis of PAD in unclear cases where the ABIs at rest are borderline or mildly reduced, and in situations when the patient presents with exertional lower extremity discomfort indistinguishable from claudication ("pseudoclaudication," see Chapter 1). They may also serve as a useful index of disease severity, to assess response to an intervention, and to serially follow patients. With exercise challenge (classically constant-speed, constant-grade treadmill testing at 2 mi/h at a 12% incline to a maximum of 5 minutes, or non–treadmill-based active pedal plantar flexion), the arterial limb pressure decreases in patients with PAD. A decrease of at least 20 mm Hg means the test is considered suggestive of hemodynamically significant PAD. The response to exercise in a patient without PAD is typified by a slight increase or no change in the ankle systolic pressures compared with resting pressures. An additional component that may be evaluated is the time for recovery of resting pressures to determine the "functional severity" of the patients' PAD.

Once the ABI has been performed, providing objective evidence of the overall severity of PAD in a limb, more specific noninvasive information may be obtained in the vascular laboratory. The use of SLPs in conjunction with PVRs can aid in localizing diseased arterial segments.

Segmental Limb Pressures

A series of limb pressure cuffs are placed on the thigh (typically two thigh cuffs–some centers prefer one in the upper thigh and the other in the lower thigh), calf, ankle, and, less commonly, the transmetatarsal region of the foot. The ABI is calculated, and then the pressure is sequentially inflated in each cuff to approximately 20 to 30 mm Hg above systolic pressure. Utilizing a continuous-wave Doppler probe and by gradually decreasing the pressure in the cuff, the pressure at each segment is measured. If a decrease in pressure between two consecutive levels of ≥30 mm Hg is identified, a stenosis in the arterial segment proximal to the cuff is inferred (Fig. 2.2). In addition,

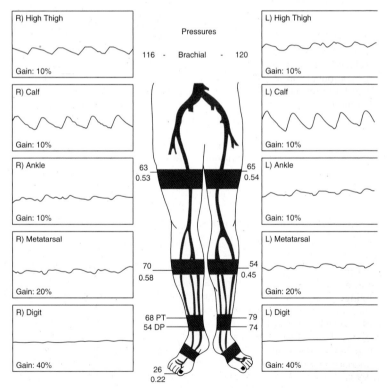

FIGURE 2-2.   SLPs and PVRs demonstrating aortoiliac disease. Note the dampened PVR waveforms in the thigh segment, as well as the decrease in thigh pressures compared to the brachial pressures (*Right*: 120–163 mm Hg; *left*: 120–165 mm Hg.)

comparing the two limbs, a 20- to 30-mm Hg discrepancy from one limb to the other at the same cuff level also suggests a significant arterial stenosis or occlusion proximal to the cuff ipsilateral to the limb with the lower pressure.

Pulse Volume Recordings

These are plethysmographic tracings that detect the changes in the volume of blood flowing through a limb. Using equipment similar to that previously described, the cuffs are inflated to 60 to 65 mm Hg, and a plethysmographic tracing is recorded at various levels. The normal PVR is similar to the normal intra-arterial pulse wave tracing and consists of a rapid systolic upstroke and rapid downstroke and a prominent dicrotic notch. With increasing severity of disease, the waveform becomes attenuated, with a widened waveform, and ultimately becomes flat or nonpulsatile. The limitations of this approach include prolonged examination time, increased cost, and difficulty in interpreting sequential or tandem lesion severity distal to a significant proximal stenosis.

Doppler Spectral Waveform Analysis

This can be used in lieu of pulse wave recordings, although they tend to be more operator dependent than PVRs. Used in conjunction with SLP, the waveform analysis provides additional information in assessing the extent and location of disease. The normal waveform is triphasic and includes forward and reverse (diastolic) components. With progression, the reverse component is lost, and the waveform becomes biphasic. When forward flow becomes continuous, the waveform is considered monophasic. With severe disease, the waveform amplitude is attenuated. Patterns of arterial flow may be recorded using a continuous Doppler over the femoral, popliteal, posterior tibial, and dorsalis pedis arteries.

Arterial Duplex Ultrasonography

Native vessel arterial DUS is widely performed. This examination is generally accepted as a precise method of defining arterial stenoses or occlusion. The sensitivity of DUS to detect occlusions and stenoses has been reported to be 95 and 92%, with specificities of 99 and 97%, respectively. Figure 2.3 illustrates a complete occlusion of the distal abdominal aorta in the same patient who underwent SLPs illustrated in Figure 2.2. Using a 5.0- to 7.5-MHz transducer, imaging of the suprainguinal and infrainguinal arteries is performed. The vessels are studied in the sagittal plane, and Doppler velocities are obtained using a 60-degree Doppler angle. Vessels are classified into one of five categories: normal, 1 to 19% stenosis, 20 to 49% stenosis, 50 to 99% stenosis, and occlusion. The categories are determined by alterations in the Doppler waveform, as well as increasing peak systolic velocities. For a stenosis to be classified as 50 to 99%, for example, the peak systolic velocity must increase by 100% in comparison to the normal segment of artery proximal to the stenosis. Arterial DUS has been used to guide the interventionist toward appropriate access to a lesion potentially amenable to endovascular therapy and

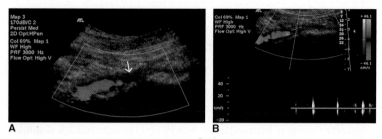

FIGURE 2-3. Duplex ultrasound of the abdominal aorta in the same patient as in Figure 2.2. **A:** Color image demonstrating occluded infrarenal aorta. **B:** Doppler analysis demonstrating preocclusive "thump" characteristic of occlusion. (*See* color insert.)

after endovascular intervention as a means of follow-up (Fig. 2.4). DUS following intervention may overestimate residual stenosis, and this may represent a limitation of this technique following intervention. However, with increasing experience, serial surveillance following endovascular intervention has been found to be quite effective in predicting anatomic regions of restenosis.

DUS is very helpful in identifying areas of vascular trauma, specifically iatrogenic trauma. Pseudoaneurysms occur in up to 7.5% of femoral artery catheterizations and can result in significant complications,

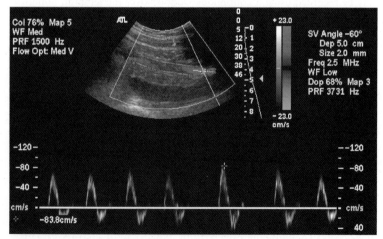

FIGURE 2-4. Duplex ultrasound analysis of an external iliac artery stent, demonstrating normal Doppler velocities and waveforms of a patent stent.

including distal embolization into the native arterial system, expansion, extrinsic compression on neurovascular structures, rupture, and hemorrhage. DUS can rapidly and accurately identify these lesions. In addition, the use of direct ultrasound-guided compression or, more recently, ultrasound-guided thrombin injection can repair these lesions without the need for more invasive surgical procedures.

Surgical Bypass Graft Surveillance

In patients who have undergone surgical bypass graft revascularization, particularly with saphenous vein, stenoses will develop in a number of cases. Once the graft becomes thrombosed, secondary patency rates are dismal. If the stenosis is detected and repaired prior to graft thrombosis, up to 80% of grafts will be salvaged (primary-assisted patency). Therefore, a well-organized graft surveillance program is crucial in preserving patency of the bypass graft (Fig. 2.5). Vein bypass grafts should be studied within 7 days of placement, at 1 month, and at 3-month intervals for the first year. If the graft remains normal after year 1, follow-up surveillance should be performed every 6 months thereafter. Ankle pressures and waveforms should also be performed at the time of each surveillance study. The development of a stenosis during a surveillance examination should prompt consideration toward x-ray contrast arteriography or magnetic resonance angiographic evaluation. The procedure for graft surveillance is performed in a similar manner as used in native vessel arterial DUS. The inflow artery to the bypass graft is initially imaged using a 5.0- to 7.5-MHz transducer at a Doppler

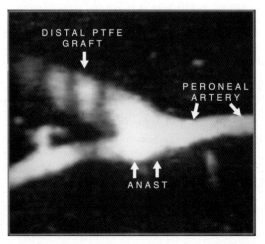

FIGURE 2-5. Duplex ultrasound demonstrating color power angiography technique of the distal anastomosis of a synthetic external iliac artery to peroneal artery bypass graft. (See color insert.)

angle of 60 degrees. Subsequently, the proximal anastomosis; proximal, mid, and distal graft; distal anastomosis; and outflow artery are interrogated. Peak systolic and end-diastolic velocities are obtained at each segment and compared to the segment of graft proximal to the area being studied. If the ratio of the peak systolic velocity within a stenotic segment relative to the normal segment proximal to the stenosis is greater than 2, this suggests 50 to 75% diameter reduction. The additional finding of end-diastolic velocities greater than 100 cm/s suggests greater than 75% stenosis.

Endovascular Intervention Surveillance

Recent data suggest that serial duplex ultrasound–based surveillance following certain interventions will translate to improved long-term patency. In one series, the ideal indicator of need for surveillance is an intraprocedural completion duplex ultrasound examination. If this examination is normal, it is unlikely that subsequent severe stenosis will be identified. In revascularization procedures where long-segment disease is treated, serial surveillance is likely beneficial.

Magnetic Resonance Angiography

MRA for the diagnosis of PAD is discussed in detail in Chapter 4.

Computed Tomographic Angiography

CT angiography using breath-hold spiral techniques is commonly used for the diagnosis of lower extremity arterial disease. 64-detector CT scanners using nongated techniques are widely used and provide for high resolution isotropic voxels ($0.5 \times 0.5 \times 0.5$ mm). Limited prior studies have demonstrated that computed tomographic angiography (CTA) using ≥16-detector systems CT angiography correctly depicted segmental occlusions and significant stenoses (greater than 50%) with a sensitivity and specificity of greater than 95% and an overall accuracy of greater than 95% compared to digital subtraction x-ray contrast arteriography. One limitation of CTA, is the presence of calcification, particularly in the infrageniculate territory that limits visualization of luminal patency. Additional considerations that impact on its routine use are contrast nephropathy, particularly in diabetics with low GFR, and increasing concern about concomitant radiation.

Noninvasive Evaluation of Extracranial Carotid Artery Disease

Duplex Ultrasonography

Direct visualization of the extracranial carotid arteries with DUS has been shown to provide excellent accuracy and reproducibility and is the initial modality of choice for noninvasive evaluation of extracranial carotid artery disease. The carotid duplex examination identifies plaque, stenoses, and occlusions in the common, internal, and external carotid arteries. The exam also identifies flow direction in the vertebral arteries. This examination is routinely indicated for patients with a history of transient

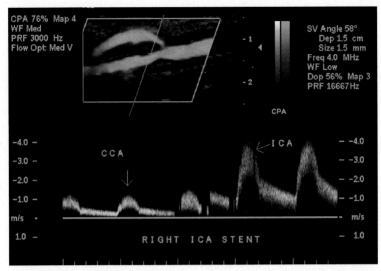

FIGURE 2-6. Duplex ultrasound of a carotid stent. Note the increase in peak systolic velocity comparing the *CCA* (common carotid artery) to the *ICA* (internal carotid artery) within the stent, suggesting a >50% stenosis.

ischemic attacks, stroke, or cervical bruits, after surgical or endovascular revascularization, and in patients deemed to be at high risk for the presence of carotid stenosis. The extracranial carotid arteries are identified in the longitudinal and transverse orientations, noting the presence of plaque and alterations in the color flow patterns. Doppler waveforms and velocity measurements are then obtained in representative segments of the common, external, and internal carotid arteries. These velocity data are obtained using a constant Doppler angle of ≤60 degrees (Fig. 2.6). Doppler-derived velocity measurements have been used to determine the severity of stenosis, based on many validation studies comparing these velocity data to the "gold standard" arteriograms (Table 2.2). Current data suggest the sensitivity of carotid duplex to be 85%, with a specificity of 90%. DUS is highly accurate in identifying a carotid artery occlusion, with a positive predictive value of 93%, and is very useful in documenting results of revascularization. However, each vascular laboratory must validate its own accuracy in order to avoid common, yet important errors in performing these exams. These limitations include overestimation of degrees of internal carotid artery stenosis due to severe contralateral internal carotid artery disease, underestimation of stenosis of the internal carotid artery due to unrecognized ipsilateral common carotid stenosis, misidentifying the external carotid artery as the internal, and interpreting severe stenoses as occlusions. Carotid DUS is useful in determining the adequacy of carotid revascularization, via either endarterectomy or stent deployment. Using similar protocols to native vessel imaging, the site of revascularization is

TABLE 2.2

DIAGNOSTIC CRITERIA FOR INTERNAL CAROTID ARTERY STENOSIS

% Stenosis	PSV	EDV	Flow Characteristics
0–19	<105 cm/s	—	Normal
20–39	<105 cm/s	—	Spectral broadening
40–59	105–150 cm/s	—	Increased spectral broadening
60–79[a]	151–240	—	Marked spectral broadening
80–99	>240 cm/s	>135 cm/s	Marked spectral broadening
Occluded	N/A	N/A	No flow. Preocclusive "thump." "Externalized" common carotid artery signal

[a]Peak systolic velocity, internal carotid artery/common carotid artery.
≥4.0 suggests >70% stenosis.
≥4.0 suggests <70% stenosis.

interrogated, and peak systolic and end-diastolic velocities are measured. Although imaging of carotid stents is straightforward, velocity criteria identifying restenosis suggest that Doppler velocities within stents are higher than in native, nonstented arteries. Many vascular laboratories compare immediate postprocedural velocities with those obtained during follow-up to assess restenosis (Fig. 2.6).

Magnetic Resonance Angiography

MRA techniques for the evaluation of the cerebral circulation are discussed in Chapter 4. MRA in conjunction with MRI of the brain provides excellent visualization of the extracranial and intracranial arterial circulation and may often be required in patients with symptomatic disease unexplained by duplex findings or in patients with suspected intracranial disease or other concomitant processes.

Computed Tomography Angiography

Similar to the techniques used in peripheral artery evaluation, CT angiography has become an important addition to the diagnostic armamentarium for patients with extracranial and intracranial carotid artery disease. When compared to diagnostic arteriography with modern CT systems (≥16-detectors), CTA performs very well. In one series of patients presenting with high-grade carotid artery stenosis with symptoms, the sensitivity and specificity of CTA were 95 and 93%, respectively. An important limitation to its routine first-line use is the presence of calcification, which occurs commonly at the bifurcation/ICA that severely limits accurate assessment of stenosis severity owing to "blooming artifact." CTA is therefore used best as an adjunct to ultrasonography particularly in cases where additional questions need to be addressed including the status of the proximal arch, great vessel origins, and high bifurcation of the carotid and intracranial stenosis. Dual-energy CT has the theoretic potential to differentiate between calcified plaques and iodinated contrast medium by exploiting the energy dependence of the CT attenuation of calcium and iodine and might therefore provide luminograms comparable to those generated by DSA. Initial studies suggest a high sensitivity for the detection of relevant stenoses, a higher correlation to DSA but frequent overestimation of high-grade stenoses as occlusions. Dual-energy CT plaque and bone removal may serve as a complementary technique to standard CTA in the near future, especially in the assessment of carotid stenosis.

Noninvasive Evaluation of Renal Artery Stenosis

Atherosclerotic renal artery stenosis (RAS) has become increasingly recognized as a contributing factor to resistant hypertension, deterioration in renal function, recurrent "flash pulmonary edema," and the long-term cardiovascular effects of poorly controlled hypertension. Patients with severe bilateral RAS or stenosis to a solitary functioning kidney are at risk for the development of end-stage renal disease. Long-term survival of patients with atherosclerotic RAS requiring dialytic support is dismal. A number of noninvasive methods of diagnosis in RAS are now available such as DUS, CT angiography, and MRA. Each "screening" test has inherent advantages and limitations and, depending on experience with the use of these modalities, has its own proponents. These techniques are increasingly being used to evaluate the renal arteries and are supplanting radionuclide scans to evaluate RAS. These techniques are discussed in some detail in Chapters 4 and 10, respectively. A reasonable algorithm for approaching RAS is provided in Figure 10.2.

Renal Artery Duplex Ultrasonography

Ultrasonography has significant advantages that make it an excellent diagnostic test when performed by experienced technologists. To provide an accurate renal artery duplex examination, both the technologist and the physician must be committed to learning all of the nuances of this examination. An important metric is based on the comparison of peak systolic velocities within the renal arteries and the abdominal aorta, referred to as the renal:aortic ratio (RAR). The peak systolic velocity is obtained in the aorta at the level of the superior mesenteric artery. The entire renal artery from the ostium to the hilum of the kidney must be interrogated (Fig. 2.7). If the RAR is ≥3.5, this corresponds with a 60 to 99% stenosis (Fig. 2.8). (For duplex criteria to diagnose RAS also see Table 10.2.) In a large prospective series of 102 consecutive patients who underwent both DUS and contrast arteriography within 1 month of each other, 62 of 63 arteries with less than 60% stenosis, 31 of 32 arteries with 60 to 79% stenosis, and 67 of 69 arteries with 80 to 99% stenosis were correctly identified by DUS. Occluded renal arteries were correctly identified by ultrasonography in 22 of 23 cases. The overall sensitivity of DUS was 98%, specificity 99%, positive predictive value 99%, and negative predictive value 97%.

DUS is the ideal method of determining the adequacy of renal artery stent revascularization. The entire renal artery can be imaged, despite the

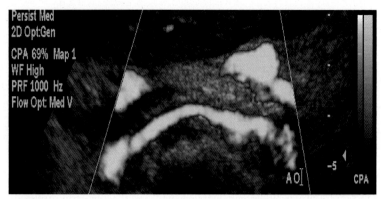

FIGURE 2-7. Color power angiography technique demonstrating the right renal artery from the aorta (*AO*) to the hilum of the kidney. (See color insert.)

presence of a metallic endoprosthesis. In addition, early or late restenosis is detected by an increase in the peak systolic velocity within the stented segment of the renal artery, as well as an increase in the RAR. Doppler velocity criteria suggesting in-stent restenosis of the renal artery is significantly higher than those seen in native renal arteries.

Limitations of renal artery duplex imaging include body habitus and overlying bowel gas obscuring identification of the renal arteries. Some

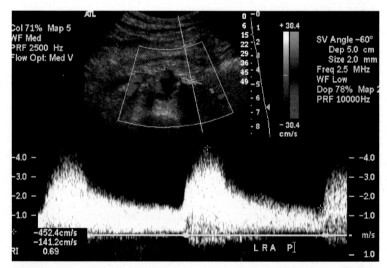

FIGURE 2-8. Duplex ultrasound analysis of the proximal right renal artery (*LRA P*). The peak systolic velocity (452.4 cm/s) and end-diastolic velocity (141.2) suggest a critical 80 to 99% stenosis.

authors have suggested that renal hilar imaging is easier and is as accurate as complete interrogation of the renal arteries. However, direct comparison of both techniques has revealed limitations of hilar scanning, including low sensitivity, inability to discriminate between stenosis and occlusion, and inadequate determination of accessory renal arteries. Given that many patients have both main renal artery disease and intraparenchymal disease, the addition of resistive indices within the parenchyma may help predict which patients will benefit from revascularization.

Magnetic Resonance Angiography

MRA is extremely useful in cases where DUS is not feasible or cannot be performed accurately. In some centers, MRA is routinely used for the diagnostic workup of secondary hypertension due to RAS. Gadolinium-enhanced MRA provides high-resolution 3D data sets in a single breath hold that permit multiplanar reformatting of the renal arteries. This is discussed in detail in Chapters 4 and 10.

Computed Tomography Angiography

Recent data using 64-slice multidetector CTA scanners have suggested that, when compared to contrast arteriography, CTA performs exceptionally well in the diagnosis of RAS. However, limitations of the technology include visualization of lumen in significantly calcified and stented arteries and those not specific to the diagnosis of renal artery disease including iodinated contrast administration (especially in those with preexisting renal dysfunction) and radiation exposure.

Noninvasive Evaluation of Aortic Aneurysmal Disease

An abdominal aortic aneurysm is suspected in the following scenarios: palpation of a pulsatile abdominal mass, a family history of aortic aneurysms in a first-degree relative, or the incidental discovery on an imaging study performed for unrelated reasons. Management decisions are based on the transverse dimension of the aneurysm, the location (e.g., suprarenal vs. infrarenal), and the overall health of the patient. Ultrasound, MRA, and CT angiographic techniques are widely used in the initial diagnosis of aneurysmal disease involving the abdominal aorta. MRA and, more commonly, CTA are preferred in the planning of endograft therapy for aneurysmal disease. CTA specifically provides exquisite anatomic and spatial detail that is essential for the endovascular management and postprocedure follow-up of these patients.

Duplex Ultrasonography

This is the preferred modality for initial screening of populations for abdominal aortic aneurysms (AAAs) and for periodic surveillance of AAA expansion, as ultrasound-based measurements are extremely reliable and reproducible. Ultrasonography is also commonly used for the assessment of aortic root aneurysms and concomitant aortic insufficiency. However, the inability of this technique to provide detailed assessment of the rest of the thoracic aorta including the arch and the great vessels is an important limitation in the comprehensive assessment of aneurysmal disease. This same limitation involving anatomic coverage and resolution of aortic branches is an important advantage for CTA and MRA.

The technique for performing duplex evaluation of the abdominal aorta involves using a low-frequency (i.e., 3.5-MHz) transducer. After an overnight fast, the patient is studied in the supine, reverse Trendelenburg position and the aorta is identified at the level of the diaphragm in the sagittal plane throughout its length. The ultrasound probe is then reoriented in the coronal plane, and transverse measurements are obtained in the suprarenal, juxtarenal, and infrarenal positions (Fig. 2.9). The normal infrarenal abdominal aortic diameter varies by sex and age. Specifically, in one series of 261 normal patients who volunteered for abdominal aortic duplex scanning, the aortic diameter in the transverse plane was 1.73 ± 0.30 cm, with males over age 50 demonstrating significantly larger aortic diameters than younger women. Although several different measurements can be obtained, most believe that the transverse measurement is the most accurate and a representative of true aortic diameter. Serial ultrasound evaluations of AAAs have demonstrated important information about rate of growth and potential for aneurysm rupture. In one series of 181 patients with the diagnosis of AAA, the median overall aneurysm growth rate was 0.21 cm/y. Estimated rupture risk was 0% per year when the last

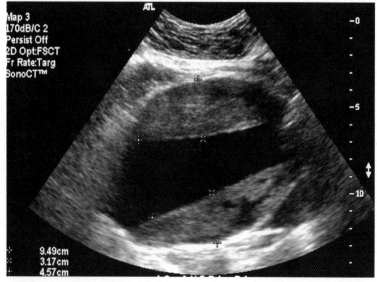

FIGURE 2-9.   Gray-scale duplex ultrasound image of an abdominal aortic aneurysm, with extensive intraluminal thrombus.

ultrasound measurement was less than 4.0 cm, 1.0% per year when 4.0 to 4.99 cm, and 11% per year when the measurement was 5.0 to 5.99 cm. Screening for AAA with ultrasonography has translated into a reduction in aneurysm rupture rate of 49%. Recently, there have been some data with the use of color DUS in the detection of AAA endoleaks although the utility of ultrasonography in assessment of endoleaks in endografts in locations other than abdominal is likely to be limited. Additional limitations include obesity and overlying bowel gas, which may preclude direct visualization of the stent graft. The administration of an intravenous echo contrast agent may enhance the sensitivity of DUS to detect endoleaks.

Computed Tomographic Angiography

CT techniques are commonly used in the diagnosis of thoracic and abdominal aortic disease, owing to the widespread availability of CT scanners. The volume coverage provided by CTA is exceptional and provides for comprehensive assessment of the arch, aorta, and iliac bifurcation in one single scan. This is a singular advantage over ultrasound-based techniques that provide limited visualization of the aorta. CTA is also superior to ultrasound techniques in assessing aneurysmal wall integrity, the location and amount of calcification within vessel walls, venous anomalies, retroperitoneal blood, and aortic dissection, infection, or inflammation, as well as the proximal and distal extent of the aneurysm. CT may also demonstrate concomitant pathology (presence of masses, concomitant stenosis, tortuosity, etc.) that may be important during planning for either an open or an endovascular approach. CT is the modality most commonly used in the diagnosis and follow-up of endoleaks (see Chapters 4b and 12). Reformatting using maximum intensity projections, curved planar reformations, and volume rendering techniques provides for visualization in an infinite number of planes.

Magnetic Resonance Imaging

MR imaging obviates the need for iodinated contrast agents and catheter-based arteriography with their associated risks of nephrotoxicity and atheroembolization, respectively. MR protocols utilized in the systematic evaluation of the thoracic aorta include 3D contrast-enhanced MRA and spin-echo techniques (black-blood techniques) in multiple planes to assess the extent of the aneurysm and provide information on the involvement of great vessels and their relationship to the aneurysm. 3D contrast data set acquisition is fast (less than 30 seconds) and provides detailed images of the thoracic and abdominal aorta. Multiplanar reformations of the image data sets aid in the display of the often complex tortuous anatomy of aneurysms. MR imaging may also be used in the follow-up of endovascular stents provided the metallic stents are made of a material that can be visualized.

CONCLUSIONS

The vascular laboratory provides accurate and noninvasive methods of determining the presence and severity of arterial disorders. An appropriate history and physical examination will often provide guidance as to the type of examination required. DUS remains the staple of modern noninvasive vascular imaging. Accuracy with this technique is dependent on a commitment to high-quality examinations and correlation with other "gold-standard" tests to provide reassurance of accuracy in the laboratory. MR and CT techniques are particularly helpful in the comprehensive evaluation of aortic aneurysmal disease and cerebrovascular disease. Each test has limitations that must be considered when interpreting the results.

PRACTICAL POINTS

■ The first test to perform in patients with suspected peripheral arterial disease is the ABI.

■ SLPs and PVRs provide information regarding location of arterial disease of the lower extremities.

■ Exercise studies are helpful in excluding disease in patients with lower extremity discomfort and "pseudoclaudication."

■ RAS may be reliably detected with renal artery DUS. A renal-to-aortic ratio (RAR) > 3.5 corresponds to a 60 to 99% stenosis.

■ DUS is useful for screening and follow-up of AAAs.

■ CT is superior to ultrasonographic techniques in assessing aortic wall integrity (dissection) calcification, venous anomalies, retroperitoneal blood, and anatomic extent of the aneurysmal disease, and in the diagnosis and follow-up of endoleaks.

RECOMMENDED READING

Bandyk DF. Ultrasonic duplex scanning in the evaluation of arterial grafts and dilatations. *Echocardiography* 1987;4:251–264.

Bandyk DP, Chauvupan JP. Duplex ultrasound surveillance can be worthwhile after arterial intervention. *Perspect Vasc Surg Endovasc Ther* 2007;19:354–359.

Berg M, Zhang Z, Ikonen A, et al. Multi-detector row CT angiography in the assessment of carotid artery disease in symptomatic patients: comparison with rotational angiography and digital subtraction angiography. *Am J Neuroradiol* 2005;26:1022–1034.

Chi YW, White CJ, Thornton S, et al. Ultrasound velocity criteria for renal in-stent restenosis. *J Vasc Surg* 2009;50:119–123.

Elsman BHP, Legemate DA, van der Heyden FWHM, et al. The use of color-coded duplex scanning in the selection of patients with lower extremity arterial disease for percutaneous transluminal angioplasty: a prospective study. *Cardiovasc Intervent Radiol* 1996;19:313–316.

Espinola-Klein C, Rupprecht HJ, Bickel C, et al. Different calculations of ankle-brachial index and their impact on cardiovascular risk prediction. *Circulation* 2008;118(9):961–967. [Epub 2008 Aug 12.]

Golledge J, Cuming R, Ellis M, et al. Duplex imaging findings predict stenosis after carotid endarterectomy. *J Vasc Surg* 1997;26:43–48.

Hadley G, Jaff MR. Duplex ultrasonography following carotid artery stent placement. *Semin Cerebrovasc Dis Stroke* 2005;5:83–92.

Olin JW, Piedmonte MR, Young JR, et al. The utility of duplex ultrasound scanning of the renal arteries for diagnosing significant renal artery stenosis. *Ann Intern Med* 1995;122:833–838.

Rademacher J, Chavan A, Bleck J, et al. Use of Doppler ultrasonography to predict the outcome of therapy for renal-artery stenosis. *N Engl J Med* 2001;334:410–417.

Reed WW, Hallett JW, Damiano MA, et al. Learning from the last ultrasound: a population-based study of patients with abdominal aortic aneurysm. *Arch Intern Med* 1997;157:2064–2068.

Ricci MA, Kleeman M, Case T, et al. Normal aortic diameter by ultrasound. *J Vasc Tech* 1995;19:17–19.

Stewart JH, Grubb M. Understanding vascular ultrasonography. *Mayo Clin Proc* 1992;67:1186–1196.

Strandness DE. Noninvasive vascular laboratory and vascular imaging. In: Young JR, Olin JW, Bartholomew JR, eds. *Peripheral vascular diseases*, 2nd ed. St. Louis: Mosby, 1996:33–64.

Whelan JF, Barry MH, Moir JD. Color flow Doppler ultrasonography: comparison with peripheral arteriography for the investigation of peripheral vascular disease. *J Clin Ultrasound* 1992;20:369–374.

Zwiebel WJ, ed. *Introduction to vascular ultrasonography*, 5th ed. Philadelphia: Saunders, 2004.

CHAPTER 3 ■ Diagnostic Catheter–Based Vascular Angiography

Debabrata Mukherjee

Angiography allows direct visualization of blood vessels in the body by the injection of iodinated contrast material via a catheter placed directly into the artery or vein. It remains the gold standard to determine the severity and extent of peripheral arterial disease. Digital subtraction angiographic technology allows high-quality images using small amounts of contrast material. The field of angiography has grown tremendously in recent years, and today we have percutaneous methods for accessing virtually every artery in the human body. A number of unique catheter shapes have been developed to facilitate intubation/cannulation of the ostium of specific arteries. However, angiography is invasive and is typically indicated only in patients in whom revascularization is being considered.

ANATOMIC CONSIDERATIONS

Access for Vascular Angiography

The choice of the appropriate arterial access site is crucial. Typically for the purposes of endovascular intervention, the access site should be as close to the intended lesion as possible. The location of the lesion determines the access site in most cases, and approach to iliac occlusive disease is most commonly made from the ipsilateral femoral artery via retrograde common femoral artery (CFA) access. Lesions of the CFA, however, must be approached from a contralateral-puncture, axillary, or popliteal approach. Lesions distal to the CFA are best approached and treated with an antegrade CFA approach. For renal, mesenteric, and cerebral angiography, the typical access site is retrograde CFA.

Retrograde Common Femoral Artery Access

This is the commonest access site used for diagnostic angiography. The CFA is palpated below the inguinal ligament, which courses between the pubis and the anterior superior iliac spine. In patients with peripheral arterial disease, one should always check the site/level under fluoroscopy prior to arterial puncture. In individuals with severe peripheral arterial disease, the femoral pulse is often not palpable, and in those instances, ultrasound-guided approach should be used or an alternative access site should be used. The SmartNeedle (Escalon Vascular Access Inc., New Berlin, WI) is a percutaneous Doppler-guided vascular access device, which uses a handheld monitor and a Doppler transducer located at the tip of an access needle to provide continuous auditory feedback and is often helpful in patients with absent or weak pulses.

Brachial/Radial Artery Access

Brachial artery access is considered in individuals with bilateral iliac artery or distal aortic occlusions. In some individuals with severely angulated origin of the visceral vessels, that is, celiac, superior mesenteric, or renal arteries, brachial approach may make selective cannulation easier. Left brachial approach is preferable to minimize the potential risk of stroke, as entry from the right exposes both the carotid and vertebral arteries to risk of embolization. The risk of injury and thrombosis is significantly higher with brachial compared to femoral access. It is recommended that the operator injects 3,000 to 5,000 units of unfractionated heparin in the sheath after brachial/radial access to minimize risk of thrombosis. If the radial artery is used for access, 50 to 100 μg of intra-arterial nitroglycerin or verapamil is administered to minimize spasm in addition to heparin.

Popliteal Artery Access

In individuals with occluded superficial femoral arteries, the popliteal artery may be cannulated for diagnostic angiography. Limitations to this access site include the requirement that the patient lies prone during the procedure and the difficulty in localizing the artery. Doppler-guided needle approach should ideally be used to access the popliteal artery. This access site is rarely used for diagnostic angiography and more commonly used for interventions.

FUNDAMENTALS

Angiography involves direct injection of iodinated contrast material into the blood vessels for their visualization. Many different contrast agents are available today for angiography. The two clinically important attributes of a contrast agent are its iodine dose and osmolality. To maintain good radiographic efficacy and safety, contrast agents must balance the somewhat paradoxical relationship between these two properties. Iodine dose refers to the amount of iodine delivered in an injected dose of contrast material. The iodine, delivered by iodinated benzene ring compounds, produces radiographic "contrast" by blocking x-rays. Visualization is typically improved by increasing the iodine load, a function of the percentage of iodine and the concentration of the compound present upon injection. Increasing the iodine load, however, results in increased osmolality. Osmolality refers to the number of dissolved particles in a solution or the concentration. Ideally, contrast agents injected into the vasculature should have an osmolality as close to that of body fluids as possible. Solutions with osmolality greater (hypertonic) or less (hypotonic) than that of body fluids can cause cells to shrink or swell, respectively, contributing to numerous hemodynamic, physiologic, and biologic adverse effects. The body also attempts to quickly dilute and excrete hypertonic solutions to maintain osmotic equilibrium. Therefore, the benefits gained from increasing the iodine load in contrast agents to improve radiographic efficacy may be offset by the adverse effects associated with higher osmolality solutions.

The goal should be to use the lowest dose and volume of contrast necessary for adequate clinical angiography. Broadly, there are two types of agents, high-osmolality and low-osmolality agents. The major resistance to the use of low-osmolality agents used to be expense, but recent price reductions have made this a relative nonissue. High-osmolality agents are rarely used in practice now. Third-generation nonionic contrast agents reduce osmolality even further by creating a dimer. Iodixanol is a dimeric contrast agent in this class and is iso-osmolal with plasma. Nonionic, low osmolal contrast agents are now routinely used for angiography. Individuals with prior significant contrast reactions, active asthma, severe congestive heart failure, active significant arrhythmia, aortic stenosis, pulmonary hypertension, or significant renal dysfunction (serum creatinine greater than 2 mg/dL) should receive a low-osmolal or preferably an iso-osmolal agent. For diagnostic vascular angiography, we use an iso-osmolal agent iodixanol (Visipaque, GE Healthcare, Little Chalfont, Buckinghamshire) that has been shown to cause significantly less discomfort for patients and also significantly reduces the relative risk of developing contrast media–induced renal failure. In individuals with prior severe allergic reaction to contrast agents, gadolinium can be used for angiography using digital subtraction angiography (DSA) provided GFR is greater than 30 mL/min. Carbon dioxide has a limited role as a vascular contrast agent because of poor opacification of the vessels despite use of DSA.

CLINICAL ASPECTS OF ANGIOGRAPHY

Knowledge of appropriate catheters, angulations, and injection rates is imperative in performing safe and optimal vascular angiography. Table 3.1 makes general recommendation for catheter selection and injection rates in different vascular territories.

Lower Extremity Angiography

Despite recent advances in the noninvasive evaluation of lower extremity vascular disease, contrast angiography remains the gold standard. A pelvic/abdominal aortogram (Fig. 3.1) is initially performed with a straight pigtail catheter (Fig. 3.2) placed at the level of L1-L2 slightly above the level of the aortoiliac bifurcation (typically L3). This allows excellent visualization of the distal aorta and the origin of the common iliac arteries and the external iliac and the common femoral vessels. Angulated views are indicated to visualize the iliac and the femoral bifurcations without overlap. A left anterior oblique (LAO 30 degrees) view allows visualization of the left common iliac and right common femoral bifurcations without overlap. Digital subtraction pelvic aortograms are performed with 10 to 15 mL of iso-osmolal contrast at a rate of injection of 15 mL/s. Following the pelvic aortogram, the pigtail catheter is withdrawn to the aortic bifurcation so that the injected contrast fills the runoff vessels bilaterally with minimal contrast diverted to the viscera. DSA with moving table and bolus chase technology to visualize the outflow (Fig. 3.3A) and the runoff vessels

TABLE 3.1

RECOMMENDATIONS FOR DIAGNOSTIC VASCULAR ANGIOGRAPHY

Artery	Catheter	Angulation	Injection
Arch aortogram	5 FR angulated pigtail at aortic root	30° LAO	10 mL/s for 3 s
Abdominal aortogram for suspected mesenteric ischemia	5 FR straight pigtail between T12 and L1	Biplane or lateral	20 mL/s for 2 s
Abdominal aortogram for suspected renal artery stenosis	5 FR straight pigtail between T12 and L1	AP	20 mL/s for 0.5 s using DSA
Pelvic/abdominal aortogram	5 FR straight pigtail between L1 and L2	AP	15 mL/s for 1 s using DSA
Distal aorta for bolus chase and runoff[a]	5 FR straight pigtail between L2 and L3	AP	8 mL/s for 10 s using DSA
Carotids and great vessels	JR4 catheter for level 1 arch	Ipsilateral oblique 30° and lateral	Hand injection with DSA
	Vitek or Headhunter catheter for level 2 arch	Ipsilateral oblique 30° and lateral	Hand injection with DSA
	Simmons 1 or 2 for level 3 arch	Ipsilateral oblique 30° and lateral	Hand injection with DSA
Renal arteries	JR4 catheter, SOS catheter	AP and ipsilateral oblique at 20°–30°	Hand injection with DSA
Celiac trunk	JR4, SOS, Cobra catheters	AP	Injection at 10 mL/s
Superior mesenteric artery	JR4, SOS, Cobra catheters	AP	Injection at 8 mL/s
Inferior mesenteric artery	JR4, SOS, Cobra catheters	AP	Injection at 3 mL/s
Pulmonary artery	Grollman catheter	LAO/RAO 30°	20 mL/s for 2 s

[a]The volume should be reduced by 50% if each leg is injected separately.
LAO, left anterior oblique; RAO, right anterior oblique; AP, anteroposterior; DSA, digital subtraction angiography.

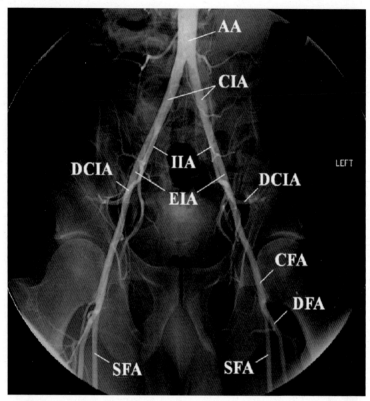

FIGURE 3-1. Pelvic aortogram showing common iliac arteries and their bifurcation. Common femoral artery and its bifurcation are also displayed. (AA, abdominal aorta; CIA, common iliac artery; EIA, external iliac artery; IIA, internal iliac artery; DCIA, deep circumflex iliac artery; CFA, common femoral artery; SFA, superficial femoral artery; DFA, deep femoral artery)

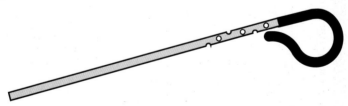

FIGURE 3-2. A straight pigtail catheter (Omniflush) is used to perform abdominal and pelvic aortograms.

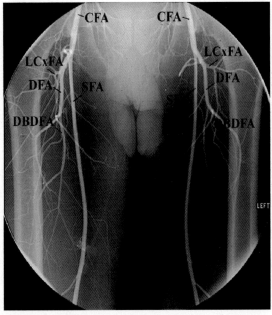

FIGURE 3-3.   A: Bilateral lower extremity outflow angiography; anteroposterior view with digital subtraction technique. (CFA, common femoral artery; DFA, deep femoral artery; SFA, superficial femoral artery; LCxFA, lateral circumflex femoral artery; DBDFA, descending branch of deep femoral artery)   (*Continued*)

is recommended (Fig. 3.3B). The bolus chase technology combines the advantages of digital subtraction and step table technology. Mask images are obtained prior to acquisition of contrast images to further accentuate the arterial tree. Figure 3.4 is a schematic of the arterial supply to the lower extremities.

Upper Extremity Angiography

Upper extremity angiography is performed significantly less often than lower extremity angiography as fewer than 5% of limb ischemia cases affect the arms. It is indicated primarily for the diagnosis of thoracic outlet syndromes and embolic disease. If upper extremity angiography is performed, one should delineate the entire circulation of the extremity from the subclavian to the digital vessels. The procedure is usually performed via retrograde femoral access with a JR4 catheter, to selectively cannulate the subclavian arteries. For older individuals with significant tortuosity of the arch, a Vitek or a Simmons catheter may be used instead. Once the proximal vessels are examined, the catheter is advanced into the axillary artery for more distal imaging. Optimal imaging of the digital vessels is performed with the catheter in the brachial artery using DSA. Knowledge of

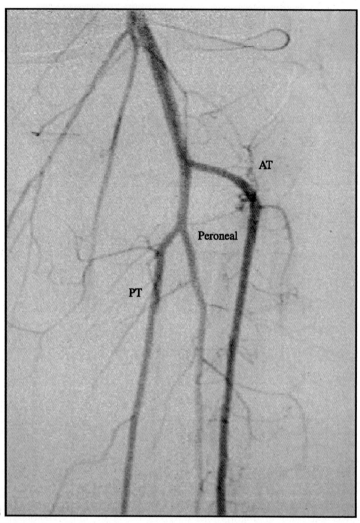

B

FIGURE 3-3. (*Continued*) **B:** angiogram of the runoff of the lower extremity. The arterial supply below the knee is via the anterior tibial (*AT*), the peroneal, and the posterior tibial (*PT*) arteries. The AT is the most lateral vessel and the PT is the most medial. The peroneal lies in the middle and gives off perforator branches.

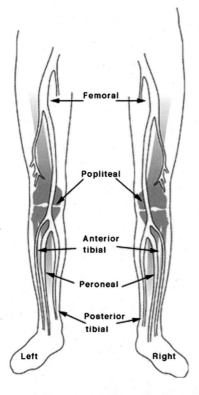

FIGURE 3-4.   Schematic of the circulation of the lower extremities.

TABLE 3.2

ANOMALIES OF THE UPPER EXTREMITY VESSELS

Common Arterial Variants	Incidence (%)
Brachial Artery	
Persistent superficial brachial artery	1–2
Radial artery origin from proximal brachial artery	12
Ulnar artery origin from proximal brachial artery	1–2
Forearm Arteries	
High origin of radial artery from brachial or axillary artery	14–17
Persistent median artery	2–4
Persistent interosseus artery	<0.1
Palmar Arch	
Incomplete deep arch of the hand	3–5
Incomplete superficial palmar arch	22

(Adapted from Kadir S. Regional anatomy of the thoracic aorta. In: *Atlas of normal and variant angiographic anatomy.* Philadelphia: WB Saunders, 1991.)

normal anatomy of the arch and upper extremity vessels as well as common anatomic variations (e.g., incomplete palmar arch) is crucial. Table 3.2 lists the common anatomic variants encountered in practice that are relevant to upper extremity angiography, and Figure 3.5 depicts several anomalies of the origin of the subclavian artery.

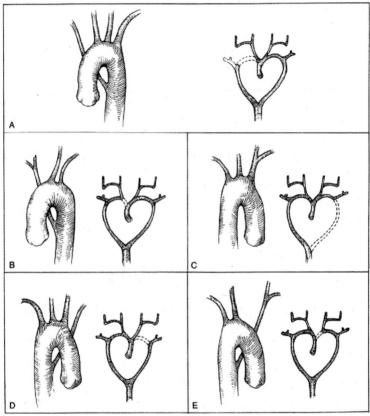

FIGURE 3-5. Diagram illustrating the development of aberrant subclavian or brachiocephalic arteries. A: Interruption of the embryonic right arch proximal to the seventh cervical intersegmental artery gives rise to the aberrant right subclavian artery. This can also be associated with other anomalies of the arch vessels. B: Interruption at a more central level gives rise to the aberrant right brachiocephalic artery. C: Persistence of the right fourth arch and regression of the left aorta give rise to the right aortic arch. D: Interruption of the left fourth arch proximal to the seventh cervical intersegmental artery gives rise to the aberrant left subclavian artery seen with a right aortic arch. E: Interruption of the left fourth arch at a more central location results in the formation of aberrant left brachiocephalic artery. (Adapted from Kadir S. Regional anatomy of the thoracic aorta. In: *Atlas of normal and variant angiographic anatomy.* Philadelphia: WB Saunders, 1991.)

Renal and Mesenteric Angiography

Renal angiography is usually performed as a prelude to renal artery revascularization in patients with refractory hypertension or renal insufficiency. Other indications for renal angiography include evaluating prospective renal donors to define arterial supply (contrast-enhanced magnetic resonance angiography is a good option as well) and assessing tumor vascularity in renal tumors. An abdominal aortogram (Fig. 3.6) is initially performed with a straight pigtail catheter (Fig. 3.2) placed at the level of the L1 vertebra. DSA is used and a total of 10 mL of contrast is injected for abdominal aortogram (20 mL/s and 0.5 s injection). This allows visualization of the origin of the main renal arteries and accessory renal arteries if present. Kidneys are typically supplied by a single artery arising from the aorta caudal to the superior mesenteric artery (SMA) origin between L1 and L2. In a significant proportion of individuals (as high as 40% in some reports), multiple renal arteries are present and may arise as caudally as the iliac arteries. Selective renal artery cannulation can usually be performed using a Judkins Right (JR4) catheter (Fig. 3.7).

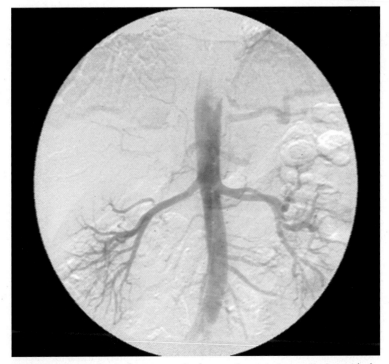

FIGURE 3-6. Abdominal aortogram in the anterior-posterior projection with the catheter at T12-L1 level. The angiogram reveals normal bilateral renal arteries.

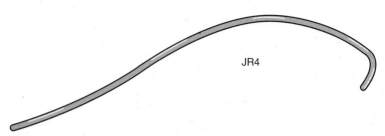

FIGURE 3-7. The Judkins Right 4 (JR4) catheter can be used to selectively cannulate the renal, the mesenteric, and the great vessels.

Arteries with unusual or angulated takeoffs may need to be cannulated with an SOS catheter (Fig. 3.8). Selective renal angiograms are performed with 3 to 4 mL of contrast, hand-injected, using DSA. One should stay on cine for delayed imaging to visualize the nephrogram and ascertain the renal size. The renal artery ostium is best visualized in the ipsilateral 30-degree oblique view (LAO 30 degrees for the left renal artery ostium). If there is significant angiographic stenosis of the renal artery, a pressure gradient should be measured prior to consideration of revascularization. A gradient more than 20 mm Hg suggests hemodynamically significant stenosis. A clinical benefit of using a 5-French SOS catheter for selective

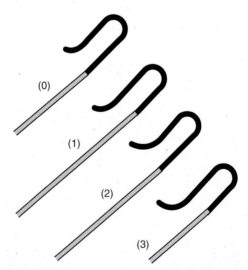

FIGURE 3-8. The SOS catheter is a unique preshaped catheter useful for selective cannulation of the renal and mesenteric vessels. The length of the catheter tip defines the catheter from 0 to 3.

cannulation is that by withdrawing the catheter slightly, the tip advances beyond the proximal portion of the renal artery and a gradient can be measured directly.

Typical indications for mesenteric angiography include chronic mesenteric ischemia or intestinal angina, acute mesenteric ischemia, and uncontrolled gastrointestinal bleeding. Lateral aortography should be performed as the initial study to identify the origin of the mesenteric vessels. Selective cannulations of the celiac, the SMA, and the inferior mesenteric artery (IMA) can usually be performed using a JR4 catheter (Fig. 3.7). In some cases, catheters with longer tips such as SOS (Fig. 3.8) or the Cobra catheter (Fig. 3.9) may be needed for selective injections. For good-quality mesenteric angiograms without streaming, the rate of injection should match the flow rate of the vessel being studied. The typical flow rates are 10 mL/s for the celiac trunk, 8 mL/s for the SMA, and 3 mL/s for the IMA. DSA acquisition is less likely to be helpful for mesenteric angiography because of the presence of bowel gas. In individuals who are being evaluated for GI bleeding, the clinically suspected vessel should be injected first.

When interpreting mesenteric angiograms, one needs to be aware of common aberrancies and anomalies. Anomalies of the celiac trunk complex are common (30 to 40%) and usually involve the origin of the hepatic arteries. The hepatic arteries may arise from a number of locations, including the abdominal aorta, left gastric, or superior mesenteric arteries. When the common hepatic artery arises from a source other than the celiac trunk, it is considered an aberrant common hepatic artery. The term "accessory" hepatic artery is used only when a right or left hepatic artery coexists with

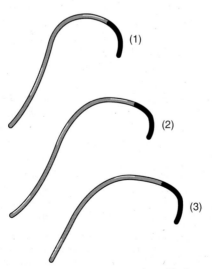

FIGURE 3-9.   The Cobra catheter is a unique preshaped catheter useful for selective cannulation of the mesenteric vessels.

a normal hepatic artery arising from the celiac trunk. In the absence of a normal right or left artery, its replacement by an aberrant vessel is called a "replaced" hepatic artery.

Cerebral Angiography

An arch aortogram should be performed prior to attempts at selective cannulation of the great vessels. Figure 3.10 is a schematic of the variations in the origins of the aortic arch vessels. A low-profile preformed catheter is advanced into the ostium of the great vessels for selective angiograms. Since even small emboli may have devastating consequences in this territory, use of gentle and meticulous technique is imperative. A minimum number of catheter exchanges are recommended, and it is useful to start

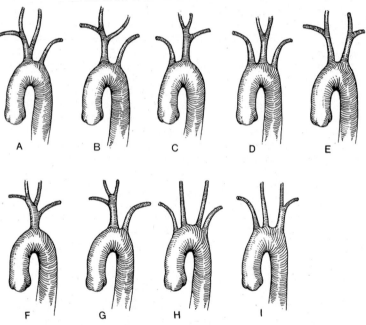

FIGURE 3-10. Variations in the origins of the aortic arch vessels. **A and B:** Account for 73% of all arch vessel anomalies. **A:** Common origin of left common carotid and brachiocephalic arteries (~15% of individuals). **B:** Left common carotid originating from mid to upper brachiocephalic artery (~7% of individuals). **C:** Common carotid trunk giving off the left subclavian artery. **D:** Common carotid trunk. **E:** Left and right brachiocephalic arteries. **F:** Single arch vessel (the brachiocephalic artery) gives off the left common carotid and left subclavian arteries. **G:** Common carotid trunk gives off the right subclavian artery, or origin of left CCA from the right CCA. **H:** Independent origin of all vessels; that is, no brachiocephalic artery is present. **I:** Left brachiocephalic artery. (Adapted from Kadir S. Regional anatomy of the thoracic aorta. In: *Atlas of normal and variant angiographic anatomy.* Philadelphia: WB Saunders, 1991.)

with an appropriate catheter for a more difficult arch in the first place. The least amount of contrast and number of injections needed for adequate visualization of the carotid and the cerebral vasculature should be used. Patients should have received aspirin therapy prior to the procedure, and it is routine to administer 3,000 to 4,000 units of unfractionated heparin to further reduce the risk of embolization for diagnostic angiography. An arch aortogram is performed in the LAO 30- to 45-degree projection to assess the origin of the great vessels and delineate the tortuosity of the arch. Typical arch anatomy or level 1 arch is seen in 70% of cases. Shared origin of the brachiocephalic trunk and left common carotid artery (CCA) is seen in 15% of cases (bovine arch), while the origin of the left CCA from the brachiocephalic trunk is seen in 8 to 10% of cases (Fig. 3.10). With increasing age, hypertension, and atherosclerotic changes in the aorta, the arch sinks deeper into the thoracic cavity and draws the origin of the great vessels along with it. Using the origin of the left subclavian artery as the landmark, the arch curvature can be classified into three levels (Figs. 3.11 to 3.13). An aortogram helps define the type or the level of the aortic arch and helps the operator choose the appropriate diagnostic catheter for the case. One should start with a catheter appropriate to the level of difficulty of the arch rather than repeatedly scraping the arch with an inappropriate catheter and thus increasing the risk of stroke and other procedural complications. It is inappropriate to try to cannulate the great vessels with a JR4 catheter in an individual with a level 3 aortic arch. A Vitek (Fig. 3.14) or a Headhunter (Fig. 3.15) catheter should be the initial catheter of choice in individuals with a level 2 arch, and a Simmons 1 or 2 catheter (Fig. 3.16) should be chosen for cannulating great vessels in an individual with a level 3 arch. The traditional angiographic views for visualizing the carotid arteries are an ipsilateral 30-degree oblique (Fig. 3.17) and a lateral view. The vertebral arteries are best visualized in an AP view, although angulated views may be needed to visualize the ostium adequately because of its posterior superior takeoff. The intracranial anterior and posterior circulation is best viewed in the AP cranial and lateral projection (Figs. 3.18 to 3.21).

Pulmonary Angiography

Pulmonary angiography is usually performed for the diagnosis of acute pulmonary embolism or for planning operative treatment of chronic pulmonary embolism. A radionuclide ventilation-perfusion (V/Q) scan or a spinal CT scan should be obtained whenever possible in a patient suspected of acute pulmonary embolism in order to be able to perform a more directed angiogram. Venous access is obtained through the common femoral vein and an 8-French sheath introduced. The catheter used for pulmonary angiogram should have a large bore (7- or 8-French catheters preferred) with multiple sideholes and a pigtail tip. It is not possible to obtain adequate vascular opacification with smaller bore catheters. A Grollman catheter (Fig. 3.22) is ideal as it has excellent torque control and has a sidearm curve that allows it to be directed through the tricuspid valve. The catheter tip is placed within the pulmonary trunk identified by the V/Q scan and 40 mL of contrast injected at the rate of 20 mL/s (Fig 3.23). Two

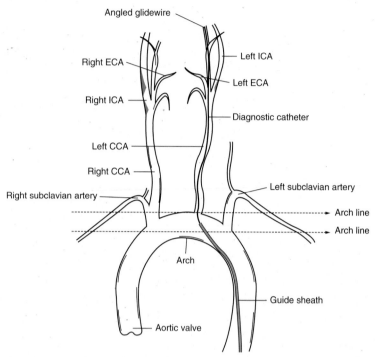

FIGURE 3-11.   The aortic arch curvature can be classified into three levels of difficulty using the origin of the left subclavian artery as a landmark. In a level 1 arch, the great vessels rise above the horizontal line drawn across the origin of the left subclavian artery or the peak of the arch, whichever is the highest point (Arch line). (CCA, common carotid artery; ICA, internal carotid artery; ECA, external carotid artery) (Adapted from Myla S. Carotid access techniques: an algorithmic approach. *Carotid Intervent* 2001;3(1):2–12.)

orthogonal views (LAO/RAO 30-degree) of each lung should be obtained. Biplane angiography may be used to minimize contrast if available. Selective and subselective angiography are indicated based on the results of the V/Q scan to definitively rule out pulmonary embolism.

LIMITATIONS/RISKS

There are potential risks with any invasive procedure. Complications associated with vascular angiography include access-site vascular injury, contrast reactions, renal failure, stroke, and rarely death. For diagnostic vascular angiography, the incidence of death is less than 0.1%, the incidence of vascular complications is less than 1%, and the risk of stroke is 0.07%. The overall complication rate with femoral access is significantly

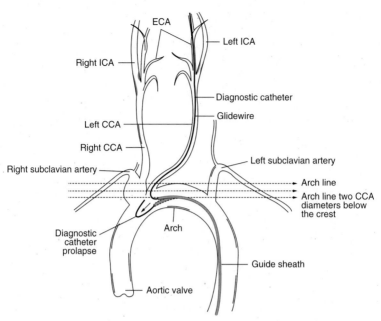

FIGURE 3-12.   In a level 2 arch, the great vessels rise below the arch line or within three CCA diameters of it. (CCA, common carotid artery; ICA, internal carotid artery; ECA, external carotid artery) (Adapted from Myla S, Carotid access techniques: an algorithmic approach. *Carotid Intervent* 2001;3(1):2–12.)

lower at 1.7% compared to the 7% complication rate seen with brachial artery access. Most of the complications with brachial artery access are local vascular complications. Although the overall risk of stroke with diagnostic angiography is 0.07%, the risk is about 10-fold higher with cerebrovascular angiography at 0.7%. Therefore, meticulous attention to detail and technique is indicated for cerebral angiography. The severity of anaphylactoid reactions to iodinated contrast agents varies from nausea, emesis, and rash to laryngeal edema, cardiovascular collapse, and death. The risk of death due to a severe contrast reaction is real and ranges from 1 in 12,000 to 1 in 75,000. The reported incidence of renal dysfunction with vascular angiography has ranged from 0.5 to 35%, which is a reflection of the patient comorbidities and criteria used to define renal dysfunction. Individuals with any degree of renal dysfunction should receive adequate intravenous prehydration prior to angiography and should be considered for *N*-acetylcysteine (600 mg orally for two doses the day prior to the contrast injection, then 600 mg orally immediately before the injection, and 600 mg 4 to 6 hours following the injection of contrast).

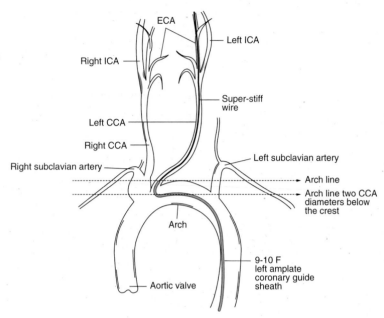

FIGURE 3-13. In a level 3 arch, the great vessels rise well below the arch line or beyond three CCA diameters of it. (CCA, common carotid artery; ICA, internal carotid artery; ECA, external carotid artery.)(Adapted from Myla S. Carotid access techniques: an algorithmic approach. *Carotid Intervent* 2001;3(1):2–12.)

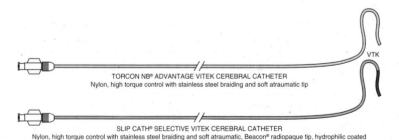

FIGURE 3-14. The Vitek catheter is a unique preshaped catheter useful for selective cannulation of the great vessels in individuals with a level 2 aortic arch.

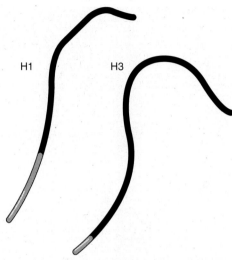

FIGURE 3-15. The Headhunter catheter is a unique preshaped catheter useful for selective cannulation of the great vessels in individuals with a level 1 or 2 aortic arch.

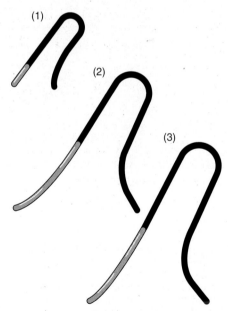

FIGURE 3-16. The Simmons catheters, H1 and H3 are unique preshaped catheters useful for selective cannulation of the great vessels in individuals with a level 3 aortic arch. (*Caution*: Significant skill level is needed to use this catheter appropriately and to reshape the reverse curve.)

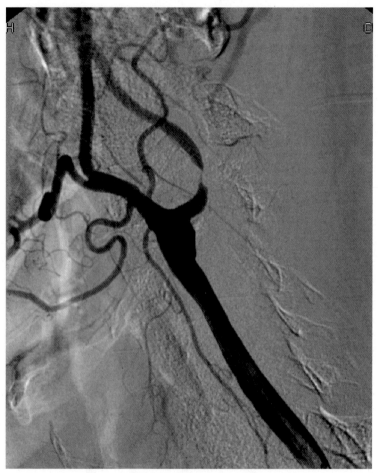

FIGURE 3-17. Left anterior oblique 30-degree projection of a severe stenosis in the left internal carotid artery.

SPECIAL ISSUES CONTRAINDICATIONS

The only absolute contraindications for diagnostic angiography are inadequate equipment or catheterization facility and an untrained operator. Relative contraindications include severe hypertension, uncorrectable coagulopathy, clinically significant iodinated contrast material sensitivity, severe renal insufficiency, congestive heart failure, and severe anemia. Clinicians should make every effort to address and correct these relative contraindications prior to the procedure.

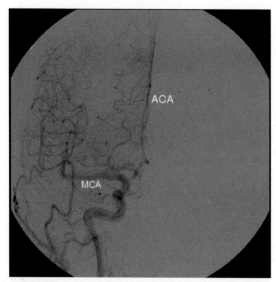

FIGURE 3-18. Anterior-posterior projection of the intracranial anterior circulation after selective injection of the right CCA. (ACA, anterior cerebral artery; MCA, middle cerebral artery.)

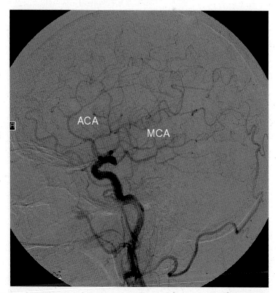

FIGURE 3-19. Lateral projection of the intracranial anterior circulation after selective injection of the right CCA. (ACA, anterior cerebral artery; MCA, middle cerebral artery.)

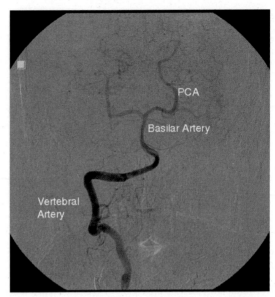

FIGURE 3-20. Anterior-posterior projection of the intracranial posterior circulation after selective injection in the right vertebral artery. (PCA, Posterior cerebral artery.)

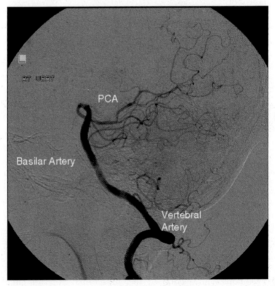

FIGURE 3-21. Lateral projection of the intracranial posterior circulation after selective injection in the right vertebral artery. (PCA, posterior cerebral artery.)

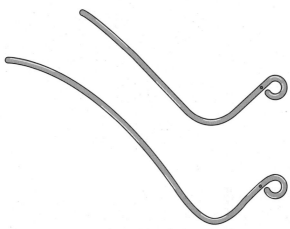

FIGURE 3-22. The Grollman catheter has a reversed secondary curve which, when introduced from the right femoral vein, passes readily from the right ventricle to the pulmonary artery and is ideal for pulmonary angiography.

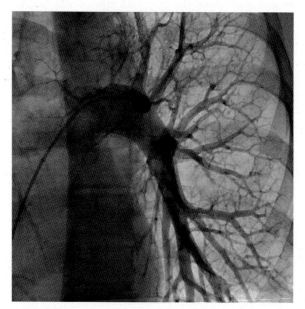

FIGURE 3-23. Pulmonary angiography of the left pulmonary artery.

CONCLUSIONS

Contrast angiography remains the gold standard for defining the extent and severity of vascular diseases. The objective of performing diagnostic angiography is to answer a clinical question, which in turn will affect management of the patient. Angiography is typically performed in individuals who are being considered for revascularization and should be preceded by a thorough preprocedure history and physical examination to identify potential contraindications to the procedure. Choosing appropriate catheters at the start of the procedure significantly reduces the duration and complications associated with angiography. A pressure gradient of more than 20 mm Hg across a stenosis is a reliable indicator of a hemodynamically significant lesion.

PRACTICAL POINTS

- Iodixanol (Visipaque) is better tolerated than high-osmolal contrast agents for vascular angiography with fewer adverse reactions.

- Adequate hydration should be administered to all patients with any degree of renal dysfunction prior to the procedure.

- Lateral aortography should be performed to identify the origins of the mesenteric vessels prior to attempts at selective cannulation.

- An arch aortogram should be performed prior to attempts at selective cannulation of the great vessels.

- Selective pulmonary angiograms based on the results of the V/Q scan or spinal CT scan are significantly better than nonselective main pulmonary artery angiograms in diagnosing pulmonary embolism.

- Choice of the appropriate arterial access site is crucial to performing safe and successful angiography.

RECOMMENDED READING

Baum S, ed. *Abrams' angiography*, 4th ed. Philadelphia: Lippincott Williams & Wilkins, 1997.

Hallett JW, Brewster DC, Rasmussen TE. *Handbook of patient care in vascular diseases*, 4th ed. Philadelphia: Lippincott Williams & Wilkins, 2001.

Kadir S. Regional anatomy of the thoracic aorta. In: *Atlas of normal and variant angiographic anatomy*. Philadelphia: WB Saunders, 1991.

Mukherjee D, Yadav SJ. Update on peripheral vascular diseases: from smoking cessation to stenting. *Cleveland Clin J Med* 2001;68:723–734.

Mukherjee D, Yadav J. Angiographic techniques and endovascular therapy for symptomatic vertebral artery stenosis. *Carotid Interv* 2002;3:13–15.

Spittell PC. Peripheral vascular disease. In: Murphy J, ed. *Mayo Clinic cardiology review*, 2nd ed. Philadelphia: Lippincott Williams & Wilkins, 2000:1013–1024.

Wojtowycz M. *Handbook of interventional radiology and angiography*, 2nd ed. St. Louis: Mosby-Year Book, 1995.

CHAPTER 4 ■ Magnetic Resonance Angiography in the Diagnosis of Vascular Disease

Paaladinesh Thavendiranathan and Georgeta Mihai

Magnetic resonance angiography (MRA) is an excellent modality that has become the noninvasive modality of choice for imaging in a number of vascular beds. MRA refers to a set of pulse sequences in magnetic resonance imaging (MRI) that have been adapted for the clinical imaging of the lumen and the walls of vascular structures. These sequences take advantage of and/or obviate specific properties of blood, blood flow, or vascular walls or use gadolinium (Gd)-based contrast agents to enable visualization of vascular structures with high resolution.

FUNDAMENTALS OF MAGNETIC RESONANCE IMAGING

The Physics of Magnetic Resonance Imaging

MRI is based on two properties of the hydrogen nucleus (called either proton or spin) to produce images of biological objects: its magnetic moment (similar to a small bar magnet) and its angular momentum or spin. When a proton is placed under a strong magnetic field B_0 (typically 10,000 times greater than the earth's magnetic field), its magnetic axis aligns itself with B_0 and experiences a motion of precession (similar to a top) around the direction of B_0. The frequency of the precession, called the Larmor frequency, is proportional to the intensity of the local magnetic field experienced by the proton. Resonance is referred to as the property of a nucleus with an odd number of protons or neutrons to selectively absorb and later release energy specific to the element and its chemical environment. When a short radiofrequency (RF) excitation pulse—B_1, with a frequency that matches the Larmor frequency of protons, is applied on an object placed under a strong magnetic field, the resonance phenomenon occurs and its protons synchronize their precession and have their magnetic axis tipped out of alignment with B_0. The angle of net magnetization–deflection created after the end of the RF pulse is referred to as the *flip angle* and is dependent on the strength of the externally applied field B_1 and the duration of the RF pulse. A 90 degrees RF pulse will rotate the net magnetization totally from longitudinal plane (z, or B_0 plane) to transversal plane (xy). It is the transversal component (M_{xy}) of the net magnetization that generates the MR signal in the form of an oscillating current induced in a receiver antenna placed perpendicular on the xy plane. After the RF excitation pulse ends, two concurrent events happen: (i) M_{xy} starts to decay (with a time constant T2 called transversal or spin-spin relaxation) due to the loss of phase coherence among spins (as each spin "feels" a different magnetic field environment dependent on the neighboring spins), and (ii) the magnetic axes of the protons realign themselves with B_0 with a time constant T1 (longitudinal or spin-lattice relaxation time). The oscillating signal produced by the decay in time of M_{xy} is called free induction decay (FID) and is dependent on the local magnetic environment surrounding each proton. The spin-spin interaction is not the only factor responsible for the loss of phase coherence among spins and the time decay of M_{xy}. Extrinsic magnetic filed inhomogeneities (magnetic field imperfections and/or susceptibility differences between adjacent tissues) accelerate the MRI signal decay that becomes characterized by a time constant T2*, which is always shorter than T2. However, in *spin-echo* sequences, the signal loss caused by static, extrinsic magnetic field inhomogenities is corrected by the use of the 180 degrees RF pulse that reverses the phase differences and reestablishes phase coherence allowing "echo formation," as such the signal decay is only T2 dependent. In *gradient-echo* imaging, where different polarity gradients instead of the 180 degrees RF pulse are used to form an echo, the T2* FID is observed. The loss of phase coherence among spins occurs more rapidly than the longitudinal magnetization recovery, as such always T1 > T2 > T2*. T1, T2, and spin (proton) density (PD, number of spins per unit tissue area) are fundamental, intrinsic properties of tissue that could be exploited by MRI to differentiate tissues.

Spatial Localization and K-Space

Field Gradients

Field gradients (linear, controlled variations in the B_0 strength) make MRI possible by allowing the MR signal to be localized in space. These linear changes in B_0 translate into linear, location-dependent changes in the Larmor frequency of the spins. By precisely controlling the strength of the magnetic field in space and time, the frequency and phase of spin precession also become a function of location and time. An image can be formed as the MR signals coming from different locations within the body can be distinguished from one another. The gradients are applied in three planes as slice select, phase encode, and frequency (readout) gradients. The exact timing, order, polarity, repetition frequency of the RF pulses, and applied gradient fields are specific to each pulse sequence (used to emphasize different types of contrast information in the tissues of the object). The specific succession of RF pulse, gradients, and echo acquisitions has to be repeated numerous times (number of repetitions = acquired matrix size). The time between successive RF pulses is referred to as repetition time (TR), while the time between RF pulse and echo is referred to as echo time (TE).

k-Space

During a pulse sequence, after each echo acquisition, the resulting echoes are digitized and stored in a data acquisition matrix using Fourier transformation methods. This data matrix is referred to as *k*-space. Tissue contrast is principally determined by the center of *k*-space (central phase encoding lines), while the periphery encodes image detail. The order in which *k*-space lines are collected can be varied (*phase reordering*) and strongly influences tissue contrast and detail. In conventional MRI, the k-space acquisition is sequential, while in fast MRI techniques for three-dimensional (3D) contrast angiography, centric or elliptic-centric acquisition is often used. The k-space data set is Fourier transformed to produce the images that are routinely seen in clinical practice.

General Magnetic Resonance Imaging Pulse Sequences and Fast Vascular Imaging

Pulse sequences that are routinely used in MRI can be classified into two main categories: gradient-recalled echo (GRE) sequences and spin-echo (SE) sequences. In GRE sequences, following the initial RF pulse, opposite polarity, same area gradients are used to dephase and rephase the protons in the transverse plane in order to obtain an echo and the MR signal. These sequences generally use an RF pulse with a flip angle less than 90 degrees. This is advantageous in fast imaging approaches such as contrast angiography as there is always residual magnetization left after application of the RF pulse, obviating the need to wait long times to allow sufficient longitudinal recovery. Even though GRE sequences are faster than SE sequences, they often result in lower signal-to-noise ratio (SNR) images due to use of low flip angle and often require T1-shortening contrast agents to enhance SNR. In SE sequences, following a 90 degrees RF pulse, 180 degrees RF pulses are applied to rephase the protons in the xy plane in order to obtain an MR signal. In fast SE techniques, multiple 180 degrees pulses can be applied for each 90 degrees pulse allowing for collection of multiple lines of k-space during a TR interval. However, generally SE sequences result in slower imaging than GRE. T1, PD, T2* weighting and a contrast based on the ratio of T1/T2 of tissues can be obtained in GRE sequences, while T1-, PD-, and T2-weighted contrast can be obtained with SE sequences. Both GRE and SE sequences are routinely utilized in vascular MRA.

A prerequisite of vascular imaging approaches is the ability to rapidly image the vasculature that often spans large territories. An approach that is commonly used to speed imaging is parallel imaging. Parallel imaging techniques use the spatial information inherent in local phased-array coils to replace time-consuming phase encoding steps and can be subdivided into the domains (k-space/image-space) in which processing is mainly performed. SMASH (simultaneous acquisition of spatial harmonics) and GRAPPA (for generalized autocalibrating partially parallel acquisition) are techniques that acquire local coil information in Fourier space that is then used to reconstruct the image. In contrast, the processing in SENSE (for sensitivity encoding) is performed in the imaging domain by acquisition of local coil data and application of correction after the Fourier transform.

Magnetic Resonance Angiography Pulse Sequences for Vascular Imaging

MRA pulse sequences can be categorized into (a) flow-dependent versus independent sequences, (b) "black-blood" versus "bright-blood" sequences, or (c) contrast-enhanced versus unenhanced sequences. The most practical classification is to consider these sequences as black-blood or bright-blood techniques based on the appearance of the vascular lumen following application of certain pulse sequences. Thinking of these sequences as contrast-enhanced (CE) versus unenhanced sequences is also important as it has practical implications in imaging patients with contraindications to Gd-based contrast administration.

Black-blood Techniques

Black-blood imaging techniques are useful for assessing vessel wall pathologies such as atherosclerosis, aneurysms, intramural hematoma, aortic dissections, and vasculitides. Generally black-blood sequences are fast SE sequences with preparation modules for blood signal suppression. These sequences are mostly two dimensional (2D), allow for depiction of lumen and vascular wall, are able to deliver all contrast types (T1, T2, and PD), and need efficient suppression of the flowing blood. The latest is accomplished either by inflow-outflow saturation bands (flowing blood experiences an extra 90 degrees RF pulse outside the imaging slice) or double inversion recovery (IR) or even triple IR to null the flowing blood. Black-blood techniques are all noncontrast sequences making them useful in patients with contraindications to Gd contrast agents.

Partial Fourier Acquisition Methods

Partial Fourier methods appeal to vascular imaging due to the speed of acquisition. Half-Fourier Acquisition Single-Shot Turbo Spin-Echo (HASTE) imaging is a rapid SE sequence where the entire 2D slice dataset data is acquired in a heart beat (TR = R − R interval) and is accomplished using very short inter-echo spacing, acquisition of slightly more that 50% of the k-space and mathematically interpolating the remaining k-space lines. For MRA applications, HASTE sequences are executed with preparatory double inversion pulses with specific inversion times, to selectively null signal from flowing blood. These sequences are typically implemented with ECG gating, with image acquisition during diastolic period to avoid flow-related artifacts. Due to the partial Fourier acquisition, spatial resolution and SNR are inferior compared to full k-space acquired fast SE methods. However, the rapidity of image acquisition reduces cardiac and respiratory motion artifacts allowing imaging of large vascular areas within 1 to 2 minutes with the patient breathing freely. Typically, coronal, axial, and sagittal HASTE images are obtained and can be used for diagnostic purposes as well as subsequent planning of contrast-enhanced MRA sequences.

Another partial Fourier approach is an ECG-gated 3D sequence which is triggered for systolic and diastolic acquisitions. This method relies on loss of signal or flow void during systole as a result of fast arterial flow. The diastolic acquisition is characterized by slow flow and high-signal intensity on T2-weighted images. Bright-blood angiography can then be accomplished by simple Fourier subtraction of the images.

Bright-blood Techniques

While dark-blood techniques focus on signal loss due to flow, bright-blood imaging uses flow-related enhancement or Gd-based contrast agents to enhance signal from blood. Bright-blood sequences are generally GRE sequences. Time-of-flight (TOF) MRA, phase-contrast (PC) imaging, and steady-state free precession (SSFP) imaging with navigator gating are noncontrast techniques, while 3D CE-MRA and time-resolved MRA (TR-MRA) require the use of contrast.

Balanced Steady-state Free Precession Magnetic Resonance Angiography. Balanced SSFP imaging is a GRE technique where the image contrast is determined by the intrinsic T2/T1 differences between blood and tissue. In this sequence, RF pulses of alternating direction are applied with a TR much shorter than T1, hence maintaining residual M_{xy}. This residual magnetization is used to increase final signal intensity resulting in bright-blood images with no reliance on flow. The high SNR of this sequence allows it to be well suited for parallel imaging. Balanced SSFP imaging can be used to obtain 2D datasets, cine images, or 3D datasets using navigator-gated free breathing techniques. In the latter application, 3D-MRA is acquired using ECG gating to trigger for diastolic acquisitions, as well as respiratory triggering to obtain 3D datasets in 5 to 10 minutes. These sequences are however susceptible to field inhomogeneities including air-tissue interfaces, metallic implants, and stents. Additionally, these sequences are not specific for veins or arteries, as both structures appear bright in the images.

Time-of-flight Magnetic Resonance Angiography. In TOF imaging, a series of RF pulses is used to "saturate" all protons in an imaging volume and suppress the signal from all stationary tissue within that volume. Blood flowing into the imaging volume brings "unsaturated" protons that have not experienced the prior excitation pulses of the other protons stationary in the imaging plane and produce higher signals. In 2D-TOF, thin slices are excited, whereas in 3D-TOF, thicker volumes are excited. The application of 2D or 3D techniques is dependent on velocity of blood flow. In general, flow that is too slow to cross the entire volume between excitations may partly saturate with parts of it producing no signal. Thinner slices, as used in 2D-TOF, are therefore better suited to image slow-flowing blood. Additional saturation pulses immediately above or below the plane of imaging can be used to selectively suppress signals from either veins or arteries, allowing the respective production of MRA and MR venograms (MRV).

Phase-contrast Imaging. In PC imaging, bipolar magnetic gradient fields perpendicular to the plane of imaging are used to quantify the speed of spatially moving protons. PC method relies on velocity of the moving spins to produce signal, and as such, there is excellent background suppression. A short-duration gradient is applied to a vessel followed by an opposite and equal gradient for the same duration. As a consequence, stationary protons do not gain a net phase. However, for protons moving perpendicular to the plane of imaging, the effect of the first gradient field is not perfectly counteracted by the second gradient field, resulting in a phase offset. The greater the velocity of the moving protons, the greater the resulting phase offset. These phase offsets can then be used to calculate velocity. Given that phase can only take values between –180 and +180 degrees, a net offset in phase of 200 degrees is identical to an offset of –160 degrees.

The intensity of the bipolar gradient fields must thus be adjusted according to the maximum expected velocity (V_{max} or VENC, velocity encoding) to maintain all phase offsets within the −180- to +180-degree interval and avoid aliasing.

3D Contrast-enhanced-Magnetic Resonance Angiography. 3D CE-MRA uses a 3D spoiled gradient-echo (SPGR) pulse sequence (rapid imaging) to optimize imaging of the first pass of a Gd-based contrast agent in vessels. The contrast agent shortens the T1 of blood, increasing the natural contrast between the blood and the surrounding tissues. A large enough dose of contrast agent must be administered to lower the T1 of blood below that of the surrounding fat for good signal contrast between vessels and perivascular tissue. A typical dose of Gd contrast is 0.1 to 0.3 mmol/kg and is injected at a rate of at least 2.0 mL/s. Timing of the contrast bolus with respect to imaging is important. A technical trick can be used where the central part of k-space (reflecting the global contrast in an image) alone is acquired during the peak of concentration of the bolus in the arteries of the targeted anatomy, thus shortening the time of acquisition. High-resolution arterial phase images of the lumen with high contrast delineation may be obtained when combined with parallel imaging techniques.

Time-resolved Magnetic Resonance Angiography. TR-MRA is a technique of assessing the kinetics of contrast enhancement in a chosen vascular bed. It uses fast imaging methods to acquire multiple MRA images with high temporal resolution to demonstrate the dynamics of contrast enhancement during first-pass of the contrast bolus. There is repetitive filling of the center of k-space as the contrast bolus is injected, followed by later filling of the remainder of k-space. TR-MRA techniques when used in conjunction with parallel imaging can effectively reduce temporal resolution to 200 to 300 ms/3D imaging slab. The rapid image acquisition obviates the need for precise arterial contrast timing and provides selective arterial enhancement. However, the downside of performing rapid imaging is the compromised (low) spatial resolution of the images.

Noncontrast Approaches

These approaches may provide either black-blood or bright-blood images, depending on the sequence. These include Sampling Perfection with Application of optimized Contrast using different flip angle Evolution (SPACE) (see below), SSFP (bright-blood approach described above), and 3D ECG-gated partial Fourier fast-spin echo approaches and arterial spin labeling (both, typically dark blood). The application of these in various beds is described in Table 4.1. For detailed reviews on noncontrast approaches, the reader is referred to detailed reviews on the topic.

3D-sampling Perfection with Application of Optimized Contrast Using Different Flip Angle Evolution

The SPACE technique is a new 3D dark-blood method used for vascular imaging that belongs to the family of turbo-spin echoes and is still used mainly for investigational purposes. This sequence utilizes variable refocusing flip

TABLE 4.1

PREFERRED NONCONTRAST MRA TECHNIQUES BY LOCATION

Vascular Bed	Technique	Specifics
Carotid/vertebral	3D-SPACE, TOF, partial Fourier 3D-FSE, balanced SSFP ± ASL, TOF	3D-SPACE may provide atherosclerotic plaque characterization as well
Thoracic aorta/ pulmonary artery	3D-SPACE, partial Fourier 3D-FSE, balanced SSFP ± ASL	—
Abdominal aorta and branches (renals)	SPACE, balanced SSFP ± ASL, PC-MRA (renals)	3D PC-MRA may provide flow and significance of renal artery stenosis
Lower extremity	Balanced SSFP, TOF, 3D-SPACE (thigh)	—

SPACE=Sampling Perfection with Application of optimized Contrast using different flip angle Evolution; TOF=Time of Flight; SSFP=Steady State Free Precession; PC-MRA=Phase Contrast MRA; ASL=Arterial Spin Labeling.

angles allowing for longer echo train duration and nonselective refocusing pulses to minimize echo spacing. This significantly improves its time efficiency over conventional 3D fast-spin echo sequences. Additionally, flowing blood is dephased and blood signal is suppressed without the need for double inversion preparation pulses, hence allowing the use of thick 3D slabs and efficient coverage of large vascular territories. To acquire large slabs of vascular structures such as the thoracic and abdominal aorta, respiratory gating is used with the patient breathing freely during acquisition as the acquisition can take 10 to 15 minutes. SPACE can achieve any of the SE contrasts (T1, T2, PD). Other than for vessel wall pathology, SPACE can be used when significant stent susceptibility artifact precludes the use of GRE sequences, as it allows imaging outside of the stent without any signal loss.

Magnetic Resonance Imaging Approaches for Tissue Characterization

These can be part of MRA protocols and may help with interrogation of pathology in the arterial wall and are helpful in characterization of atherosclerotic plaque and complications such as thrombosis, which may occur as part of diverse arterial and venous disorders. Tissue characterization relies on the intrinsic signal characteristics of pathology such as iron, methemoglobin, or thrombus and can be discerned by their image characteristics on specific pulse sequences. These include T1-weighted SE or GRE sequences with and without IV contrast, T2* images, or T2-weighted SE imaging.

Magnetic Resonance Digital Subtraction Angiography

Image contrast can be improved by digital subtraction of precontrast image data from dynamic, arterial, or venous phase image data. This subtraction is typically performed prior to the Fourier transform by using a complex subtraction method. The improvement in contrast achieved with DSA may reduce the Gd dose required. However, there must be no change in the patient position between the precontrast and dynamic/post–contrast-enhanced imaging. This requirement for no motion is easily met in the pelvis and legs, which can be sandbagged and strapped down. It is more difficult to achieve in the chest and abdomen, where respiratory, cardiac, and peristaltic motions are more difficult to avoid.

CLINICAL APPLICATIONS OF MAGNETIC RESONANCE ANGIOGRAPHY IN VASCULAR DISEASE

Carotid and Verterbral Magnetic Resonance Angiography

Indications

MRA can delineate carotid bifurcation disease, aortic arch branch vessel disease, stenosis and occlusion, atherosclerotic disease, fibromuscular dysplasia, carotid and vertebral artery dissection, vascular neoplasms, and carotid artery aneurysms. A more contemporary application of MRA (using mostly dark-blood techniques) that is likely to become a valuable tool for therapeutic planning in the future is carotid plaque characterization to detect high-risk components within atherosclerotic plaques. This is however still experimental at present.

Approach

3D CE Angiography

3D CE-MRA has revolutionized noninvasive examination of the carotid and aortic arch vessels and has replaced intra-arterial angiography in many institutions. Figure 4.1 illustrates an MRA of the extracranial carotid arteries, revealing a tight stenosis at the origin of the left internal carotid artery. 3D CE-MRA of the carotid is usually obtained in the coronal plane and does not require breath-holding. The acquisition is performed with centric k-space weighting from the beginning of the scan to avoid jugular venous enhancement. Arterial-venous transit time in the cerebral circulation is rapid, necessitating split-second timing typically executed with a timing bolus.

Flow Measurements. PC imaging can be performed in areas identified to assess hemodynamic significance of stenosis or flow direction using in-plane acquisitions as well as to quantify the severity by using through plane acquisitions.

Tissue Characterization. For vessel wall and plaque imaging, other more standard MRI sequences such as double and triple IR, T1-weighted pre-IV and post-IV contrast, and T2-weighted sequences can also be performed in chosen areas. Many of these however have to be performed precontrast administration.

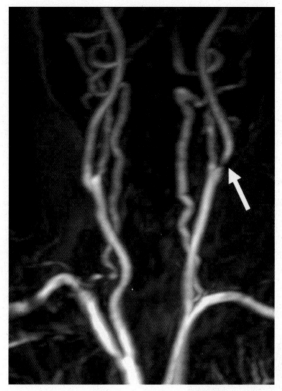

FIGURE 4-1. Maximal intensity projection display of a carotid 3D CE-MRA angiogram illustrating tight stenosis at the origin of the left internal carotid artery (*arrow*).

Typical Protocols

A typical MRA of the extracranial circulation begins with anatomic localizers in the transverse, sagittal, and coronal planes. Dark-blood 3D T1- or T2-weighted SPACE imaging of the carotids can be subsequently performed for plaque characterization (however, this is mainly a research tool at present). This is followed by coronal 3D CE-MRA through the extracranial carotids in a single injection. Inclusion of the arch and the origins of all supra-aortic arteries in the field of view is important. If an area of stenosis is detected, sagittal 2D PC slabs positioned on the right or left carotid can be performed to assess for presence of turbulence. Maximum intensity projections (MIP) reconstructions are typically performed for global assessment of carotid pathology. In cases of subclavian artery stenosis, an axial PC MRA at the level of the proximal neck may be informative to deduce direction of flow in the ipsilateral vertebral artery.

Thoracic Magnetic Resonance Angiography

Noninvasive techniques of computed tomographic angiography (CTA) and MRA have completely replaced diagnostic catheter angiography of the thoracic vessels. The ability to obtain physiologic information and vessel wall information is a particular advantage of thoracic MRA.

Indications

MRA is able to accurately assess pathology of the great vessels in the chest. This includes the thoracic aorta and its branches, the pulmonary arteries and their branches, and the large veins of the chest. Imaging of the coronary arteries and veins is possible by MRI but is not widely used clinically.

Aortic Disease

MRA is able to evaluate normal anatomy as well as congenital and acquired diseases of the thoracic aorta. Congenital aortic diseases regularly assessed by MRA include coarctation, right-sided aorta, vascular rings, supra-aortic membranes, anomalous origins of the head and neck vessels, double arches, and connective tissue diseases (Marfan's syndrome, Ehlers-Danlos syndrome, etc.). Acquired aortic diseases include aneurysms, dissection, trauma, postsurgical complications, and inflammatory diseases (giant cell arteritis). Figure 4.2 illustrates a normal thoracic aortic CE-MRA in a young patient. Figure 4.3 illustrates a thoracic aortic dissection.

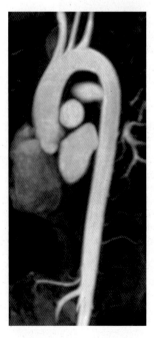

FIGURE 4-2. Maximal intensity projection display of a normal 3D CE-MRA of the thoracic and proximal abdominal aorta.

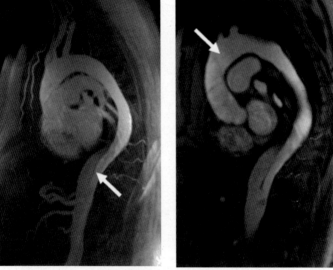

FIGURE 4-3. **A:** Maximal intensity projection display of 3D CE-MRA of the thoracic aorta in a sagittal view showing a dissection flap in the descending aorta (*arrow*). **B:** Multiplane reformat of the same image illustrating that the dissection flap begins in the ascending aorta (*arrow*).

Pulmonary Disease

MRA can assess the anatomy and diseases of the pulmonary arteries and veins. Anatomic abnormalities such as pulmonary atresia, pulmonary slings, and arteriovenous malformations are well characterized by MRA. Acquired disease such as pulmonary hypertension or postoperative complications can be assessed by MRA. Figure 4.4 illustrates large pulmonary arteries in a patient with a pulmonic valve stenosis resulting in poststenotic dilatation of the pulmonary arteries. MRA also shows high sensitivity and specificity in the evaluation of pulmonary embolism but the PIOPED-3 trial suggests that the technique is useful for PE evaluation only if performed with care. Compression and invasion of the pulmonary arteries by tumor are also well characterized by MRA.

Venous Diseases

MRV of the large veins of the chest has proven clinically useful to assess thoracic inlet syndrome, superior vena cava syndrome, and the presence of thrombus in the superior vena cava and branches. Figure 4.5 illustrates a thrombus in the left brachiocephalic vein on an MRV. Pulmonary vein anatomy can be assessed by MRV before and after RF ablation therapy for refractory atrial fibrillation (Fig. 4.6).

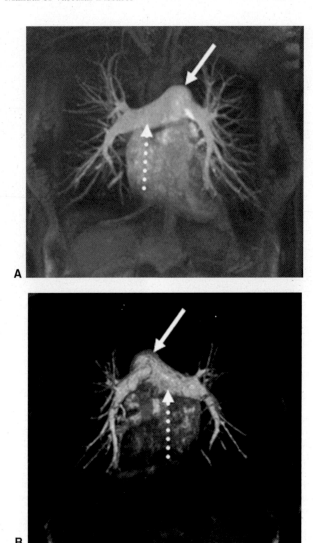

FIGURE 4-4. **A:** Maximal intensity projection display (anterior view), **B:** volume-rendered display (posterior view) of a dilated main pulmonary artery (*solid arrow*) and right pulmonary artery (*broken arrow*) secondary to underlying pulmonic stenosis.

Approach

Dark-blood Sequences

HASTE sequence (Fig. 4.7) allows rapid assessment of the entire thoracic aorta without the need for breath hold. Images can be obtained in any of the three standard planes although blood nulling is best

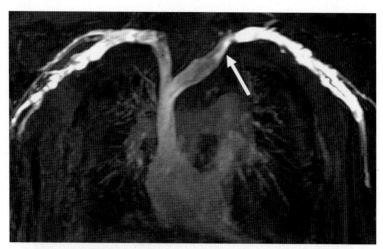

FIGURE 4-5. Maximal intensity projection display of an upper extremity 3D CE-MR venogram showing a thrombus in the left brachiocephalic vein. Simultaneous injection of both arms was performed (*arrow*).

achieved in the axial planes. This sequence is usually applied with fat suppression. *SPACE* sequence (Fig. 4.8) can be performed precontrast administration for assessment of vessel wall pathology or in circumstances where known stents (e.g., at site of coarctation) will affect GRE imaging. This is performed with respiratory gating allowing patient to breathe freely and can often take 10 to 15 minutes to image the entire thoracic aorta.

Bright-blood Techniques. ***Balanced SSFP*** is a bright-blood technique with high SNR that provides excellent contrast between blood pool and vessel wall. Single-shot SSFP images in the axial plane can be obtained similar to

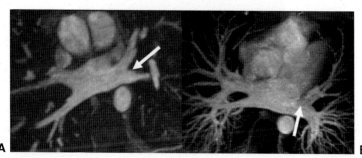

FIGURE 4-6. Multiplane reformat **A:** and maximal intensity projection **B:** displays of the pulmonary veins illustrating right upper and lower pulmonary veins and a left common pulmonary vein (*arrows*).

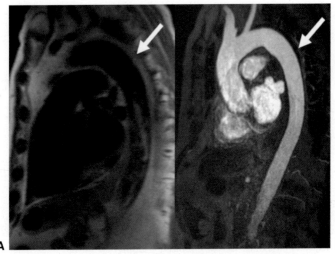

FIGURE 4-7.   A: Sagittal HASTE image illustrating intramural hematoma (*arrow*) involving the aortic arch and descending aorta. **B:** Sagittal CE-MRA of the same patient showing the same.

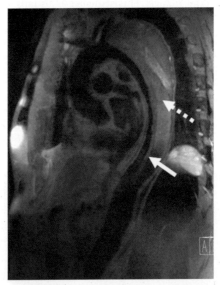

FIGURE 4-8.   Sagittal view of a 3D-SPACE image illustrating a Type B dissection beginning just distal to the subclavian artery and extending into the proximal abdominal aorta. Dissection flap (*solid arrow*) and partially thrombosed lumen (*broken arrow*) seen in the image.

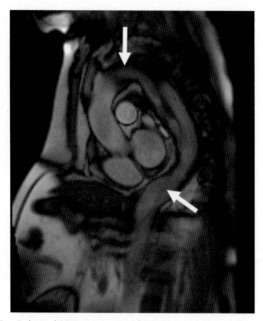

FIGURE 4-9.   Balanced SSFP cine image of a patient with Type A dissection ("candy cane" view) with the dissection beginning at the distal ascending aorta and extending into the proximal abdominal aorta (*arrows*).

axial HASTE images for luminal assessment. Cine-SSFP sequences can be used to depict functional abnormalities of the entire thoracic aorta throughout the cardiac cycle in a single "candy cane" plane (Fig. 4.9). This may be useful in patients with aortic dissection for the evaluation of the dynamic behavior of the intimal flap or the pulsatility of the true or false lumens. This may be limited in patients who have tortuous aortas where a single plane is unable to illustrate the entire thoracic aorta. Respiratory- and cardiac-gated balanced SSFP images can be used to obtain 3D datasets of the entire thoracic aorta or pulmonary artery in patients where contrast administration is contraindicated or in cases where the 3D CE-MRA evaluation is suboptimal. *3D CE-MRA* is the dominant imaging method for the evaluation of the thoracic aorta (Figs. 4.2 and 4.3) and pulmonary arteries (Fig. 4.4). It involves rapid acquisition following the administration of a bolus of IV contrast. Again, timing is of paramount importance in thoracic imaging and a timing bolus, or CareBolus, can be used for appropriate timing to either the aorta or the pulmonary artery. In either technique, breath hold during image acquisition is essential as both breathing motion and cardiac motion degrade the acquired images. Cardiac gating techniques are not commonly used for thoracic MRA. Precontrast images should be acquired for the purpose of displaying subtracted images. Pulmonary MRA is at times supplemented by an axial 2D or 3D gradient sequence of the pelvis and thighs to assess for intravascular thrombus if the DVT/PE is of clinical concern.

Flow Measurement. PC imaging is used in specific cases to assess for turbulence and to quantify blood flow. A V_{max} of at least 150 cm/s is used to image the aorta. It can also be used to determine the presence and direction of flow (e.g., in a communication between the true and false lumen through an intimal tear in cases of dissection). PC imaging can be acquired in an "in-plane" direction or through plane direction. The in-plane assessment allows visualization of large areas of the aorta and its branches and allows identification of gross areas of flow acceleration (Fig. 4.10). Targeted "through plane" assessment can be subsequently performed at areas of increased velocity to accurately measure peak flow velocities (e.g., coarctation).

Tissue Characterization. *General axial MRI* sequences can be used for targeted assessment of vascular wall and mediastinal structures. They include double- or triple-IR T2 sequences without contrast and T1 sequences before and after contrast administration. The use of double-IR SE sequences may allow interrogation of regional and subtle abnormalities of the vessel wall including intra-aortic hematoma, focal dissection, or the assessment of thrombus.

Typical Protocols

A typical exam for the thoracic aorta includes coronal, axial, and sagittal HASTE images, and single-shot SSFP axial stacks for luminal assessment. This can be followed by segmented SSFP cine sequences in the "candy cane" view for depiction of anatomy and pathophysiologic events of the aortic lumen. In cases of suspected aortic pathology, single-slice T1-weighted spin-echo images with or without fat suppression can be performed coupled with SPACE imaging if necessary. This can be followed by a sagittal CE-MRA from the base of the neck to below the diaphragm in a single injection following a timing bolus. Delayed imaging is performed in some cases, as for the evaluation of thrombus. A PC sequence can be used to assess for flow in false lumen in cases of dissection, peak velocities across stenosis, etc. A typical exam for the pulmonary arteries includes a coronal CE-MRA through the pulmonary arteries in a single injection following a timing bolus. Imaging in both the arterial phase and the equilibrium phase is performed. In some cases, a sagittal CE-MRA through each lung, requiring two different injections, is performed instead of a coronal approach. Alternatively, a 3D TR-MRA can be performed, with some trade-off in image resolution.

Abdominal and Pelvic Magnetic Resonance Angiography

Although CTA is still the preferred modality for imaging the abdominal aorta and its branches at many institutions, MRA is beginning to surpass CTA in many aspects of abdominal and pelvic vascular disease imaging. Abdominal MRA may be performed as several variations that are

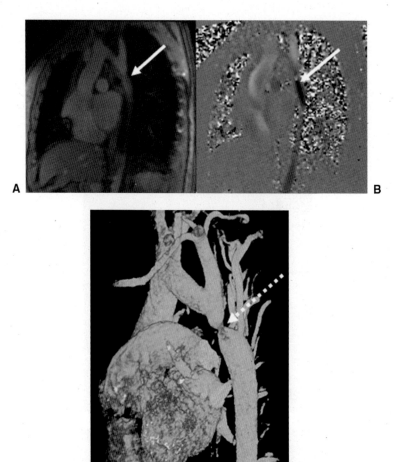

FIGURE 4-10. Sagittal PC images **A:** magnitude image **B:** phase image showing flow acceleration at the site of coarctation (*arrows*). **C:** Volume-rendered display of the coarctation site (*broken arrow*).

specifically designed to provide information on the arterial bed in question. Thus, an abdominal aorta protocol may include overall evaluation of the abdominal vessels with imaging from above the celiac trunk to the iliac arteries or may include sequences that are meant to provide additional information on specific vascular beds (organ-specific protocols such as renal, mesenteric, and portal vein protocols).

Indications

Abdominal Aortic Disease

Abdominal aorta can be evaluated for the same pathologies as the thoracic aorta, such as aneurysm, stenosis, occlusion, dissection, inflammation, and postoperative complications. MRA can play a role in abdominal aneurysm surveillance, intervention planning, and postintervention monitoring. Figure 4.11 illustrates a large aneurysm of the distal abdominal aorta with layered thrombus.

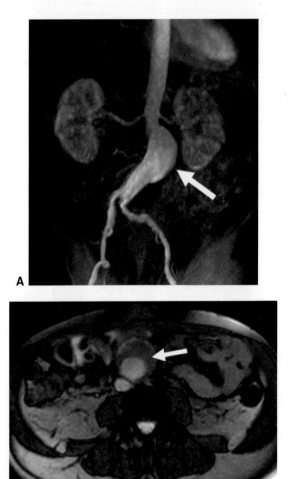

FIGURE 4-11.   A: Maximal intensity projection display of a coronal CE-MRA image of the abdominal aorta illustrating an infrarenal abdominal aortic aneurysm. **B:** An SSFP axial image of the same patient at the site of the aneurysm showing layered thrombus (*arrows*) in the aneurysm.

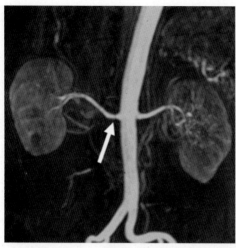

FIGURE 4-12. Maximal intensity projection display of 3D CE-MRA of the renal arteries showing mild stenosis near the origin of the right renal artery (*arrow*).

Renal Arterial Disease

MRA is very useful in the evaluation of renal artery stenosis, aneurysms, dissection, and fibromuscular disease. Renal anatomy and function can be assessed concurrently with MRA, which is a clear advantage over traditional angiography. Figure 4.12 illustrates mild stenosis in the right renal artery. MRA is excellent for the evaluation of renal donors to determine anatomical variations in the renal vasculature and structure and the evaluation of the renal allograft after transplantation to assess the patency of the anastomosis, as well as global function of the allograft. Atherosclerotic renal arterial stenosis is a good indication for MRA as it allows assessment of concomitant arterial beds and often provides information on renal perfusion as well.

Mesenteric Arterial Disease

This can be assessed by MRA in cases of mesenteric ischemia for aneurysm, dissection, anatomic variations, collateral circulation, and encasement by tumor. Figure 4.13 illustrates a normal MRA of the mesenteric arteries.

Systemic and Portal Venous Disease

MR can image both the systemic and portal venous systems. The inferior vena cava and branches can be evaluated for occlusion, tumor encasement, and the presence of thrombus. Figure 4.14 illustrates a normal MRV of the mesenteric and portal veins. MRA is very good for assessing occlusive disease of the renal veins and the extent of tumor thrombus in renal cell

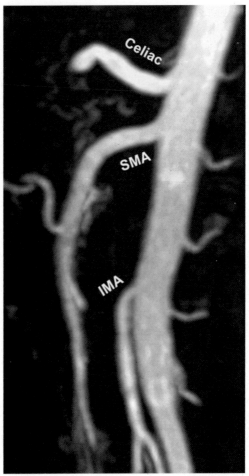

FIGURE 4-13. Maximal intensity projection display of the 3D CE-MRA of normal mesenteric arteries. (SMA, superior mesenteric artery; IMA, inferior mesenteric artery.)

carcinoma, for mesenteric vein thrombosis, and for acute thrombosis of the ovarian veins.

Approach

Morphology and Function

Dark-blood sequences such HASTE and SPACE sequences similar to that described for the assessment of thoracic aorta can be used for both vessel wall pathology and luminal assessment. Bright-blood techniques such

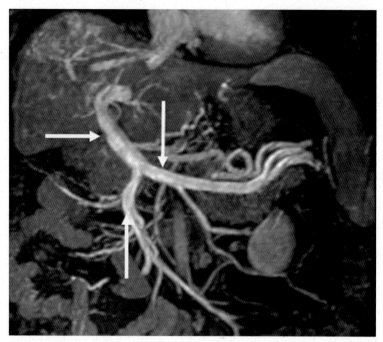

FIGURE 4-14. Maximal intensity projection display of a mesenteric 3D CE-MR venogram in the portal venous phase. There is normal confluence of the mesenteric vein and the splenic vein to form the portal vein (*arrows*).

as single-shot SSFP images in the axial plane can be used for luminal assessment followed by Cine-SSFP sequences to depict functional abnormalities of the entire abdominal aorta. Respiratory- and cardiac-gated balanced SSFP images can also be obtained similar to the thoracic aorta if noncontrast imaging is needed.

CE-MRA of the Abdominal Aorta (Renal/Mesenteric)

3D Gd-enhanced MRA using dynamic SPGR imaging is performed with breath hold in the coronal plane, taking care to include the origins of the abdominal vessels in the imaging volume. During imaging for renal or mesenteric vasculature, it is important to optimize the spatial resolution of the scans to obtain submillimeter spatial resolution whenever possible. The sequence is repeated three times: precontrast (mask images), during the arterial phase, and during the venous or equilibrium phase of contrast administration. The precontrast images are checked to ensure that the imaging volume has been positioned properly and for the purposes of digital subtraction. In order to obtain arterial phase images, a central k-space data set may often be required (especially with renal MRA).

Delayed venous imaging after contrast administration is also performed, after a 5- to 10-second breathing interval following the arterial phase. Portal venous flow and hepatic veins are imaged during this delayed phase. Aortic endoleaks may also be detected during the delayed phase acquisition.

Time-resolved-MRA

Time-resolved exam at high frame rates (3D frame rate of 5 to 10 seconds per image) can be performed for the assessment of the abdominal aorta. This may be useful in assessing differential blood flow in true versus false lumen or for the evaluation of endoleaks in aortic stent grafts.

PC-MRA

PC imaging is useful in renal, portal, and mesenteric imaging, where it is used for assessment of flow (portal vein) and stenosis severity (renal/mesenteric) and typically follows a 3D CE-MRA protocol to take advantage of residual contrast. Areas of hemodynamic severity are detected as a signal void ("dephasing"). In general, PC-MRA is acquired at a plane perpendicular to the artery measurement. A V_{max} or VENC (velocity-encoded value) of 30 to 60 cm/s is used for renal imaging. A V_{max} of 40 cm/s is used to assess flow in the portal veins.

Tissue Characterization

Sequences identical to that described for thoracic MRA can be used for targeted tissue characterization as necessary.

Typical Protocols

A typical exam for the abdominal aorta includes axial, coronal, and sagittal HASTE and/or SSFP images to provide a global assessment of vascular and nonvascular structures as well as assessment of vessel wall pathology. This can be followed by a breath held coronal or sagittal CE-MRA from above the celiac axis to the femoral heads in a single injection following a timing bolus. Delayed venous images should be obtained to assess venous structures and to assess complications such as false lumen assessment, endoleaks, etc. PC-MRA can be performed after the CE-MRA sequence to assess for turbulence and stenosis if indicated. To assess the renal arteries, a coronal acquisition is performed before and after IV contrast. This is supplemented by axial 2D or 3D PC to assess for turbulence in areas of stenosis, as well as more traditional axial sequences, such as gradient echo with fat saturation before and after IV contrast and T2 with fat saturation. Assessment of a pelvic renal allograft uses similar sequences, although the imaging planes need to be optimized depending on the orientation of the allograft. To assess the portal mesenteric circulation, a coronal 3D CE-MRA is used in the arterial and portal venous phases. In cases where contrast is contraindicated owing to advanced CKD (GFR less than 30), noncontrast approaches outlined in Table 4.1 may be used.

Peripheral Vascular Magnetic Resonance Angiography

The principal role of diagnostic MRA is provision of a roadmap of peripheral vessels for diagnostic and planning purposes. The need for extensive anatomic coverage at high resolution mandates specific modifications in sequences.

Indications

MRA is useful to assess peripheral arteries of the upper and lower extremities when they are involved by a variety of diseases including atherosclerosis (native and graft disease), aneurysms, inflammatory vasculitis, and embolic disease. MRA is useful in the investigation of arteriovenous malformations and in the assessment of dialysis fistulas in the upper extremities. MR venography of the upper and lower extremities is used to assess deep venous thrombosis, vascular malformations, and postthrombotic venous disease. Figure 4.15 illustrates a normal three-station lower extremity MRA; Figure 4.16 illustrates a patent femoral-to-femoral bypass graft with occlusion of the right common iliac artery.

Approach

Single-shot SSFP images are performed extending from the infrarenal aorta to the toes in multiple planes. Due to the large field of view, three different localizers are usually needed. In addition PC imaging is occasionally used for localization of vessels in order to ensure that they are not excluded from the 3D volumes used for CE-MRA.

Angiography

CE-MRA is the mainstay of peripheral lower extremity vascular imaging as other approaches are usually more time-consuming. However, with

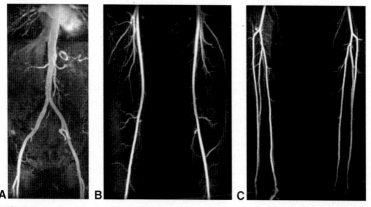

FIGURE 4-15. Maximal intensity projection display of a lower extremity runoff 3D CE-MRA. Three different stations are illustrated: **A:** the abdominal aorta and iliac arteries down to the femoral heads, **B:** the thigh arteries, and **C:** the lower leg arteries.

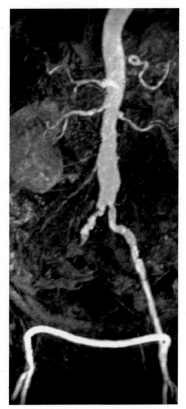

FIGURE 4-16. Maximal intensity projection display of a lower extremity runoff 3D CE-MRA illustrating occlusion of the right common iliac, with a patent femoral to femoral bypass graft supplying the right femoral artery after the obstruction.

limitations with use of Gd contrast, noncontrast MRA approaches may be another option. The main challenge with extremity imaging is that it involves imaging of a large field of view. Given magnet design limitations, this large field of view is covered in three or four (minimally) overlapping imaging stations in the lower extremity (abdomen/pelvis; thigh; legs/feet). The rapid arteriovenous transit time especially in the distal upper extremity requiring rapid imaging together with the high-spatial resolution (less than 1 mm) required to image the smaller vessels of the distal extremity may often require imaging separately as one discrete station. TR-MRA is especially helpful in the distal lower extremity to provide a "quick look" at the status of runoff vessels and is often performed using 3 to 5 mL of contrast agent.

Noncontrast Imaging Approaches

Table 4.1 provides alternatives in the event that the patient is unable to receive contrast agents.

Typical Protocols

A typical exam for the lower extremity arteries begins with localizers for planning of the 3D CE-MRA. This is followed by coronal 3D CE-MRA at three different imaging stations: the abdominal aorta down to the femoral heads, the thighs, and the lower leg. Imaging before contrast is performed for subtraction purposes. The timing of the contrast bolus is extremely important and is achieved by use of a timing bolus or a bolus-triggering method (e.g., CareBolus). Delayed imaging (venous phase) is utilized in dissection, obstruction, and large aneurysms and to assess the veins. Similar sequences are used for the examination of the upper extremities, which can require one or two imaging stations. In cases where more detailed information is warranted such as in the case of digital vessel involvement of the upper extremity, a dedicated examination may be warranted.

Nephrogenic Systemic Fibrosis with Gadolinium Contrast Agents

A recent concern in the use of Gd CE-MRA is nephrogenic systemic fibrosis (NSF). This rare but debilitating and largely untreatable disease varies in severity and is hypothesized to be related to the deposition of Gd in the skin after dissociation from the chelated form of Gd used in MRI contrast agents. Several factors have been reported to contribute to the development of NSF including the type of Gd chelate; the total dose administered and factors including renal failure; inflammatory state (lupus, recent major vascular surgery, recent thrombosis); and comorbidities of renal failure including acidosis, elevated phosphate levels, and high-dose erythropoietin therapy. Although the overwhelming majority of cases have been reported in patients on dialysis, a GFR less than 30 mL/min is a relative contraindication for administration of Gd-based contrast. These facts have led to widespread screening of MRI patients for renal dysfunction and using caution in administering Gd-based contrast agents when GFR is estimated to be less than 30 mL/min. As a result, NSF has been virtually eliminated with only a handful of new cases discovered in the past 2 years. When the need to establish a diagnosis outweighs the risk of NSF, steps should be taken to ensure that the patient is well hydrated, that acute inflammatory states have resolved before MRA is performed, that low-dose or noncontrast protocols are attempted first, and that patients on dialysis are dialyzed immediately after receiving Gd contrast.

Image Display Techniques

Postprocessing techniques have been developed to improve image contrast or to combine the information on these source images into a much smaller set of images offering a more global view of large vascular beds.

(i) *Multiplanar reformation*. Multiplanar reformation enables the user to reconstruct 3D datasets in any desired plane allowing structures of interest to be analyzed from multiple different planes (Figs. 4.3B and 4.6A).

(ii) *Maximal intensity projection*. This is the most commonly used tool for angiographic rendering of source images (Figs. 4.1, 4.2, and 4.4). MIP images summarize a whole stack of source images into projection images where each pixel represents a projection of the most intense pixels along a specified direction in the stack of images. It is important to correlate any abnormality seen on the MIP images with the original source images, to avoid false-positive findings due to artifacts (Fig. 4.3A vs. B).

(iii) *Surface shaded display*. This technique uses ray-casting algorithm to make surfaces of vessels appear opaque. Furthermore, simulated virtual light source is used to provide visual clues about the relative positions of vessels based on shading. The endoluminal fly-through technique is an application of SSD that can often be used to assess origins and tortuosity of vessels.

(iv) *Volume rendering*. This technique displays the entire data set in a way that 3D relationship between structures are preserved (Fig. 4.10C). The image can be manipulated to obtain a preliminary understanding of the 3D relationship between various vascular structures.

LIMITATIONS

There are a large number of artifacts that can degrade data and influence findings on MRA. Knowledge of the most common artifacts is crucial to the correct interpretation of MR angiograms.

Susceptibility Artifacts

These are T2* effects due to the presence of metal, such as surgical clips, shrapnel, and stents; the presence of high concentration of IV contrast agent, such as in the draining veins of injection sites; or at air-tissue interfaces, such as at lung-vessel or at bowel-vessel interfaces. These produce focal signal dropout (dark areas in the image) that can obscure image details, decrease visualization of surrounding vessels, and simulate stenoses or obstructions. This artifact can be minimized (but not eliminated) by using short TE and high receiver bandwidth.

Motion Artifacts

MR imaging involves excitation protocols that are performed over seconds or even minutes, and image reconstruction algorithms assume stationary tissue. If there is gross body motion by an uncooperative patient or breathing motion, the resulting images are degraded and blurred. These artifacts can be minimized by breath-holding during the exam, shorter acquisition times, and navigator gating. Motion artifacts that cannot be controlled by patients include peristalsis and vessel pulsation, which cause ghosting artifacts in the phase-encoding direction. These artifacts can be minimized by ECG gating, respiratory gating, or selective preparative pulses.

Coverage Artifacts

If parts of the vessels are not included in the acquired images, they appear occluded on MIP images. This happens, for example, in patients with a tortuous aorta. Localizer images must be procured carefully with examination of precontrast images to confirm inclusion of the complete anatomy of interest. Vessels included near the edges of the field of view can show signal drop-off, as the coil sensitivity drops off near the edges of the coil. Similar effects are noted in vessels outside the imaged slab of tissue during TOF sequences. Although present on the acquired images, vessels can be cut off during postprocessing, such as in the production of MIP images. Additional postprocessing artifacts include excessive filtering and subtraction artifacts. Evaluation of the source images is always necessary to confirm a finding on MIP images.

Timing Artifacts

This is one of the most common artifacts with MRA that occurs due to suboptimal contrast timing. If image acquisition occurs too late with respect to the peak arterial enhancement, venous opacification may obscure visualization of arterial vessels (venous contamination). Conversely, if the peak concentration of the bolus has not been reached during acquisition of the central portion of k-space and the T1 value of arterial blood is still changing during imaging, a ringing artifact with intraluminal dark longitudinal stripes of signal may occur and can simulate a dissection (Gibbs artifact).

Resolution Artifacts

Limited spatial resolution limits sensitivity to detect subtle lesions. In such cases, indirect findings, such as bowel mucosal enhancement on delayed images, can be used as surrogates for perfusion. Partial volume effects that may occur due to thick slices can give the appearance of stenosis or fail to detect intraluminal lesions, partially obstructing flow.

SPECIAL ISSUES

Contraindications to MRI exams include patients with pacemakers, epicardial pacer wires, aneurysm clips, metal fragments in the eyes, or some metallic implants. Many metallic implants, such as hip prostheses, are compatible with MRI. Endovascular stents are MR compatible, although manufacturer's guidelines must be respected. Nitinol stents are totally nonmagnetic and are very safe for MRI. A good source of information about MRI safety of various material is the Web site **www.mrisafety.com**. Pregnant patients may be scanned but without the administration of IV contrast agents.

MR Protocols

A good source of information about MRA is the Web site **www.mrprotocols. com** by Dr. Martin Prince, which has extensive reference information on multiple protocols for MRA. Other general MRI Web site resources include **www.mr-tip.com** and **www.imaios.com**. Table 4.2 summarizes some of the suggested protocols for MRA.

TABLE 4.2

SUGGESTED MRA PROTOCOLS BY TERRITORY[a]

	Carotid Arteries	Aortic Arch/Carotids	Thoracic Aorta
Black blood (wall)	3D-SPACE	HASTE (axial/sag/cor) or 3D-SPACE[b]	HASTE (axial/sag/cor) or 3D-SPACE[b]
Bright blood (lumen)	Coronal 3D CE-MRA (arterial/venous)	Coronal 3D CE-MRA (arterial/venous)	Oblique 3D CE-MRA (arterial/venous)
Flow/function	PC-MRA[b]	PC-MRA[b]	PC-MRA[b]
Stand-alone noncontrast	3D-SPACE or HASTE[b]	3D-SPACE or HASTE[b]	3D-SPACE or HASTE[b]
MRA option	3D-SSFP ± ASL or 2D-SSFP[b]	3D-SSFP ± ASL or 2D-SSFP[b]	3D-SSFP ± ASL or 2D-SSFP[b]

	Pulmonary Arteries	Abdominal Aorta	Renal Arteries
Black blood (wall)	HASTE (axial/sag/cor)	HASTE (axial/sag/cor) or 3D-SPACE[b]	HASTE (axial/sag/cor) or 3D-SPACE[b]
Bright blood (lumen)	Coronal 3D CE-MRA	Coronal 3D CE-MRA	Coronal 3D CE-MRA (arterial and venous)
Flow/function	PC-MRA (optional)	PC-MRA (optional)	PC-MRA (optional)
Thrombus		VIBE (selected area)	VIBE (selected area)

	Peripheral (Abd/pelv/thigh/legs)	MRA Upper Extremity	MR Venography
Black blood (wall)	3D-SPACE (abd/pelvic/thigh)	—	HASTE or 3D-SPACE
Bright blood (lumen)	TR-MRA (legs/feet)	TR-MRA	Coronal 3D CE-MRA
	Coronal 3D CE-MRA (abd/pelvic/thigh)	3D CE-MRA (unilateral)	
Stand-alone noncontrast	3D-SSFP ± ASL or 2D-SSFP[b]	3D-SPACE or HASTE[b]	3D-SPACE or HASTE[b]
MRA option	3D-SPACE (Abd/thigh) 2D-TOF (legs)	3D-SSFP ± ASL or 2D-SSFP[b]	3D-SSFP ± ASL or 2D-SSFP[b]
Thrombus	3D VIBE (infrarenal abdominal aorta and popliteal fossa)		3D VIBE

[a]Planning localizers are not included.
[b]Optional.
CE-MRA, contrast-enhanced MRA; VIBE, T1-weighted volumetric interpolation with breath hold (postcontrast); SPACE, sampling perfection with application of optimized contrast using different flip angle evolution; SSFP, steady-state free precession; ASL, arterial spin labeling; HASTE, Half-Fourier acquisition single-shot turbo spin-echo; PC-MRA, phase-contrast MRA; TR-MRA, time-resolved MRA.

CONCLUSIONS

MRA has become the imaging technique of choice in a number of vascular beds. The minimal risk associated with the procedure combined with its ability for high-resolution anatomical and functional assessment of the vessels and the organs supplied by these vessels is the major reason for its popularity. High-performance gradient systems in combination with paramagnetic contrast agents permit 3D CE-MRA within a single breath hold. TR-MRA exams permit assessment of a vascular bed in the arterial and venous phases. Dark-blood sequences allow assessment of various vessel wall pathologies. PC-MRA exams when used in conjunction with typical CE-MRA protocols provide functional information on flow and hemodynamic significance of a stenosis. There are a large number of artifacts that can degrade data and influence findings on MRA. Knowledge of the most common artifacts is crucial to accurate reporting on MR angiograms.

PRACTICAL POINTS

■ Vascular imaging can be broadly classified as black-blood or bright-blood techniques based on the appearance of the vascular lumen.

■ Spin-echo sequences are less susceptible to artifacts than gradient-echo sequences.

■ Contrast-enhanced MRA is currently the predominant technique to image most vascular beds.

■ Noncontrast imaging techniques are useful for assessment of vessel wall pathology and when Gd administration is contraindicated.

■ Time-resolved MRA sequences provide an assessment of the contrast flow kinetics through a vascular bed of interest.

■ PC imaging provides an assessment of the hemodynamic significance of stenosis.

■ Source images (nonsubtracted) should always be reviewed to avoid artifacts.

RECOMMENDED READING

Carroll TJ, Grist TM. Technical developments in MR angiography. *Radiol Clin North Am* 2002;40:921–951.

Dellegrottaglie S, Sanz J, Macaluso F, et al. Technology Insight: magnetic resonance angiography for the evaluation of patients with peripheral artery disease. *Nat Clin Practice Cardiovascular Med* 2007;4(12):677–687.

Edelman RR, Sheehan JJ, Dunkle E, et al. Quiescent-interval single-shot unenhanced magnetic resonance angiography of peripheral vascular disease: technical considerations and clinical feasibility. *Magn Reson Med* 2010;63(4):951–958.

Ersoy H, Rybicki FJ. MR angiography of lower extremities. *Am J Roentgenol* 2008;190:1675–1684.

Ho VB, Corse WR. MR angiography of the abdominal aorta and peripheral vessels. *Radiol Clin North Am* 2003;41:115–144.

Lee VS. *Cardiovascular MRI: physical principles to practical protocols.* Philadelphia, PA: Lippincott Williams & Wilkins; 2006.

Leung DA, Hagspiel KD, Angle JF, et al. MR angiography of the renal arteries. *Radiol Clin North Am* 2002;40:847–865.

Miyazaki M, Lee VS. Nonenhanced MR angiography. *Radiology* 2008;248(1):20–43.

Mohrs OK, Petersen SE, Schulze T, et al. High-resolution 3D unenhanced ECG-gated respiratory-navigated MR angiography of the renal arteries: comparison with contrast-enhanced MR angiography. *Am J Roentgenol* 2010;195(6):1423–1428.

Mukherjee D, Rajagopalan S. *CT and MR angiography of the peripheral circulation: practical approach with clinical protocols*. London, UK: Informa Health Care, 2007.

Prince MR, Grist TM, Debatin JF. *3D contrast MR angiography*, 3rd ed. Berlin: Springer Verlag, 2003.

Schneider G, Prince MR, Meaney JFM, et al., eds. *Magnetic resonance angiography. techniques, indications and practical applications*. Milan: Springer, 2005.

Zhang H, Maki JH, Price MR. 3D contrast-enhanced MR angiography. *J Magn Reson Imag* 2007; 25(1):13–25.

CHAPTER 5 ■ Computed Tomography Angiography in the Diagnosis of Vascular Disease

Paaladinesh Thavendiranathan, Michael Walls, and Georgeta Mihai

Imaging of the peripheral vascular system became possible in the 90s with the introduction of 4-slice multidetector scanner with 0.5-second gantry rotation speed. Ongoing advances have led to increases in z-axis coverage with a single rotation and better temporal resolution. The most contemporary scanners include those with 320 detectors, with a gantry rotation speed of 350 ms (temporal resolution 175 ms), and dual source scanners with a temporal resolution of up to 42 to 83 ms. These advances have enabled rapid scanning at superior temporal and spatial resolution, and together, radiation reduction techniques have led to establishing multidetector CT angiography (MDCTA) as a viable and accurate modality in the assessment of vascular disease.

FUNDAMENTALS OF COMPUTED TOMOGRAPHY IMAGING

Major Components of a Computed Tomography Scanner

The major components of a CT scanner are an x-ray tube and generator, a collimator, and photon detectors. These components are mounted on a rotating gantry. The x-ray tube produces the x-rays necessary for imaging. The collimator helps shape the x-ray beams that emanate from the x-ray tube in order to cut out unnecessary radiation. The detectors consist of multiple rows of detector elements (greater than 900 elements per row in the current scanners), which receive x-ray photons that have traversed through the patient. The older generation scanners only had single detector row; however, the newer scanners have as many as 320 detector rows. With the increase in detector rows, the width of each detector has also decreased from 1.5 to 0.5 mm. The most important benefit of increasing the detector rows is the increased coverage per gantry rotation (a 320-row detector CT with a detector width of 0.5 mm will have coverage of 160 mm). Decreased detector width improves spatial resolution in the z axis, while increased coverage shortens scan time. The gantry rotation times determine the temporal resolution of the images with older scanners having a rotation time of 0.75 second, while the more contemporary scanners have a rotation time of 0.33 second. The temporal resolution of the CT image is half the time it takes for the gantry to rotate 360 degrees.

Attenuation Data for Image Reconstruction

Similar to other x-ray techniques, cardiac CT uses differences in attenuation in order to map and display anatomy. The gantry rotates around the patient collecting attenuation data from different angles. The attenuation data obtained between 0 and 180 degrees will be identical, hence negating the necessity to obtain 360 degrees of data. The images displayed are a map of differences in relative attenuation that the x-ray beam experiences as it passes through the area of interest. Different objects have different attenuation properties described by its attenuation coefficient μ. This is an indicator of the likelihood that the x-ray photons will interact with an atom of the tissue rather than passing through it. This attenuation coefficient varies depending on the thickness of the material and the energy of the photons (measured in keV) that pass through them. The measured intensity of photons at the CT detector can be expressed using a formula (below) describing the relationship between the photon flux coming through the x-ray tube and that detected at the detector elements. "I" is the intensity measured at the detector, "I_o" is the photon flux from the x-ray tube measured in milliamperes (mA), "e" is the exponent, and "μ" is the attenuation coefficient.

$$I = I_o e^{-m}$$

Therefore, as the attenuation of the tissue increases, the fraction of photons that are detected at the detector element decreases. As these photons strike the scintillation crystals at the detector array, they are converted into light, which then strike photodiodes that convert light into digital signals. Therefore, during CT imaging, the photon energy (keV) and the photon flux (mA) are set by the user, the photon intensity at the detector is measured with the scintillation data, and using the formula described about the attenuation coefficient is back-calculated. This attenuation data is then "referenced" to the attenuation coefficient of water to generate a CT number, which is expressed in Hounsfield units. By default the CT value of water is set at 0, while CT value of air is –1,000.

$$\text{CT number} = \left[(\mu_{tissue} - \mu_{water}) / u_{water} - \mu_{air} \right] \times 1,000$$

These CT values are "number behind the images" and are used to fill a "matrix" that consists of pixel elements. The most commonly used matrix size is 512×512 pixels in the x and y directions. This process of projecting these CT values into the matrix is referred to as back projection. Combination of multiple back projections with filtering is necessary to reduce noise and to increase the sharpness of an image. This process is referred to as filtered back projection. A grayscale window is then applied to this matrix generating tissues of different brightness depending on the CT values and the window settings. Where the CT values are higher, the image will be brighter and where the CT values are lower, it would be darker.

Scanning Modes

The two scanning modes used in CT are the axial mode and the spiral/helical mode. The major differences between these modes include (i) differences in table movement during image acquisition, (ii) differences in assignment of data to each channel, and (iii) need for interpolation for data reconstruction. Each mode has its benefits; however, the mode used for vascular CTA is the spiral/helical mode. For coronary CTA, there has been a shift toward using axial mode due to its benefit in significantly reducing radiation exposure. In the axial mode, images are acquired at particular selected points in the cardiac cycle (ECG based) with the tube being turned off between images.

Spiral/Helical Mode

During spiral scanning, there is continuous table movement and the tube is on the whole time; however, the tube current can be made to fluctuate. Since the table is moving during the acquisition, the detector channels are not dedicated to a slice of the patient and hence it receives data from multiple contiguous slices of the patient. An interpolation algorithm would be necessary to reconstruct "virtual" axial slices with some loss in image quality. Spiral imaging is fast and can provide infinite reconstruction of data, however, at the cost of higher radiation.

Pitch

Pitch is an expression of the relationship between the table speed of the scanner per gantry rotation and the coverage of the scanner. Pitch = [table feed per rotation (mm)/coverage (mm)]. If the pitch is 1, then there would be no gaps between the data set. However, if the pitch is greater than 1, gaps would be present, and if the pitch is less than 1, there would be overlap in the data acquisition. The pitch for ECG-gated cardiac scanning is 0.2 to 0.3. For most vascular CT, the pitch ranges between 0.5 and 1.2.

ECG Gating

ECG gating is a method of correlating changes in the heart or vascular structure to the cardiac cycle. It is mainly used for cardiac CTA and often for thoracic aortic imaging. The two most common ECG gating methods are retrospective and prospective gating. With traditional spiral scanning, the ECG gating is performed retrospectively where the data and ECG information are acquired and subsequent reconstructions can be performed at various time points in the RR interval. Whereas in prospective ECG gating, the scanner is usually triggered at the R wave and image acquisition occurs at a fixed point in the cardiac cycle. This is the method used for axial scanning. However, with recent advances in CT imaging, it is also now possible to perform prospectively ECG-triggered helical scans using high pitch with extremely low radiation exposure. These have been referred to as "flash" scans and are gaining significant popularity for coronary imaging.

General Acquisition Parameters

The selection of the specific acquisition parameters of imaging depends on the employed scanner model, the patient's body habitus, and the clinical question. The two main adjustable parameters are the tube voltage and current. The voltage is typically set at 120 kilovolts (kV) although 100 kV provides acceptable images with significantly reduced radiation and can be employed in most individuals who are not obese for vascular imaging.

Tube current is usually 200 to 300 mA and again can be adjusted upward if the patient is very large. Breath-holding is required only for the chest and abdomen CTA acquisitions in order to reduce motion artifact. In MDCT spiral scans, the volume coverage speed (v, cm/s) can be estimated by the following formula:

$$v = \frac{Ms_{coll}p}{t_{rot}}$$

where M = number of simultaneous acquired slices, s_{coll} = collimated slice width, p = pitch, and t_{rot} = gantry rotation time. Although current generation scanners offer improved spatial resolution, their increased coverage and rotation speeds pose the risk of "outrunning" the bolus of contrast in CTA applications. Accordingly, adjustments in both the pitch and the gantry rotation speed must be made in order to achieve a table translation speed of no more than 30 mm/s for CTA applications. In a 64-slice scanner, this usually is achieved by a reduction in t_{rot} to 0.5 second and a decrease in pitch to ≤0.8.

Contrast Administration

Low-osmolar nonionic iodinated contrast agents are most commonly used for CTA applications. Patients' renal function should be assessed prior to administration of contrast and decisions regarding prophylactic medication use should be made if necessary. The contrast agent is administered intravenously using a power injector into an antecubital vein, preferably on the right side. Since contrast arrival time may vary, appropriate timing could be determined using a small test bolus or an automated bolus–triggered technique. For most CTA applications, 100 to 120 mL of contrast (with an iodine concentration between 320 and 370 mg/mL) is administered at a rate of 4 mL/s followed by a saline flush. Although, the use of higher iodine concentration (370 to 400 mg/mL) contrast agents yields improved enhancement, there is likely no difference in diagnostic ability for vascular applications. When an automated bolus–detection algorithm is used for CTA, the region of interest (ROI) is placed in the part of the aorta close to the area of interest. A repetitive low-dose acquisition is performed at the monitoring location (e.g., ascending aorta for thoracic aorta CTA and suprarenal aorta for distal abdominal and lower extremity CTA) and is started approximately 5 to 10 seconds after contrast injection begins. The actual angiographic acquisition is started when the contrast enhancement reaches a prespecified Hounsfield unit threshold (e.g., 110 HU).

Image Reconstruction at the Scanner Console

Various image reconstruction filters are offered by each manufacturer. These filters are referred to as "sharp" or "soft" filters. Sharper reconstruction filters will provide more details but also more noise and are best for assessment of stents and areas of calcifications. Softer reconstruction filters provide less image detail but less noise as well. Soft to medium filters are usually used for most CTA applications. Image reconstruction can also be performed at different phases in case of cardiac-gated acquisitions and may be important in assessment of coronary anatomy in cases of dissections or concomitant assessment of coronary artery/graft anatomy in cases of thoracic aortic aneurismal disease. This is most important for cardiac CTA where coronary anatomy may need to be assessed at different phases to ensure accurate delineation of coronary stenosis. When ECG-gated thoracic aortic image is performed, various phases can be reconstructed to assess the aorta.

Slice width and slice increment used for image reconstruction at the scanner console depend on the anatomy being assessed and scanner capabilities. Reconstruction thickness for vascular imaging can be performed at the same width (thin) or several times the detector width (thick) to reduce noise (thinner slices are associated with higher image noise compared to thicker slices and take longer time to review). A slice increment of approximately 50% of the slice thickness is used.

Image Postprocessing

Similar to vascular MRA (Chapter 4), multiple postprocessing techniques can be used in vascular CTA to assess the thousands of images that are generated. Usually, two data sets are reconstructed including "thick" and "thin" sets. The thick set (5.0 mm) is used for general assessment, whereas the thin set (0.6 to 0.75 mm) is more suited for detailed evaluation. Image formats used for evaluation include (i) multiplanar reformats (MPR), (ii) maximal intensity projections (MIPs), (iii) curved planer reformats (CPRs), (iv) volume rendering (VR), and (v) shaded surface display. Please refer to the vascular MRA section for description of these techniques. For CTA, the evaluation of the data set begins with review of the axial images to assess gross anatomy and scan quality. This is followed by use of a MIP format in traditional projections as well as in oblique projections. Care must be taken in viewing MIP images when calcium is present, as it can overestimate the severity of stenotic lesions. For detailed evaluation, especially when calcium and stents are present, the raw MPR images should be reviewed. Curved planar reconstruction is a unique technique that makes it possible to follow the course of any single vessel and displays it in nontraditional plane where the entire vessel can be seen in a single image. 3D-VR images can also be reviewed to define anatomic course and anatomic variations if necessary. Each of these reconstruction methods has its pitfalls and it is important to assess an abnormality identified in a systematic manner, in multiple different planes, using different techniques, and different phases of the cardiac cycle if available.

Radiation

Radiation exposure of the patient during a CT exam and the resulting potential radiation hazards has gained considerable attention in the public and the scientific literature. The Bier VII committee states that "there is a linear no-threshold dose response relationship between exposure to ionizing radiation and cancer risk." This has resulted in the adoption of the ALARA

(As Low as Reasonable Achievable) principle in the use of radiation-based diagnostic studies. Typical effective dose of radiation for CT protocols vary from 1 to 2 mSv for a head examination, 2 to 3 mSv for CT pulmonary angiography, 4 to 6 mSv for a nongated thoracic CTA, and 6 to 10 mSv for a coronary CT (64 detector scanners, with ECG dose modulation). This must, however, be considered in the context of the average annual background radiation exposure worldwide of approximately 2.4 mSv/y and the radiation exposure from an alternative diagnostic modality. The radiation exposure depends on many factors including scan factors such as coverage, slice thickness, pitch, ECG gating, tube voltage, and tube current, and patient factors such as BMI and heart rate. It is therefore incumbent upon the physician supervising the study to individualize scan protocols to ensure a diagnostic study while minimizing radiation exposure.

CLINICAL APPLICATIONS OF COMPUTED TOMOGRAPHY ANGIOGRAPHY IN VASCULAR DISEASE

Computed Tomography Angiography of the Extra Cranial Circulation

Technical Considerations

To perform CTA of the cervicocranial arteries, the patient is placed in the supine position with upper arms along the body. A topogram is first performed to assist planning of the imaging volume. The scan volume should include the aortic arch to the level of the circle of Willis. A submillimeter detector collimation is preferable. Tube current and voltage is vendor dependent. A test bolus or a bolus tracking algorithm can be used for synchronizing contrast arrival and initiation of scanning. Thin collimation (= minimal detector width) should be used whenever possible to achieve high z-axis spatial resolution. The pitch can range between 0.5626 and 1.0 depending on the vendor and the number of detector rows. Breath-holding is recommended especially for better assessment of the aortic arch vessels, and the patient should be asked to not swallow during the study. Reconstruction of the acquired images should be performed using a smooth reconstruction kernel (e.g., Siemens B20f). Reconstructions slice thickness of 0.6 to 1.0 mm with a 50 to 80% reconstruction increment is often used for assessment of the carotid circulation.

Clinical Application

Atherosclerotic and Nonatherosclerotic Disease

The most common indication for CTA of the extracranial circulation is for the evaluation of suspected carotid stenosis due to atherosclerosis (Fig. 5.1A). CTA is also an important component of the comprehensive evaluation of a patient with acute stroke coupled with nonenhanced brain CT and perfusion imaging. Other nonatherosclerotic diseases such as fibromusclar dysplasia, carotid aneurysms or pseudoaneurysms, or dissection in the carotid, subclavian, or vertebrobasilar systems can also

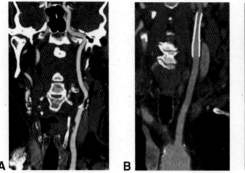
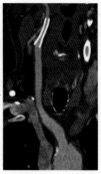

FIGURE 5-1.   A: Curved planar reconstruction from the left carotid artery illustrating stenosis with a mixed plaque at the bifurcation and an ulcerated plaque at the common carotid. (**B**) Postprocedural CT angiography of another patient showing curved planar reformations of stents in the right external carotid artery (**C**) and in the left internal carotid artery (Reprinted from Berg M, Kangasniemi M, Manninen H, et al. CT angiography of the extracranial and intracranial circulation with imaging protocols. In: Mukerjee D, Rajagopalan S, eds. *CT and MRI angiography of the peripheral circulation: practical approach with clinical protocols.* London, UK: Informa Health Care, 2007:67–69, with permission.)

be assessed with high spatial resolution. CTA also has a unique role for the follow-up after carotid endovascular stenting (Fig. 5.1B and C) over MRA due to its ability to assess complications such as dissection and in-stent restonosis and the lack of susceptibility artifacts that would be seen with MRA. CTA is accurate compared to digital subtraction angiography for the identification of total or near occlusions of the carotid artery, and for the identification of location of the stenosis; however, it may underestimate and sometimes overestimate stenosis severity. There are also other limitations with CTA including assessment of calcified segments and their associated artifacts and inability to assess flow dynamics.

Computed Tomography Angiography of the Pulmonary Artery

Technical Consideration and Clinical Applications

CT of the pulmonary arteries (CTPAs) is the diagnostic test of choice for the assessment of pulmonary thromboembolic disease. Specifically when combined with CT venography of the proximal lower extremities, CTPA has high sensitivity and specificity for the diagnosis of pulmonary embolus (Fig. 5.2). To perform a CTPA, the patient is placed in the supine position with the hands above the head. Following a topogram, the field of view is prescribed to include the adrenals to the lung apices. The voltage, current, and pitch will vary depending on vendor and patient characteristics. For contrast timing, the pulmonary trunk is used. The pulmonary arteries are imaged with the first pass of intravenous contrast, while the pelvis

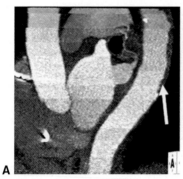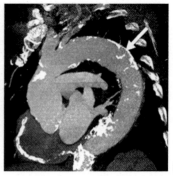

A   B

FIGURE 5-2. Sagittal MIP display of the thoracic aorta illustrating diffuse atherosclerotic plaques (*arrow*) (**A**) and significant calcification (**B**) (*arrow*).

and lower extremity veins are imaged later with a scan delay of 2.5 to 3.5 minutes. CTPA images can be reconstructed using several techniques; however, one suggested method is 1.25 mm slice thickness slices with a 50 to 60% slice increment. Large slice thickness is used for reconstruction of the pelvis and lower extremity veins. Multiple artifacts can mimic pulmonary emboli, and hence, careful scrutiny of the acquired images with active scrolling in and out of each main, lobar, segmental, and subsegmental arteries is necessary, to avoid overcalling or missing pulmonary emboli. Similarly, CT venography of the proximal lower extremities is fraught with artifacts that can mimic deep vein thrombosis and hence has to be evaluated thoroughly.

Other clinical applications of CTPA includes assessment of pulmonary artery aneurysms and pseudoaneurysms, congenital anomalies such as pulmonary artery atresia, assessment of congenital palliative shunts, arteriovenous malformations, and preprocedure planning for percutaneous pulmonary valve replacement or stenting of branch pulmonary artery stenosis.

Computed Tomography Angiography of the Thoracic Aorta

Technical Considerations

With current generation scanners, the speed of acquisition, and the outstanding spatial resolution (0.6 × 0.6 × 0.6 mm) CTA examination of the thoracic aorta is the method of choice both in the acute setting (dissection, rupture, and intramural hematoma) and in chronic diseases both preintervention and postintervention. Furthermore, CTA is an excellent modality for the assessment of congenital vascular anomalies of the thoracic aorta or its branch vessels. For thoracic CTA, a wide field of view (50 cm) is used including the ribs laterally and extending from the thoracic inlet to the aortic bifurcation. A 120-keV tube setting is most commonly used and the tube current is individualized. ECG gating is preferred for most thoracic aortic evaluation especially if the coronary arteries are simultaneously evaluated and to assess subtle abnormalities involving the proximal ascending aorta. The minimal detector collimation should be used to obtain high resolution isotropic images. A higher pitch is used for nongated studies compared to gated studies where coronary arteries may be assessed. Bolus tracking or timing bolus timed to the distal ascending aorta or arch is used with contrast administration. Images can be reconstructed at a slice thickness of 1.5 mm width with 50% slice increments and soft filter kernel. Precontrast and postcontrast studies may be performed for the assessment of hemorrhage, intramural hematoma, and slow leaks.

Clinical Application

Atherosclerotic Disease

The clinical indications and utility of CTA closely mirror that of MRA. Applications include aortic atherosclerotic disease, inflammatory disease, aneurismal disease, acute aortic syndromes, and chronic dissection. CTA can demonstrate calcified plaques, plaque ulceration, thrombus formation, and protruding atheroma (Fig. 5.2) in addition to subtle abnormalities of the aortic wall including intra-aortic hematoma. Also, CT attenuation properties can sometimes be used to assess the composition of plaque, delineation of hemorrhage, thrombus, and calcification.

Acute Aortic Syndromes

CTA plays an important role in the assessment of acute aortic syndromes which comprise of penetrating aortic ulcer, aortic dissection, and intramural hematoma. With penetrating ulcer the protrusion of the plaque through the intima and internal elastic membrane of the aorta can be seen when the lumen is filled with contrast. This appears as a focal contrast out-pouching. Occasionally, aortic wall enhancement and contrast extravasation can be seen. With acute aortic dissection, the rapidity of imaging and the high spatial resolution make it possible to perform studies safely and obtain essential information such as the dissection entry and exit points, size of the aorta, patency of the false lumen, degree of compression of the true lumen, and the involvement of the coronary arteries, head and neck vessels, or abdominal vessels (Fig. 5.3). Intramural hematoma appears as a focal thickening of the aortic wall with high attenuation and may be better appreciated in noncontrast images.

Aortic Aneurysms

Another clinical application of CTA of the thoracic aorta includes assessment of thoracic aortic aneurysms to delineate the size, spatial extent, tortuosity, and morphological features (Fig. 5.4). This information is essential for decision regarding surgical intervention and surgical planning. Also, in the postoperative state, CTA is used for the assessment of graft patency and other postoperative complications. Knowing the surgical history is essential in making the correct diagnosis in the postoperative setting as surgical changes may mimic dissection and pseudoaneurysms. In emergency

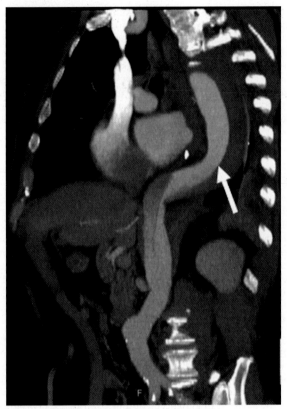

FIGURE 5-3. MIP display of a Type B aortic dissection with extension into the abdominal aorta.

settings or when surgical intervention is not possible, CTA can play an important role in planning endovascular aortic repair (EVAR) by providing an assessment of diameter of the vessels, the status of the aortic branches, and the sizes of the iliac and femoral arteries for vascular access. Stent graft diameter is determined based on CT findings. Also, postprocedure CTA is performed at discharge and during follow-up to assess the EVAR integrity and presence of endoleaks (Fig. 5.5).

Congenital Anomalies and Inflammatory Diseases

CTA can be used for the assessment of congenital anomalies such as aortic coarctation (Fig. 5.6) and anomalous origin of the head and neck vessels. However, MRA is more useful in this circumstance as it provides additional hemodynamic data that is not possible with CTA. Also, in patients with congenital heart disease with multiple previous surgeries

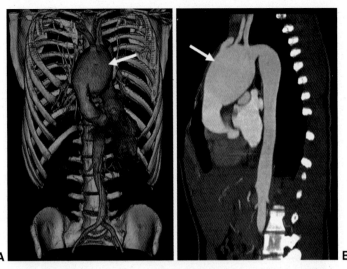

FIGURE 5-4. Volume rendered (**A**) and MIP (**B**) display of a large ascending thoracic aortic aneurysm. (See color insert.)

who are planned for a repeat sternotomy, CT has a unique role in assessing the relationship of vascular structures such as main pulmonary artery, ascending aorta, and mammary arteries to the sternum. Finally, CTA can be used for the assessment of aortic inflammatory diseases that involve the aorta and its proximal branches including giant cell arteritis. Wall thickness can be easily assessed and arterial phase wall enhancement has been at times used as a marker of ongoing inflammatory disease activity.

Computed Tomography Angiography of the Abdominal Aorta

Technical Considerations

CTA has an important role in abdominal aortic imaging due to its ability to assess intrinsic vessel pathology and branches such as the renal and mesenteric arteries with high degree of accuracy. The protocols for image acquisition vary significantly based on the clinical question and the CT scanner used for imaging. The patient is placed in the supine position, with imaging collimation set at the lowest possible by the scanner. The scanning volume can range from the upper limit of the 12th rib to the femoral heads or the iliac crest inferiorly. Scanning is performed in the craniocaudal direction without cardiac gating. Breath-holding will improve image quality especially of the upper abdominal vessels and is suggested whenever possible. A noncontrast study may be performed using larger collimation to assess for hemorrhage or aortic hematoma. This is followed by a contrast study with triggering at the diaphragmatic

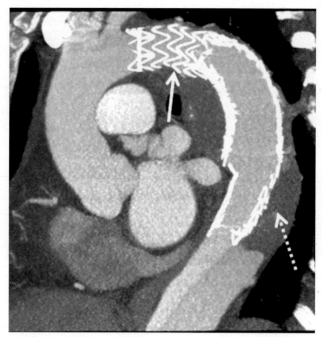

FIGURE 5-5.   MIP display of a Type B thoracic aortic dissection postendovascular stenting (*solid arrow*). Ongoing type B dissection with thrombus still present (*broken arrow*).

or supraceliac aorta. A postcontrast study may be performed to evaluate venous anatomy, renal perfusion, or slow bleeding. Images can be reconstructed using a softer filter at submillimeter slick thickness with 50% slice increments.

Clinical Applications

Acute Aortic Syndrome

MDCT is a facile noninvasive technique that is an excellent diagnostic tool for the assessment of acute abdominal aortic dissection. Acute dissection occurs either due to a ruptured abdominal aortic aneurysm or extension of thoracic aortic dissection (Fig. 5.7). CTA in addition to assessing the vasculature can also provide information on soft tissue structures including complications such as hemorrhage. A noncontrast study may illustrate acute hemorrhage within an aortic dissection plane, peri-aortic or retroperitoneal structures. In addition, this precontrast study allows for comparison of subtle changes in thrombus opacification postcontrast suggesting a slow bleed. Furthermore, delayed acquisitions 1 to 2 minutes postcontrast can help identify slow hemorrhage and venous abnormalities.

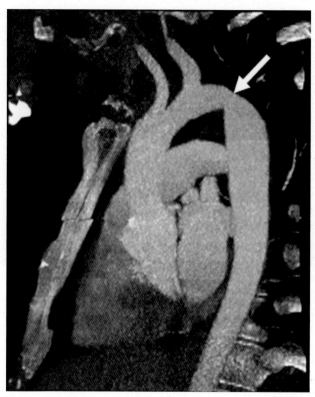

FIGURE 5-6.   MIP display of a patient with juxtaductal coarctation (*arrow*) with poststenotic dilatation of the descending thoracic aorta.

Contrast-enhanced study will provide assessment of mesenteric and renal arteries that may be involved in the dissection.

Abdominal Aortic Aneurysm

CTA may not have a role in screening for abdominal aortic aneurysms; however, it can be performed for assessment of the extent of the aneurysm, involvement of aortic branches, presence of mural thrombus, and dissections (Fig. 5.8). Ultrasound, however, remains the screening test of choice. However, in patients with pre-existing abdominal aortic aneurysms, CTA has a role in surgical planning and endovascular stenting. Specifically, in endovascular stenting, several features such as proximal neck diameter, location of the branch vessels, size of the aneurysm, and distal neck length necessary for planning of the intervention can be easily obtained using CTA. Also poststenting, CTA is used for periodic surveillance for stent graft migration and/or endoleak.

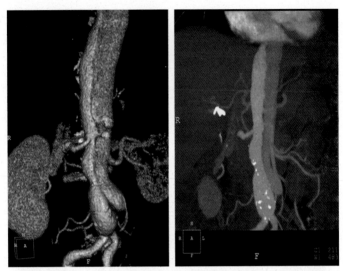

FIGURE 5-7. An aortic dissection with extension into the abdomen. A: Three-dimensional volume reconstruction. B: A maximum intensity projection with a 60-mm thickness (slab-MIP) demonstrates calcium in the abdominal aorta and reveals segments of the celiac, superior mesenteric, and lumbar arteries (See color insert.)

Vessel Wall Disease

In the abdomen, CTA also has a role in assessing vascular wall and branch vessel changes associated with large vasculitis such as Takayasu's arteritis and medium vessel vasculitis such as polyarteritis nodosa, and Behcet's disease. Furthermore, aortic atherosclerosis, penetrating ulcers, and pseudoaneurysm can be readily identified using CTA.

Renal Artery Disease

The superb isotropic spatial resolution (0.5 × 0.5 × 0.5 mm) provides excellent assessment of the renal arteries disease unsurpassed by any other imaging modality. Thus CTA is well suited for the assessment of atherosclerotic renal stenosis, fibromuscular dysplasia, aneurysms, dissection involving the renal arteries, or the presence and number of accessory branches. In addition, CTA has a role in the follow-up of patients after renal artery stenting. However, the biggest limitation is the fact that a large proportion of patients with renal artery disease also have advanced renal dysfunction, hence precluding a contrast-enhanced CTA study. Also, unlike MRI, the hemodynamic consequences of the stenosis cannot be evaluated using CTA. Fibromuscular dysplasia is an excellent indication for CTA as this provides for spatial resolution

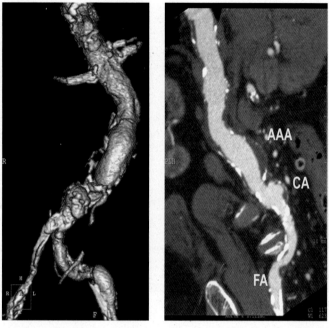

FIGURE 5-8. The volume-rendered image (**A**) of this aorta does not adequately reveal diffuse aneurysmal involvement. A curved multiplanar reconstruction (**B**) of this tortuous area enables electronic linearization of the aorta perpendicular to the flow of blood and provides a more reliable assessment of abdominal aneurysm length. (Reprinted from Goldman C, Sanz J. *CT Angiography of the abdominal aorta and its branches with protocols.* In: Mukerjee D, Rajagopalan S, eds. *CT and MRI angiography of the peripheral circulation: practical approach with clinical protocols.* London, UK: Informa Health Care, 2007:117, with permission.) (See color insert.)

currently not possible with MRA allowing evaluation of distal branches of the renal artery which are often not adequately assessed by MRA techniques.

Mesenteric Arterial Disease

The celiac and/or superior mesenteric arteries may be involved with mesenteric ischemia (Fig. 5.9). The proximal celiac trunk or the branch vessels may be involved in either an acute thrombotic, embolic, vasospastic process or dissection. In a more chronic setting mesenteric ischemic could be due to a stenotic process from atherosclerosis typically involving at least 2/3 mesenteric vessels. The site of stenosis, the severity, and length can be delineated using CTA. Median arcuate ligament syndrome is easily diagnosed using CTA (see Chapter 15).

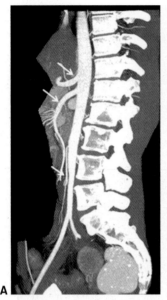 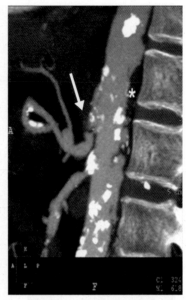

FIGURE 5-9.   A: MIP display of a CTA of the abdominal aorta and the mesenteric arteries. Celiac artery, and superior and inferior mesenteric arteries (*arrows*). **B:** Severe celiac artery stenosis on a MIP of an abdominal aortogram (*arrow*). Note calcifications and severe ulcerated plaques in the supraceliac segment (denoted by the *asterisk*). (Reprinted from Goldman C, Sanz J. CT Angiography of the abdominal aorta and its branches with protocols. In: Mukerjee D, Rajagopalan S, eds. *CT and MRI Angiography of the peripheral circulation: practical approach with clinical protocols*. London, UK: Informa Health Care, 2007:122, with permission.)

Peripheral Vascular Magnetic Resonance Angiography

Technical Considerations

Contemporary MDCT scanners are capable of adequately assessing the distal vessels in lower extremities. In order to image vessels less than 1 mm in diameter as is the case in pedal vessels, submillimeter detector collimation is necessary. Patients are placed in a supine position on the scanner table in a feet-first orientation. The typical field-of-view (FOV) should extend from the diaphragm to the toes with an average scan length of 110 to 130 cm. The scanning protocol begins with a scout image of the entire FOV followed by a test bolus or bolus triggering acquisition. Breath-holding may be necessary for the more proximal abdominal station, but not for the distal stations. This is followed by a contrast-enhanced angiographic acquisition during arterial contrast phase. With newer scanners, care must be taken to set the gantry rotation times and pitch appropriately to avoid the risk of "out running" the contrast bolus. A second late acquisition of the calf vessels can be prescribed in the event of inadequate pedal opacification during the arterial phase. Images can be reconstructed using a smooth kernel into one data set of thicker slices at 5.0 mm slice thickness for general assessment, and another data set of thinner slices of 0.6 to 0.75 mm with a 25 to 50% overlap.

Clinical Application

Atherosclerotic Peripheral Artery Disease

Atherosclerotic disease is the most common indication for CTA evaluation of the peripheral arterial system (Fig. 5.10). MDCTA can provide assessment of stenosis location, length, number, and severity all of which have a direct bearing on the choice of therapy. Furthermore, other conditions that may mimic atherosclerotic disease such as endovascular fibrosis of the external iliac artery, fibromuscular dysplasia, popliteal cyst, etc. can be assessed in the same exam. CTA assessment of the degree of stenosis in the distal vessels in diabetics and patients with long standing end-stage renal disease may be limited by calcification which is often present.

Vasculitis

Buerger's disease typically affects the small-to-medium sized arteries of the extremities and primarily affects young male smokers. The distal nature of the disease may favor CTA over MRA in light of the submillimeter resolution of the technique. Polyarteritis nodosa typically presents with nonspecific vascular symptoms and involves the visceral vessels. CTA hence may be well suited in light of superior spatial resolution giant cell arteritis and Takayasu's arteritis may involve the aorta, arch, and its branches. The age of the patient and the pattern and type of vessels involved are often crucial in differentiation (Fig. 5.11).

Endovascular Stent Evaluation

CTA may be used for evaluation of in-stent restenosis particularly in proximal vessels such as the iliac and femoral arteries. This may require reconstruction with alternate kernels and adjustment of window-levels. There is currently no prospective or accumulated retrospective evidence evaluating peripheral stents. From clinical experience, CTA has a good negative predictive value for in-stent stenosis, but its specificity for the degree of narrowing, when present, is lacking. When the radiation dose is not prohibitive, increasing the tube current can reduce the metallic artifact.

Other Indications

A variety of other conditions may represent less common indications for the use of a peripheral CTA including persistent sciatic artery (Fig. 5.12) popliteal entrapment (Fig. 5.13) and cystic medial adventitial disease. Also, arteriovenous malformations and fistulas may be well delineated by acquiring images during the arterial and venous phase. CTA imaging may significantly contribute to the characterization of congenital abnormalities with direct or indirect involvement of the peripheral vessels.

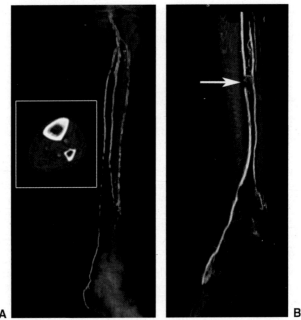

FIGURE 5-10. A volume-rendered display of lower extremity atherosclerotic disease (**A**). Axial CTA image (**inset**) illustrates calcification within the walls of the anterior tibial, posterior tibial, and peroneal arteries with poor luminal visualization. Occlusive disease (**B**). Three-dimensional CTA volume-rendered image (*left anterior oblique view*) shows a segmental occlusions of the anterior tibial artery (*arrow*) with small bridging collateral arteries. (Reprinted from Cohen E, Doshi A, Lookstein, R. CT angiography of the lower extremity circulation with protocols. In: Mukerjee D, Rajagopalan S, eds. *CT and MRI angiography of the peripheral circulation: practical approach with clinical protocols*. London, UK: Informa Health Care, 2007:139, with permission). (See color insert.)

Computed Tomography Angiography Artifacts and Pitfalls

There are several artifacts that can be seen with CT imaging that one should be aware of to avoid erroneous interpretation. Artifacts could include those that are patient related, procedure related, or reconstruction related. Three of the most common artifacts include motion artifact, beam hardening, and partial volume effects. Motion artifacts can occur due to body motion during scanning or inability to hold breath. Beam hardening artifacts occur due to the passage of photons through structures such as pacemaker leads, metal clips, or calcium resulting in lower energy photons being filtered out. As a consequence dark areas are created next to these structures that can affect assessment of lumen patency. Partial volume effects occur when parts of the voxel representing a structure has other structures with different attenuation properties resulting in averaging of the CT values for that voxel. As a consequence the image appears distorted.

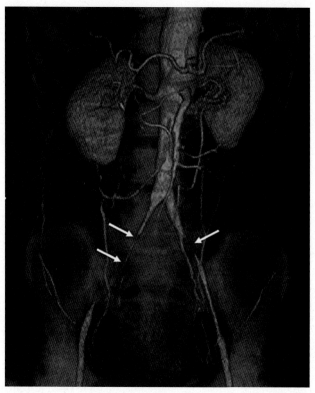

FIGURE 5-11. Volume-rendered image illustrating occlusion of bilateral common iliac arteries (*arrows*) and the proximal portion of the right external iliac artery secondary to giant cell arteritis. (Reprinted from Cohen E, Doshi A, Lookstein R. CT angiography of the lower extremity circulation with protocols. In: Mukerjee D, Rajagopalan S, eds. *CT and MRI angiography of the peripheral circulation: practical approach with clinical protocols*. London, UK: Informa Health Care, 2007:141, with permission). (See color insert.)

The most frequent pitfall encountered during the interpretation of CTA images is represented by the difficulty in the evaluation of vascular segments affected by moderate-to-severe calcification or occupied by a stent. The selection of the adequate windowing set (~1,500 window width) may help in reducing the unavoidable blooming effect produced by structures with high signal attenuation. Cross-sectional MPR images of the vessel of interest are very helpful in visualizing, at least in part, the underlying lumen in the presence of intense calcification or stent. Other interpretation pitfalls such as pseudostenoses or pseudo-occlusions may potentially be generated by inadequate image postprocessing (e.g., partial or total vessel removal during MIP image editing and inaccurate centerline definition in CPR images).

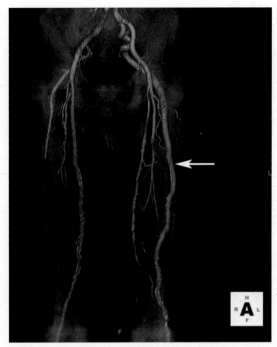

FIGURE 5-12. Persistent sciatic artery. Three-dimensional CTA volume-rendered image (*anteroposterior view*) shows occlusion of the distal left superficial femoral artery. The left popliteal artery is supplied by a persistent left sciatic artery fed by the internal iliac artery (*arrow*). (Reprinted from Cohen E, Doshi A, Lookstein R. CT angiography of the lower extremity circulation with protocols. In: Mukerjee D, Rajagopalan S, eds. *CT and MRI angiography of the peripheral circulation: practical approach with clinical protocols.* London, UK: Informa Health Care, 2007:143, with permission). (See color insert)

SUMMARY

CT technology has continued to evolve and its application for the diagnosis of vascular disease has gained significant momentum. There are multiple publications of clinical studies documenting its accuracy when compared with other modalities. Although the attenuation from severe calcium deposition and stents are potential limitations, the high spatial resolution, ability to use alternate software kernels, and rapid throughput of CTA have enabled its widespread acceptance into evaluation of such patients. CTA is now routinely used in clinical practice and rivals MR angiography for the evaluation of vascular disease.

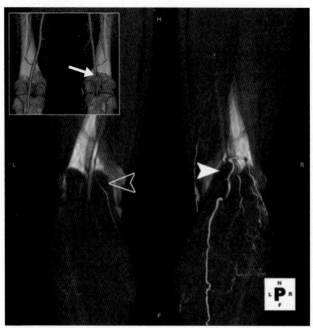

FIGURE 5-13. Popliteal artery entrapment. Three-dimensional CTA volume-rendered image (*posteroanterior view*) of a young patient with right calf pain on exertion. The medial head of the right gastrocnemius muscle demonstrates an abnormal origin lateral to the popliteal artery (*closed arrowhead*). *Inset* image shows complete occlusion of the right popliteal artery (*arrow*) with multiple superficial collateral arteries originating just proximal to this level. The normal origin of the medial head of the left gastrocnemius medial to the popliteal artery (*open arrowhead*) is shown for comparison. (Reprinted from Cohen E, Doshi A. Lookstein R. CT angiography of the lower extremity circulation with protocols. In: Mukherjee D, Rajagopalan S, eds. *CT and MRI angiography of the peripheral circulation: practical approach with clinical protocols.* London, UK: Informa Health Care, 2007:143, with permission). (See color insert.)

Choice of Imaging Modality—Magnetic Resonance Angiography Versus Computed Tomography Angiography

The choice between MRA versus CTA often depends on the disease entity being studied, comorbidities (e.g., renal dysfunction), prior endovascular intervention (e.g., stents), technical expertise available at the institution, patient tolerability, and finally physician familiarity. The image interpretation time required for CTA may be higher than for MRA, largely due to the presence of calcification within the vessels of interest. Calcifications are not a problem in MR, nor are the bony structures. On the other hand, stent artifacts (nonnitinol) continue to create artifacts with MR imaging. Similarly, patients with pacemakers are effectively excluded from having an MRA.

At the present time, the choice of MRA or CTA depend largely on scanner availability, with MR preferred in general, particularly in patients with pre-existing mild to moderate renal insufficiency or iodinated contrast allergy. Recently, the issue of NSF has mandated that Gd be used with caution in patients with advanced renal disease (GFR < 30). In most of these same cases, CTA is also relatively contraindicated, unless the patient is already on dialysis. MRA has an additional advantage in light of newly available non-contrast imaging approaches that may provide the required information.

PRACTICAL POINTS

- Adequate patient preparation and education is a critical step in the acquisition of good quality images.

- Consider the ALARA principle when planning CTA examinations. ECG dose modulation should be used whenever it is deemed appropriate.

- Use thinnest detector collimation to obtain high spatial resolution in the z-direction and approach isotropic resolution whenever possible.

- Vessel dimensions should always be measured wall-to-wall using the MPR mode after ensuring appropriate orientation.

- Multiple artifacts can mimic pulmonary emboli and hence careful scrutiny of the acquired images with active scrolling in and out of each main, lobar, segmental, and subsegmental arteries is necessary to avoid overcalling or missing pulmonary emboli.

- When evaluating a suspected acute aortic syndrome, a precontrast scan may aid in the detection of hemorrhage.

- Gated thoracic aorta should be performed whenever possible in order to avoid artifacts as well to be able to assess the coronary arteries if desired.

- Attenuation characteristics may help differentiate aortic thrombus from intra-mural hematoma.

- Multiple image postprocessing methods should be used to assess the data set as each has its own strengths and pitfalls.

- Vessels that are calcified may be better assessed by CTA in the MPR mode with appropriate windowing and thresholding, and reconstruction with sharper kernels.

- Always review sources images in axial orientation and as MPR images especially when vessels are calcified.

RECOMMENDED READING

Almandoz JED, Romero JM, Pomerantz SR, et al. Computed tomography angiography of the carotid and cerebral circulation. *Radiol Clin North Am* 2010;48(2):265–281.

Berg M, Zhang Z, Ikonen A, et al. Multi-detector row CT angiography in the assessment of carotid artery disease in symptomatic patients: comparison with rotational angiography and digital subtraction angiography. *AJNR* 2005;26(5):1022–1034.

Budovec JJ, Pollema M, Grogan M. Update on multidetector computed tomography angiography of the abdominal aorta. *Radiol Clin North Am* 2010;48(2):283–309.

Cademartiri F, Nieman K. Contrast material injection techniques for CT angiography of the coronary arteries. In: Schoepf UJ, ed. *CT of the heart: principles and applications.* New Jersey: Humana Press, 2005.

Chung JH, Ghoshhajra BB, Rojas CA, et al. CT angiography of the thoracic aorta. *Radiol Clin North Am* 2010;48(2):249–264.

Cody DD. AAPM/RSNA physics tutorial for residents: topics in CT image processing in CT. *Radiographics* 2002;22:1255–1268.

Fleischmann D. CT angiography: injection and acquisition technique. *Radiol Clin North Am* 2010;48(2):237–247.

Fleischmann D, Hallett RL, Rubin GD. CT angiography of peripheral arterial disease. *J Vasc Interv Radiol* 2006;17:3–26.

Flohr TG, Schaller S, Stierstofer K, et al. Multi-detector row CT systems and image-reconstruction techniques. *Radiology* 2005;235:756–773.

Foley WD, Stonely T. CT Angiography of the lower extremities. *Radiol Clin North Am* 2010;48(2):367–396.

Fraioli F, Catalano C, Napoli A, et al. Low-dose multidetector-row CT angiography of the intra-renal aorta and lower extremity vessels: image quality and diagnostic accuracy in comparison with standard DSA. *Eur Radiol* 2006;16:137–146.

Gruden JF. Thoracic CT performance and interpretation in the multi-detector era. *J Thorac Imag* 2005;20(4):253–264.

Horton KM, Fishman EK. CT Angiography of the mesenteric circulation. *Radiol Clin North Am* 2010;48(2):331–345.

Kumamaru K, Hoppel BE, Mather RT, et al. CT angiography: current technology and clinical use. *Radiol Clin North Am* 2010;48(2):213–235.

Kuriakose J, Patel S. Acute pulmonary embolism. *Radiol Clin North Am* 2010;48(2):31–50.

LePage MA, Quint LE, Sonnad SS, et al. Aortic dissection: CT features that distinguish true lumen from false lumen. *Am J Roentgenol* 2001;188:207–211.

Liu PS, Platt JF. CT Angiography of the renal circulation. *Radiol Clin North Am* 2010;48(2): 347–365.

Mukherjee D, Rajagopalan S. *CT and MR angiography of the peripheral circulation: practical approach with clinical protocols.* London, UK: Informa Health Care, 2007.

Patel S, Kazerooni EA. Helica CT for the evaluation of acute pulmonary embolism. *Am J Roentgenol* 2005;185:135–149.

Vasbinder GB, Nelemans PJ, Kessels AG, et al. Accuracy of computer tomographic angiography and magnetic resonance angiography for diagnosing renal artery stenosis. *Ann Intern Med* 2004;141(9):674–682.

Yee J, Galdino G, Urban J, et al. Computed tomographic angiography of endovascular abdominal aortic stent-grafts. *Crit Rev Comput Tomogr* 2004;45(1):17–65.

Yoo SM, Lee HY, White CS. MDCT evaluation of acute aortic syndrome. Current technology and clinical use. *Radiol Clin North Am* 2010;48(2):67–83.

CHAPTER 6

Approach to and Management of Intermittent Claudication
Rekha Durairaj and Sanjay Rajagopalan

INTRODUCTION

Incidence and Prevalence of Peripheral Artery Disease

Lower extremity atherosclerotic peripheral artery disease (PAD) is commonly encountered in clinical practice. Although prevalence figures vary widely, assessment of ankle/brachial systolic pressure index (ABI) indicates that prevalence increases to 20% in individuals greater than 70 years. Of those with PAD, 10% have classic claudication, 50% have atypical leg pain, and the remaining 40% did not have exercise-induced leg pain. The relative risk of PAD in women versus men is 0.7. PAD seems to occur more frequently in Hispanics (relative risk, 1.5) and African Americans (relative risk, 2.5).

Risk Factors for Peripheral Arterial Disease and the Risk Conferred by Peripheral Artery Disease

The risk factors for claudication are the same as those for atherosclerosis as outlined in Figure 6.1. Smoking, male gender, age, diabetes, dyslipidemia in particular ratio of total to high-density lipoprotein (HDL) cholesterol (TC/HDL-C) and low HDL have strong associations with lower extremity atherosclerosis. Given the commonality of risk factors and the systemic nature of atherosclerosis, it is not surprising that patients with PAD have concurrent coronary artery and cerebrovascular disease.

Cardiovascular Risk with PAD

The 10-year risk of death in people diagnosed as having PAD is 40% and has remained largely unchanged since 1950. After multivariate adjustment for age, sex, and other risk factors for cardiovascular disease, patients with PAD had a threefold higher risk of all-cause death and a sixfold higher risk of cardiovascular-related death. Patients with an anklebrachial index (ABI) of less than 0.9 were found to have hazard ratios of 1.7 and 2.5 for all-cause and cardiovascular mortality, respectively. In patients with an ABI greater than 1.4 (indicative of poorly compressible vessels), the hazard ratios was 1.8 and 2.1 for all-cause and cardiovascular mortality, respectively. The REACH registry, an international consortium of practices examined the morbidity/mortality associated with vascular disease. The study involved 55,814 patients, the majority of whom were on evidence-based risk-reduction therapy. The 1-year incidence of cardiovascular death, MI, stroke and hospitalization was highest in patients with established PAD (21%) compared to 15% for CAD patients. The event rates increased with the number of symptomatic arterial disease locations, ranging from 5.3% for patients with risk factors only

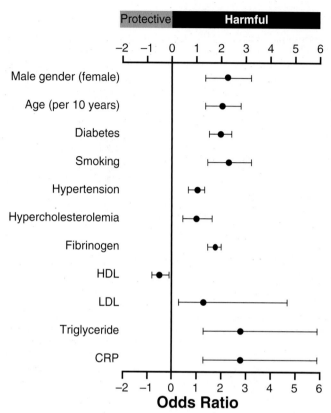

FIGURE 6-1.   Risk factors for the development of peripheral arterial disease and IC. (Adapted from TASC Working Group. *J Vasc Surg* 2000;31(1 Suppl):S1–S296 and Ridker PM, et al. *Circulation* 1998;97:425–428.)

to 13% for patients with one, 21% for patients with two, and 26% for patients with three arterial disease locations.

Progression to Limb Threat and Chronic Critical Limb Ischemia

The vast majority of patients with intermittent claudication (IC) (~70%) do not alter their symptoms. Progression of symptoms occurs in 25% of cases over a 5-year period. The deterioration is most often during the first year after identification of cases (7 to 9%) compared with 2 to 3% per annum thereafter. Major amputation is relatively rare in IC, with 1 to 3% needing major amputation over a 5-year period. A changing ABI is possibly the best individual predictor of deterioration of PAD (e.g., need for arterial surgery or major amputation). In patients with IC in the lowest strata of ankle pressure (i.e., 40 to 60 mm Hg), the risk of progression to severe ischemia or actual limb loss is 8.5% per year.

Impact on Quality of Life

PAD does impact quality of life negatively, especially in patients with CLI. In a number of cases, the patients adapt subconsciously to a new work-routine to avoid provocation of symptoms.

CLINICAL FEATURES

Presenting Features

IC is classically defined as pain in one or both legs that occurs with walking or exertion, does not resolve with continued activity, and abates shortly (within 10 minutes) upon rest or a reduction in walking pace. Symptoms vary depending on the extent and levels of disease involvement but are commonly described as a cramping pain with or without muscle weakness. Recent observational studies demonstrate that greater than 50% of individuals with PAD are asymptomatic or report lower extremity symptoms that are atypical.

Pathophysiology

Regardless of the location of PAD within the lower extremity vasculature, claudication symptoms are most frequently localized to the muscles of the calf. This may be on account of the relatively greater metabolic demand and the common affliction of the superficial femoral artery (SFA) in atherosclerosis. The pathophysiology of IC is multifactorial and includes hemodynamic factors akin to coronary stenosis (e.g., a 70% stenosis may produce no symptoms at rest but may be flow-limiting with exercise). Other factors include deconditioning, metabolic changes including accumulation of acylcarnitines, impaired synthesis of phosphocreatine, and skeletal muscle injury characterized by a distal axonal denervation leading to muscle fiber loss and atrophy of affected muscles.

DIAGNOSIS

History and Physical Examination

Features that should be elicited include (a) the location of the pain or discomfort and duration of the symptoms, (b) the distance before (i) experiencing the discomfort (initial claudication distance) and (ii) being forced to stop (absolute claudication distance), (c) the elapsed time after exercise is stopped before the pain is relieved, and (d) the position of patient (standing at rest, sitting, lying) necessary to relieve the pain. Examination of the entire vascular system (looking for carotid and abdominal bruits) is mandatory with palpation of the radial, carotid, femoral, popliteal, dorsalis pedis, and posterior tibial artery pulses being crucial. In up to 10% of cases, pedal pulses may not be palpable. In such cases, the lateral tibial artery (branch of the peroneal) may be palpated below the ankle medial to the bony prominence of the fibula. Conversely, detection of arterial pulses does not preclude severe ischemia in cases of very distal occlusions, which may occur as part of the cholesterol embolization syndrome or in diabetic patients.

Differential Diagnosis

IC may mimic other conditions and vice versa. Chapter 1 (Table 1.1) lists the most common conditions that may present as hip, calf, or foot claudication. Although PAD is the most common etiology for IC, occasionally other conditions may present with IC (Table 6.1). IC should be distinguished from pseudoclaudication secondary to lumbar spinal canal stenosis. Features that distinguish true claudication from pseudoclaudication include sharp and paresthetic nature of the discomfort, pain with variable walking distance and relief with sitting or leaning forward.

Laboratory Testing in the Claudicant

The following tests should be routinely performed in all patients with claudication: CBC with platelets, fasting blood glucose, HbA1c levels, renal function (creatinine and BUN), fasting lipid profile, urinalysis (for microalbuminuria), and a 12-lead EKG. Concomitant testing (if indicated) for carotid stenosis (duplex exam) and coronary disease (if indicated) may be performed. In the atypical patient (premature disease, personal, or family history of thrombosis), one should consider a comprehensive workup for premature vascular disease including hypercoagulability as outlined in Table 6.2.

Diagnostic Modalities and Approach to Intermittent Claudication

Figure 6.2 provides an initial diagnostic approach toward PAD. An ABI is often the first screening test in suspected PAD. Indices between 0.4 and 0.9 are associated with increasing disease severity. The ABI may be defined as the highest ankle pressure although recent studies suggest that the adoption of the lower of the two ankle pressures may provide for even better prognostic information. Segmental limb pressures, which may be obtained readily in the noninvasive vascular lab, may help localize the disease in the majority of patients with abnormal ABI. Exercise ABIs may be obtained in situations where the diagnosis is uncertain. Imaging with magnetic resonance angiography (MRA) and computed tomographic angiography (CTA) may provide additional information in patients who are candidates for endovascular or surgical revascularization. In addition, these studies may be indicated where the diagnosis is uncertain. A false high normal ABI of greater than 1.3 can be associated with PAD in patients with diabetes mellitus when calcification of the media prevents compression of the artery by the cuff. In this situation, a toe brachial index of less than 0.7 will confirm the presence of PAD.

MANAGEMENT

The goals of treatment and management of patients with IC is to reduce cardiovascular risk, to relieve lower extremity symptoms, and to improve functional walking capacity and quality of life.

Risk Factor Modification

All patients with IC need intensive risk factor modification with careful attention paid to the factors outlined in Table 6.3. Patients with PAD

TABLE 6.1

CAUSES OF IC OTHER THAN ATHEROSCLEROSIS

Diagnosis	Clinical Features
Buerger's disease	Typically presents with ulcers and foot claudication; may progress to involve calf vessels and cause IC.
Hypoplasia and acquired coarctation of the abdominal aorta ("mid-aortic syndrome")	Hypoplastic abdominal aorta is nonhereditary and associated with renal artery involvement. Acquired coarctation may occur with focal atherosclerosis in women 30–60 y in the celiac aorta ("coral reef atherosclerosis"), neurofibromatosis (usually with renal artery involvement), and radiation treatment.
Vasculitis (Takayasu's)	May involve abdominal aorta and iliac branches.
Collagen vascular disease (GCA, SLE), pseudoxanthoma elasticum (PXE)	GCA typically involves subclavian or femoral arteries, bilaterally >50 y, SLE typically involves smaller vessels but can cause IC. PXE may present with IC.
Remote trauma or irradiation injury	Consequence of radiation treatment of abdominal/pelvic cancers with iliofemoral lesions.
Peripheral embolization from proximal aneurysm (popliteal/femoral/abdominal)	Distal embolization may result in foot claudication.
Popliteal etiologies (adventitial cystic disease, entrapment)	*Entrapment*: Young patients; abnormal origin of the medial head of the gastrocnemius muscle usually bilateral but may present unilaterally. *Adventitial cystic disease*: "Ganglion" cyst involving the popliteal artery (popliteal most common artery followed by femoral). Young males afflicted.
Fibrodysplasia (external iliac artery)	Third common vessel involved after renal and carotid.
Persistent sciatic artery (thrombosed)	Rare congenital anomalies where sciatic artery persists as the major inflow artery.
Iliac syndrome of the cyclist	Narrowing of the external iliac artery owing to trauma; unilateral buttock symptoms usually provoked with cycling in professional male cyclists.

cover the gamut of risk with some individuals carrying disproportionate risk compared to others. Appropriate identification of individuals at "high-risk" may be beneficial with the intention of more aggressive targets in such individuals. However, data demonstrating a survival benefit for PAD patients who have received aggressive risk modification are lacking. PAD at "very high risk" may be defined as the involvement of multiple

TABLE 6.2

RECOMMENDED HYPERCOAGULABILITY WORKUP IN INDIVIDUALS WITH PREMATURE PAD AND IC

Test	Condition
Lipid Levels with detailed workup indicated if lipid abnormalities	Hyperlipidemia
Homocysteine levels	Homocystinuria
Plasma fibrinogen	Hyperfibrinogenemia
Antiphospholipid antibodies and Lupus anticoagulant	Antiphospholipid antibody syndrome

Factor V Leiden, Protein C, Protein S, Anti-thrombin III evaluation is not recommended in patients presenting primarily with arterial disease unless there is a predilection to venous thromboembolic disease as well. In general, the association with arterial thrombosis with these disorders is extremely uncommon.

vascular beds (with a direct increase in risk based on the number of vascular beds involved); established PAD plus multiple ongoing major risk factors especially poorly controlled diabetes and smoking; PAD with prior intervention(s), especially surgical revascularization.

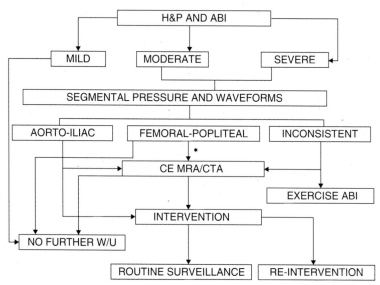

FIGURE 6-2. Diagnostic approach to the patient with IC. *Asterisk* indicates a patient with appropriate revascularizable targets and with disabling IC unresponsive to exercise and pharmacotherapy. (Adapted from Dellegrottaglie, Sans J, Macaluso F et al. Technology insight: Magnetic resonance angiography for the evaluation of patients with peripheral artery disease. *Nat Clin Pract Cardiovasc Med* 2007;4(12):677–687).

TABLE 6.3

RISK FACTOR MODIFICATION IN PERIPHERAL ARTERIAL DISEASE

Risk Factor	Goals	Therapy
Tobacco smoking	Complete cessation	Counseling/drugs
Lipoproteins	LDL-C < 70[a] mg/dL Non–HDL-C < 130 mg/dL	Statin (first line). Ezetimibe or BAR added if LDL not at goal or statin intolerant Niacin 500–2,500 mg/fibric acid/ BAR
Antiplatelet therapy	Recommended in symptomatic PAD especially those with prior CAD and CVD	Aspirin/clopidogrel
Blood pressure	<140/90 mm Hg	ACEI (first line) BB (with CAD)
Diabetes mellitus	HbA1C of ~7.0% to reduce microvascular complications	Avoid hypoglycemia

[a]Preferable as a goal in PAD but suggested in ALL patients with high-risk PAD.
LDL, low density lipoprotein; HDL, high density lipoprotein; BAR, bile acid resin; ACEI, angiotensin converting enzyme inhibitor; BB, beta-blocker; CAD, coronary artery disease; CVD, cerebrovascular disease.

Smoking Cessation

Smoking cessation slows the progression of IC to critical limb ischemia, reduces need for revascularization, improves graft patency, and reduces cardiovascular events. All patients with IC should be referred to a smoking cessation program with use of nicotine replacement therapies (NRTs) and intensive counseling. NRT is dispensed as a gum (2 or 4 mg), nasal spray (0.5 mg/dose), patch (7, 14, and 21 mg), lozenge (2, 4 mg, typically), or inhaler (10 mg/cartridge with 4 mg/ delivered dose). In general, various forms of NRT increase the likelihood of smoking cessation when used alone at least in the short-term. Evidence also indicates that the nicotine patch combined with another NRT is more effective than any single NRT. An advantage of NRT over other pharmacotherapy is their over-the-counter availability and flexible dosing. NRT can also be combined with other pharmacotherapy such as Bupropion. Bupropion is begun at 150 mg q.d. for 3 days, then increasing to b.i.d. for 6 to 10 weeks and longer if needed. Treatment with sustained-release bupropion in combination with NRT may not necessarily result in higher rates of cessation.

Varenicline is a non-nicotinic partial agonist of the $\alpha 4\beta 2$ nicotinic receptors. Varenicline binding to these receptors leads to partial stimulation of receptor-mediated release of dopamine in the reward center in the brain and competitive inhibition of receptor binding by nicotine delivered from cigarettes. Data from three trials suggest that varenicline is more effective than sustained-release bupropion at least at 12 weeks of therapy. The recommended dosage schedule for varenicline is 0.5 mg q.d. for 3 days then twice daily for 4 days, increased to 1 mg twice daily for 7 to 12 weeks. Caution should be exerted with this drug in patients with neuropsychiatric conditions and seizures.

Correction of Hyperlipidemia

Treatment of hyperlipidemia prevents the progression of peripheral vascular atherosclerosis. Lipid lowering therapy may improve claudication distance at least on the basis of small trials. Statins are mandatory in patients with PAD by virtue of their effects in reducing CV events as shown initially in the Heart Protection Study that enrolled 6,748 patients (out of 20,500 patients) with PAD. The target LDL for PAD patients is less than 70 mg/dL. Additional medications (Table 6.3) may be required alone (e.g., individuals intolerant of statins) or in combination therapy to achieve LDL-C goals. Insulin resistance typified by an elevated triglyceride level in the setting of a low HDL-C is common in PAD. A secondary lipid goal in the IC patient is to achieve an appropriate target non–HDL-C level (total cholesterol—HDL-C) of less than 130 mg/dL in such patients. Patients who require the addition of niacin or fibric acid therapy to statins (Table 6.3) to achieve goals should undergo appropriate monitoring of liver function tests. Statins have been shown in small trials to improve claudication symptoms and objective parameters of treadmill walking. Niaspan (sustained release niacin) in conjunction with statin did not, however, appear to improve claudication distance in PAD over a duration of 6 months. The benefit of Niaspan in Type II DM patients and in metabolic syndrome (with Lapropripant) is being tested in AIM-HIGH and HPS-THRIVE studies, respectively.

Hypertension Control

The presence of PAD is evidence of cardiovascular "target organ disease" that should prompt acceleration of the pace of pharmacologic antihypertensive therapy with blood pressure goals of less than 140/90 mm Hg in most patients and perhaps a goal of less than 130/80 mm Hg in the diabetic (although ACCORD-BP questions this goal, the low event rates in these trials and the sample size complicates definitive interpretation). A goal of less than 130/80 may also be reasonable in the CKD patient. The effect of BP control on PAD progression or IC symptoms remains uncertain. The addition of an ACE inhibitor/ARB, especially in the PAD patient with concomitant diabetes, is reasonable. The Heart Outcomes Prevention Evaluation trial showed that ramipril protected against cardiovascular events beyond the extent expected from blood pressure lowering alone. There is also evidence that ACE inhibition may increase pain-free and maximum walking time in patients with symptomatic PAD. The typical PAD patient may require multiple medications and a combination of ACEI with calcium channel blockers may be particularly beneficial in both diabetics and nondiabetics. The use of beta-blocker medications may also be indicated in the PAD patient with concomitant coronary artery disease and/or angina. There is no contraindication to using beta-blockers in these patients.

Glycemic Control

Diabetics with IC have an overall amputation risk of 20% and a 5-year mortality of 50%. These patients have not been formally studied as a group in clinical trials and thus information is based on Type II DM patients. Intensive blood glucose control (HbA1c < 7) while beneficial for microvascular complications, may not provide macrovascular benefits in Type II DM within 5-years. A tighter goal may be reasonable in specific patients who are not on hypoglycemia-inducing drugs, do not have evidence of advanced disease, and are involved in their own care. In most PAD patients, a goal of 7 may be reasonable. Meticulous attention to foot care is necessary to reduce the risk of skin ulceration, necrosis, and subsequent amputation. The role of newer therapies such as GLP-1 analogues and DPP-IV inhibitors needs to be studied.

Antiplatelet Therapy and Anticoagulation for Cardiovascular Risk Reduction

Aspirin should be used in dosages between 81 and 325 mg daily in patients with symptomatic PAD as part of overall cardiovascular prevention. On the basis of data from the Antiplatelet Trialists' meta-analysis, aspirin may also reduce the need for peripheral revascularization and increase graft patency postsurgery. Compared to aspirin treatment, use of clopidogrel (an ADP receptor antagonist) results in a relative risk reduction of 24% for major adverse cardiovascular events compared to ASA alone in a prespecified subgroup of PAD in the CAPRIE trial. The data for antiplatelet therapy in the primary prevention of events in the asymptomatic patient population or in those with Type II diabetes or risk factors alone (absence of PAD) are more controversial. Table 6.4 summarizes the data from trials since 2008 that have attempted to address this question. A key issue with a number of these trials, at least in Type II diabetes and PAD is their small sample size and that a lower dose of ASA was typically used. Ongoing clinical trials, such as A Study of Cardiovascular Events in Diabetes, which involves 10,000 patients with diabetes, and the Aspirin and Simvastatin Combination for Cardiovascular Events Prevention Trial in Diabetes (ACCEPT-D) may have adequate statistical power to detect a significant treatment effect of aspirin beyond contemporary background therapy.

There is no indication to use systemic anticoagulation therapy in patients with PAD without bypass grafts based on the WAVE trial that also showed increased fatal bleeding in this population (Table 6.4).

Antithrombotic/anticoagulation in Peripheral Artery Disease Post Lower Extremity Bypass Grafting

Postoperatively, treatment with aspirin at 325 mg is recommended in all patients to decrease graft occlusion, as well as for its cardio protective effects. A study comparing infrainguinal autologous bypass with and without adjunctive ticlopidine has shown superior graft patency rates in those receiving this antiplatelet agent. In the more recent CASPAR, although there was no benefit of clopidogrel + ASA (75 to 100 mg) in below-knee bypass grafts in the main trial compared to ASA. In a prespecified subgroup of below-knee prosthetic grafts, there was a benefit of dual antiplatelet therapy in patients with prosthetic (HR, 0.65; 95% CI, 0.45–0.95;

TABLE 6.4

SUMMARY OF EVIDENCE FOR ANTIPLATELET AND ANTITHROMBOTIC THERAPY IN PAD. RESULTS FROM TRIALS AND SELECT META-ANALYSIS IN PAD

Author	Trial	Results
POPADAD study	1,276 patients with Type II DM and asymptomatic PAD randomized to ASA (75–100 mg) or placebo	No evidence of benefit from ASA on cardiovascular disease events and mortality. (HR 0.98, 95% CI 0.76–1.26)
AAA trail, Fowkes G et al.	3,350 patients with asymptomatic PAD randomized to ASA 100 mg/d or placebo	Risk of using aspirin for primary prevention outweighed any benefit among participants at high vascular risk (HR 1.03, 95% CI 0.84–1.27)
Ogawa H et al.	2,539 Japanese patients with Type II DM randomized to aspirin(80–100 mg/d) or placebo	ASA did not reduce the risk of cardiovascular events (HR 0.80, 95% CI 0.58–1.10, $P = 0.16$) or mortality (HR 0.90, 95% CI 0.57–1.14, $P = 0.67$)
Berger et al.	Meta-analysis of ASA alone or in combination with dipyridamole among 5,269 patients with PAD enrolled in 18 prospective randomized studies	No benefit of aspirin on CV events (HR 0.88, 95% CI 0.76–1.04). Inadequate evidence to support aspirin prophylaxis in patients with symptomatic PAD who do not have coronary or cerebrovascular events. No benefits established diabetes mellitus
De Berardis G et al.	Meta-analysis of six studies that included 10,117 patients with Type II DM randomized to ASA or placebo	No reduction in major cardiovascular events (RR 0.90, 95% CI 0.81–1.0); cardiovascular mortality (HR 0.94, 95% CI 0.72–1.23)
ANTICOAGULATION AND ANTIPLATELET TRIALS		
Cacoub et al.	Post hoc analysis of 3,096 patients with symptomatic or asymptomatic PAD from CHARISMA	Primary endpoint 7.6% in the clopidogrel plus ASA vs. 8.9% in the placebo plus ASA (HR, 0.85; 95% CI, 0.66–1.08; $P = 0.18$). MI and hospitalization lower in the dual antiplatelet arm than ASA alone. Rate of major bleeds no different in groups with PAD, whereas minor bleeding was increased with clopidogrel
WAVE trial.	ASA/ticlopidine/clopidogrel vs. Vit K antagonist +antiplatelet therapy randomly assigned to 2,161 patients with PAD and carotid artery disease	Combination therapy not more effective than antiplatelet therapy alone in preventing cardiovascular events. Significant increase in major bleeding with combination therapy
CASPAR trial.	Clopidogrel +ASA vs. ASA + Placebo randomly assigned to PAD patients who underwent recent below-knee bypass graft	Primary endpoint (graft occlusion, revascularization, amputation, or death); no difference in groups(HR 0.98, 95% CI 0.78–1.23). Clopidogrel plus ASA conferred benefit in patients receiving prosthetic grafts without increase in bleeding

TABLE 6.5

RECOMMENDATIONS FOR EXERCISE THERAPY IN IC

Type of exercise
    Treadmill and track walking is the most effective form for IC
    Should incorporate warm up and cool down periods
Initiation of exercise program
    Should be supervised
    Initial Gardner protocol determines intensity that brings on moderate claudication
        (3–4 on a 5 scale)
    Patient walks to this workload and then rests until claudication subsides
    The initial session should include 35 min of intermittent walking
Maintenance
    Goal should be to increase the duration of walking by 5 min every visit
    Increases in grade if patient can walk 10 min at the lower work load
    Additional goal is to increase the walking speed to 3.0 mph from the average 1.5 mph
        in the PAD patient
    The exercise regimen should be at a frequency of three to five times a week

$P = 0.025$), but not venous, grafts. It may be beneficial to anticoagulate patients with a vitamin K antagonist, such as warfarin, in high-risk grafts prone to thrombosis, such as those with grafts to below the knee locations, at least for the first 3 months following bypass with continued therapy mandated by the presence of other risk factors for continuing thrombosis. In the BOA trial, however, there was no benefit of oral anticoagulation in infrainguinal grafts with a particular lack of benefit in prosthetic grafts (also see section on anticoagulation in Chapter 7).

Nonpharmacologic Therapy for Intermittent Claudication

Exercise Rehabilitation

Exercise has been shown to improve symptoms, functional capacity, and quality of life for PAD patients. Pooled analysis from multiple studies suggests a significant beneficial effect of exercise on pain-free (139 m increase) and total walking (179 m increase) distance. Data from individual studies support the efficacy of scheduled, supervised exercise programs over home-based programs. The biologic mechanisms mediating the improved walking distance and reduction of symptoms of IC by exercise training remain unclear but potential pathways include increased leg muscle oxygen utilization and metabolism, improved collateral blood flow, decreased blood viscosity, enhanced walking efficiency, and an increased pain threshold. Table 6.5 provides key elements of an exercise prescription.

Weight reduction: Patients who are overweight (BMI 25 to 30) or obese (BMI 30) should receive counseling on how to achieve weight reduction.

TABLE 6.6

PHARMACOLOGIC TREATMENT OF IC

Drug	Dose	Mechanism of Action	Side Effects	Interactions
Cilostazol	50–100 mg b.i.d.	Inhibition of phosphodi-esterase III	Headache, diarrhea, flatulence, palpitations, and dizziness	Drugs that inhibit CYPA4 or CYP2C19 including macrolide antibiotics, ketoconazole, grapefruit juice, and omeprazole, respectively
Pentoxifylline	400 mg t.i.d.		Nausea, bloating, and dizziness	Theophylline (increases levels)
Beraprost	40 μg t.i.d.	Oral prosta-glandin I2 analogue	Headache, flushing	—

Pharmacologic Therapy for Intermittent Claudication

Several medications can be prescribed for symptomatic relief and/or to improve functional capacity (Table 6.6).

Cilostazol

Cilostazol is a Type III phosphodiesterase inhibitor that increases intracellular cAMP levels. Other mechanisms include release of prostaglandin I_2, inhibition of platelets and vascular smooth muscle proliferation, and modest improvements in serum lipoproteins (10% decrease in triglycerides and 4% increase in HDL). Cilostazol (100 mg b.i.d.) results in a 129 m increase in maximal walking distance at 6 months following initiation of treatment. Cilostazol is contraindicated for patients with congestive heart failure of any severity or an ejection fraction of less than 40%. Side effects include headache (most common), diarrhea, abnormal stools, and palpitations. The inhibition of vascular smooth muscle proliferation is clinically significant. In a small multicenter open label trial performed in Japan, the rate of restenosis and freedom from target lesion revascularization favored cilostazol-treated patients undergoing femoropopliteal intervention.

Naftidrofuryl

This is a 5-hydroxytryptamine type 2 antagonist and has been available for treating claudication in several European countries. It may improve muscle metabolism, as well as reduce erythrocyte and platelet aggregation. Naftidrofuryl at 600 mg/d improves pain-free walking distance (26% vs. placebo) and quality of life. Side effects include mild gastrointestinal discomfort. This is not available in the US or Canada.

Pentoxifylline

Pentoxifylline provides marginal benefits on walking ability and symptom relief and should not be used.

Endovascular Treatment of Intermittent Claudication

Endovascular procedures are indicated for individuals with a vocational or lifestyle-limiting disability due to IC when clinical features suggest a reasonable likelihood of symptomatic improvement with endovascular intervention and (a) there has been an inadequate response to exercise or pharmacological therapy and/or (b) there is a favorable risk-benefit ratio. The TASC (Transatlantic Inter-Society Consensus) classification is helpful in guiding therapy and is outlined in Table 6.7 and Figure 6.3.

Periprocedural Antithrombotic Use

There are no controlled data to define optimal antithrombotic management in patients who have undergone lower extremity intervention. All patients should receive aspirin 81 to 325 mg orally prior to the procedure. A common practice is to front-load patients undergoing interventions with 300 to 600 mg of clopidogrel at least 12 hours prior to the procedure. The role of newer P2Y12 inhibitors, that is, prasugrel and ticagrelor has not been studied in this setting. Adjunctive glycoprotein IIb/IIIa inhibitors have limited or no role in lower extremity interventions. Unfractionated heparin 50 to 70 U/kg to achieve an ACT 200 to 250 seconds is the anticoagulant most commonly used but bivalirudin has also been used successfully.

Factors that Determine Patency

Anatomic factors that affect the patency include severity of disease in run-off arteries and the TASC class (length of the stenosis/occlusion and the number of lesions treated). Clinical variables impacting the outcome include diabetes, renal failure, and smoking.

Percutaneous Treatment of Aortoiliac Disease

Revascularization of aortoiliac occlusive disease has shifted from a predominantly surgical to an endovascular-based therapeutic approach. The basis for this change is the less invasive nature of PTA/stenting and its durable clinical success, in both immediate and long-term patency of the stented vessel. Endovascular therapy currently has been established as the treatment of choice for localized aortoiliac occlusive disease (TASC-A and B). With evolution of endovascular techniques and widespread availability of re-entry devices, many class D lesions are now amenable to an endovascular approach. Surgical patency rates for standard aortobifemoral bypass (AFB) grafting at 5-years remain superior to percutaneous therapy (see below, Table 6.8).

Aortic Bifurcation Disease. Based on current evidence, endovascular procedures are favored over surgical revascularization in TASC class

TABLE 6.7

TASC II CLASSIFICATION OF AORTOILIAC AND FEMORAL–POPLITEAL LESIONS FOR GUIDING INTERVENTIONAL THERAPY

	Iliac Disease	Femoral Lesions
TASC A	1. Unilateral or bilateral stenoses of CIA 2. Unilateral or bilateral single short (≤3cm) stenosis of EIA	1. Single stenosis ≤ 10 cm 2. Single occlusion ≤ 5 cm
TASC B	1. Short (≤ 3 cm) stenosis of infrarenal aorta 2. Single or multiple stenosis totaling 3–10 cm involving the EIA not extending into the CFA 3. Unilateral CIA occlusion 4. Unilateral EIA occlusion not involving the origins of internal iliac or CFA	1. Multiple lesions (stenoses or occlusions), each ≤5 cm 2. Single stenoses or occlusions ≤ 15 cm not involving the infrageniculate popliteal artery 3. Single or multiple lesions in the absence of continuous tibial vessels to improve inflow for a distal bypass 4. Heavily calcified occlusion ≤ 5 cm 5. Single popliteal stenosis
TASC C	1. Bilateral CIA occlusions 2. Bilateral EIA stenoses 3–10 cm long not extending into the CFA 3. Unilateral EIA stenosis extending into CFA 4. Unilateral EIA occlusion that involves the origins of internal iliac and/or CFA 5. Heavily calcified unilateral EIA occlusion with or without involvement of origins of internal iliac and/or CFA	1. Multiple stenoses or occlusions totaling > 15 cm with or without heavy calcification 2. Recurrent stenoses or occlusions that need treatment after two endovascular interventions
TASC D	1. Diffuse, multiple stenoses involving the unilateral CIA, EIA, and CFA 2. Unilateral occlusion involving both the CIA and EIA 3. Bilateral EIA occlusions 4. Diffuse disease involving the aorta and both iliac arteries requiring treatment 5. Infrarenal aortoiliac occlusion 6. Iliac stenoses in patients with AAA requiring treatment and not amenable to endograft placement or other lesions requiring open aortic or iliac surgery	1. Chronic total occlusions of CFA or SFA(>20 cm, involving the popliteal artery) 2. Chronic total occlusion of popliteal artery and proximal trifurcation vessels

Endovascular procedure is the treatment of choice for type A, and surgery the procedure of choice for type D. At present, endovascular treatment is more commonly used in type B lesions, and surgical treatment is more commonly used in type C lesions. There is insufficient evidence to make firm recommendations, particularly in the case of types B and C. (Adapted from Norgren L, Hiatt WR, Dormandy JA, et al. Inter-Society Consensus for the Management of Peripheral Arterial Disease (TASC II). *J Vasc Surg* 2007;45[Suppl S]:S5–S67.)

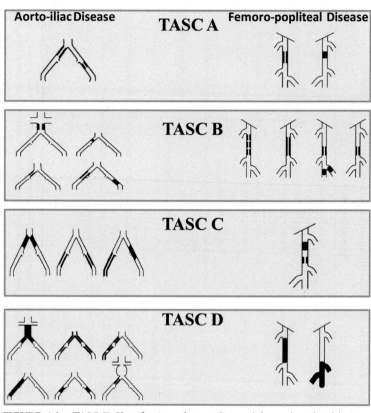

FIGURE 6-3. TASC II Classification of aorto-iliac and femoral-popliteal lesions. (Adapted from Norgren L, Hiatt WR, Dormandy JA, et al. Inter-Society Consensus for the Management of Peripheral Arterial Disease (TASC II). *J Vasc Surg* 2007;45(Suppl S):S5–S67).

A and B lesions and perhaps now for class C lesions, while patients with class TASC D are generally considered surgical candidates. However, selective TASC D lesions may also be considered for an endovascular approach. Excellent results are seen even with PTA alone in TASC A and B lesions with or without stenting with 5-year patency rates that exceed 80%. The "kissing" technique, involves simultaneous deployment of two balloon-expandable stents across the origins of both iliac arteries to reconstruct the aortic bifurcation.

Iliac Disease. Iliac arteries are ideally suited for endovascular intervention with current guidelines recommending primary stent placement. When long-term outcomes are combined from recent trials in patients with iliac stents, the acute procedural success rate exceeds 90%. Risks with percutaneous therapy are generally minor and include access complications

TABLE 6.8

SUMMARY OF DATA OBTAINED FROM A DECADE OF ENDOVASCULAR STUDIES IN AORTO-ILIAC DISEASE

First Author	Year	N	eAIOD	1 year		3 year		5 year	
				PP	SP	PP	SP	PP	SP
Nyman	2000	30	21						
Scheinert	2000	212	212[a]	97	100[b]				
Ali	2001	22	22	84	88	78	86	66	80
Greiner	2003	25	23						
Rzucidlo	2003	34	29		91[b]				
Domanin	2003	42	28	70	88				
Lagana	2005	19	11	70	88				
Ballzer	2006	89	89	89	100				
De Roeck	2006	38	26			90	96		
Park	2006	218	66	94	100	89	94	77	94
Piffaretti	2007	43	43	C 94	C 97	C 94	C 97	C 78	C 74
				D 93	D 94	D 74	D 85	D 74	D 85
Bjorses	2008	173	88	97	100	83	95	65	83
Chang	2008	171	171					60	98
Gandini	2008	138	138	95	97	91	94	86	90
Hans	2008	40	40			69[d]	89[d]		
Sixt	2008	375	179	C 86	C 98				
				D 85	D 98				
Sharafuddin	2008	66	47			81[d]	94[d]		
Kashyap	2008	83	65	90	97	74	95		
Moise	2009	31	31	85	100	66	90		
Average				**87%**	**95%**	**82%**	**93%**	**71%**	**89%**

Primary and secondary patency rates for extensive aorto-iliac disease are reported.
[a]Primary assisted patency.
[b]Limb salvage rate.
[d]Four-year patency rates.
C, Results for patients with TASC type C lesions; D, results for patients with TASC type D lesions; PP, primary patency; SP, secondary patency.
(Adapted from Jongkind V, Akkersdijk GJ, Yeung KK, et al. A systematic review of endovascular treatment of extensive aortoiliac occlusive disease. *J Vasc Surg* 2010;52(5):1376–1383).

and rarely, lower extremity embolization (it seems like the list of potential complications should be expanded, especially since surgical complications occupy at least a few pages below. Bottom line: endovascular therapy is safe but not entirely without risk). The 3-year primary patency rates range from 74 to 87% and secondary patency rates from 84 to 95%. The 5-year primary patency rates exceed 75%, while secondary patency rates are >85%. Thus, patency rates of primary stenting compare favorably to surgical patency rates, while carrying a lower risk of mortality and morbidity. The overall complication rates are usually access site-related and minor, and the mortality rate is less than 0.5% at 30 days.

Percutaneous Treatment of Femoropopliteal Disease

The femoropopliteal segment remains the most challenging area with respect to recurrence of disease after endovascular treatment. The SFA is the longest artery in the human body and is fixed between two major flexion points, the hip and the knee. During movements, tremendous mechanical forces are exerted on this vessel, particularly at the adductor canal. In contrast to the iliac arteries, the SFA is a muscular artery and thus has a more robust restenotic response to injury. Traditionally, balloon angioplasty alone was advocated as the treatment of choice for the femoropopliteal segments. Primary success rates were good but results at 1 year were disappointing, with restenosis rates of 40 to 75% (Table 6.8). Particularly poor results were encountered after PTA of extensive SFA disease with failure rates greater than 70% at 1 year after angioplasty of lesions longer than 10 cm. Endovascular stents (self-expanding) in the femoropopliteal segment resolved the problems of early elastic recoil, residual stenosis and flow-limiting dissections after balloon angioplasty and enabled treatment of longer and more complex lesions even in heavily calcified arteries. The current indications for percutaneous therapy include those with disabling IC or RP who have failed medical therapy. A percutaneous approach may be considered in patients with TASC A, most type B lesions and select TASC C lesions, provided that the approach preserves potential future landing zones for a bypass graft. Bypass grafting must still be considered the most durable revascularization technique for patients with chronic limb ischemia and extensive disease in the SFA (TASC D).

Femoro-popliteal PTA. This may still be considered in individuals with disabling claudication refractory to other therapy with short TASC A lesions in the common femoral, SFA, or popliteal artery. Selected patients with TASC B may also be candidates for an initial approach with PTA. There is general agreement that if PTA fails in the SFA, provisional stent placement is indicated.

Stenting for Femoropopliteal Lesions. Stenting for SFA disease has evolved from not being recommended in TASC-I guidelines to being a definite consideration in patients with femoropopliteal disease. The indications for primary stenting for above-knee femoropopliteal disease continue to expand with contemporary trials suggesting a benefit with such an approach in carefully selected patients including as provisional therapy in cases of residual stenosis greater than 30%, flow-limiting dissection, thrombus/poor flow after angioplasty. There are several randomized controlled trials comparing self-expanding nitinol stents with PTA alone for femoropopliteal disease that are listed in Table 6.9. There is still a residual concern with fracture rates in some of these studies owing to mechanical forces acting on the stent, although the rates are lower in current generation of stents. The

TABLE 6.9

RESULTS OF CONTEMPORARY TRIALS IN FEMOROPOPLITEAL DISEASE

	Characteristics of Patients in Trial	Restenosis at 12 mo[a]	Other Results
Vienna ABSOLUTE Trial	Severe IC/CLI due to AK-FP disease to primary self-expanding nitinol stents ($n = 55$) or BA ($n = 55$) with optional stenting (residual stenosis, early recoil, or dissection). Mean lesion length 13 cm in stent and BA groups	37 and 63.5% ($P < 0.01$) by ultrasound in stent and PTA groups. Results significant at 24 mo follow-up	24 and 43% ($P > 0.05$) at 6 mo by angiography (primary-endpoint)
FAST trial	Severe IC/CLI due to AK-FP randomized to BA ($n = 121$) vs. self-expanding nitinol stent ($n = 123$); Mean lesion length was 45 mm in both groups	Restenosis rates 32% vs. 39% in the stent vs. BA ($p = $ NS)	Small sample size with trends favoring restenosis in all subgroups
RESILIENT Trial	Severe IC/CLI secondary to AK-FP; 2:1 randomization to self-expanding nitinol stent ($n = 134$) vs. BA ($n = 72$). Mean lesion length 6.5 cm	12 mo, freedom from TVR was 87% in stent group vs. 45% for PTA group ($P < 0.0001$). Duplex derived primary patency at 12 mo was 81% vs. 37% in stent and PTA groups; $P < 0.0001$	High-cross-over rate of 40% in the BA group to stenting arm. Fractures in 3.1% of stents. No fractures resulted in loss of patency or TVR.
ASTRON Trial	73 patients with AK-FP randomized to self-expanding nitinol stenting ($n = 34$) or BA with optional stenting ($n = 39$); mean lesion length 8.4 cm	Restenosis rate 34 vs. 61% with BA	
Drug eluting stents or drug-coated balloons			
SIROCCO 1 Trial	36 patients severe AK-FP disease randomized to sirolimus-eluting self-expanding stents or uncoated self-expanding stents. Mean lesion length of 8.6 cm	6-mo restenosis of 23% in sirolimus-eluting stent vs. 31% in uncoated stent ($P = 0.3$)	Fractures in 31%; all fractures occurred in three overlapping stents

(Continued)

TABLE 6.9

RESULTS OF CONTEMPORARY TRIALS IN FEMOROPOPLITEAL DISEASE (Continued)

	Characteristics of Patients in Trial	Restenosis at 12 mo[a]	Other Results
SIROCCO 2 Trial	57 patients with SFA lesions limited to 7–15 cm stenosis or 4–15-cm occlusion	6-mo restenosis of 3.8% in sirolimus-eluting stent vs. 0% in uncoated. 24-mo restenosis of 22.9 and 21.1%, respectively	4 stent fractures (2 in each arm)
THUNDER Trial	Severe AK-FP disease (n = 154) randomized to PTA with paclitaxel coated balloons, PTA with paclitaxel dissolved in contrast or uncoated balloons (control); the mean lesion length was 7.4 ± 6.5 cm	6-mo re-stenosis of 17% in paclitaxel coated balloons vs. and 54% in uncoated balloons with paclitaxel in contrast and 44% in uncoated balloons (P = 0.01 for paclitaxel balloon vs. control)	Rate of TVR at 6-mo 4% in paclitaxel-coated balloons (P < 0.001) 29% in paclitaxel contrast medium and 37% in uncoated balloon Rates of TVR lower at 12 mo and 24 mo
ZILVER Trial (TCT 2010)	Severe AK-FP disease (n = 479): Polymer-free paclitaxel coated self-expanding stents, n = 241; PTA, n = 238). In PTA, group 50% had suboptimal angioplasty and underwent secondary randomization to stenting with paclitaxel coated (n = 61) or BMS (n = 59)	12-mo patency 83% with paclitaxel stent and 67% with angioplasty with BMS. In the provisional stenting group patency was 90% with the paclitaxel coated and 73% with BMS	Fracture rate of 0.9% at 12 mo. Clinically significant reduction of major adverse events (death, amputation, TVR, or worsening Rutherford score in paclitaxel group vs. PTA group

STRIDES Dynalink-E, Everolimus Eluting Peripheral Stent System	Severe FP disease (78% TASC C), 17% with CLI	A retrospective comparison to the historical VIENNA. Absolute trial suggested improved patency rate of DYNALINK-E vs. bare metal at 6 mo. However, the improved patency rate was not sustained at 12 mo	
PaRADISE Preventing leg amputation in critical limb ischemia with below the knee drug eluting stents	Critical limb ischemia	The efficacy and safety of coronary drug eluting stents (83% Cypher, 17% Taxus) when deployed in the infrapopliteal vessels to prevent amputation was evaluated	The 3-y cumulative rate of amputation was 6% ± 2 and the restenosis rate was low at 12%

(Schilling M, et al. Balloon angioplasty versus implantation of nitinol stents in the SFA. N Engl J Med 2006;354:1879 and Circulation 2007;15:2745–2749; Krankenberg H, et al. Nitinol stent implantation versus percutaneous transluminal angioplasty in SFA lesions up to 10 cm in length: the femoral artery stenting trial (FAST). Circulation 2007;116:285–292; Duda SH, et al. Sirolimus eluting versus bare nitinol stent for obstructive SFA disease: the SIROCCO II trial. J Vasc Interv Radiol 2005;16:331–338; Tepe G, et al. Local delivery of paclitaxel to inhibit restenosis during angioplasty of the leg. N Engl J Med 2008;358:689–699; ASTRON (Balloon Angioplasty vs. Primary Stenting of Femoropopliteal Arteries Using Self-Expandable Nitinol Stents). Unpublished observations; Laird JR, Katzen BT, et al. Nitinol stent implantation versus balloon angioplasty for lesions in the superficial femoral artery and proximal popliteal artery: twelve-month results from the RESILIENT randomized trial. Circ Cardiovasc Interv 2010;3(3):267–276; ZILVER Trial Results presented at the Transcatheter Cardiovascular Therapeutics (TCT) 2010 scientific symposium in Washington, DC. STRIDES Trial Results presented at the CIRSE 2009, September 19–23, Lisbon, Portugal; Feiring, AJ, Krahn M, Nelson L, et al. Preventing leg amputations in critical limb ischemia with below-the-knee drug-eluting stents: the PaRADISE (PReventing Amputations using Drug eluting StEnts) trial. J Am Coll Cardiol 2010;55:1580–1589).

results from contemporary trials suggest improving short-term (6 months) and intermediate restenosis rates (12 or 24 months) with reduction in target vessel revascularization. It must be kept in mind that short-term success rates as evidenced by improvement in binary restenosis rates at 6 months is not an adequate measures of success. At the very least, 12-month or even 24-month patency rates should also be reported.

Drug-eluting Stents in Femoropopliteal Lesions. Early studies with drug-coated (Sirolimus) nonexpanding stents have noted very good early success (6 months) with waning success at intermediate time points resulting in no differences over nondrug eluting nitinol stents. Stent/strut fractures were also a concern in SIROCCO-1 and were reported in greater than 30% in this trial with these events occurring exclusively in patients receiving multiple stents (≥3 stents with mean stent length of 8.5 cm). There were no clinically significant events reported for any of these patients. Lesion length is however only one factor in stent fracture, with stent design perhaps being a more important variable. In keeping with this newer generation of stents have seen fewer rates of failure even on longer term follow-up (Table 6.9).

Restenosis in Stented Femoropopliteal Disease. The wide-spread use of stents in the femoropopliteal region has seen an increase in restenotic lesions with recurrence of symptoms. Recurrent restenosis after balloon angioplasty of a nitinol stent ISR occurs in up to 60% within only 6 months after retreatment. Treatment of restenoses with balloon angioplasty alone has a high rate of recurrent failure. The optimal treatment approach remains to be determined. Alternative technologies, such as cutting balloon angioplasty and cryoplasty, have not proven effective. Close follow-up with early intervention are important especially in patients who undergo stenting over long segments. In such patients it may be far easier to intervene on a focal restenotic lesion even on a relatively asymptomatic individual rather than having to intervene on extensive thrombosis. This is however entirely untested.

Infrapopliteal Interventions. There is a limited role for primary infrapopliteal PTA in patients with IC. Medical therapy for IC patients is appropriate. However, for patients with severe claudication, PTA may be considered. Endovascular intervention may be useful either as adjunctive therapy in patients undergoing bypass surgery or PTA directed at inflow vessels, in an attempt to improve the outflow. Encouraging preliminary results using combined PTA and surgery have been reported.

Surgical Revascularization Approaches in Intermittent Claudication

General Principles

Firm indications for surgical revascularization in IC is relief of symptoms that are disabling and significantly interfere with quality of life and vasculogenic impotence. The following are general caveats to be considered in the decision-making process: (a) long-term patency rates for aortoiliac

> femoropopliteal reconstructions > infrapopliteal bypass procedures; (b) surgery for infrainguinal disease in IC should be resorted to only if all other options have been exhausted; (c) autologous conduits (saphenous vein segments) are strongly preferred for below-knee procedures, while prosthetic materials are fully acceptable alternatives for above-knee bypasses if vein grafts are not available; and (d) establishing good inflow to the affected area by proximal revascularization is critical for achieving optimal results in distal procedures.

Surgical Bypass for Aortoiliac Disease

Results for surgical bypass for aortoiliac disease are excellent with operative mortality rates of less than 3% and long-term patency rates of greater than 90% at 5 and greater than 70% at 10 years for both aortofemoral bypass and aortic endarterectomy.

Aortobifemoral Bypass. The AFB is considered the reference standard for treatment of aortoiliac disease as it consistently offers the most reliable results (Fig. 6.4). The prosthetic material used most commonly is polytetrafluoroethylene (PTFE). Limb-based patency rates in this analysis are 91 and 87% at 5 and 10 years, respectively.

Choice of Graft. Prosthetic grafts for inflow disease are constructed from polyester (Dacron) or PTFE. Numerous modifications depending on the method of fabrication (knitted vs. woven, external velour vs. double velour) and addition of various biologic coatings (collagen or albumin) have been devised. Currently "zero porosity" biologically coated grafts dominate the market because of their ease of use (no need to preclot) and probably lower

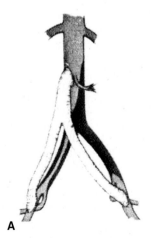
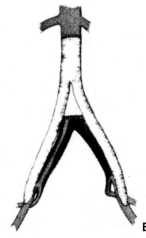

FIGURE 6-4. Illustration of end-to-side aorto-femoral bypass graft (**A**) and end-to-end aorto-femoral bypass graft (**B**).

associated blood loss. At present, there is no hard evidence to favor use of one material over the other, and the single most important predictor of success is operative technique and the choice of the correct size prosthesis (i.e., avoidance of graft-outflow vessel mismatch). A 16×8 mm bifurcated graft is most often employed. The size may be reduced to 14×7 mm in the female patient. The limb length is adjusted to match the femoral arteries or those of the SFA.

Anastomotic Considerations. Patency rates do not seem to differ with an end-to-side versus an end-to-end anastomosis (Fig. 6.4). However, anatomic considerations may often influence the type of anastomosis (preservation of blood flow to the internal iliac and hypogastric arteries). The avoidance of the hypogastric plexus minimizes the risk of sexual dysfunction. The following reasons are often propounded as advantages of the end-end anastomosis: (a) aortic blood flow is directed to the graft directly without the native aorta competing for blood flow, (b) a portion of the infrarenal aorta is resected with this procedure and therefore the anastomosis origin is higher from a less diseased portion of aorta, (c) the end-side graft protrudes more anteriorly than the end-end anastomosis and has therefore been thought to be less frequently associated with tendency to adhere to bowel and cause an aorticenteric fistula, and (d) application of partially occluding tangential clamps required for the creation of the end-side anastomosis theoretically carries a risk of dislodgement of clot to the pelvic and lower extremity circulation. The end-side technique is favored under the following circumstances: (a) when performance of the end-end anastomosis will jeopardize other circulatory beds (renals, mesenteric, or pelvic circulation), (b) patent and enlarged IMA or accessory renal arteries arising from the distal aorta, (c) occlusive disease confined mostly to the external iliac with the common iliac and internal iliac mostly preserved (most common indication for end-side) where in retrograde flow through the external iliac cannot be expected to perfuse the hypogastric arterial plexus and will result in a high percentage of sexual dysfunction, and (d) collaterals originating from the distal aorta and supplying the pelvis that may be compromised by an end-end anastomosis and increase the risk of postoperative colon ischemia, spinal ischemia, and hip claudication on recovery.

There are five types of distal anastomosis (Fig. 6.5): (a) type 1 (to the CFA) is preferred in those with widely open profunda femoris artery (PFA) and SFA; (b) type 2 extends the hood of the graft to the proximal SFA, is recommended in those with stenosis involving the origin of the SFA, but the distal SFA and PFA are patent; (c) type 3 extends the hood to the PFA (provided the caliber of the PFA is at least greater than 3 mm and the length is at least 15 to 20 cm); (d) type 4 extends the graft to the PFA alone and is done when the SFA and the CFA are extensively obliterated; and (e) type 5; the hood of the graft is split to patch proximal stenosis involving the SFA and PFA.

Postoperative Complications

Early Complications. These include *Bleeding*: Major bleeding from an arterial graft anastomosis is usually manifested as hypotension and shock with intra-abdominal anastomotic sites and with a groin hematoma with

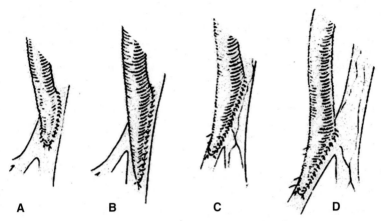

FIGURE 6-5.   Types of distal anastomosis (aorto-femoral grafts).

femoral or popliteal anastomosis. Prompt recognition and early reoperation is required. The most common acquired coagulation deficiency leading to oozing or serious bleeding is dilution of coagulation factors with transfusion of avascular fluids and banked bloods. This is reversed by fresh frozen plasma. *Limb ischemia*: This could result either from thrombosis of the graft or from distal embolization. These cases are recognized by the loss of previously detected pulses, signs of acute limb ischemia, or the failure of expected pulses to appear after surgery. The patient should be promptly returned to the operating room, for assessment of the cause. Thromboembolic complications of the graft or the larger outflow vessels may be generally treated with embolectomy catheters. However, more distally lodged debris (in the pedal and digital arteries) may require administration of heparin or intra-arterially administered thrombolytics. *Renal failure*: Renal failure in the absence of preoperative renal dysfunction is unusual with elective surgery. The low rates in contemporary surgery, reflect due diligence in the avoidance of hypotension through maintenance of adequate intravascular volume and avoidance of declamping hypotension. Intraoperative embolization of atheromatous debris may occur during aortic clamping in patients with juxta or pararenal atherosclerotic plaque. In such cases, aortic clamping at a suitable distance, (e.g., supraceliac), with some duration of renal and mesenteric ischemia, may be preferable to embolization with a clamp below the level of the renal arteries. *Colonic ischemia*: This most commonly involves the rectosigmoid and is more common after surgery for aneurysms than for occlusive disease. The etiology is most often secondary to interruption of primary or collateral flow to the bowel in combination with atheromatous embolization and/or perioperative hypotension. Recognition of predisposing circumstances is crucial to its avoidance. These includes the presence of significant disease involving the celiac and the superior mesenteric vessels and a patent and enlarged IMA, sacrifice of which by an end-end anastomosis, would lead to colonic ischemia. Arterial reconstruction with either reimplantation of the IMA or concomitant bypass to the SMA and/or celiac may be required. The postoperative manifestations of colonic ischemia include (a) liquid brown diarrhea or hematochezia, (b) abdominal distension, and (c) signs of peritonitis and unexplained metabolic acidosis. Mild cases may merely require supportive care. More severe cases may require resection of bowel.

Late Complications.
Anastomotic pseudoaneurysm. This may occur in 2 to 5% of patients and most commonly involves the femoral anastomotic site, where it may present as a pulsatile mass. Retroperitoneal aortic or iliac anastomotic aneurysms are asymptomatic and may present with acute rupture or erosion in to a hollow viscus. A CT scan or duplex scan to assess graft size is therefore mandatory in the late follow-up of these patients. Aneurysms that are asymptomatic and less than 2.5 cm may be serially followed.

Sexual dysfunction. Approximately 25% of individuals who undergo proximal aortic reconstructive surgery may experience sexual dysfunction, which may manifest as impotence or lack of ejaculation after normal coitus. It is important to document sexual function preoperatively. Paying meticulous attention to the following caveats may minimize the risk for sexual dysfunction: (a) Minimal dissection at the area of the bifurcation of the aorta and avoidance of the nerve fibers along the left lateral wall of the aorta. (b) Preservation of hypogastric artery flow. *Infection*: The incidence of this complication is less than 1% in most modern series. The most common site is the inguinal portion of an aortofemoral graft. Staphylococcus remains the commonest pathogen. The treatment comprises removal of the infected graft.

Surgical Treatment of Infrainguinal Disease

Infrainguinal disease even if extensive, very rarely justifies surgical intervention for IC. If the disease is strictly localized to the superficial femoral arteries, is associated with disabling claudication and is nonamenable to percutaneous intervention, bypass may be justified in select patients.

Femoropopliteal Bypass Grafting. In view of the comparative long-term patency rates for prosthetic grafts with saphenous veins in the above-knee position, most surgeons would advocate synthetic material for the above-knee position. Five-year patency rates for above-knee anastamosis range from 60 to 75% for vein and are lower for prosthetic grafts. For bypass grafting to below-knee locations, a saphenous graft is advocated. A variety of other procedures (e.g., femoro-femoral or extra-anatomic axillofemoral bypass) are undertaken when necessitated by unfavorable anatomy or concomitant disease.

Complications of Infrainguinal Bypass. Perioperative morbidity ranges from 1 to 5% most often secondary to concomitant CAD. Local complications include bleeding, infection, graft thrombosis, lymphatic leaks, wound infection, and delayed healing. Early graft thrombosis may occur secondary to poor outflow and small caliber vein, technical defects (kinks, intimal flaps, injury by valvotome) and idiopathic thrombosis. Hypercoaguable states such as HIT, antiphospholipid syndrome, protein C and protein S deficiency may be potential etiologies and should be investigated. Wound infection is aggravated by persistent lymph leaks (lymphocele/lymphorrhea) at the groin site, owing to inadvertent transection of lymphatics. Most lymph leaks respond to immobility, leg elevation, and local care; some require re-exploration and ligation of lymph channels.

Extra-anatomic Bypass Grafting in Intermittent Claudication. In general, these techniques are reserved for the patient with limb threat and ought to be employed in IC only when all percutaneous options have been exhausted. The indications for these operations are diminishing.

Femoro-femoral bypass grafting. This may be considered in the setting of a long unilateral iliac occlusion not amenable to percutaneous intervention. This operation should only be performed provided the SFA is patent. In the presence of limited stenosis of the donor iliac artery, adjunctive PTA and stenting may be employed with this approach. Long-term patency rates (5 year) with this procedure are greater than 70% at 5 years (provided SFA intact on the recipient side).

Axillo-femoral bypass. This procedure has patency rates ranging from 20 to 80% and should rarely be performed for the treatment of claudication.

CONCLUSIONS

Peripheral arterial disease confers a marked increased future cardiovascular risk. Aggressive management of risk factors, lifestyle interventions including exercise rehabilitation, smoking cessation, and pharmacologic therapy have a central role in reducing future cardiovascular events. Percutaneous revascularization for aortoiliac disease is preferable over surgery as it provides durable treatment for individuals with disabling symptoms without the risk. Surgical treatment may be considered for the treatment of aortoiliac disease and femoropopliteal disease not amenable to other options The availability of newer stents and therapies to prevent restenosis may extend the applicability of endovascular therapy to difficult to treat infrainguinal lesions in the future.

PRACTICAL POINTS

- Normal ABIs do not exclude PAD in a patient with IC. Consider distal disease (diabetes atheroembolism) and aortoiliac disease with good collateral support.
- Normal thigh pressures (on segmental limb pressures) may not exclude aortoiliac disease owing to overestimation of pressures.
- Improvements with cilostazol take time (2 to 3 months). Patient education is important to improve compliance.

- Exercise rehabilitation in supervised setting preferable and regular walking more effective than strength training

- Long-term patency rates of bypass: aortoiliac > femoropopliteal > infrapopliteal bypass

- Extra-anatomic bypass grafts are reserved for the patient with limb threat and ought to be employed in IC only when all percutaneous options have been exhausted.

- The 5-year patency rate for AFB grafts are better than endovascular approaches in TASC C and D. However, endovascular approaches may be considered for these patients when symptoms are debilitating with an eye to repeat revascularization in the future.

RECOMMENDED READING

Baigent C, Blackwell L, Emberson J, et al. Efficacy and safety of more intensive lowering of LDL cholesterol: a meta-analysis of data from 170,000 participants in 26 randomised trials. Cholesterol Treatment Trialists' (CTT) Collaboration. *Lancet* 2010;376(9753):1670–1681.

Bhatt DL, Flather MD, Hacke W, et al. Patients with prior myocardial infarction, stroke, or symptomatic peripheral arterial disease in the CHARISMA trial. *J Am Coll Cardiol* 2007;49(19):1982–1988.

Cacoub PP, Bhatt DL, Steg PG, et al. Patients with peripheral arterial disease in the CHARISMA trial. *Eur Heart J* 2009;30(2):192–201.

CAPRIE. A randomised, blinded, trial of clopidogrel versus aspirin in patients at risk of ischaemic events (CAPRIE). CAPRIE Steering Committee. *Lancet* 1996;348(9038):1329–1339.

Creager MA, White CJ, Hiatt WR, et al. Atherosclerotic Peripheral Vascular Disease Symposium II: executive summary. *Circulation* 2008;118(25):2811–2825.

Fowkes FG, Murray GD, Butcher I, et al. Ankle brachial index combined with Framingham Risk Score to predict cardiovascular events and mortality: a meta-analysis. Ankle Brachial Index Collaboration, *JAMA* 2008;300(2):197–208.

Gray BH, Conte MS, Dake MD, et al. for Writing Group 7 Atherosclerotic Peripheral Vascular Disease Symposium II: lower-extremity revascularization: state of the art. *Circulation* 2008;118(25):2864–2872.

Hiatt WR, Hirsch AT, Creager MA, et al. Effect of niacin ER/lovastatin on claudication symptoms in patients with peripheral artery disease. *Vasc Med* 2010;15(3):171–179.

Jongkind V, Akkersdijk GJ, Yeung KK, et al. A systematic review of endovascular treatment of extensive aortoiliac occlusive disease. *J Vasc Surg* 2010;52(5):1376–1383.

Mohler E III, Hiatt W, Creager M. Cholesterol reduction with atorvastatin improves walking distance in patients with peripheral arterial disease. *Circulation* 2003;108(12):1481–1486.

Mondillo S, Ballo P, Barbati R, et al. Effects of simvastatin on walking performance and symptoms of intermittent claudication in hypercholesterolemic patients with peripheral vascular disease. *Am J Med* 2003;114(5):359–364.

McDermott MM, Greenland P, Liu K, et al. Leg symptoms in peripheral arterial disease. *JAMA* 2001;286(13):1599–1606.

Norgren L, Hiatt WR, et al. Inter-Society Consensus for the Management of Peripheral Arterial Disease (TASC II). *J Vasc Surg* 2007;45(Suppl S):S5–S67.

Resnick HE, Lindsay RS, McDermott MM, et al. Relationship of high and low ankle brachial index to all-cause and cardiovascular disease mortality: the Strong Heart Study. *Circulation* 2004;109(6):733–739.

Soga Y, Yokoi H, Kawasaki T, et al. Efficacy of cilostazol after endovascular therapy for femoropopliteal artery disease in patients with intermittent claudication. *J Am Coll Cardiol* 2009;53(1):48–53.

Steg PG, Bhatt DL, Wilson PW, et al. One-year cardiovascular event rates in outpatients with atherothrombosis. REACH Registry Investigators. *JAMA* 2007;297(11):1197–1206.

CHAPTER 7

■ Management of the Patient with Acute Limb Ischemia

Michael R. Go

INTRODUCTION

Acute limb ischemia (ALI) is one of the most common and difficult problems encountered by vascular surgeons and endovascular specialists, and the incidence will likely increase with the aging of the population. The potential outcome of this disease is limb loss or death, and it represents a significant burden on the health care system, with cost estimates ranging from $10,000 to $45,000 per admission. Paramount in the treatment of this condition is prompt recognition followed by rapid restoration of blood flow to the ischemic extremity to minimize the risk of limb loss and subsequent reperfusion-related local and remote organ injury. ALI typically occurs in elderly patients with concomitant coronary artery disease and can be associated with significant morbidity or death, even after successful limb revascularization. The average hospital length of stay for ALI is 10 days. Overall amputation rate is 13% and mortality approaches 20%.

Demographic Profile

The incidence of ALI is estimated to be 14 per 100,000 with men and women being equally affected. Most patients with peripheral arterial disease (PAD) present with chronic symptoms such as claudication, rest pain, or gangrene rather than ALI. However, patients who have had previous bypass surgery may present with ALI if their bypass graft occludes.

CLINICAL FEATURES

The underlying cause of ALI is a sudden and complete blockage of an axial artery in the affected extremity. The distal tissue beds become ischemic, with energy metabolism shifting from an aerobic to an anaerobic phase. Progressive ischemia leads to cell dysfunction and death, with nervous tissue, followed by muscle, being most susceptible. Typically, a patient without underlying vascular disease and therefore minimal preexisting collateralization who develops an acute arterial blockage will develop irreversible functional damage within 6 hours. Thus, an attempt at revascularization within this time frame is critical. Successful revascularization after a period of profound ischemia may result in reperfusion injury, causing secondary remote organ dysfunction partly related to factors released from the ischemic limb into the systemic circulation.

TABLE 7.1

LIMB ISCHEMIA CATEGORIZATION

Class	Description	Neuromuscular Findings	Doppler
I	Viable	No sensory or motor loss	Audible arterial and venous
IIa	Threatened (marginally)	Some sensory loss, no motor loss	Often inaudible arterial, audible venous
IIb	Threatened (immediately)	Sensory loss and some motor loss	Usually inaudible arterial, audible venous
III	Irreversible	Paralyzed and insensate	No signals

Classification

A useful limb ischemia categorization system has been put forth by the Society for Vascular Surgery/International Society for Cardiovascular Surgery joint council (Table 7.1) and is also known as the Rutherford Classification for ALI. Class I represents a viable limb that is not immediately threatened. No sensory deficit or muscle weakness is present, and arterial and venous Doppler signals are audible. Chronic ischemic rest pain is an example of Class I ischemia. Class IIa is a marginally threatened limb, with minimal to no sensory loss, normal motor function, and inaudible arterial Doppler signals, but audible venous Doppler signals are present. Class IIb is an immediately threatened limb that requires rapid revascularization and is associated with sensory loss and muscle weakness with inaudible arterial signals. Class III is irreversible limb ischemia, with major tissue loss or permanent nerve damage and an insensate and paralyzed limb with rigor and inaudible arterial or venous signals. Patients with class III ischemia usually require primary amputation. These categories are a simple and useful way for clinicians to communicate with each other about ALI patients and their urgency and also represent a reporting standard for clinical research.

Etiology

The most common etiology of ALI is embolization. Seventy five percent of embolic ALI is cardiogenic. In this context, left atrial appendage thrombus developing in the setting of atrial fibrillation and left ventricular mural thrombus formation after myocardial infarction are the most clinical scenarios and may often occur after recent infarction or postcardioversion, but thrombi forming in a left ventricular aneurysm or in the setting of valvular disease (mitral) are also not uncommon. Proximal aneurysm of a major artery or plaque atheroembolization accounts for 25% of embolic ALI. Rarely, embolic material may pass from the right-sided circulation to the left through a patent foramen ovale or may be related to a mechanical valve, endocarditis, or myxoma. Emboli usually lodge at arterial bifurcations, including the aortic bifurcation, the femoral bifurcation, or the tibial trifurcation. The other primary pathophysiologic mechanism of ALI is *in situ* thrombosis. Whereas in many cases embolization occurs in patients who may not have preexisting vascular disease, thrombosis is typically seen in patients with underlying PAD who sustain a thrombotic event involving a chronically stenosed axial vessel, a large collateral pathway, or perhaps a previously placed bypass graft. Other less common etiologies of ALI include trauma, for example, popliteal artery disruption with posterior knee dislocation, or dissection, such as in the aorta with propagation of a dissection flap causing occlusion of an iliac artery.

DIAGNOSIS

History and Physical Examination

Common presenting features of the two primary entities that cause ALI are listed in Table 7.2. Clinically, the diagnosis of ALI may be obvious, and the six Ps apply: pain, poikilothermia, pulselessness, paresthesias, paralysis, and pallor. However, some patients may present with subtle changes or a primary neurologic complaint such as numbness or acute paralysis without pain. If a careful history and thorough pulse exam are not obtained, this may lead to a fatal outcome as the patient is sent for consultation and other diagnostic measures, delaying reestablishment of limb blood flow.

History and physical examination often will identify the etiology and location of ALI as well as make the diagnosis and, therefore, are critical in directing therapy in the most efficient manner. Patients with embolic ALI tend to have a more abrupt onset of pain and present with a very cold and mottled extremity with a clear demarcation, usually one level below where the embolus is lodged. While some patients with embolic ALI may have preexisting PAD and robust collateral pathways, most do not, and therefore their ischemia is often profound and may fall into the IIb or III category. Other clues that embolism is the cause of ALI may include a recent cardiac event (such as a recent anterior wall myocardial infarction or a recent cardioversion), a recent history of palpitations, recent discontinuation of anticoagulation, a lack of antecedent claudication, and the presence of normal pulses in the unaffected limb.

TABLE 7.2

COMMON PRESENTATION FEATURES

	Embolism	*In Situ* Thrombosis
History	Rapid onset	Vague onset
	Prior cardiac event	No recent cardiac event
	No prior PAD history	History of PAD
Physical exam	Cold, mottled, paralyzed	Cool, bluish, paresthesias
	Normal contralateral limb pulse exam	Abnormal contralateral limb pulse exam
	Clear demarcation	No distinct demarcation
Prior vascular surgery	Usually no	Often yes
Rapid anticoagulation	Yes—heparin	Yes—heparin
Most common ischemic class	IIb	IIa

By contrast, patients with *in situ* thrombosis may have a vaguer onset of pain, with no recent cardiac events, though typically they do have coronary artery disease. An antecedent history of claudication or other symptoms of PAD is present, the limb is cool and more bluish than mottled, and no distinct demarcation is present. Pulses in the unaffected limb are often not palpable and only can be heard with a continuous-wave handheld Doppler. *In situ* thrombosis is much more likely if the patient has had a prior surgical or endovascular revascularization. These patients usually fall in the IIa category, as collateral pathways are often already developed, mitigating the effect of acute occlusion of a diseased axial vessel.

The special situation of aortic dissection deserves mention. A severely hypertensive patient or a patient with risk factors for a connective tissue disorder whose initial presentation includes chest or back pain prior to the onset of ALI must expeditiously be worked up for aortic dissection, which dramatically alters treatment if present.

Laboratory Evaluation

Laboratory evaluation should include determination of potassium, creatine kinase, renal function, and acid-base status. An electrocardiogram should be obtained to assess rhythm and identify myocardial infarction. A prothrombin time and partial thromboplastin time (PT and PTT) should be obtained in all patients along with standard hematology and transfusion screening. Creatinine phosphokinase level should also be measured to assess muscle damage. Patients with a suspected hypercoagulable state will need additional studies seeking anticardiolipin antibodies, elevated homocysteine concentration, and antibodies to platelet factor IV.

MANAGEMENT OF THE PATIENT

Patient management begins with appropriate resuscitation, immediate anticoagulation, and then a decision to proceed with thrombolytic therapy versus open revascularization. A useful therapeutic algorithm is shown in Figure 7.1. Limb viability should be confirmed at the outset. If the patient has true class III ischemia, a primary amputation should be considered, as revascularizing the nonviable limb may produce systemic complications and may prove to be fatal. Finally, consideration must be given to the patient's comorbidities, especially cardiac and pulmonary diseases. A patient with a questionably salvageable limb and significant operative risk may be best served with a primary amputation rather than a sustained and complex revascularization attempt.

General Measures

Regardless of ALI etiology, the patient should be appropriately resuscitated with intravenous (IV) fluids, preferably without potassium supplementation until renal function is determined, and all patients should receive aspirin. IV mannitol will induce an osmotic diuresis and may have free radical scavenging properties and should be considered in patients at risk for renal compromise or when significant myoglobinuria or reperfusion

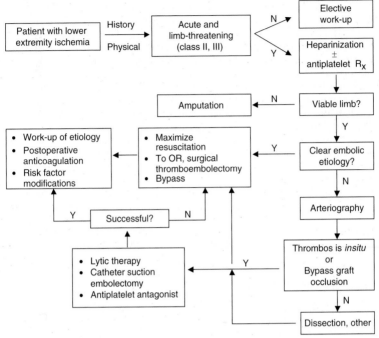

FIGURE 7-1.   Treatment algorithm for patients with ALI.

injury is expected. The patient should be therapeutically heparinized with a 100 U/kg bolus and a maintenance infusion of 12 to 15 U/kg/h to keep the PTT 2 to 2.5 times baseline value. If the patient has a known history of heparin-induced thrombocytopenia or an antithrombin III deficiency, alternative agents such as the direct thrombin inhibitors, for example, argatroban (100 µg/kg IV bolus followed by a 2 µg/kg/min infusion), can be used, and the PTT can be used to titrate the medication. In patients without renal impairment, bivalirudin is an option (1 mg/kg IV bolus followed by a 2.5 mg/kg/h infusion). No reversal agents are available for direct thrombin inhibitors and if major bleeding occurs, fresh frozen plasma may need to be given.

Approach to the Patient

The decision whether to proceed with thrombolytic therapy versus open revascularization depends largely on the etiology of the ALI and the severity of ischemia. Patients with class I ischemia typically have rest pain but a viable limb. They have severe chronic PAD and typically have multilevel arterial occlusions that require open bypass or in select cases endovascular reconstruction. Often, they can be worked up electively, but expeditiously, with angiography, perioperative risk stratification, and subsequent surgery.

Patients with class IIa ischemia usually also have preexisting PAD and often are in need of open bypass for multilevel arterial occlusions or have suffered acute thrombosis of a preexisting bypass. They have a marginally threatened limb from acute *in situ* thrombosis and elective treatment is inappropriate. These patients should be heparinized and urgent angiography performed to guide subsequent therapy. Thrombolysis should be considered in some of these patients who do not have an immediately threatened limb and can afford the extra time needed to administer this therapy.

Patients with class IIb ischemia have an immediately threatened limb. Thrombolytics or diagnostic angiography may require too much time in this situation, and immediate revascularization is indicated. Often, patients with such profound ischemia have an embolic etiology, and the location can be discerned by physical exam (e.g., a palpable external iliac pulse and a nonpalpable femoral pulse signifying femoral bifurcation embolization). These patients should be taken immediately to surgery and an open embolectomy performed, as will be described later. If the patient *does not* have a clear embolic etiology in the setting of class IIb ischemia, the patient should proceed to the operating room immediately with an on-table arteriogram performed to delineate the anatomy and likely cause. The surgeon should be prepared to proceed right away with embolectomy, thrombectomy, or attempt at a surgical or endovascular revascularization depending on the angiographic findings.

Surgical Versus Thrombolytic Therapy

Two landmark articles were published in the 1990s that suggested thrombolytic therapy had equivalent outcomes to surgical therapy in patients with ALI. These were the Surgery or Thrombolysis in Lower Extremity Ischemia (STILE) and Thrombolysis Or Peripheral Artery Surgery (TOPAS) trials, which randomized patients to arteriography and lytic therapy with urokinase versus arteriography and embolectomy or urgent bypass. Although these data are robust and the conclusions sound, it is important to note that a majority of patients in both of these trials had class I and IIa ischemia, with less than 25% having class IIb or III limb ischemia, as evidenced by including patients with up to 14 days of symptoms for the trial. Thus, many of these patients had prior extensive PAD and occluded bypass grafts, for which thrombolytic or other endovascular therapies are most appropriate. A recent national hospital administrative database review suggested that risk for an amputation with embolic ALI is significantly lower with surgical embolectomy, whereas thrombolytic therapy was not associated with fewer amputations in this setting. Thus, the choice of surgical versus thrombolytic therapy must be made very carefully and often is determined by the underlying etiology.

Surgical Therapy

The patient is widely prepped and draped to facilitate the performance of an inflow bypass (e.g., femoral-to-femoral or axillofemoral bypass) if an embolectomy or thrombectomy to restore inflow is unsuccessful. Typical lower-extremity embolic ALI may be approached through a standard femoral artery exposure and Fogarty balloon thromboembolectomy from the

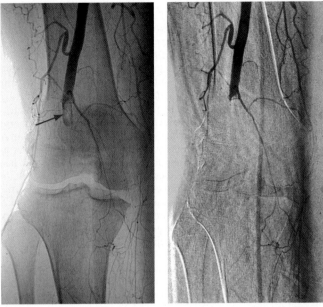

A   **B**

FIGURE 7-2. Typical digital subtraction angiography of a patient with embolic ALI. **A:** Note lucent ovoid embolus that has lodged in the distal superficial femoral artery (*arrow*). **B:** Same patient with a later contrast view. Few collaterals are present. This patient underwent a successful open embolectomy with limb salvage.

aortic bifurcation to the ankle can be performed (Fig. 7.2). Occasionally, below-knee trifurcation arterial exposure with tibioperoneal thromboembolectomy may be required. Thrombectomy of an occluded bypass graft often will require exposure of both the proximal and distal anastomoses. Care with balloon catheter extraction is important as vessel dissection and injury may occur if catheter pullback and balloon insufflation do not occur coincidentally. If signals are not present at the ankle after retrieval of thrombus, an arteriogram should be performed to document any residual thrombi or native arterial lesions. Most modern operating suites have endovascular capabilities with a high-quality C-arm or even a fixed fluoroscopy unit and a full array of catheters, wires, and balloons, allowing for endovascular treatment of residual arterial disease after surgical thromboembolectomy. Intraoperative lysis by flushing thrombolytic agent [e.g., 10-mg tissue plasminogen activator (tPA) in 100 mL of saline] in the femoral artery and occluding the outflow and inflow for several minutes has shown mixed results in the literature in terms of improved limb salvage. Rarely, emergent open bypass is needed if thromboembolectomy alone in the setting of multilevel disease does not restore limb viability. Patients who are critically ill may undergo a thromboembolectomy under local anesthesia if necessary. Postoperatively, the patient is maintained on heparin, and further medical management ensues.

Thrombolytic Therapy

Arteriography and thrombolysis should be considered in patients in whom the etiology of ALI is unclear or the history and physical exam strongly suggest a diagnosis of *in situ* thrombosis (Fig. 7.3), as long as the limb is not immediately threatened. Several well-written reviews and consensus statements have been published regarding the use of thrombolytic therapy for ALI, and surgical therapy is recommended for most patients with profound ischemia (IIb) as mean thrombus lysis times may be too long, typically 18 to 24 hours. However, thrombolytic therapy is appropriate in many instances of class IIa ALI. Therapeutic thrombolysis with agents such as tPA or urokinase works by activating plasmin, which breaks down fibrin, allowing thrombus dissolution. Table 7.3 has the recommended medications and doses that are typically used. Standard endovascular access and catheter techniques are involved. Usually, the contralateral femoral artery is cannulated and an aortic outflow arteriogram performed to define the exact location and extent of blockage. A guide wire is passed through the segmental thrombus. A multi side hole catheter follows and the entire thrombus is laced with an infusion of lytic agent. Heparin is given at a low dose through the side port of the sheath to prevent catheter-associated thrombus development. The infusion is maintained for 6 to 12 hours and reimaging done to determine success of thrombus dissolution. Success of the thrombolytic therapy can also be followed by clinical exam as evidenced by improvement in limb temperature, capillary refill, and patient symptoms. It should be noted that a patient's symptoms may transiently worsen as the thrombus fragments and travels distally. Thrombolysis typically requires 12 to 24 hours and infusions longer than 48 hours may incur higher bleeding risk. Fibrinogen levels should be checked every 6 hours, as a level less than 100 mg/dL is associated with systemic fibrinolysis and increased risk of bleeding. Once lysis is complete, the sheaths are removed and heparinization is continued at full dose. Absolute contraindications to thrombolysis are well known and include active bleeding, CNS injury, or recent major surgery. Relative contraindications include uncontrolled hypertension, recent eye surgery, pregnancy, and intracranial neoplasms.

Occluded Bypass Grafts

Thrombolytic therapy has been used extensively in the setting of acutely occluded arterial bypass grafts. This strategy is reasonable if the ischemia is class I or IIa, and often thrombolysis will uncover a causative lesion responsible for graft thrombosis such as a stenosis at the distal anastomosis, progression of disease distal to the bypass, or inflow compromise. Action can then be taken to address such lesions, including angioplasty or surgical revision. Certain clinical characteristics portend a successful outcome of thrombolysis of occluded bypass grafts: (i) if the occlusion is less than 14 days old; (ii) if the guide wire and lysis catheter can easily traverse the occluded graft; (iii) if the graft has been in place for more than 1 year; and (iv) if a defined anatomic etiology for the failure can be unmasked and treated. Factors portending poor outcomes after thrombolysis include

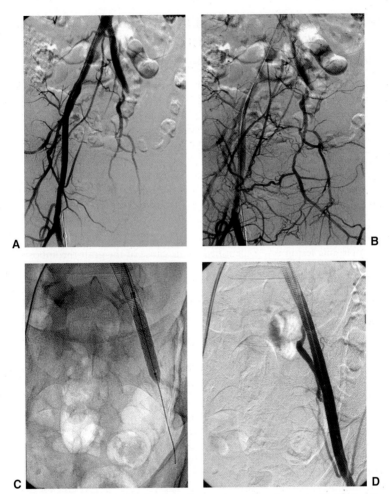

FIGURE 7-3. Typical digital subtraction angiography of a patient with *in situ* thrombosis as a cause for ALI. This patient had a long history of iliac occlusive disease and had undergone left distal common iliac angioplasty and stenting a year prior. **A:** He presented with left lower-extremity ALI, and the initial arteriogram shows complete occlusion of his external iliac system and distally. **B:** A later contrast view shows extensive preformed collaterals that reconstitute his femoral system. **C:** Catheter directed thrombolytic therapy was used for 8 hours and a tight distal CIA lesion was found. Angioplasty was performed and an additional stent was placed. **D:** Post treatment, the arteriogram shows a normal caliber external iliac artery and free outflow. This patient had successful limb salvage.

TABLE 7.3

RECOMMENDED MEDICATIONS AND DOSES OF THROMBOLYTICS

Medication	Route	Dosage	Laboratory
Aspirin	PO/PR	325 mg	None
Heparin	IV	100 U/kg bolus then 12 U/kg/h	PTT, plt, Hct
Mannitol	IV	12.5–25 g	Creatinine
Plasminogen activator	IA	Depends on the agent[a]	Hct, fibrinogen, FSP

[a]Retaplase 0.25–1.0 U/h; alteplase 0.2–1.0 mg/h; tenecteplase 0.25–0.5 mg/h.
FSP, Fibrin split products; Hct, hematocrit; IA, intra-arterial; IV, intravenous; plt, platelet count; PO, orally; PR, rectally.

diabetes and ongoing tobacco use. Overall postlysis graft patency rates are between 10 and 40% at 2 years and have led some to suggest that replacement of a failed graft is better for long-term outcome, especially if an anatomic lesion is not identified as the cause of the graft thrombosis.

Pharmacomechanical Thrombolysis

New endovascular mechanical thrombolysis techniques include catheter suction thrombectomy and rheolytic thrombus fragmentation and aspiration. These devices are guide wire directed and function to physically remove thrombus burden using mechanical thrombus disruption. Rheolytic registry data have been published with promising results in native arteries, the pulmonary artery circulation, and prosthetic dialysis access grafts. Many of these catheter devices allow concurrent pulse spray of lytic agent as well. Other technology includes the use of ultrasonic energy concurrently delivered with lytic agent through the same catheter to increase the efficiency of fibrin degradation by plasminogen activators. A larger clinical experience with these techniques is necessary before they become a standard of care, but these technologies have the potential to minimize the two main drawbacks of thrombolytic therapy, namely, the long duration of lytic infusion needed to establish full arterial perfusion and hemorrhagic complications.

SPECIAL ISSUES AND COMPLICATIONS

Complications from a surgical thromboembolectomy include the usual gamut of infectious, hemorrhagic, and cardiac events and are primarily determined by the patient's comorbidities. Thrombolytic therapy has the potential for decreasing open operative risks with the trade-off of serious hemorrhagic complications. The most feared complication of thrombolytic therapy is intracranial hemorrhage, which may be fatal. An emergent CT scan should be obtained in all patients who develop neurologic changes while undergoing thrombolysis. The lytic agent should be stopped and supportive measures taken if a stroke is confirmed. Lower-extremity four-compartment fasciotomies should be performed to prevent compartment syndrome after reperfusion in the setting of class IIb and III ischemia regardless of whether revascularization is achieved surgically or with thrombolysis. Thus, frequent neurovascular exams are essential during ongoing lytic therapy. The benefit of four-compartment fasciotomy in limb salvage has been difficult to prove by retrospective analysis and, indeed, has been associated with increased limb loss and mortality. A policy of selective prophylactic fasciotomy in those at greatest risk for compartment syndrome or close neurovascular observation and therapeutic fasciotomy, rather than routine fasciotomy, seems appropriate.

CONCLUSION

Good patient outcomes depend on the rapidity and completeness with which arterial blood flow to the limb can be reestablished. Endovascular therapy, including thrombolysis, has an important role in the treatment of ALI, but surgical therapy remains preferred in class IIb and III ischemia. The general approach to an acutely ischemic limb should include (i) rapid diagnosis, determination of ischemic class, and prompt institution of anticoagulation; (ii) determination of appropriate therapeutic approach: surgical thromboembolectomy and/or revascularization versus arteriogram and thrombolysis; and (iii) remembering to save life over limb: emergent amputation is sometimes required to save a patient's life.

PRACTICAL POINTS

- History and physical exam are essential for determining the etiology of ALI and guiding therapy.

- A bilateral pulse exam is essential, and a handheld Doppler is an extension of the standard physical exam.

- Immediate anticoagulation and careful IV hydration are recommended for all ALI patients.

- Surgical embolectomy is best for embolic ALI in most cases.

- Angiography, on table if necessary in cases of immediately threatened limbs, is important in cases where etiology of ALI is unclear.

- Thrombolysis is best for most cases of in situ thrombosis of native axial vessels or bypass grafts, provided that the limb is not immediately threatened.

RECOMMENDED READING

Ansel GM, George BS, Botti CF, et al. Rheolytic thrombectomy in the management of limb ischemia: 30-day results from a multicenter registry. *J Endovasc Ther* 2002;9:395–402.

Blaisdell FW, Steele M, Allen RE. Management of acute lower extremity ischemia due to embolism and thrombosis. *Surgery* 1978;84:822–834.

Braithwaite BD, Buckenham TM, Galland RB, et al. Prospective randomized trial of high-dose bolus versus low-dose tissue plasminogen activator infusion in the management of acute limb ischemia. *Br J Surg* 1997;84:646–650.

Dormandy J, Heeck L, Vig S. Acute limb ischemia. *Semin Vasc Surg* 1999;12:148–153.

Drescher P, Crain MR, Rilling WS. Initial experience with the combination of reteplase and abciximab for thrombolytic therapy in peripheral arterial occlusive disease: a pilot study. *J Vasc Intervent Radiol* 2002;13:37–43.

Greenberg R, Ouriel K. The role of thrombolytic therapy in the management of acute and chronic lower extremity ischemia. *J Endovasc Ther* 2000;7:72–77.

Korn P, Khilnani NM, Fellers JC, et al. Thrombolysis for native arterial occlusions of the lower extremities: clinical outcome and cost. *J Vasc Surg* 2001;33:1148–1157.

Nackman GB, Walsh DB, Fillinger MF, et al. Thrombolysis of occluded infrainguinal vein grafts: Predictors of outcome. *J Vasc Surg* 1997;25:1023–1032.

Ouriel K, Gray B, Clair DG, et al. Complications associated with the use of urokinase and recombinant tissue plasminogen activator for catheter-directed peripheral arterial and venous thrombolysis. *J Vasc Intervent Radiol* 2000;11:295–298.

Ouriel K, Veith FJ, Sarahara AA. A comparison of recombinant urokinase with vascular surgery as initial treatment for acute arterial occlusion of the legs. *N Engl J Med* 1998;338:1105–1111.

Palfreyman SJ, Booth A, Michaels JA. A systematic review of intra-arterial thrombolytic therapy for lower limb ischemia. *Eur J Vasc Endovasc Surg* 2000;19:143–157.

Panetta T, Thompson JE, Talkington CM, et al. Arterial embolectomy: a 34-year experience with 400 cases. *Surg Clin North Am* 1986;66:339–352.

Rutherford RB, Baker JD, Ernst C, et al. Recommended standards for reports dealing with lower ischemia: revised version. *J Vasc Surg* 1997;26:517–538.

STILE investigators. Results of a prospective randomized trial evaluating surgery versus thrombolysis for ischemia of the lower extremity. *Ann Surg* 1994;220:251–268.

Working Party of Thrombolysis in the Management of Limb Ischemia. Thrombolysis in the management of lower limb peripheral arterial occlusion—a consensus document. *Am J Cardiol* 1998;81:207–218.

Zehnder T, Birrer M, Do DD, et al. Percutaneous catheter thrombus aspiration for acute or subacute arterial occlusion of the legs: how much thrombolysis is needed? *Eur J Vasc Endovasc Surg* 2000;20:41–46.

CHAPTER 8 ■ Management of Chronic Critical Limb Ischemia

David Paul Slovut and Timothy M. Sullivan

Chronic critical limb ischemia (CLI), defined as greater than 2 weeks of rest pain, ulcers, or tissue loss attributed to arterial stenosis, affects approximately 1% of patients with peripheral arterial disease.

Definition of CLI: Based on the consensus document published by the Joint Council of the Society of Vascular Surgery and the North American Chapter of the International Society for Cardiovascular Surgery, CLI is characterized by persistent rest pain with or without ongoing tissue loss (Table 8.1). In general, CLI patients are characterized by low ankle (less than 70 mm Hg) and/or toe (less than 50 mm Hg) systolic pressures and/or reduced transcutaneous tissue oxygen concentration ($TcPO_2$) of less than 50 mm Hg. Ischemic rest pain most commonly occurs with an ankle pressure less than 50 mm Hg or a toe pressure less than 30 mm Hg.

CLINICAL FEATURES

Prognosis

Prognosis for patients with CLI is poor. One year following presentation, 25% of patients have resolved CLI, 20% have ongoing CLI, 30% are alive with amputation, and 25% are dead. The degree of ischemia, when classified by Fontaine and Rutherford stage (Chapter 1), correlates with outcome: the greater the ischemic burden, the worse the outcome. The concept that all patients who require an amputation have steadily progressed through increasingly severe claudication to rest pain/ulcers and, ultimately, amputation is incorrect. It has been shown that more than 50% of patients having a below-knee major amputation for ischemic disease had no symptoms of leg ischemia whatsoever as recently as 6 months prior to presentation.

Risk Factors

Risk factors for CLI are well-defined and are identical to those associated with systemic atherosclerosis although the associations with some risk factors are stronger than others. All epidemiological studies of PAD have confirmed that besides age, cigarette smoking and diabetes are the strongest risk factors for the developing CLI (OR greater than 3). Diabetes was traditionally associated with exceptionally high rates of amputations, but recent clinical trials suggest a lower rate compared to nondiabetics. In a recent double-blind placebo trial in poor option patients evaluating fibroblast growth factor-1 (TAMARIS), diabetics with CLI had death and major amputation rates of 15 and 17% at 12 months compared to 8 and 26% in nondiabetics.

TABLE 8.1

FEATURES OF CRITICAL LIMB ISCHEMIA

Physical Exam

Dry skin, thickened nails, loss of hair, loss of subcutaneous fat, or muscle atrophy

Coolness to palpation

Decreased or absent pulses

Elevation pallor or dependent rubor

Nonhealing wound or ulcer, especially over bony prominences, distally, and on the plantar surface of the foot

Noninvasive Vascular Laboratory

Ankle-brachial index ≤ 0.4

Ankle systolic pressure ≤ 50 mm Hg

Toe systolic pressure ≤ 30 mm Hg

Measures of skin microcirculation

Capillary density ≤ 20 mm^2

Absent reactive hyperemia on capillary microscopy

$TcPO_2$ < 10 mm Hg

(Adapted from Slovut DP, Sullivan TM. Critical limb ischemia: medical and surgical management. *Vasc Med* 2008;13:281–291.)

Physical Examination

Examination of the lower extremities and pulses is of paramount importance in the patient with CLI and, when used in conjunction with a careful history and testing, can provide diagnostic and prognostic information. Table 8.1 provides physical exam and vascular laboratory features that are consistent with a diagnosis of CLI.

Differential Diagnosis

Particularly in patients with diabetes, nonhealing wounds often occur due to a combination of ischemia and neuropathy with additional mechanical insults (neuroischemic ulcers). Ischemic ulcers should be distinguished from neuropathic ulcers in patients with neuropathy (see Chapter 1).

DIAGNOSTIC EVALUATION

Multiple tests are often used to confirm the diagnosis of limb-threatening ischemia, assess revascularization options, and predict wound healing (Table 8.1). The ankle-brachial index (ABI) provides important prognostic and diagnostic information in CLI. In patients with a falsely elevated ABI, the toe-brachial index or toe pressure may be diagnostic.

Imaging in Critical Limb Ischemia

Once a decision has been made to proceed to revascularization, imaging of the aorta and runoff vessels may be performed using computed tomographic angiography (CTA), magnetic resonance angiography (MRA), or x-ray digital subtraction angiography (DSA). X-ray DSA is the most common procedure performed to guide intervention planning in CLI. Although x-ray DSA has long been considered the gold standard of lower extremity arterial imaging, 3D gadolinium-based MRA techniques are increasingly used for intervention planning in CLI but must involve dedicated assessment of pedal vessels. Assessment by MRA as a routine strategy is tempered by its contraindication in advanced CKD and rapid arterial venous transit in CLI. If experience in performing high-quality exams by MRA is unavailable, x-ray DSA should be performed. Use of carbon dioxide and intravascular ultrasound limits the need for iodinated contrast in patients with impaired renal function who require intervention. CTA is particularly useful for assessing aortoiliac disease, but in some cases, extensive calcification of infrageniculate vessels and suboptimal imaging at the level of the foot reduce enthusiasm for this modality. Figure 8.1 provides an initial approach to the patient with CLI.

Cutaneous microcirculation may be assessed using capillary microscopy, laser Doppler perfusion, or transcutaneous oxygen pressure ($TcPO_2$). These techniques are often used predominantly as research modalities, although measures of microcirculation predict amputation risk in CLI. Patients with poor microcirculation, defined as capillary density less than $20/mm^2$, absent reactive hyperemia by capillary microscopy and laser Doppler, $TcPO_2 < 10$ mm Hg, experienced 1-year limb survival of only 15%. In contrast, patients with good microcirculation (capillary density

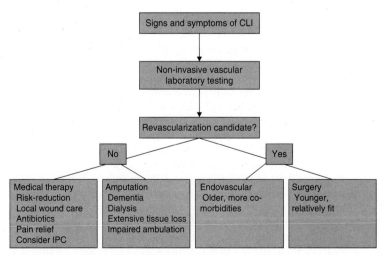

FIGURE 8-1.   Approach to patients with CLI.

$\geq 20/mm^2$, reactive hyperemia in capillary microscopy and laser Doppler, $TcPO_2 \geq 30$ mm Hg) achieved a 1-year limb survival of 88%.

MANAGEMENT

Optimal therapy for CLI patients includes reducing cardiovascular risk factors, relieving ischemic pain, treating ulcers, preventing major amputation, and improving quality of life and survival. These aims may be achieved through medical therapy, revascularization, or amputation, or a combination of therapies. A clinically driven algorithm for patients with CLI is shown in Figure 8.1.

Medical Therapy

Medical therapy for CLI patients includes modification of atherosclerotic risk factors, providing pain relief, local ulcer care, treatment of infection, and pressure mitigation.

1. *Atherosclerosis risk reduction.* Atherosclerosis care is of great importance in the patient with CLI owing to these patients' high risk for cardiovascular events. All patients with CLI should be considered to be candidates for antiplatelet agents and statins unless contraindicated.
   a. *Antiplatelet drugs*: There is a case for treatment of all patients with CLI with long-term antiplatelet therapy, such as with aspirin or clopidogrel, based on the pathophysiologic importance of the platelet in thrombus propagation, which undoubtedly is a component in CLI. Recent small randomized trials in PAD and a more recent meta-analysis of previous prospective randomized trials that included PAD patients as a subset have questioned the efficacy of aspirin in PAD in reducing overall mortality or recurrent cardiovascular events except for stroke (Table 6.4). However, none of these studies specifically address the CLI population. In the absence of such data and in light of the critical importance of ongoing thrombosis in many patients with CLI, antiplatelet therapy with ASA (81 to 325 mg daily) alone or clopidogrel 75 mg daily is recommended. At this time, there are no data supporting one agent over the other or a combination except in post hoc analysis from CHARISMA in non-CLI patients with PAD. A small double-blind randomized controlled trial ($n = 108$) from the United Kingdom in CLI patients undergoing infrainguinal revascularization demonstrated that a preoperative regimen of clopidogrel (600 mg prior to surgery, and 75 mg daily for 3 days; $n = 50$) with ASA 75 mg reduced platelet activation and troponin release both before and after surgery.
   b. *Statins*: Post hoc data from statin trials suggest a reduction in the need for amputations in subjects with a diagnosis of PAD. In the PREVENT-III trial of 1,404 patients with CLI, the use of statins was associated with reduced 1-year mortality rate. The NCEP-ATP III

guidelines support PAD as a risk equivalent with LDL and non-HDL goals similar to those with coronary heart disease. It is prudent to lower LDL to less than 70 mg/dL and non-HDL cholesterol as a secondary goal to less than 100 mg/dL in these patients.

c. *Anticoagulation*: The role of systemic anticoagulation in the setting of CLI remains controversial. Small trials have demonstrated benefits mainly in the subset of CLI patients undergoing peripheral bypass grafting. Based on post hoc analysis of the Dutch Bypass Oral Anticoagulants or Aspirin trial, patients who have undergone infrainguinal bypass graft surgery using autologous vein may benefit from oral anticoagulation with warfarin. The main trial did not show an advantage of oral anticoagulation, but the subset of patients receiving venous bypass grafts benefited from anticoagulation and a target international normalized ratio of 3.0 to 4.0; aspirin appeared better for prosthetic grafts. However, patients treated with oral anticoagulants had nearly twice the rate of major bleeding than patients taking aspirin. Anticoagulation for 3 months following bypass grafting is generally accepted to prevent acute graft thrombosis and thromboembolic complications in the acute phase. However, the decision to continue treatment long-term should be made on an individual basis. In general, anticoagulation for preserving graft patency may be considered in specific high-risk situations such as bypasses with comorbidities that increase the risk for thromboembolization, such as atrial fibrillation or low ejection fraction. There is some evidence that low-molecular-weight heparin administered for 3 months at 2,500 IU is better than aspirin and dipyridamole in maintaining femoropopliteal graft patency in patients with CLI undergoing salvage surgery. The CASPAR trial evaluated the efficacy of clopidogrel 75 mg + ASA 325 mg in comparison with ASA alone following below-knee bypass grafts. The primary composite outcome (death/index-graft occlusion/revascularization/above-ankle amputation) occurred in an equal number of patients in both groups (Table 6.4). In a pre-specified subgroup analysis, patients who underwent a prosthetic bypass graft demonstrated a benefit with the combination of ASA and clopidogrel without an increase in bleeding.

2. *Pain control*. Treatment of pain in the CLI patient is an important aspect of care. Pain should be assessed at every clinic visit and documented (a simple pain scale between 1 and 10 is useful). Although ultimate pain relief comes with improvement in blood flow with revascularization or amputation (if indicated), pain control is essential when these therapies are being planned. Narcotics are often required for complete pain relief.

3. *Treatment of infection*. Systemic antibiotics may be indicated for superadded infection or cellulitis. Infection may be suspected with the onset of rubor and tenderness in a wound. The use of antibiotics should

not delay more definitive treatment, which often requires a combination of prolonged antibiotic administration and surgical debridement of the infected bone. Osteomyelitis should be suspected if the ulcer area is greater than 2 × 2 cm, a probe can pass through tissue to bone, or the erythrocyte sedimentation rate is greater than 70 mm/h. Plain radiographs should be employed as the first imaging modality. Computed tomography may detect the presence of sequestrum, foreign body, or gas formation. Nuclear studies and magnetic resonance imaging offer the most sensitive and specific means of detecting osteomyelitis. Infections are often polymicrobial, especially in diabetics. *Staphylococcus aureus* is the most common pathogen cultured from bone samples, followed by *S. epidermidis*. Common Gram-negative pathogens include *Escherichia coli*, *Klebsiella pneumoniae*, *Proteus* sp., and *Pseudomonas aeruginosa*.

4. *Wound care.* The basic tenets of wound healing include assurance of adequate perfusion to the ischemic limb, adequate nutrition, and eradication of infection and mechanical features that inhibit healing. Table 8.2 presents guidelines for ischemic ulcer care. In general, adherence to these principles alone obviates the need for more expensive topical therapies. Debridement of infected wounds may be achieved by surgery, biosurgery (i.e., myiasis), hydrotherapy, negative pressure therapy, and wound dressings. Negative pressure wound therapy (Vacuum Assisted Closure, Kinetic Concepts Inc., San Antonio, TX) is a technique that uses subatmospheric pressure to remove excess fluid from the wound, which leads to improved oxygenation and blood flow. The technique is contraindicated in patients with thin, friable skin and in those with wounds secondary to neoplasm.

5. *Footwear.* Each CLI patient should be evaluated by a podiatrist to ensure that footwear is appropriate and not causing repetitive foot trauma.

6. *Specific pharmacotherapy in CLI.* Currently, no pharmacologic agent is approved by the Food and Drug Administration for the treatment of CLI. Prior trials using a number of drugs have been disappointing in their ability to reduce limb loss and overall morbidity and mortality associated with CLI.

   a. *Prostanoids and vasodilator therapy*: Nine double-blind studies have demonstrated significant reductions in pain and ulcer size and three

TABLE 8.2

GENERAL PRINCIPLES OF ISCHEMIC ULCER CARE

Keep area assiduously clean
Saline dressings three or four times a day when the ulcer is "weeping"
Transition to dry dressings once ulcer is dry
Avoid excessive debridement and topical antibiotics

studies have shown a reduced need for amputation with parenterally administered vasodilator prostaglandins such as prostaglandin E1. In general, the responses tend to be greater when these drugs are administered for 4 weeks rather than for shorter periods. Iloprost, a stable analogue of prostacyclin, is the most extensively investigated prostanoid. In one trial, patients who received iloprost were less likely to undergo a major amputation compared with patients in the placebo group (23 vs. 39%; $P < 0.05$) during treatment and follow-up, supporting its usage in patients with CLI, in patients who are unsuitable for a revascularization procedure, or in patients in whom such procedures have failed. These findings have not been replicated by more recent studies using oral iloprost or parenteral lipo-ecraprost as destination therapy or as adjunctive therapy immediately following distal revascularization. Based on available data, prostaglandins cannot be recommended as therapy for patients with CLI.

Evidence from randomized controlled studies to support the use of vasoactive drugs, such as cilostazol, in CLI is lacking.

b. *Angiogenic growth factors and stem cell therapy*: Single growth factor approaches including those delivered via plasmid or adenoviral approaches including VEGF-A and Hepatocyte Growth Factor were evaluated as part of early Phase I/IIa trials but are not being pursued owing to lack of convincing effect. A recent large trial in 525 patients with CLI comparing FGF-1 delivered as a plasmid versus placebo showed that FGF-1 was not effective in reducing amputations or deaths in patients with CLI. Early phase I data involving delivery of transcription factors such as hypoxia inducible growth factor (HIF-1α) appear promising. These need to be rigorously tested in randomized controlled clinical trials. A large number of open-label Phase I trials with bone marrow mononuclear cells have demonstrated benefit in small numbers of patients. The benefit of these approaches needs to be tested in larger Phase II/III trials.

c. *Mechanical therapies*: Intermittent pneumatic compression (IPC) may provide symptom relief and wound healing for CLI patients who are not candidates for vascular reconstruction. A retrospective study of CLI patients with nonhealing wounds in whom all means of additional revascularization had been exhausted found that the below-knee amputation (BKA) rate for IPC patients was 42 versus 83% for controls at 18-months follow-up. IPC requires an intensive time commitment; patients in the active treatment group received 6 hours of IPC (ArterialFlow, DJO, Vista, CA) each day in addition to standard wound care.

d. *Spinal cord stimulation (SCS) and sympathectomy*: The use of SCS remains controversial. A Cochrane review concluded that SCS was superior to medical management for treating CLI patients with unreconstructable vascular disease. However, a meta-analysis of five randomized trials showed that SCS was no better than medical therapy alone in preventing amputations; at least 14 patients must be treated to avoid one amputation at a cost of more than $150,000 per limb saved. Another option for selected patients is surgical or chemical lumbar sympathectomy, which improves skin blood flow in the leg and foot and is associated with 1-year limb-salvage rates of 58 to 61%. Because of high cost and uncertain benefit, use of hyperbaric oxygen may be limited to reducing the risk of major amputation in patients with diabetic foot ulcers.

Revascularization

Even with aggressive local wound care, patients with severe limb ischemia who do not undergo revascularization often progress to amputation. Revascularization to reestablish continuous in-line flow from the aorta to the pedal arch represents the preferred treatment for patients with limb-threatening ischemia. The multilevel, multisegment nature of disease in CLI and the presence of numerous complicating illnesses render it difficult to make generalizations about the optimal form of therapy; rather, revascularization decisions need to be tailored to individual patients' needs. Both percutaneous and surgical options have appropriate roles in the management of patients with CLI. Although one or the other method may be appropriate initially and in some cases used exclusively, CLI frequently lends itself to multimodal treatment. The procedure(s) chosen should strike a balance between maximizing durability and minimizing risk. Extremely high-risk patients, particularly if they are nonambulatory with large areas of tissue loss, may be best treated with primary amputation. On the other hand, a minimally invasive approach in an otherwise stable patient may not be appropriate if durability is inferior to a more invasive surgical option.

Outcome following revascularization is related to the degree of ischemia. A study of 2,240 consecutive limb revascularizations (approximately 1/3 endovascular and 2/3 open surgery) demonstrated that for every outcome studied—primary patency, secondary patency, limb salvage, survival, amputation-free survival, and maintenance of ambulation—patients with claudication outperform those with ischemic rest pain, and patients with rest pain outperform those with ischemic tissue loss (Table 8.3).

Revascularization Trials in Critical Limb Ischemia

Revascularization trials in CLI to assess optimal approach (surgery vs. endovascular) are intrinsically difficult to execute owing to the considerable comorbidity of CLI patients and the fact that randomized trials are not strictly a comparison of one strategy versus the other owing to significant crossover rates. Although there have been multiple single-center studies evaluating various revascularization options in CLI, to date, only one prospective, randomized trial, Bypass versus Angioplasty in Severe Ischemia of the Leg (BASIL), has compared outcome of a surgery-first with an angioplasty-first strategy (no stents were allowed) in patients with severe limb ischemia due to infrainguinal disease. Most patients were not on

TABLE 8.3

OUTCOMES OF 2,240 CONSECUTIVE LIMB REVASCULARIZATIONS (BOTH SURGICAL AND PERCUTANEOUS) PERFORMED AT A SINGLE CENTER STRATIFIED ACCORDING TO PREOPERATIVE INDICATION

	1 Year		3 Year		5 Year	
Patency Rate (1° = Primary; 2° = Secondary)						
	1°	2°	1°	2°	1°	2°
IC	85	97	69	94	60	93
Rest pain	65	88	54	81	50	80
Tissue loss	54	74	46	67	43	66
Maintenance of Ambulation						
IC	99		98		96	
Rest pain	91		81		78	
Tissue loss	83		75		68	
Amputation-free Survival						
IC	96		87		78	
Rest pain	75		55		42	
Tissue loss	61		41		25	
Survival						
IC	96		88		78	
Rest pain	79		61		46	
Tissue loss	66		46		30	

All values are in %.
IC, intermittent claudication.
(Adapted from Taylor SM, Cull DL, Kalbaugh C, et al. Comparison of interventional outcomes according to preoperative indication: a single center analysis of 2,240 limb revascularizations. *J Am Coll Surg* 2009;208:770–778.)

evidence-based pharmacotherapy with only 58 and 34% of patients receiving an antiplatelet drug and statin, respectively. The use of β-blockers was not reported. Only 10% of screened patients were eventually randomized due to exclusions based on need for aortoiliac intervention, lack of targets, significant comorbidity, or a pattern of disease that was technically unsuitable for angioplasty or surgery. The primary outcome measure was amputation-free survival, which was no different between the two groups at 2 years. Twenty percent of patients assigned to angioplasty suffered immediate technical failures; stents were not utilized. Angioplasty was associated with a higher rate of reintervention than surgery with 50% of patients meeting evidence of clinical failure. Of those, 54% underwent a second intervention, which in most instances was surgery. In the short-term (30-day), both strategies had similar mortality but surgery-first strategy was associated with a twofold greater incidence of myocardial infarction and threefold greater rate of stroke, longer hospital stay, and greater utilization of the intensive care unit. At medium-term follow-up (all patients followed at least 3 years), outcome of vein bypass was better for amputation-free survival ($P = 0.003$) but not overall survival ($P = 0.38$, log rank tests) than outcome of prosthetic bypass. Amputation-free survival ($P = 0.006$) but not overall survival ($P = 0.06$, log rank test) was significantly worse after bypass following failed angioplasty than after bypass as a first revascularization attempt. The BASIL authors suggested that patients who are expected to live less than 1 to 2 years and have significant comorbidity should be offered angioplasty first, whereas patients who can withstand the rigors of an open procedure and are expected to live more than 2 years should undergo surgery first.

Endovascular Approaches

In the past decade, endovascular therapy has supplanted surgery as the initial approach for patients with CLI. Endovascular revascularization is appealing as it is minimally invasive and is associated with low morbidity and mortality, reduced hospital costs, and decreased length of hospitalization. Furthermore, if this approach fails, surgical revascularization may be an option in the future.

The TASC classification is helpful in assessing feasibility of endovascular versus surgical therapy (Fig. 6.3). TASC A and B lesions are ideal for percutaneous intervention. However, in contemporary practice, a large percentage of patients with TASC-C and TASC-D lesions undergo endovascular treatment. Select patients with TASC-D lesions, particularly those with concomitant aneurysms or long-segment complete occlusions of the aorta, may benefit from an initial surgical approach.

Aortoiliac PTA and stenting: Aortoiliac disease may be treated with percutaneous transluminal angioplasty (PTA) alone or with a stent. Technical success rates exceed 90%. A meta-analysis of data from six PTA studies (1,300 patients) and eight stent placement studies (816 patients) showed decreased risk of long-term failure with stent placement. For patients with CLI, the risk of long-term failure was reduced by 39% after stent placement compared with PTA. Current guidelines support use of primary stenting for suitable lesions in the distal aorta and common and external iliac arteries. The primary patency rates for aortoiliac lesions is excellent (Table 6.7). Several factors may influence long-term patency including stent placement, lesion length, morphology, and outflow. Patency rates following external iliac artery stenting appear lower in women. The Dutch Iliac Stent Trial, a randomized study comparing primary stenting with provisional stent placement in aortoiliac disease, has shown similar late patency for both groups, with lower costs in the selective stenting group. Despite this, primary stenting is preferred by most practitioners for patients with extensive aortoiliac lesions.

Femoropopliteal intervention: Most lesions in the superficial femoral and popliteal artery are treated with PTA alone or PTA with stenting. A meta-analysis of 19 studies (923 PTA, 473 stent implantations) showed combined 3-year patency rates after balloon dilation of 43% for stenoses and 30% for occlusions in CLI patients. The 3-year patency rates after stent implantation were 63 to 66% and were independent of clinical indication and lesion type. A more recent meta-analysis incorporating data from 10 trials (greater than 1,400 patients) found similar patency, target vessel revascularization, amputation rate, and mortality in patients treated with PTA alone versus those treated with a stent. Technical failure following PTA is often readily treated by stent placement. Factors associated with procedural failure include lesion length greater than 10 cm, extensive calcification, and diffuse distal disease. Self-expanding stents are prone to strut fracture, an event that nearly doubles the chance of developing severe in-stent restenosis. Recent developments the in-stent design have reduced the incidence of strut fractures, but this remains a concern in the femoropopliteal location. Numerous adjunctive therapies have been utilized in an effort to improve patency of infrainguinal reconstruction including the cutting balloon (Boston Scientific Corporation), cryoplasty catheter (PolarCath, Boston Scientific Corporation), excimer laser (CLiRPath, Spectranetics, Inc., Colorado Springs, CO), atherectomy (Silverhawk, Excision System, ev3, Plymouth, MN; Pathway Jetstream G2, Kirkland, Washington), drug-eluting stents, and covered stents. Although each of these adjunctive therapies adds substantially to the cost of intervention, none appears superior to PTA and/or stenting. Table 6.8 provides data from contemporary trials (mostly in IC patients) with some of these devices.

Tibioperoneal intervention: With the development of balloons and self-expanding stents tailored to the trifurcation vessels, endovascular therapy is becoming the initial treatment of choice for infrapopliteal lesions. This is especially the case in individuals with limited conduit and/or substantial medical comorbidity. In the case of infrapopliteal angioplasty, technical success may approach 90% with resultant limb salvage rates of greater than 85% (Table 8.4). To date, no studies have been conducted comparing open surgery and endovascular therapy for infrapopliteal occlusive disease. For follow-up periods of 1 to 3.3 years, target limb revascularization ranged from 21 to 42%, limb salvage from 80 to 91%, and death from 9 to 46%.

TABLE 8.4

INFRAPOPLITEAL INTERVENTION TRIALS

Trial	*N*	TVR	Limb Salvage	Death	Follow-up
BTK chill	108	21	80	9	1
Chromis deep	50	NR	91	21	1
Bosiers (Xpert)	94	42	91	29	2
Siablis (BMS)	41	30	80	29	3
Siablis (SES)	62	23	82	32	3
Conrad	144	38	86.2	46	3.3

(Das T, et al. *J Endovasc Ther* 2009;16(Suppl II):II19–II30; Deloose K, et al. *Eurointervention* 2009;5:318–324; Bosiers M, et al. *Vascular* 2009;1:1–8; Siablis D, et al. *J Vasc Interv Radiol* 2009;20:1141–1150; Conrad MF, et al. *J Vasc Surg* 2009;50:799–805.)
BMS, bare metal stent; SES, sirolimus-eluting stent.

Drug-eluting stents in infrainguinal disease: The PARADISE trial was a nonrandomized trial of 106 CLI patients who underwent placement of drug-eluting coronary stents (DES) in the infrageniculate vessels conducted in patients presenting with CLI. The trial enrolled 106 patients who received balloon expandable DES [83% received Cypher (Cordis, J&J, NJ), while 17% received Taxus (Boston Scientific, MN)]. The average number of stents per limb was 1.9 and 35% of limbs received overlapping DES (length of 60 mm). There were no procedural deaths, and 96% of patients were discharged within 24 hours. The 3-year cumulative incidence of amputation was 6%, survival was 71%, and amputation-free survival was 68%. Target limb revascularization occurred in 15% of patients, and repeat angiography in 35% of patients revealed a binary restenosis rate of 12%. This early study is promising but must be tested in a randomized controlled trial.

Subintimal angioplasty in infrainguinal disease: Subintimal angioplasty was first described in 1987 as a method of performing an endovascular arterial bypass. The subintimal space at the start of the occlusion is entered with a catheter and a wire loop is used to cross the occlusion and reenter the vessel lumen distally. Reentry devices such as the Outback Re-Entry Catheter (Cordis, J&J, NJ) may be required in up to 15% of cases to regain the true lumen. In patients with CLI, there is evidence from prospective nonrandomized trials suggesting that the limb salvage rate for SIA performed primarily for superficial femoral artery (SFA) disease may be superior to PTA alone. In a meta-analysis of all trials with SIA performed till 2008 [37 studies (prospective and retrospective in 2,810 limbs)], the primary patency at 12 months was 56% with a limb salvage rate of 89%. More recent trials suggest that these rates may be even higher. A 5-year observational study comparing SIA with bypass for CLI patients with infrainguinal disease suggested nearly comparable 5-year amputation-free survival. Compared with patients who underwent bypass, patients who underwent SIA had a shorter hospitalization, substantially lower cost, greater freedom from major adverse events, and improved quality of life.

Hybrid Revascularization

An increasing number of CLI patients undergo a combination of endovascular and open surgery to achieve complete revascularization. Hybrid therapy represents an attractive revascularization option in patients who are older, frail, or have limited autologous conduit for bypass. In a hybrid procedure, the endovascular portion may consist of restoring inflow, outflow, a combination of inflow and outflow, or revising a bypass graft. Endovascular repair may be performed percutaneously using the crossover technique from the contralateral common femoral artery (CFA) or via cut down over the ipsilateral CFA, which permits reconstruction using femoral artery endarterectomy and patch angioplasty or placement of an interposition graft. The use of an endovascular inflow procedure—whether of the aortoiliac segment or the SFA—does not appear to compromise long-term patency of the downstream bypass graft. A recent series examined outcomes in

171 patients who underwent combined common femoral endarterectomy and either iliac stenting or iliac stent grafting for rest pain (32%), tissue loss (22%), or claudication (46%). Median length of hospital stay was 2 days. The 30-day mortality was 2.3% with perioperative complications seen in 22%. Five-year primary, primary-assisted, and secondary patencies were 60, 97, and 98%, respectively.

Surgical Approaches

Surgical therapy may be considered in patients who are not candidates for a percutaneous option based on the severity of disease and comorbidities. Surgical revascularization may be considered as a first-line approach in patients with excellent conduit and a single-vessel target where bypass may restore in-line flow from the aorta. The durability of bypass, especially in the suprainguinal segment, in patients who are otherwise relatively fit and have a life expectancy greater than 2 years, is a consideration that support such a strategy. Table 8.5 provides approximate patency rates for bypass grafting in the setting of CLI.

Aortoiliac Revascularization: Currently, the most frequently performed surgical procedures for aortoiliac disease are aortobifemoral bypass and extra-anatomic (axillofemoral and femorofemoral) bypass. Five-year primary patency of aortobifemoral bypass performed for CLI is approximately 80% (Table 8.5).

TABLE 8.5

PATENCY RATES OF BYPASS GRAFTING IN CLI/SEVERE LIMB ISCHEMIA

Procedure	5-Year Patency
Aortobifemoral bypass	87 (80–88)[a]
Axillounifemoral bypass	51 (44–79)[a]
Axillobifemoral bypass	71 (50–76)[a]
Femoropopliteal vein	69 (60–82)[b]
Femoropopliteal above-knee (Dacron)	49 (46–53)[c]
Femoropopliteal above-knee (PTFE)	38 (32–45)[c]
Femoropopliteal below-knee	47

Note: Evidence from trials.
[a]Data adapted from TASC; Norgren L, Hiatt WR, Dormandy JA, et al. Inter-Society consensus for the management of peripheral arterial disease (TASC II). *J Vasc Surg* 2007;45(Suppl S):S5–S67; S54A for patients with CLI.
[b]Klinkert P, Post PN, Breslau PJ, et al. Saphenous vein versus PTFE for above-knee femoropopliteal bypass. *Eur J Vasc Endovasc Surg* 2004;27(4):356–357; Analysis of studies between 1966 to 2002 and 25 articles selected.
[c]Takagi H, Goto SN, Matsui M, et al. A contemporary meta-analysis of Dacron versus polytetrafluoroethylene grafts for femoropopliteal bypass grafting. *J Vasc Surg* 2010;52(1):232–236 (Randomized Controlled Trial Evidence only). No statistically significant difference in outcomes between PTFE and Dacron were reported despite the mean effect estimates being lower with PTFE.

Surgical considerations: A number of different technical variations of aortobifemoral bypass exist (also refer to Chapter 6). In general, an end-to-side approach is favored when preservation of antegrade flow to either the inferior mesenteric artery or internal iliac arteries is necessary. An end-to-end configuration is favored when the aorta has associated aneurysmal changes or is a source of emboli. No differences in patency rates have been shown between these two approaches. Debate continues on the optimal approach, that is, transperitoneal versus retroperitoneal with no real differences in outcome between the two. A potential disadvantage of aortobifemoral bypass is the associated morbidity and mortality, which range from 2 to 10% and from 1 to 3%, respectively. In high-risk patients for whom endovascular treatment is not an option, extra-anatomic bypass, that is, axillobifemoral bypass for bilateral disease and femorofemoral bypass for unilateral disease, is a reasonable alternative. Patients who undergo extra-anatomic repair are generally older, more likely to have advanced ischemia, previous aortofemoral inflow operation, renal insufficiency, and severe chronic obstructive pulmonary disease. Mortality and systemic morbidity for anatomic bypass have decreased over time, even as the complexity of cases has increased. Contemporary 30-day operative mortality is 2.3% after aortobifemoral bypass, 5.6% after femorofemoral bypass, and 12% after axillofemoral bypass. The late patency is 82 to 92% for aortofemoral grafts, 52 to 83% for femorofemoral grafts, and 45 to 62% for axillofemoral grafts. At 5 years, limb salvage rates following surgical revascularization for aortoiliac occlusive disease are 90 to 94% for anatomic bypass procedures and 60 to 90% for extra-anatomic procedures. Other methods of aortoiliac reconstruction, such as aortoiliac endarterectomy, have specific indications but overall play a limited role in the treatment of aortoiliac occlusive disease in CLI.

Adjunctive profundaplasty: The profunda femoris and its collaterals are a major source of blood flow to the lower leg in individuals with SFA occlusion (50% of patients with CLI have occluded SFA). Involvement of the profunda most often occurs proximally. Visualizing profunda stenosis requires oblique views on angiography because of the posterolateral origin of the vessel from the CFA. Profundaplasty is a low-morbidity procedure that is indicated in the presence of a profunda stenosis with SFA occlusion, in the setting of aortoiliac disease requiring aortobifemoral bypass, and in the case of failure of a distal bypass to improve limb salvage.

Infrainguinal revascularization: Outcomes following infrainguinal revascularization have steadily improved largely as a result of improved operative technique, patient selection, and perioperative care. Since most patients with CLI have multilevel disease, prior to addressing "outflow" vessels the adequacy of "inflow" must be assessed carefully and significant stenosis treated. In some situations, a combined approach with dilatation of proximal lesions and bypass of distal lesions may be warranted (see "Hybrid Revascularization," above). Patients who have reasonable operative risk and adequate conduit may benefit from surgical revascularization.

Conduit Considerations: The type of conduit used exceeds all other factors as the primary determinant of long-term patency of infrainguinal bypass grafts. Wherever possible, autogenous vein is preferred. In experienced hands, reversed autogenous vein and *in situ* vein bypass are equally effective in terms of patency and limb salvage. The greater saphenous vein is the primary choice for autogenous vein conduit. When the greater saphenous vein is not available, other veins that may be used include the cephalic or basilic veins in the arm, lesser saphenous vein, and superficial femoral veins. The use of prosthetic conduits for bypass grafting is significantly inferior and is reserved for those instances where no vein is available. Duplex vein mapping is useful for the preoperative assessment of potential venous conduits in both the arms and legs. Veins as small as 3 mm in external diameter may be used, but 4-mm veins are preferred.

Anastomotic considerations: The site for the proximal anastomosis is often chosen based largely on the length of the available vein. The only requirement for the proximal anastomosis is that of unimpeded pulsatile flow. The CFA is the most common origin of femoral-distal bypass graft. Use of the superficial or profunda femoral arteries as inflow is frequently necessary to permit use of shorter vein grafts. It is crucial to ensure that vessels proximal to the eventual takeoff of the graft are uncompromised as even minor stenosis proximal to a graft origin has been correlated with eventual graft failure. The choice of distal anastomosis is based on preoperative arteriography. Any distal artery may serve as a touchdown site for a bypass graft. The choice of distal anastomosis site should be based on the quality of the distal artery and its runoff rather than on the length of the bypass or simply because one site is more proximal than the other. Femoral-to-below-knee bypass grafting yields comparable results to a more distal bypass site, with the major consideration being the quality of the target vessel. The popliteal artery is chosen over tibial sites if the artery appears minimally diseased and distal runoff unimpeded. Infrapopliteal arteries are chosen over the popliteal artery if there is significant disease in the popliteal artery and/or at the tibial artery origins. Bypass to an isolated popliteal segment is rarely performed and only when a more distal target is unavailable or venous conduit is limited. If the tibial arteries are chosen as the distal site, the choice of which tibial artery to use depends on which one appears best on the arteriogram. CLI patients who lack a patent outflow vessel for distal anastomosis may undergo "blind bypass" to a collateral artery, although the limb salvage rates are lower than the rates when bypass is performed to a patent outflow vessel.

Alternate conduit bypass grafting: Lower extremity revascularization for limb salvage in the absence of a suitable autogenous vein conduit is a frequent challenge associated with a high failure rate. Options for an alternative bypass conduit are few but include human umbilical vein, preserved venous and arterial allografts, and prosthetic grafts. The most widely used alternate conduit is prosthetic graft, which is most frequently made from polytetrafluoroethylene. In situations where the bypass is required below the knee, prosthetic grafts perform significantly worse than autologous veins in terms of patency and limb salvage. Cryopreserved saphenous vein allografts have been used for lower extremity bypasses in patients in whom autogenous vein is unavailable and an above-knee prosthetic bypass cannot be performed. Since cryopreserved vein grafts are considerably more expensive than prosthetic grafts and patency results are comparable, the use of cryopreserved vein grafts for bypass should be limited to patients without autogenous vein who are at too high an infection risk for placement of a prosthetic graft.

Postoperative Follow-up

Diligent follow-up following lower extremity revascularization is critical since CLI patients have a high frequency of limb-specific and cardiovascular events. Palpation of pulses, rest and exercise ABIs, and duplex ultrasonography provide the best means for detecting a failing graft. The purpose of periodic duplex ultrasound surveillance is to recognize impending graft failure by identifying areas of stenosis within the graft or within the native artery proximal to or distal to the graft. Graft stenosis, which can result from fibrointimal hyperplasia, fibrosis at valve sites, or atherosclerosis, may lead to graft thrombosis and failure. Once thrombosed, vein grafts can rarely be salvaged. When a graft occludes, the patient may be left with worse ischemia than existed prior to bypass. To avoid this outcome, noninvasive vascular laboratory follow-up is recommended at 3-month intervals through the first year after bypass and every 6 months thereafter. Early detection of graft stenosis is an indication for graft revision. Findings consistent with a significant vein graft stenosis include peak systolic velocity over 300 cm/s or a prestenotic to intrastenotic velocity ratio greater than 3.5 on duplex or an ABI decrease ≥ 0.15. Patients impending graft failure should be considered for PTA or surgical repair (i.e., patch angioplasty, segmental vein resection, and interposition vein graft).

Although duplex ultrasound for postoperative graft surveillance has been the standard of care, its utility was called into question by results from the Vein Graft Surveillance Randomized Trial, which randomized 594 patients with a patent vein graft at 30 days after surgery to either clinical or duplex ultrasound follow-up at 6 weeks and then at 3, 6, 9, 12, and 18 months postoperatively. The two groups had similar amputation rates (7% for each group) and vascular mortality rates (3 vs. 4%) over 18 months. Although more patients in the clinical group had vein graft stenosis at 18 months (19 vs. 12%, $P = 0.04$), primary, primary-assisted, and secondary patency rates, respectively, were similar in the clinical group (69, 76, and 80%) and the duplex group (67, 76, and 79%). Costs for patients followed by duplex were substantially higher than for patients followed clinically.

SPECIAL ISSUES

Primary Amputation

Amputation is indicated after failed attempts at revascularization, if the patient is unfit or unable to undergo revascularization, or in the presence of extensive tissue loss or infection. Predictors of adverse functional outcomes following revascularization that suggest primary amputation should be performed include impaired ambulatory status at baseline, dementia, end-stage renal disease, and extensive necrosis. According to the TASC II guidelines, "…amputation may offer an expedient return to a useful quality of life, especially if a prolonged course of treatment is anticipated with little likelihood of recovery." Amputation level is determined clinically, although objective data such as $TcPO_2$, fluorescein angiography, or skin thermography may supplement the surgeon's judgment. Based on data from PREVENT III, a risk score has been devised to stratify patients according to their risk of death or major amputation. The PIII score includes dialysis (4 points), tissue loss (3 points), age greater than 75 (2 points), and presence of coronary artery disease (1 point). The 1-year amputation-free survival for PIII score ≤3 was 87.7%, PIII 4 to 7 was 63.7%, and PIII ≥8 was 45%. The 30-day mortality for BKA is 5% and for above-knee amputation (AKA) 17.5%. It is thought that preservation of the knee joint helps preserve patient mobility and improve outcome; a recent study suggested little difference in ability to ambulate independently following BKA or AKA. For purposes of perioperative cardiac risk stratification, it is reasonable to consider BKA an intermediate-risk procedure and AKA a high-risk operation. Use of perioperative β-blockers may decrease cardiovascular mortality. Long-term survival is markedly reduced with higher amputation level (5-year survival after AKA 31 vs. 48% after BKA).

The use of myocutaneous flaps for necrotic muscle in conjunction with revascularization usually involves multiple procedures and recuperative periods in excess of 6 months. In spite of this aggressive effort, a functional foot is obtained in only 50 to 75% of cases. Thus, aggressive vascular reconstructive efforts are not beneficial in gaining functionality in patients with extensive necrosis.

Functional Outcomes

Following Revascularization

Traditionally, results of lower extremity revascularization have been reported using standard parameters including graft patency, limb salvage, and patient survival. While reports of modern series confirm ever-improving graft patency and limb salvage, these parameters assess only the technical success of peripheral revascularization and limb salvage and may not always translate to a good functional outcome for the patient. Nonambulatory patients suffer from extensive comorbid conditions. They are accompanied with an increased occurrence of adverse events, unplanned reinterventions, and poor long-term survival rates. Successful revascularization may not necessarily improve functional status (Fig. 8.2). This emphasizes the fact that attempts for limb salvage must be carefully considered in patients with CLI and decisions made on a case by case basis. No specific functional outcome measures have been validated in this population, although several are under investigation. Based on contemporary series less than 50% of patients who undergo bypass for limb salvage are completely cured and achieve the ideal surgical result (i.e., uncomplicated operation with elimination of symptoms, maintenance of functional status, and recurrence of ischemia or need for repeat operations). A high percentage of patients have perioperative complications and need repeat hospitalizations for wound care, redo revascularization, and amputation.

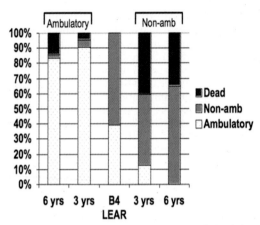

FIGURE 8-2. Functional status of CLI patients stratified by functional status before lower extremity arterial revascularization (LEAR) and during follow-up at 3 years and 6 years. (Adapted from Flu HC, Lardenoye JH, Veen EJ, et al. Functional status as a prognostic factor for primary revascularization for critical limb ischemia. *J Vasc Surg* 2010;51:360–371, e361, with permission.)

Following Amputation

Postoperative ambulation following amputation is higher following BKA than AKA. However, the ability to predict precisely which patients will gain ambulation after BKA in the vascular population is poor. Despite the availability of improved prostheses, functional outcomes based on contemporary series following both BKA and AKA in CLI remain poor. Seventeen months after either BKA or AKA, only one third of CLI patients are able to ambulate while the remainder remain nonambulatory.

CONCLUSION

Whenever possible, functional, ambulatory patients with CLI should undergo revascularization. All patients need to be on optimal medical therapy. The decision to perform surgery, endovascular therapy, or a combination of the two modalities must be individualized. Patients who are relatively fit and able to withstand the rigors of an open procedure may benefit from the long-term durability of surgical repair. In contrast, patients with a limited life expectancy may experience better outcomes with endovascular reconstruction. Primary amputation should be considered for patients who are nonambulatory, demented, or unfit to undergo revascularization. For patients who are not candidates for revascularization, or who are unwilling or unable to undergo amputation, medical therapy that may offer symptom relief and promote wound healing may be pursued. Regardless of which treatment strategy is employed, clinicians must redouble their efforts to place CLI patients on appropriate medication regimens to reduce risk of myocardial infarction, stroke, and death.

RECOMMENDED READING

Adam DJ, Beard JD, Cleveland T, et al. Bypass versus angioplasty in severe ischaemia of the leg (BASIL): multicentre, randomised controlled trial. *Lancet* 2005;366:1925–1934.

Arain SA, White CJ. Endovascular therapy for critical limb ischemia. *Vasc Med* 2008;13: 267–279.

Biondi-Zoccai GGL, Sangiorgi G, Lotrionte M, et al. Infra-genicular stent implantation for below-the-knee atherosclerotic disease: clinical evidence from an international collaborative meta-analysis on 640 patients. *J Endovasc Ther* 2009;16:251–259.

Blevins WA Jr, Schneider PA. Endovascular management of critical limb ischemia. *Eur J Vasc Endovasc Surg* 2010;39:756–761.

Chang RW, Goodney PP, Baek JH, et al. Long-term results of combined common femoral endarterectomy and iliac stenting/stent grafting for occlusive disease. *J Vasc Surg* 2008;48: 362–367.

Chung J, Bartelson BB, Hiatt WR, et al. Wound healing and functional outcomes after infrainguinal bypass with reversed saphenous vein for critical limb ischemia. *J Vasc Surg* 2006;43(6):1183–1190.

Conte MS, Bandyk DF, Clowes AW, et al. Risk factors, medical therapies and perioperative events in limb salvage surgery: observations from the PREVENT III multicenter trial. *J Vasc Surg* 2005;42:456–464.

Davies AH, Hawdon AJ, Sydes MR, et al. Is duplex surveillance of value after leg vein bypass grafting? Principal results of the Vein Graft Surveillance Randomised Trial (VGST). *Circulation* 2005;112:1985–1991.

Dorros G, Jaff MR, Dorros AM, et al. Tibioperoneal (outflow lesion) angioplasty can be used as primary treatment in 235 patients with critical limb ischemia: five-year follow-up. *Circulation* 2001;104:2057–2062.

Dosluoglu HH, O'Brien-Irr MS, Lukan J, et al. Does preferential use of endovascular interventions by vascular surgeons improve limb salvage, control of symptoms, and survival of patients with critical limb ischemia? *Am J Surg* 2006;192:572–576.

Dutch Bypass Oral anticoagulants or Aspirin (BOA) Study Group. Efficacy of oral anticoagulants compared with aspirin after infrainguinal bypass surgery (The Dutch Bypass Oral Anticoagulants or Aspirin Study): a randomised trial. *Lancet* 2006;355:346–351.

Eginton MT, Brown KR, Seabrook GR, et al. A prospective randomized evaluation of negative-pressure wound dressings for diabetic foot wounds. *Ann Vasc Surg* 2003;17:645–649.

Feiring AJ, Krahn M, Wesolowski A, et al. Preventing leg amputations in critical limb ischemia with below-the-knee stents (PARADISE trial). *JACC* 2010;55;1580–1589.

Flu HC, Lardenoye JH, Veen EJ, et al. Functional status as a prognostic factor for primary revascularization for critical limb ischemia. *J Vasc Surg* 2010;51:360–371, e361.

Hertzer NR, Bena JF, Karafa MT, et al. A personal experience with direct reconstruction and extra-anatomic bypass for aortoiliofemoral occlusive disease. *J Vasc Surg* 2007;45: 527–535.

Kasapis C, Henke PK, Chetcuti SJ, et al. Routine stent implantation vs. percutaneous transluminal angioplasty in femoropopliteal artery disease: a meta-analysis of randomized controlled trials. *Eur Heart J* 2009;30:44–55.

Kavros SJ, Delis KT, Turner NS, et al. Improving limb salvage in critical limb ischemia with intermittent pneumatic compression: a controlled study with 18-month follow-up. *J Vasc Surg* 2008;47:543–549.

LaMuraglia GM, Conrad MF, Chung T, et al. Significant perioperative morbidity accompanies contemporary infrainguinal bypass surgery: an NSQIP report. *J Vasc Surg* 2009;50: 299–304, e291–e294.

Lawall H, Bramlage P, Amann B. Treatment of peripheral arterial disease using stem and progenitor cell therapy. *J Vasc Surg* 2011;53(2):445–453.

Markose G, Miller F, Bolia A. Subintimal angioplasty for femoro-popliteal occlusive disease. *J Vasc Surg* 2010;52:1410–1416.

Nehler MR, Coll JR, et al. Functional outcome in a contemporary series of major lower extremity amputations. *J Vasc Surg* 2003;38:7–14.

Norgren L, Hiatt WR, Dormandy JA, et al. Inter-Society consensus for the management of peripheral arterial disease (TASC II). *J Vasc Surg* 2007;45(Suppl S):S5–S67.

Pereira CE, Albers M, Romiti M, et al. Meta-analysis of femoropopliteal bypass grafts for lower extremity arterial insufficiency. *J Vasc Surg* 2006;44:510–517.

Second European consensus document on chronic critical leg ischaemia. *Eur J Vasc Surg* 1992;6(Suppl A):1–32.

Slovut DP, Sullivan TM. Critical limb ischemia: medical and surgical management. *Vasc Med* 2008;13:281–291.

Stone PA, Flaherty SK, Aburahma AF, et al. Factors affecting perioperative mortality and wound-related complications following major lower extremity amputations. *Ann Vasc Surg* 2006;20:209–216.

Sultan S, Hynes N. Five-year Irish trial of CLI patients with TASC II type C/D lesions undergoing subintimal angioplasty or bypass surgery based on plaque echolucency. *J Endovasc Ther* 2009;16:270–283.

Taylor SM, Cull DL, Kalbaugh C, et al. Comparison of interventional outcomes according to preoperative indication: a single center analysis of 2,240 limb revascularizations. *J Am Coll Surg* 2009;208:770–778.

Ubbink DT, Spincemaille GH, Jacobs MJ, et al. Prediction of imminent amputation in patients with non-reconstructible leg ischemia by means of microcirculatory investigations. *J Vasc Surg* 1999;30:114–121.

CHAPTER 9 ■ Buerger's Disease (Thromboangiitis Obliterans)

Shane Parmer and Marc E. Mitchell

Buerger's disease (thromboangiitis obliterans) is a nonatherosclerotic inflammatory vasculitis of small- and medium-sized arteries, veins, and nerves of the upper and lower extremities. Most commonly noted among young male smokers, recently the disease has been increasing in prevalence in women. Although the classic patient is a heavy smoker, there may be an association with passive exposure to smoke. Patients typically present with distal digital ischemia involving the lower extremities often requiring amputation. Presentations involving multiple extremities and venous involvement are not uncommon.

Though the etiology of Buerger's disease remains elusive, a very strong association with tobacco use has been well documented. Other causal factors have been postulated, but none demonstrate as strong an association as smoking. Buerger's disease tends to be a chronic and progressive process, with limited long-term treatment successes in the absence of smoking cessation. Despite its relatively dismal prognosis, those afflicted with Buerger's disease have normal life expectancies.

The pathologic entity that later became known as Buerger's disease was originally described in a single patient in 1879 by the Austrian surgeon Felix von Winiwarter. Von Winiwarter described a case of presenile spontaneous gangrene, which he believed to be due to intimal proliferation he called "endarteritis obliterans." It was not until 1908 that Leo Buerger, a New York surgeon, reported the clinical and pathological characteristics in 11 cases of the disease that would eventually bear his name. Buerger described the highly cellular nature of the thrombus and perivascular inflammation that would prompt him to suggest the term "thromboangiitis obliterans."

EPIDEMIOLOGY

Buerger's disease occurs throughout the world, though it is more prevalent in Asian and Mediterranean populations. Black populations are only rarely affected. Buerger's disease was once thought to only occur in men typically below 45 years of age, with historical data demonstrating only 1 to 2% of all Buerger patients to be women. More recent series have revealed a notable increase in the number of women affected, with 8 to 23% of Buerger patients being women. The exact reason for this change is uncertain, although there has been a significant increase in the use of tobacco by women over the past several decades.

Furthermore, a substantial decline in the prevalence of Buerger's disease has also been noted over the past few decades, in both the United States and Japan. A Mayo clinic series noted that despite an increase in patient enrollment overall, the rate of Buerger's disease steadily decreased from 104 per 100,000 in 1947 to only 13 cases per 100,000 in 1986. In Japan, Matsushita et al. have noted a similar trend. In a review of their extensive national registry of Buerger patients from 1989 to 1996, they noted that 46 new cases were diagnosed between 1985 and 1989, while during the period between 1990 and 1996, only 12 new cases were diagnosed. This decline likely represents refinements in the diagnosis of Buerger's disease with the widespread use of angiography, though other causative factors may exist, including the general trend toward decreased use of tobacco.

ETIOLOGY

Although the cause of Buerger's disease remains unknown, there is a clear and well-established association between Buerger's disease and tobacco exposure. In fact, many experts believe that nonexposure to tobacco (smoking or chewing) effectively excludes the diagnosis of Buerger's disease. Even passive exposure to tobacco may trigger disease activity and progression. In keeping with this history, a number of patients with Buerger's disease have poor oral hygiene and periodontal infections typically with anaerobic bacteria.

The exact mechanism by which tobacco causes Buerger's disease is not known. There is some suggestion that tobacco use may damage the vascular endothelium with subsequent development of autoantibodies to the endothelium. In addition, deposition of autoantibodies, complement C3, and immune complexes have been demonstrated within vessel walls of patients with Buerger's disease, as have T-lymphocytes exhibiting cellular sensitivity to type II and type III collagens, further suggesting an immune-mediated pathogenesis. Buerger's disease has also been linked to exposures to other substances including arsenic, cocaine, and cannabis, though the exact nature of these associations remains uncertain. The prothrombin gene mutation 20210 and the presence of anticardiolipin antibodies are associated with an increased risk of the disease. Thromboangiitis obliterans patients with high anticardiolipin antibody titers tend to be younger and are thought to be at an increased risk for major amputation.

CLINICAL PRESENTATION

Buerger's disease patients typically tend to be male, between 20 and 45 years of age at the time of onset. Though previously thought to be uncommon, women are increasingly being diagnosed. Exposure to tobacco products is universal, with most being heavy smokers but chewing exposure to tobacco as well as marijuana use has been reported. Patients typically present with evidence of arterial insufficiency affecting the extremities. Though the clinical presentation can vary depending on the severity of disease, a review of three large clinical series (Table 9.1) concludes that claudication, rest pain, and ulceration are often the initial manifestations of this disease. Disease

TABLE 9.1

CLINICAL CHARACTERISTICS OF PATIENTS WITH BUERGER'S DISEASE IN LARGE CLINICAL SERIES

	Olin et al.	Sasaki et al.	Shionoya
Demographic data			
Mean age at presentation (years)	42	40	36
Gender			
Male (%)	77	91	98
Female (%)	23	9	2
Clinical presentation			
Raynaud's phenomenon (%)	44	—	37
Claudication (%)x	62	38	31
Rest pain (%)	81	24	16
Gangrene or ulceration (%)	76	45	18–72
Superficial thrombophlebitis (%)	38	16	3–43
Upper extremity involvement (%)	54	25	90

(Data compiled from Olin JW, Young JR, Graor RA, et al. The changing clinical spectrum of thromboangiitis obliterans (Buerger's disease). *Circulation* 1990;82:IV3; Sasaki S, Sakuma M, Kunihora J, et al. Current trends in thromboangiitis obliterans (Buerger's disease) in women. *Am J Surg* 1999;177:316; Shionoya S. Buerger's disease (thromboangiitis obliterans). *Vasc Surg* 1999;1:235.)

begins in the small vessels, resulting in symptoms of distal ischemia. In fact, claudication is most commonly seen in the foot and instep as compared to the classic calf claudication seen in patients with peripheral arterial disease. Ulceration is also a common initial presenting symptom, with ischemia involving the distal tip of the effected digit. Proximal disease progression or the development of superinfection are typical scenarios.

In contrast to atherosclerotic arterial disease, the upper extremities are often involved in Buerger's disease. Involvement of multiple limbs is also a frequent finding. Shionoya evaluated 255 patients with Buerger's disease seen over 12 years, and found that more than 84% of patients had involvement of three or four extremities and no cases had single extremity involvement. Venous involvement is highly variable and may precede arterial manifestations in a minority of patients, with migratory phlebitis being the most common presentation.

CLINICAL COURSE

Although Buerger's disease typically presents with distal manifestations, proximal progression is the rule in the face of continued exposure to tobacco. Abstinence from all tobacco products ensures a benign course. Amputation may often be required, occurring in up to 25% of affected patients. Although Buerger's disease is primarily localized to the extremities, in isolated cases visceral, coronary, and cerebral thromboangiitis have been described and are more often associated with fatal outcomes. Although previously considered to have a normal prognosis following tobacco cessations recent retrospective data analysis by Cooper et al. from the Mayo Clinic have suggested that Buerger patients have higher risk for dying compared to the average US population. In this series, the risk of amputation continues in ongoing smokers up to a median of 15 years after initial diagnosis. The risk of amputation in previous smokers is eliminated by 8 years after smoking cessation.

DIAGNOSIS

The diagnosis of Buerger's disease is based principally on clinical findings. Five clinical criteria have been proposed by Shionoya to diagnose the presence of Buerger's disease: (a) smoking history, (b) onset before the age of 50 years, (c) infrapopliteal arterial occlusive disease, (d) either upper or lower limb involvement or phlebitis migrans, and (e) the absence of atherosclerotic risk factors other than smoking. Patients with all five clinical criteria in the appropriate clinical setting are highly likely to have Buerger's disease. The presence of ischemic heart disease, cerebrovascular disease, hypercoagulable states, or collagen vascular disease argues against the diagnosis of Buerger's disease.

CT angiography may be used initially for the evaluation of patients with Buerger's disease, provides for superior resolution at the level of the foot and helps exclude proximal atherosclerotic and nonatherosclerotic causes of distal disease. MR angiography although useful as an initial screening strategy may not provide adequate detail at the level of the foot. If the diagnosis of Buerger's disease is entertained, dedicated imaging of the pedal vasculature as a separate station may be required.

The use of routine x-ray contrast angiography in Buerger's disease has helped refine its diagnosis and appreciate the fact that no finding is pathognomonic. Typical findings however include severe segmental occlusive disease involving the distal lower- and upper-extremity vessels. Proximal involvement of iliac and femoral vessels occurs in approximately 10% and usually only in advanced cases. Multiple focal areas of stenosis are noted bilaterally with areas of normal appearing intervening artery. Collaterals are abundant and often described as "corkscrew" or "tree-root" in appearance (Fig. 9.1). More distally, the vessels appear attenuated and may have abrupt occlusion. There should be no evidence of aneurysms or atherosclerosis that may lead to distal emboli.

Laboratory data play a limited role in diagnosing Buerger's disease, as there are no consistently elevated serologic or immunologic markers. Other vasculopathies and hypercoagulopathic states should be ruled out by appropriate serologic and coagulation profiles. Biopsy and histologic evaluation have a limited role in the diagnosis of Buerger's disease. When available, typical findings include a highly inflammatory thrombus in both the arteries and veins, inflammation of all three cell layers of the arterial wall and adjacent veins, and preservation of the integrity of the internal elastic lamina. More advanced, chronic cases will demonstrate extensive fibrosis of the vessel and perivascular areas.

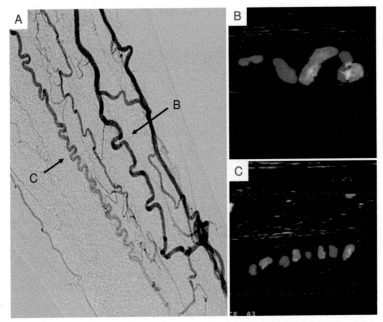

FIGURE 9-1. A: Digital subtraction angiography shows corkscrew collaterals around the area of occlusions in the right lower leg. Continuous-wave Doppler ultrasound shows corkscrew collaterals as color Doppler flows of a snake sign [A (*arrow B*), and **B**] and a dot sign [A (*arrow* C) and **C**]. (From Fujii Y, Nishioka K, Yoshizumi M, et al. Corkscrew collaterals in thromboangiitis obliterans (Buerger disease). *Circulation* 2007;116:e539–e540, with permission.) (See color insert.)

GENERAL TREATMENT

The cornerstone to any treatment of Buerger's disease is strict abstinence from smoking tobacco and exposure to all tobacco-containing products. Without that commitment from the patient, all therapies are destined to fail. Even exposure to passive smoke and smokeless tobacco must be avoided as they may lead to continued active disease and this includes nicotine containing cessation products. Smoking cessation alone may result in disease regression. In a large series from the Cleveland Clinic, 89 patients were followed, 43 of whom (48%) stopped smoking. Of those who stopped smoking only two (5%) required major amputation, while 22 (42%) of those who continued to smoke had amputations due to disease progression. These results were echoed in a recent retrospective review of 850 patients performed by Sasaki et al. They noted that failure of abstinence from smoking resulted in significantly higher rates of ulcer formation (42% vs. 58%, $P < 0.005$) and amputation (21% vs. 42%, $P < 0.0001$). Every effort should be made to encourage patients to stop smoking. Counseling or inpatient psychiatric support may be required in particularly difficult cases. Measuring urinary nicotine and cotinine in patients who continue to have active disease despite claims of tobacco cessation is often helpful. Tobacco cessation counseling including the use of pharmacologic therapy is very helpful (Varnecline and Bupropion).

In addition to smoking cessation, patients should be educated to avoid injury to the distal upper and lower extremities. Protective footwear should be used to prevent pressure injuries to the heels and soles. Avoidance of cold environments and medications that may lead to vasoconstriction is recommended. Once injury occurs, even if minor, aggressive treatment to prevent wound progression and infection should be undertaken.

MEDICAL THERAPY

Analgesics

Control of the disabling ischemic pain of Buerger's disease can be a challenge, often requiring narcotic analgesics until disease progression can be controlled by smoking cessation. In patients with severe recalcitrant ischemic pain, epidural analgesia may provide relief of pain, allowing these patients the ability to elevate the involved extremity, permitting improved healing as edema improves. In addition, the response to epidural analgesia can often provide insight into how the patient may respond to sympathectomy should the disease persist.

The use of spinal cord stimulators has been reported for severe limb ischemia. Although only a few patients with Buerger's disease were included in these studies, this modality seems to relieve pain and improve circulation in the affected dermatomes. The end result is improved pain control, wound healing, and limb salvage.

Immunosuppression

Several studies have suggested an autoimmune etiology of Buerger's disease. Though the use of corticosteroids has never been shown to be of therapeutic benefit except in care reports, recent data have shown a role for immunosuppression with cyclophosphamide. In a relatively small, nonrandomized trial, Saha et al. demonstrated that 8 weeks of immunosuppression using cyclophosphamide resulted in marked improvement in claudication and rest pain. In addition, significant improvements were noted in ulcer healing. The exact mechanism by which these clinical improvements occurred is uncertain as there were no changes in objective measurements, including angiographic findings, pulse volume recordings, or skin temperature measurements. Despite this, there were significant decreases in inflammatory cells within the vessel walls and possibly autoantibody formation, thus preventing further immune-mediated injury. The use of immunosuppressants is not recommended currently in Buerger's disease.

Prostaglandin Therapy and Adjunctive Antiplatelet Treatment

Although there are few data to suggest that the routine use of aspirin provides any significant therapeutic benefit in patients with Buerger's disease, because of its low cost and favorable side-effect profile, it is often used. Prostaglandins are also known to be potent inhibitors of platelet aggregations as well as providing significant vasodilation. In a prospective, randomized double-blind trial of 152 patients with Buerger's disease, Fiessinger and Schafer compared iloprost, a stable prostaglandin analogue, with low-dose aspirin. Patients received either daily 6-hour intravenous infusions of iloprost or low-dose aspirin for 28 days. At the conclusion of the study, 85% of the iloprost-treated patients had pain relief or healing of ischemic ulcers, compared to only 28% of those receiving aspirin. Of those who received iloprost, 35% had complete ulcer healing versus only 13% in the aspirin group. In addition to the therapeutic benefit of iloprost being persistent for 6 months post treatment, the amputation rate at 6 months was significantly less in the iloprost group (6%) versus the aspirin group (18%). Unfortunately, oral iloprost has not been demonstrated be as effective, thus obligating patients to intravenous therapy.

Thrombolytic Therapy

The role of thrombolytic therapy in the treatment of Buerger's disease is controversial and is currently on recommended. However, in the setting of an acute presentation due to definitive thrombosis, thrombolytics may provide some benefit. In a series of 11 Buerger patients treated for acute onset of limb ischemia, 58% underwent successful thrombolysis with streptokinase, resulting in improvement of ischemic symptoms, limb salvage, or a less extensive amputation. As is typical with thrombolytic therapy, those who responded most favorably were those who presented more acutely.

Cell Transplantation and Gene Therapy Approaches

In the past decade there has been an increase in the interest in stem cell and gene therapy for the treatment of vascular diseases. Gene therapy approaches to deliver growth factor approaches in general have not been successful, with early trials including a few patients with Buerger's disease. Recent data with bone marrow derived mononuclear cells have suggested promise although these data are yet to be replicated in other centers.

SURGICAL THERAPY

Revascularization

In light of the distal, diffuse and segmental nature of Buerger's disease surgical revascularization is not typically feasible. In the rare event that a distal target vessel is available, attempts at revascularization can be of benefit, provided the patient has stopped smoking. Because of the distal nature of the disease, thromboendarterectomy has no role and is not used. The role of endovascular therapies will also likely be limited for similar reasons. When bypass is possible, autogenous vein is the conduit of choice. Because of the frequent involvement of venous structures, the greater saphenous and lesser saphenous may be diseased. In that instance, any available vein should be used. In a review of their experience, Sasajima et al. concluded that arterial bypass is effective with reasonable long-term patency when combined with smoking cessation. They performed 71 autogenous vein bypasses for claudication (41%) or ischemia and gangrene (59%). Their primary and secondary patency rates at 5 years were 49 and 63%, respectively, achieving an 85% limb salvage rate. They noted that patients who continued to smoke had significantly worse patency rates 35% versus 67% in nonsmokers.

Sympathectomy

Historically, sympathetic denervation was performed for severe atherosclerotic arterial occlusive disease prior to the development of advanced vascular reconstructive techniques. As there are often no reconstructive options in patients with Buerger's disease, sympathectomy remains a viable treatment alternative for patients with refractory pain and ischemia despite maximal medical therapy. The goal of sympathetic denervation is to eliminate the vasoconstrictor tone in the region of concern. Following sympathectomy, blood flow increases preferentially to the cutaneous vascular beds, while no significant change is noted in the blood flow to the muscles. Because of this phenomenon, there is no role for sympathectomy in patients with claudication, and this procedure should be reserved for those who have superficial ulcerations or vasospastic manifestations. Once performed, the effects may only last for a few months to 1 to 2 years. This, however, may be sufficient time to allow for wound healing.

For upper-extremity disease, a thoracic sympathectomy should be performed by dividing T2, T3, and the lower half of the stellate ganglion. This is classically performed through either an open axillary or a supraclavicular approach. Thoracoscopic sympathectomy is now considered the approach of choice.

In a series of nonrandomized patients, Komori et al. reported less operative blood loss, less pain, fewer preoperative complications, and a shorter hospital stay for patients undergoing thoracoscopic versus open thoracic sympathectomy. The safety and efficacy of thoracoscopic sympathectomy has been further verified in a recent study of 15 patients that demonstrated short hospital stays, few complications, and clinical benefit and should be the preference if warranted. Lumbar sympathectomy is the preferred approach for patients with lower extremity ischemia. An anterior approach is used, with entry into the retroperitoneal space and division of L2-L4 sympathetic ganglia. When care is taken complications are uncommon for either thoracic or lumbar sympathectomy. Of most concern would be the development of a Horner's syndrome or postsympathectomy neuralgia for the thoracic approach and retrograde ejaculation after lumbar sympathectomy. Endoscopic approaches for lumbar sympathectomy have not been evaluated in Buerger's disease.

Amputation

If disease is detected early and the patient strictly avoids exposure to tobacco products, outcomes are favorable with little limb loss. However, in the face of advanced disease and continued smoking, a significant number of patients will require minor or major amputation. In the Cleveland Clinic experience, amputations were rarely required for those patients

TABLE 9.2

DISTRIBUTION OF AMPUTATIONS REQUIRED IN 24 PATIENTS WITH BUERGER'S DISEASE

Finger	6 (15%)
Toe	13 (33%)
Transmetatarsal	4 (10%)
Below knee	14 (36%)
Above knee	2 (5%)

(Adapted from Olin JW, Young JR, Graor RA, et al. The changing clinical spectrum of thromboangiitis obliterans (Buerger's disease). *Circulation* 1990;82:IV3.)

who stopped smoking. Those who did not adhere to smoking cessation frequently required amputation. Although most amputations were distal, more than 40% of patients required major amputations (Table 9.2). In the more recent Mayo Clinic retrospective analysis by Cooper et al., the risk of any amputation was 25% at 5 and 38% at 10 years while the risk of major amputation was 11% at 5 and 21% at 10 years.

CONCLUSION

Buerger's disease is a nonatherosclerotic inflammatory vasculitis of small- and medium-sized arteries, veins, and nerves of the upper and lower extremities that occurs most commonly in young male smokers. The etiology is uncertain; however, there exists a strong association with the use of tobacco products. Although medical and surgical treatment options do exist, the mainstay of treatment is smoking cessation. Without complete abstinence from tobacco products, the prognosis for limb salvage is dismal.

PRACTICAL POINTS

- Buerger's disease (thromboangiitis obliterans) is a nonatherosclerotic inflammatory vasculitis of small- and medium-sized arteries, veins, and nerves of the upper and lower extremities.

- There is a well-established strong association between Buerger's disease and tobacco exposure (smoking and chewed).

- Venous involvement is highly variable and may precede arterial manifestations in a minority of patients, with migratory phlebitis being the most common presentation.

- Typical angiographic findings include severe segmental occlusive disease involving the distal lower- and upper-extremity vessels. Collaterals are abundant and often described as "corkscrew" or "tree-root" in angiography.

- The cornerstone to treatment of Buerger's disease is complete abstinence from smoking and exposure to all tobacco-containing products.

RECOMMENDED READING

Adar R, Papa MZ, Halpern Z, et al. Cellular sensitivity to collagen in thromboangiitis obliterans. *N Engl J Med* 1983;308:1113.

Buerger L. Thromboangiitis obliterans: a study of the vascular lesions leading to presenile spontaneous gangrene. *Am J Med Sci* 1908;136:567.

Campello Morer I, Capablo Liesa JL, Guelbenzu Morte S, et al. Thromboangiitis obliterans with cerebral involvement. *Neurologia* 1985;10:384.

Fiessinger JN, Schafer M. Trial of iloprost versus aspirin treatment for critical limb ischemia of thromboangiitis obliterans. The TAO Study. *Lancet* 1990;335:555.

Komori K, Kawasaki K, Okazaki J, et al. Thoracoscopic sympathectomy for Buerger's disease of the upper extremities. *J Vasc Surg* 1995;22(3):344–346.

Lie JT. Diagnostic histopathology of major systemic and pulmonary vasculitic syndromes. *Rheum Dis Clin North Am* 1990;16:269.

Marder VJ, Mellinghoff IK. Cocaine and Buerger disease: is there a pathogenetic association? *Arch Intern Med* 2000;160:2057.

Matoba S, Tatsumi T, Murohara T, et al. TACT Follow-up study investigators. Long-term clinical outcome after intramuscular implantation of bone marrow mononuclear cells (Therapeutic Angiogenesis by Cell Transplantation [TACT] trial) in patients with chronic limb ischemia. *Am Heart J* 2008;156(5):1010–1018.

Matsushita M, Shionoya S, Matsumoto T. Urinary cotinine measurement in patients with Buerger's disease—effects of active and passive smoking on the disease process. *J Vasc Surg* 1991;14:53.

Miyamoto K, Nishigami K, Nagaya N, et al. Unblinded pilot study of autologous transplantation of bone marrow mononuclear cells in patients with thromboangiitis obliterans. *Circulation* 2006;114(24):2679–2684. (Epub 2006 Dec 4.)

Olin JW. Thromboangiitis obliterans (Buerger's disease). *N Engl J Med* 2000;343:864.

Piazza G, Creager MA. Thromboangiitis obliterans. *Circulation* 2010;121(16):1858–1861 (Review).

Rutherford R, Shannon R. Lumbar sympathectomy: indications and technique. *Vasc Surg* 1999;1:874.

Saha K, Chabra N, Gulati SM. Treatment of patients with thromboangiitis obliterans with cyclophosphamide. *Angiology* 2001;52:399.

Sasajima T, Kudo Y, Dhaba M, et al. Role of Infra-inguinel bypass in Buerger's disease: an eighteen year experience. *Eur J Vasc Endovasc Surg* 1997;13(2):186–192.

Sasaki S, Sakuma M, Kunihara T, et al. Current trends in thromboangiitis obliterans (Buerger's disease) in women. *Am J Surg* 1999;177:316.

Sasaki S, Sakuma M, Yasuda K. Current status of thromboangiitis obliterans (Buerger's disease) in Japan. *Int J Cardiol* 2000;75(Suppl 1):S175.

Shionoya S. Buerger's disease (thromboangiitis obliterans). *Vasc Surg* 1999;1:235.

Shionoya S. Diagnostic criteria of Buerger's disease. *Int J Cardiol* 1998;66(Suppl 1):S243.

Swigris JJ, Olin JW, Mekhail NA. Implantable spinal cord stimulator to treat the ischemic manifestations of thromboangiitis obliterans (Buerger's disease). *J Vasc Surg* 1999;29:928.

Von Winiwarter F. Über eine eigenthumliche Form von Endarteritis und Endophlebitis mit Gangran des Fusses. *Arch Klin Chir* 1879;23:202.

CHAPTER 10 ■ Approach to and Management of Renovascular Disease

Quinn Capers IV, Joshua Joseph, and Debabrata Mukherjee

Renal artery stenosis (RAS) is a common cause of secondary hypertension, and the incidence appears to be rising because of increased atherosclerosis in an aging population. The prevalence of atherosclerotic RAS increases with age, presence of diabetes, peripheral arterial disease, coronary artery disease, hypertension, and dyslipidemia. The most common cause is atherosclerosis, which is the etiology in over 90% of cases, that is, atherosclerotic renal artery stenosis (ARAS). Fibromuscular dysplasia (FMD) accounts for approximately 10% of cases of RAS and is typically seen in young and middle-aged females. RAS may cause renal insufficiency, uncontrolled hypertension, and recurrent congestive heart failure and "flash" pulmonary edema and is associated with increased cardiovascular morbidity and mortality. There have been significant improvements in noninvasive detection of RAS and revascularization techniques have evolved, such that most renal artery (RA) revascularization is now performed percutaneously. Patients with ARAS should also be treated with the same measures that reduce cardiovascular risk in patients with atherosclerosis in any location: statins or other lipid-lowering drugs, drugs that inhibit the renin-angiotensin system, antiplatelet drugs, tobacco avoidance, and regular physical activity, among other treatments.

ETIOLOGY

ARAS is by far the most common form of RAS (~90%). ARAS occurs when atherosclerotic plaque deposition in the renal arteries results in a critical narrowing, restricting blood flow to the renal parenchyma. Most commonly located at the ostia, it is often associated with significant atheromatous disease of the abdominal aorta and is thought to result from "creeping" of atherosclerotic material from the aortic wall into the renal arteries. This predilection for the ostia is an important consideration for the interventionalist when placing stents. A proper technique for stent placement in the case of atherosclerotic RAS at the ostium is to position the stent so that it protrudes very slightly into the aorta. Failure to do so will result in incomplete coverage and scaffolding of the offending plaque.

FMD is a nonatherosclerotic, noninflammatory arterial disease of the musculature of the arterial wall leading to stenosis of small- and medium-sized vessels in the medial to distal segments. FMD most commonly affects the renal and carotid arteries but has been shown to affect arteries throughout the body. It causes 10 to 20% of all RA stenoses and is found in about 1 to 2% of hypertensive patients. FMD is more than four times more common in women and is usually diagnosed from the ages of

15 to 50, although there is a male predominance of intimal FMD. The exact cause of the condition is unknown with a cadre of hormonal, genetic, and environmental factors postulated. Similar to atherosclerosis, there is a proven association with smoking and hypertension. The disease is also more common in first-degree relatives of patients with FMD and patients with angiotensin-converting enzyme allele ACE-I, suggesting a possible genetic link.

Other rarer causes of RAS are arteritis (Takayasu's disease, polyarteritis nodosa, Kawasaki's disease, other systemic vasculitides), renal artery aneurysm (RAA), extrinsic compression (neoplasm, Wilms' tumor, neuroblastoma), syndromic (neurofibromatosis, tuberous sclerosis, Williams' syndrome, Marfan's syndrome), radiation induced, and fibrous bands.

Prevalence of ARAS

Although, incidentally discovered RAS is quite common, renovascular hypertension is the etiology in only 1 to 5% of all patients with hypertension. The presence of anatomic RAS does not necessarily establish that the hypertension or renal failure is caused by the RAS. Essential (primary) hypertension may exist for years prior to the development of atherosclerotic RAS later in life. Several series have assessed the prevalence of renovascular disease in patients who have atherosclerotic disease elsewhere. High-grade bilateral RA disease was present in approximately 5 to 15% of patients in series examining patients with other manifestations of disease. A significant proportion (greater than 20%) of patients with lower extremity peripheral arterial disease may have significant RAS. RA disease is detected incidentally at the time of cardiac catheterization in 10 to 30% of patients, and approximately 50% of theses patients may have greater than 50% stenosis.

CLINICAL FEATURES

More than 90% of cases of RAS are atherosclerotic in nature and involve the ostium and the proximal portion of the main RA with plaque extending into the perirenal aorta. As opposed to atherosclerotic RAS, FMD often affects the distal two thirds of the main RA and the RA branches. Medial fibroplasia is the most common type of FMD and has a characteristic beaded angiographic appearance.

RAS may be associated with any degree of hypertension and is present in a third of patients with malignant or uncontrolled hypertension despite multiple antihypertensive agents. Dustan also noted that as many as 50% of patients with RAS may actually have normal blood pressure (BP). RAS may present with chronic renal insufficiency or end-stage renal failure with or without hypertension with a bland urinary sediment and usually non–nephrotic-range proteinuria. Patients with bilateral RAS or stenosis of an artery to a solitary functioning kidney may present with acute renal failure after administration of an angiotensin-converting enzyme inhibitor (ACEI) or angiotensin receptor blocker (ARB). Table 10.1 enumerates clinical clues suggestive of RAS.

TABLE 10.1

CLINICAL CLUES SUGGESTIVE OF RAS

- Young or middle-aged females with severe hypertension and no family history (FMD)
- Uncontrolled hypertension despite at least three antihypertensive agents in adequate doses (regimen includes a diuretic)
- Worsening BP control in compliant, long-standing hypertensive patient
- Acute renal failure or elevation in creatinine with ACEIs or ARBs
- Chronic renal insufficiency with mild proteinuria and bland urinary sediment
- Recurrent flash pulmonary edema
- >1.5-cm difference in renal sizes
- Epigastric bruit
- Hypertension and concomitant peripheral arterial disease
- Severe hypertensive retinopathy

Chronically reduced blood flow to the kidney may lead to renal atrophy and diminished glomerular filtration rate (GFR). Severe RAS has been identified in 15 to 25% of patients with end-stage renal failure requiring hemodialysis. While not proof of a cause and effect relationship, RAS is considered an important reversible cause of renal failure. It has been reported that percutaneous RA stenting in selected dialysis patients can salvage renal function and obviate the need for dialysis.

The most common cause of death in patients with ARAS is ischemic heart disease and its complications. This is true of patients with atherosclerosis in any location of the body. However, patients with ARAS carry the additional vascular burdens of severe hypertension; supraphysiologic levels of the proatherogenic, prothrombotic vasoconstrictor angiotensin II; and possibly diminished renal function with its cardiovascular consequences. The presence of RAS is an independent risk factor for cardiovascular and all-cause mortality, and a "dose-dependent" effect has been described, with a graded increase in mortality in patients with severe compared to moderate narrowing of the renal arteries.

Pathophysiology of Hypertension

Preclinical studies for renovascular hypertension have helped us understand the pathophysiology of hypertension in RAS. The renin-angiotensin-aldosterone system plays a critical role in this scenario. In animal models, the two kidney–one clip (2_{Kidney}-1_{Clip}) model is considered the representative model for renin-mediated hypertension and is analogous to unilateral RAS clinically. The one kidney–one clip (1_{Kidney}-1_{Clip}) model of renovascular hypertension is a model for volume-mediated hypertension and is similar in pathophysiology to either bilateral RAS or RAS in a solitary functioning kidney clinically. The acute phases of both of these models are quite similar; however, different events occur in the late phase. In the 2_{Kidney}-1_{Clip} model (unilateral RAS), there is decreased renal blood flow to the kidneys that stimulates the production of renin. Renin cleaves the proenzyme angiotensinogen to form angiotensin I, and in the presence of angiotensin-converting enzyme, it is converted to angiotensin II. Angiotensin II elevates BP directly by causing systemic vasoconstriction, stimulates aldosterone secretion causing sodium reabsorption and potassium and hydrogen ion secretion in the cortical collecting duct, and diminishes glomerular filtration by decreasing glomerular capillary surface area and redistributing intrarenal blood flow. The salt and water retention related to excess aldosterone production is rapidly excreted by the contralateral (normal) kidney by pressure natriuresis in the 2_{Kidney}-1_{Clip} model. This produces a cycle of renin-dependent hypertension. In the 1_{Kidney}-1_{Clip} model of renovascular hypertension, there is a similar decrease in blood flow to the affected kidney(s), causing the production of renin and synthesis of angiotensin II and aldosterone, which causes salt and water retention. In this model without a normal kidney, pressure natriuresis does not occur. The increased aldosterone causes sodium and water retention and volume expansion, which suppresses plasma renin activity, thus changing from renin-mediated hypertension to one of volume-mediated hypertension. During this stage, administration of an ACEI or ARB does not decrease BP or change renal blood flow. Dietary restriction of sodium or administration of diuretics will convert the patient to a renin-mediated form of hypertension and restore sensitivity to ACEIs or ARBs, which then become effective antihypertensive agents. Renal insufficiency may be precipitated in patients when ACEIs/ARBs are administered to patients with bilateral RAS or RAS to a solitary kidney especially in the volume-contracted state.

Mechanism of ACEI/ARB-mediated Azotemia in RAS

Two potential mechanisms exist by which renal function may worsen with the use of ACEs/ARBs. One mechanism may occur with any antihypertensive agent when it lowers the critical perfusion pressure and affects renal perfusion. This mechanism has been validated by infusing sodium nitroprusside in patients with high-grade bilateral RAS, which led to worsening renal function. Below the critical perfusion pressure, which may vary with the degree of stenosis and among individuals, the urine output, renal blood flow, and GFR decline. They return to normal when the BP increases above the critical perfusion pressure. The second mechanism is related to the direct effects of blocking angiotensin II on intraglomerular perfusion pressures. Patients with high-grade bilateral RAS or RAS to a solitary kidney may be highly dependent on angiotensin II for glomerular filtration. Under these circumstances, the vasoconstrictive effect of angiotensin II on the efferent arteriole maintains normal transglomerular gradient, thus allowing glomerular filtration to remain normal despite markedly diminished blood flow. When an ACEI/ARB is given, the efferent arteriolar tone is decreased, leading to reduction in glomerular filtration. A similar clinical scenario may be seen in patients with decompensated heart failure who are sodium depleted.

Progression of ARAS. Knowledge of the natural history of ARAS is extremely important in the management of these patients. Most natural history studies reported in the literature are retrospective studies. The rates of progression ranged from 36 to 71%.

Angiographic Progression. In Schreiber's series, only 16% of patients went on to total occlusion over a mean follow-up of 52 months. However, the rate of progression to total occlusion occurred more frequently (39%) when there was greater than 75% stenosis on the initial renal arteriogram. Zierler et al. utilized renal duplex ultrasound to prospectively study anatomic progression of atherosclerotic renovascular disease. If the renal arteries were normal, only 8% progressed over 36 months. However, at 3 years, 48% of patients progressed from less than 60% stenosis to ≥60% stenosis. The renal arteries that progressed to occlusion all had ≥60% stenosis at the initial visit. Progression of RAS occurred at an average rate of 7% per year for all categories of baseline disease combined.

Renal Atrophy. The effect of RAS on kidney size has been well studied. Using duplex ultrasound, Caps and colleagues prospectively followed up 204 kidneys in 122 patients with known RAS for a mean of 33 months. The 2-year cumulative incidence of renal atrophy was 5.5, 11.7, and 20.8% in kidneys with a baseline RA disease classification of normal, less than 60% stenosis, and ≥60% stenosis ($P = 0.009$, log rank test), respectively.

Prognosis with RAS. The mere presence of atherosclerotic RAS, even prior to developing end-stage renal disease, portends a poor prognosis. Patient survival decreases as the severity of RAS increases with 2-year survival rates of 96% in patients with unilateral RAS, 74% in patients with bilateral RAS, and 47% in patients with stenosis or occlusion to a solitary functioning kidney. As the serum creatinine increases, the survival decreases in patients with atherosclerotic RAS. The 3-year probability of survival in one study was $92 \pm 4\%$ for patients with a serum creatinine less than 1.4 mg/dL, $74 \pm 8\%$ for patients with a serum creatinine of 1.5 to 1.9 mg/dL, and $51 \pm 8\%$ for patients with a serum creatinine ≥ 2.0 mg/dL.

DIAGNOSIS

The decision to evaluate patients for RAS should be based on the clinical likelihood of the individual patient having RAS. The clinical clues listed in Table 10.1 will help identify individuals with high pretest likelihood of RAS. Although a systolic abdominal bruit is common and nonspecific, the presence of a systolic/diastolic bruit especially over the epigastrium may point to underlying RA disease, especially in individuals with FMD. The presence of a diastolic component to the bruit indicates that the degree of narrowing of the artery is severe since there is continued flow during diastole. Once having made the decision to screen an individual for RAS, there are multiple options available as listed below. The screening test of choice depends on the equipment and expertise that are available at a given institution. In experienced hands, duplex ultrasonography, computed tomographic angiography (CTA), and MRA are all excellent diagnostic tests.

Anatomic Considerations

The renal arteries arise just below the SMA. The right RA arises anterolaterally, while the left RA arises posterolaterally. The right RA lies behind the IVC. Accessory renal arteries supplying the poles of the kidneys and duplicated main renal arteries are seen in 10 to 30% of individuals. The left renal vein is a large structure that lies between the SMA and the aorta, usually crosses the aorta anteriorly and demonstrates phasic flow (varies with respiration). The RA is a low-resistance vascular bed and demonstrates flow in both systole and diastole under normal circumstances.

Duplex Ultrasound

Ultrasonography is an ideal imaging modality in patients with RAS. In experienced centers, it can predict the presence or absence of RAS with a high degree of accuracy, identify patients likely to achieve a beneficial response after revascularization (PTA, stent, surgery), follow the course of disease and kidney size in patients followed medically, and follow patients for the presence of restenosis after PTA and stent implantation. Duplex ultrasound is associated with a steep learning curve. It becomes difficult in obese patients and those with excess bowel gas. It is important to visualize the entire RA from the origin to the kidney parenchyma. This is accomplished by scanning from both an anterior approach and an oblique approach. By performing the duplex in this fashion, one is assured of detecting RAS from both atherosclerosis and FMD. The sensitivity of identifying accessory renal arteries is only approximately 60 to 70%.

Diagnostic Criteria for RAS

Blood flow in the renal arteries normally demonstrates a low resistance pattern (broad systolic waveforms and forward flow during diastole). Peak systolic velocity (PSV) ranges from 75 to 125 cm/s in adults and children. The principal criterion for the diagnosis of RAS is Doppler flow based. The most universally accepted velocity criteria for significant RAS (70% stenosis) are (a) PSV > 200 cm/s measured in the area of stenosis and/or (b) Renal-aortic ratio ≥ 3.5. If the end-diastolic velocity is ≥150 cm/s, the stenosis is usually greater than 80%. Table 10.2 lists a well-accepted algorithm using these criteria.

Renal Resistive Index

A renal resistive index (RRI) greater than 80 may help identify patients with intrinsic renal disease who may not benefit from percutaneous revascularization.

TABLE 10.2

DUPLEX VELOCITY AND RATIO CRITERIA TO ASSESS HEMODYNAMIC SIGNIFICANCE

Stenosis (%)	Peak Systolic Velocity	Peak Diastolic Velocity	Renal artery/ Aorta Ratio
0–50	<200 cm/s	<100 cm/s.	<3.5
50–70	>200	<100 cm/s	>3.5
>70	>200	>100	>3.5

The RRI is determined by measuring the PSV (V_{max}) and end-diastolic velocities (V_{min}) in cm/s from an intrarenal artery (usually the cortical vessels). RRI = [1 − ($V_{min} \div V_{max}$)] × 100. The measurements are obtained from the upper, middle, and the lower third of each kidney and the measurements averaged.

In 2008, De Bruyne et al. performed a comparison of invasive angiography with pressure measurements using the pressure wire technique versus duplex ultrasound. They found that when using the Pd/Pa ratio of 0.90 (see below) as the standard for significant RAS, the classic criteria for hemodynamic significance using duplex ultrasound, PSV greater than 180 cm/s, end-diastolic velocity greater than 90 cm/s, and renal-to-aortic velocity ratio greater than 3.5 were 45, 77, and 79% accurate, respectively. The respective false-positive rates of 55, 11, and 15% for these criteria indicate the possibility of an overestimation of the severity of RAS by duplex ultrasound. They proposed new cutoff values of PSV greater than 318 cm/s, end-diastolic velocity greater than 73 cm/s, and renal-to-aortic velocity ratio greater than 3.74. Overall, renal arterial duplex scanning is a very useful tool for establishing the diagnosis of severe RAS and is useful for following patients after RA stenting to detect restenosis.

Captopril Renal Scans

Captopril renal scanning (CRS) is an indirect noninvasive method for detecting RAS. It relies on a decrease in renal blood flow and GFR after the administration of an ACEI. Although this test has historically been popular, its sensitivity and specificity decline substantially in patients with bilateral disease, those with disease to a solitary functioning kidney, or patients with significant azotemia (serum creatinine greater than 2.0 mg/dL). Since other imaging modalities are so accurate, CRS should not be used as an initial screening test for diagnosing RAS, even among patients with high clinical likelihood of disease.

Computed Tomographic Angiography

CTA provides excellent anatomical images of the renal arteries but does not provide physiological information such as blood flow velocities. Disadvantages include exposure to ionizing radiation and potentially nephrotoxic iodinated contrast. In selected patients, when RA duplex scanning is not available, or when the patients have been treated with stainless steel stents, CTA is an excellent choice for the detection of RAS or in-stent restenosis. CTA is also excellent in the diagnosis of FMD.

Magnetic Resonance Angiography

Contrast-enhanced Magnetic Resonance Angiography (MRA) provides high-resolution 3D data sets (up to 0.9 × 9.9 × 0.9 mm) in a single breath hold, which permits multiplane reformatting of the renal arteries. Such an exam has been shown to have a sensitivity and specificity equal to digital subtraction angiography. MRA approaches are valuable in atherosclerotic RAS as they provide visualization of the aorta and peripheral vasculature as well in one exam. MRA can accurately identify accessory renal arteries, provide for an assessment of renal perfusion and renal sizes, and even provide for an assessment of GFR. In light of concerns regarding nephrogenic systemic fibrosis, a variety of noncontrast techniques are being evaluated for the assessment of RAS. These approaches include bright-blood techniques such as 3D-balanced SSFP (steady-state free precession) and dark-blood 3D-SPACE (see Chapter 4 for details). Both these could provide delineation of the renal arteries, but the value of these approaches in the diagnosis of RAS continues to evolve.

Contrast Angiography

Contrast angiography remains the gold standard for diagnosing RAS and is widely available. There is a risk of worsening renal function related to contrast agent or atheroemboli. In individuals with marked renal insufficiency, either carbon dioxide or gadolinium may be used for digital subtraction aortography in lieu of an iodinated contrast agent. Selective renal angiography is usually performed as a prelude to RA revascularization. Other indications for renal angiography include evaluating prospective renal donors to define arterial supply and assessing tumor vascularity. An abdominal aortogram is initially performed with a straight pigtail catheter (Fig. 10.1) placed at the level of the L1 vertebra. We typically use DSA and inject a

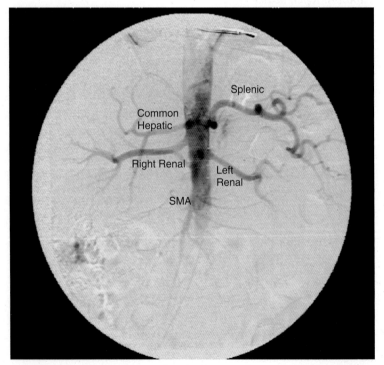

FIGURE 10-1.   Anteroposterior abdominal aortogram to visualize the mesenteric and renal arteries. (SMA, superior mesenteric artery)

total of 10 mL of contrast for abdominal aortogram (20 mL/s and 0.5 s injection). This allows visualization of the origin of the main renal arteries that typically arise at the L1/L2 level and accessory renal arteries if present. The AP abdominal aortogram is a good scout shot, useful to get orientation of the renal ostium but can miss true focal ostial stenosis as renal ostia come off a few degrees posterior. Selective RA angiograms can usually be performed using a Judkins Right (JR4) catheter by placing the catheter adjacent to the ostium without actually intubating it ("no touch technique") to minimize atheroembolization. However, arteries with unusual or angulated takeoffs may need to be cannulated with an SOS or a Cobra catheter. For renal arteries with a downward takeoff, a LIMA catheter may be used. Selective renal angiograms are performed with 3 to 4 mL of contrast hand injected using DSA in an ipsilateral oblique projection (RAO 20 to 30 degrees for right RA, etc.). One should stay on cine for delayed imaging to visualize the nephrogram and ascertain the renal size. If there is significant angiographic stenosis of the RA, a pressure gradient should be measured prior to consideration of revascularization. A systolic gradient more than 15 to 20 mm Hg suggests hemodynamically significant stenosis. A clinical benefit of using a 5-French SOS catheter for selective cannulation is that by withdrawing the catheter slightly, the tip advances beyond the proximal portion of the RA and a gradient can be measured directly. Renal angiograms can be performed from either the brachial or the femoral approach, although the femoral approach is preferred by most operators. The brachial approach may be the preferred approach in very steep downward takeoff of the renal arteries particularly if intervention is planned. Techniques to minimize embolization and other complications during renal angiogram include using a 5-French system and reforming the SOS catheter in the suprarenal aorta to minimize scraping of the renal arteries.

Renal Arteriography at the Time of Cardiac Catheterization

Some clinicians perform an aortogram on the "way out" after performing a cardiac catheterization. We strongly discourage such *routine* "drive-by angiography" at the time of cardiac catheterization. It adds time, contrast, and risk to the procedure. In addition, the quality of the image is often suboptimal. Knowing that the patient has RAS adds nothing to the patients overall management other than to tempt the angiographer to stent this RA lesion in the absence of accepted clinical indications ("oculostenotic reflex"). If the patient has a clear-cut indication for intervention (inability to control the BP with a good medical regimen, progressive renal failure, or recurrent episodes of congestive heart failure), and the clinician is prepared to perform angioplasty and stenting at a later date should significant RAS be discovered, then an aortogram at the time of cardiac catheterization is not unreasonable. The 2006 Science Advisory statement of the AHA/ACC concludes that "it is reasonable to perform screening renal arteriography at the time of cardiac catheterization in patients at increased risk for ARAS who are candidates for revascularization as defined in the ACC/AHA peripheral arterial disease management guideline document."

Pressure Wire Evaluation

In 2006, De Bruyne et al. described a new criterion for the invasive diagnosis of hemodynamically significant RAS. During renal arteriography, these investigators advanced guidewire across the stenosis with a lumen to measure pressure and compared the mean arterial pressure distal to the lesion (Pd) to the mean arterial pressure proximal to the lesion (Pa). Utilizing a technique that had previously been refined in coronary arteries, they showed that a Pd/Pa ratio less than 0.90 was associated with increased plasma renin activity in humans. The invasive nature of catheter angiography and pressure gradient measurements makes them unsuitable for a screening. However, in a patient in whom revascularization is indicated, invasive evaluation is cost-efficient and time efficient; once confirmation is obtained that an intervention is warranted, the intervention can be performed in the same setting.

In the current health care environment where cost containment is an ever present concern, several factors should be considered in the choice of a screening test for RAS. The accuracy of the screening test, local expertise in performing and interpreting the test, and the cost of the test are all important considerations. If the local expertise in RA duplex scanning is adequate, it is reasonable to start with this test unless the individual is obese, dyspneic, or has heavy arterial calcifications. In such cases, MRA may be appropriate. If an individual with indications for RA screening is scheduled for cardiac catheterization, it is reasonable to perform renal angiography with or without pressure wire readings at the time of the cardiac procedure.

MANAGEMENT

Medical Therapy

In addition to consideration of revascularization, patients with RAS should be targeted for appropriate secondary prevention for cardiovascular events as they are at high risk. Optimal therapy in these patients includes good BP control (ACEIs and/or ARBs are especially useful for patients with unilateral RAS). Cardiovascular risk factor reduction therapies should be instituted aggressively (use of antiplatelet and lipid-lowering therapy and β-blockers when indicated). Patients undergoing peripheral arterial and RA interventions have significantly improved outcomes if treated with appropriate evidence-based secondary preventive therapy.

Percutaneous Revascularization

The currently accepted indications for renal revascularization are listed in Table 10.3. Surgical revascularization is rarely performed except in the presence of abdominal aortic aneurysms, dissections, or aneurysm of the renal arteries. Angioplasty and stenting have become the revascularization modality of choice since they have demonstrated improvements in BP control in multiple trials and has been associated with attenuation of renal failure progression and preservation of renal size.

TABLE 10.3

CURRENT INDICATIONS FOR RA REVASCULARIZATION

- Percutaneous revascularization is indicated for patients with hemodynamically significant RAS and recurrent, unexplained congestive heart failure or sudden, unexplained pulmonary edema. (*Class I*, Level of Evidence: B)
- Percutaneous revascularization is reasonable for patients with hemodynamically significant RAS and accelerated hypertension, resistant hypertension, malignant hypertension, hypertension with an unexplained unilateral small kidney, and hypertension with intolerance to medication. (*Class IIa*, Level of Evidence: B)
- Percutaneous revascularization is reasonable for patients with RAS and progressive chronic kidney disease with bilateral RAS or a RAS to a solitary functioning kidney. (*Class IIa*, Level of Evidence: B)
- Percutaneous revascularization is reasonable for patients with hemodynamically significant RAS and unstable angina. (*Class IIa*, Level of Evidence: B)
- Percutaneous revascularization may be considered for treatment of an asymptomatic bilateral or solitary viable kidney with a hemodynamically significant RAS. (*Class IIb*, Level of Evidence: C)

Role for Percutaneous Renal Angioplasty

Percutaneous transluminal renal angioplasty (PTRA) alone is recommended in patients with FMD. Restenosis rates in this population are less than 15%. PTRA alone for the management of atherosclerotic disease is not recommended. Van Jaarsveld et al. conducted the DRASTIC trial, the largest trial to date comparing balloon angioplasty versus medical therapy for RAS. This was a prospective, randomized, multicenter trial of patients (N = 106) with greater than 50% stenosis of one or both renal arteries, creatinine of ≤ 2.3 mg/dL, diastolic BP ≥ 95 mm Hg on ≥ 2 antihypertensive medications, and an increase in 0.2 mg/dL of serum creatinine during treatment with an ACEI. On intention-to-treat analysis, renal angioplasty provided little advantage over antihypertensive drug. This trial suffered from major limitations including a small sample size, inferior technology (angioplasty alone with a 48% restenosis rate), and high crossover rates from medical therapy to the angioplasty arm. The STAR trial (Stent placement in Patients with Atherosclerotic Renal Artery Stenosis and Impaired Renal Function) compared stenting to medical therapy in 140 patients with a creatinine clearance of less than 80 mL/min/1.73 m^2, RAS greater than 50%, and well-controlled BP < 140 < 90. Sixteen percent of patients in the stent placement group and 22% in the medication group reached the primary end point of a drop in creatinine clearance 20% or greater, a difference that failed to reach statistical significance. In this small study, stent placement had no clear effect on progression of impaired renal function but led to a small number of significant procedure-related complications. The ASTRAL trial (Angioplasty and Stenting for Renal Artery Lesions) randomized 806 patients with atherosclerotic RA disease to angioplasty with stent placement combined with medical therapy or medical therapy alone. The primary outcome was renal function, as measured by the reciprocal of the serum creatinine level (a measure that has a linear relationship with creatinine clearance). Secondary outcomes were BP, the time to renal and major cardiovascular events, and mortality with follow-up of 34 months. RA stenting was associated with improvement in the rate of progression of renal impairment (a difference of 0.06×10^{-3} L/μmol/y) and higher mean serum creatinine levels. There were no differences in systolic BP, cardiovascular and renal events, or death. Serious complications associated with revascularization occurred in 23 patients including 2 deaths and 3 amputations of toes or limbs. The authors concluded that stent placement has no worthwhile clinical benefit but substantial risks. The third of the contemporary randomized trials of RA stenting versus medical therapy in RAS, the CORAL (Cardiovascular Outcomes in Renal Atherosclerotic Lesions) trial, concluded randomization in January, 2010. This multicenter trial with more than 1,000 randomized RAS patients randomized to optical medical therapy alone versus optimal medical therapy with RA stenting is unique in that its primary end point is survival free of cardiovascular and renal adverse events and results are awaited.

Percutaneous Renal Angioplasty and Stenting

In contrast to the results with PTRA alone, contemporary trials with stenting have demonstrated improvements in BP control (Table 10.4) and stabilization or improvement in renal function. Since not all patients demonstrate improvement in BP or renal function, Radermacher et al. used RA resistance index to help to identify patients most likely to respond favorably to PTA/stent or surgery. They demonstrated that a resistance index (RRI) value of ≥80 reliably identifies patients with RAS in whom angioplasty/stent/surgery will not improve renal function, BP, or kidney survival. Mukherjee et al. subsequently demonstrated that a preprocedural end-diastolic velocity greater than 90 and resistance index less than 75 may potentially identify individuals who are likely to benefit with improvement in creatinine or reduction in BP after renal revascularization. In both these studies, a resistance index greater than 80 was a very strong predictor for lack of benefit after revascularization. The increased RRI is a measurement of the resistance within the renal circulation and thus underlying parenchymal

TABLE 10.4

EFFECTS OF PERCUTANEOUS TRANSLUMINAL RENAL ANGIOPLASTY AND STENTING ON BP CONTROL

Author (Year)	Patients	Arteries	Cure (%)	Improvement (%)
Blum U, et al. (1997)	68	74	16	78
Tuttle KR, et al. (1998)	129	148	2	57
Rocha-Singh KJ, et al. (1999)	150	180	6	56
White CJ, et al. (1997)	100	133	N/A	76
Dorros G, et al. (1998)	163	202	1	42
STAR Investigators (2009)	140	64	0	NA
ASTRAL Investigators (2009)	806	403	0	3
Average				**52**

renal disease. Up to 20% of patients may demonstrate worsening of renal function after percutaneous revascularization. This may be in part due to atheromatous embolization. Henry et al. have reported on the initial success of the use of emboli protection devices to prevent this complication, and this may be the standard of care in the future. Figure 10.2 depicts a simplified algorithm for the screening and treatment of RAS.

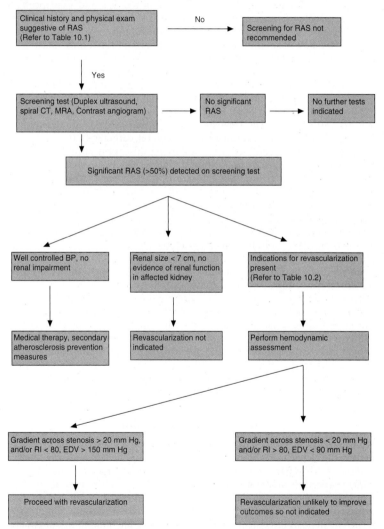

FIGURE 10-2. Algorithm for the diagnosis and treatment of RAS. (RAS, renal artery stenosis; CT, computerized tomography; MRA, magnetic resonance angiography; BP, blood pressure; RI, renal artery resistance index ([1 – end-diastolic velocity divided by maximal systolic velocity] × 100); EDV, end-diastolic velocity)

Percutaneous transluminal renal angioplasty and stenting (PTRAS) can be performed using either the femoral or the brachial approach, with the femoral approach being the preferred one. Currently, the most commonly employed technique is that of a guiding catheter as it considerably facilitates stent implantation. Available guide catheters include the Hockey Stick, Multipurpose, Renal Double Curve 1, and Renal Double Curve catheters in 6 to 8 French sizes. With improvements in balloon and stent profiles, most operators use a 6-French guide catheter. Using a smaller size catheter may decrease access-site vascular complications and may also potentially reduce RA embolic complications. Initial reports of renal angioplasty and stenting used a 0.035 or a 0.018 guidewire to allow advancement of bulky balloon catheters and stents, but currently the preferred wire is a 0.014 guidewire. A 0.014 guidewire minimizes traumatization of small branch vessels. Once an appropriate guide is seated in the ostium, unfractionated heparin is administered at 60 U/kg to achieve an activated clotting time of 200 to 250 seconds. The stenosis is crossed with a 0.014 guidewire and predilated with an appropriately sized balloon catheter (5.0- to 5.5-mm diameter for most renal arteries). Following dilatation, an appropriately sized stent (typically 6.0- to 7.0-mm diameter) is advanced and deployed to cover the entire lesion, with 1 to 2 mm of the stent extending into the aorta to ensure complete coverage of the ostium. One should choose a stent with good radial strength to prevent recoil of the ostium and we have successfully used several currently available balloon-expandable stents (Genesis, Herculink, Bridge, X3, etc.) for RA stenting (Fig. 10.3). The ostium is typically postdilated with the stent balloon partially in the aorta at higher atmosphere to flare the ostium. One should be careful to align the balloon catheter coaxially during postdilatation to avoid creating aortic dissections. Potential complications of RA stenting include renal atheroembolization, aortic dissections, blue toe syndrome from peripheral embolization, and perinephric hematomas related to branch vessel perforation. Avoiding larger diameter wires and hydrophilic guidewires significantly reduces the risk of perinephric hematomas. Postprocedure, patients should receive aspirin lifelong and clopidogrel from 1 to 12 months. Restenosis rates are less than 20% in most contemporary series. Clinical trials using drug-eluting stents will be starting in the near future. Table 10.5 lists factors that may predict an unfavorable outcome in PTRAS.

Surgical Revascularization

Surgical revascularization is now rarely used for RAS. This is due in a large part to the excellent technical results that can be achieved with angioplasty and stents. Most patients can now undergo RA stent implantation as an outpatient procedure at a fraction of the cost of surgical revascularization. Current indications for surgical revascularization are limited and include branch disease from FMD that cannot be adequately treated with balloon angioplasty, recurrent stenosis after stenting (this is extremely uncommon in our experience), or simultaneous aortic surgery (abdominal aortic aneurysm repair). Even in this circumstance, it may be advisable to stent the RA first and then proceed with aortic reconstruction. Mortality rate of RA revascularization

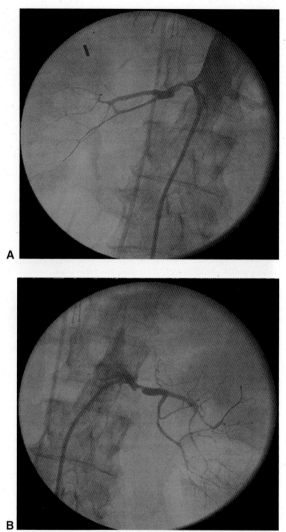

FIGURE 10-3. Two cases of severe RAS treated with RA stenting. Case 1 was a 69-year-old female who was transferred from an outside hospital for recurrent episodes of pulmonary edema requiring mechanical ventilation, a non-Q wave myocardial infarction and rising creatinine. She was severely hypertensive despite four antihypertensive drugs. Her creatinine at presentation was 1.9. Coronary angiogram revealed mild coronary disease without any significant high-grade lesion. She underwent aortography/renal angiography on the following day, which revealed severe bilateral RA stenoses. **A:** shows right RA 95% stenosis with 96-mm Hg gradient across the stenosis; **B:** shows 70% left RAS with 54-mm Hg gradient across this lesion. She underwent successful bilateral renal stenting   (*Continued*)

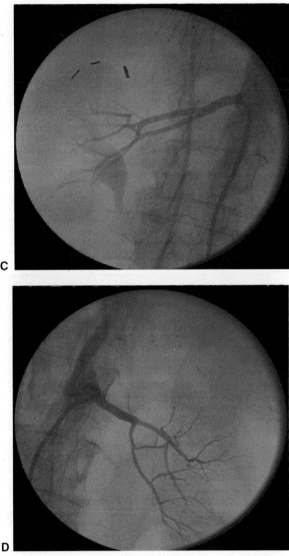

FIGURE 10-3. (*Continued*) **C:** and **D:** with complete resolution of the gradients. Over the next few days, her creatinine stabilized at 1.1 and her episodes of pulmonary edema completely resolved. She was discharged home on postprocedure day 3. Case 2 was a 59-year-old male with dyslipidemia and refractory hypertension despite five antihypertensive agents. Renal angiography revealed a severe left renal ostial stenosis

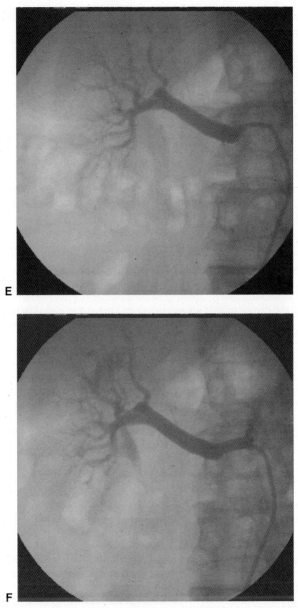

FIGURE 10-3. (*Continued*) **E:** Renal angiography revealed a severe right renal ostial stenosis and mild atherosclerosis of the left RA without hemodynamically significant stenosis. This was successfully treated with renal stenting **F:** On follow-up, his BP was well controlled on two antihypertensive agents.

TABLE 10.5

FACTORS PREDICTING POOR OUTCOME FROM PTRAS

Renal size < 8.0 cm
Serum creatinine > 3.5 mg/dL
Elevated renal resistive indices (>80)
Long-standing renal dysfunction from diabetes or hypertension
Extensive atherosclerosis

is 2 to 4%, with simultaneous aortic replacement and RA revascularization having higher rates than either procedure alone. Most studies have indicated a high technical success rate for surgical vascular reconstruction with postoperative thrombosis or stenosis rates of less than 10%. The BP response to surgical revascularization is similar to that of PTA/stent.

SPECIAL ISSUES/MISCELLANEOUS CONDITIONS

The absence of a consistent benefit across studies and the occasional increase in creatinine after endovascular intervention may potentially be attributed to atheroembolism due to debris generated during the intervention. Previous studies have demonstrated atheroembolism after either endovascular or surgical revascularization of renal arteries. It has also been demonstrated that atheroembolic renal disease after revascularization for ARAS is associated with decreased survival and an increased incidence of atherosclerotic morbid events. Preliminary results with emboli protection devices during PTRAS suggest that protected PTRAS may be a safe method to decrease the risk of renal atheroembolism and to protect against renal function deterioration. Several trials are ongoing to assess the safety and efficacy of filter-based emboli protection devices as an adjunct to RA stenting. Technological advances such as emboli-protection devices and drug-eluting stents may improve the immediate and long-term outcomes of RA stenting in the future.

Renal Artery FMD

FMD is an arterial disease of unknown etiology typically affecting the medium and large arteries of young and middle-aged women. Whereas most renovascular lesions are caused by atherosclerosis (90%), stenosis due to fibrous dysplasia remains an important disease particularly in children and young adults. FMD can be pathologically divided into three major subtypes: medial dysplasia, intimal fibroplasias, and adventitial fibroplasias. Of the medial dysplasia, medial fibroplasia is the most common type of FMD (about 70%) and occurs most often in women between the ages of 25 and 50 years. The lesion characteristically affects the distal two thirds of the main RA, often extending into its major branches. Other vessels in the body, such as the carotid, vertebral, subclavian, mesenteric, and iliac arteries, may be occasionally involved. The diagnosis of FMD is increasingly made through incidental detection of abnormalities on CTA and by MRA. X-ray contrast angiography is still used for diagnosis in many patients. MRA is also helpful although its utility in diagnosing distal forms of renal FMD is questionable. FMD is characterized on luminal angiographic techniques by a telltale "string of beads" appearance with the beads larger than the normal caliber of the artery. In perimedial fibroplasias, the beads are less numerous and smaller than the normal caliber of the artery and intimal disease is noted for concentric bandlike stenosis or smooth long stenosis. For patients with FMD, excellent results can be obtained by angioplasty. Surgical revascularization is rarely required. Because of its significantly lower morbidity and high success rate, PTRA is the treatment of choice for patients with FMD. With technically successful PTRA of FMD lesions, hypertension is cured in 33 to 63%, improved in 24 to 57%, and fails to improve in 3 to 33% of patients. Unlike atherosclerotic RA lesions, PTRA of FMD does not usually require stenting due to the low chance of restenosis after a successful dilation. The diagnosis and treatment of FMD have advanced dramatically in recent years, offering excellent prognosis for these patients.

Renal Artery Aneurysms

RAA is a rare pathological entity. The first published report in 1770 by Rouppe described the death of a sailor after a fall onto his right flank. RA is considered to be aneurismal when the diameter of that segment exceeds twice that of a normal-appearing segment. Of patients with RAAs, 20% present with bilateral pathology and 30% have multiple aneurysms. RAAs occur equally in men and women, although ruptures are more common in reproductive-aged women. Most RAAs are asymptomatic and are found incidentally while investigating other intra-abdominal pathologies using diagnostic imaging studies such as computed tomography (CT), duplex ultrasonography, angiography, magnetic resonance imaging (MRI), or MRA. Current indications for intervention include rupture (emergency surgery), symptomatic RAA with flank and/or abdominal pain, aneurysms associated with significant RAS and renovascular hypertension, RAAs in females who are pregnant or in those contemplating pregnancy, and diameter greater than 2 cm. Complete calcification of the wall of the aneurysm sac was previously believed to confer protection against rupture, even for larger aneurysms; however, more recently, this theory has been questioned and should not be used to defer surgery if an indication for repair exists. Renal ischemia or infarction secondary to embolization from the aneurysm sac and RAA associated with acute dissection are other indications for repair. Surgical correction with tangential excision with primary repair or patch angioplasty remains the cornerstone of therapy but refinements in endovascular techniques may allow more RAAs to be treated in this manner with covered stents.

RA Dissections

This is a rare entity and is typically associated with blunt trauma, iatrogenic catheter–induced dissections, and spontaneous dissections. Many spontaneous dissections are actually associated with FMD and are considered a complication of FMD. Symptoms may include flank pain, hematuria, and accelerated hypertension. Early angiography is indicated in the appropriate clinical setting for diagnosis and treatment. Some of these patients can be treated medically, while others require percutaneous revascularization or surgical therapy. Accepted criteria for revascularization include existence of technically correctable dissections causing hemodynamically significant occlusions of the main or major segmental renal arteries, documented renovascular hypertension, or significant worsening of renal function.

CONCLUSIONS

- ARAS is a common cause of difficult to treat hypertension and chronic kidney disease.
- The identification of RAS may be accomplished with a variety of modalities including duplex ultrasound, CTA, MRA, and x-ray contrast angiography.
- Accepted indications for revascularization include hemodynamically significant RAS and recurrent, unexplained congestive heart failure or sudden, unexplained pulmonary edema; accelerated hypertension, resistant hypertension, malignant hypertension, hypertension with an unexplained unilateral small kidney, and hypertension with intolerance to medication; and progressive chronic kidney disease with bilateral RAS or a RAS to a solitary functioning kidney.
- PTRAS is the procedure of choice for most patients with atherosclerotic RAS, while PTRA alone without stenting is appropriate in FMD.
- Renal function (15 to 20%) and BP (20 to 50%) may not improve or may even worsen in patients after intervention with PTRAS.
- Emerging advances in the field are more accurate ways to predict response to therapy and protection of the kidneys (emboli protection devices).

PRACTICAL POINTS

- Accessory, duplicated main renal arteries (10 to 30%) may not be visualized adequately by duplex.
- An RRI > 80 may help identify patients with intrinsic renal disease who may not benefit from percutaneous revascularization.
- CTA may be better than MRA for distal forms of FMD owing to better spatial resolution (0.5 × 0.5 × 0.5 mm).
- The benefit of revascularization for preservation of renal function in unilateral RAS is not established.
- For PTRAS, the stent must be fully expanded and extend 1 to 2 mm into the aorta in patients with ostial disease; a common flaw early on in experience is to underdeploy the stent (worthwhile to do the first 15 to 20 cases with IVUS).
- It is important to assure that no postprocedure pressure gradient exists after renal stenting.

RECOMMENDED READING

Caps MT, Zierler RE, Polissar NL. Risk of atrophy in kidneys with atherosclerotic renal artery stenosis. *Kidney Int* 1998;53:735–742.

Gross CM, Kramer J, Weingartner O, et al. Determination of renal arterial stenosis severity: comparison of pressure gradient and vessel diameter. *Radiology* 2001;220:751–756.

Harding MB, Smith LR, Himmelstein SI, et al. Renal artery stenosis: prevalence and associated risk factors in patients undergoing routine cardiac catheterization. *J Am Soc Nephrol* 1992;2: 1608–1616.

Henry M, Klonaris C, Henry I, et al. Protected renal stenting with the PercuSurge GuardWire device: a pilot study. *J Endovasc Ther* 2001;8:227–237.

Hirsch AT, Haskal ZJ, Hertzer NR, et al. ACC/AHA guidelines for the management of patients with peripheral arterial disease (lower extremity, renal, mesenteric, and abdominal aortic): executive summary: a collaborative report from the American Association for Vascular Surgery/ Society for Vascular Surgery, Society for Vascular Medicine and Biology, Society of Interventional Radiology, and the ACC/AHA Task Force on Practice Guidelines (Writing Committee to Develop Guidelines for the Management of Patients With Peripheral Arterial Disease [Lower Extremity, Renal, Mesenteric, and Abdominal Aortic]). *Circulation* 2006;113:e463–e465.

Huot SJ, Hansson JH, Dey H, et al. Utility of captopril renal scans for detecting renal artery stenosis. *Arch Intern Med* 2002;162:1981–1984.

Krishnamurthi V, Novick AC, Myles JL. Atheroembolic renal disease: effect on morbidity and survival after revascularization for atherosclerotic renal artery stenosis. *J Urol* 1999; 161:1093–1096.

McLaughlin K, Jardine AG, Moss JG. ABC of arterial and venous disease. Renal artery stenosis. *BMJ* 2000;320:1124–1127.

Mukherjee D. Renal artery stenosis: who to screen and how to treat? *ACC Curr J Rev* 2003;12(3):70–75.

Mukherjee D. Renal artery revascularization: is there a rationale to perform? *JACC Cardiovasc Interv* 2009;2(3):183–184.

Mukherjee D, Bhatt DL, Robbins M, et al. Renal artery end-diastolic velocity and renal artery resistance index as predictors of outcome after renal stenting. *Am J Cardiol* 2001;88:1064–1066.

Olin JW, Begelman SM. Renal artery disease. In: Topol E, ed., *Textbook of Cardiovascular Medicine*, 2nd ed. Philadelphia: Lippincott Raven, 2002:2139–2159.

Olin JW, Melia M, Young JR, et al. Prevalence of atherosclerotic renal artery stenosis in patients with atherosclerosis elsewhere. *Am J Med* 1990;88:46N–51N.

Olin JW, Piedmonte MR, Young JR, et al. The utility of duplex ultrasound scanning of the renal arteries for diagnosing significant renal artery stenosis. *Ann Intern Med* 1995;122: 833–838.

Radermacher J, Chavan A, Bleck J, et al. Use of Doppler ultrasonography to predict the outcome of therapy for renal-artery stenosis. *N Engl J Med* 2001;344:410–417.

Safian RD, Textor SC. Renal artery stenosis. *N Engl J Med* 2001;344:431–442.

Schreiber MJ, Pohl MA, Novick AC. The natural history of atherosclerotic and fibrous renal artery disease. *Urol Clin North Am* 1984;11:383–392.

Schoenberg SO, Rieger J, Johannson LO, et al. Diagnosis of renal artery stenosis with magnetic resonance angiography: update 2003. *Nephrol Dial Transplant* 2003;18(7):1252–1256. (No abstract available.)

van Jaarsveld BC, Krijnen P, Pieterman H, et al. The effect of balloon angioplasty on hypertension in atherosclerotic renal-artery stenosis. Dutch Renal Artery Stenosis Intervention Cooperative Study Group. *N Engl J Med* 2000;342:1007–1014.

Watson SP, Hadjipetrou H, Cox S, et al. Effect of renal stenting on renal function and size in patients with atherosclerotic renovascular disease. *Circulation* 2000;102;1671–1677.

White CJ, Ramee SR, Collins TJ, et al. Renal artery stent placement: utility in lesions difficult to treat with balloon angioplasty. *J Am Coll Cardiol* 1997;30:1445–1450.

Zierler RE, Bergelin RO, Davidson RC, et al. A prospective study of disease progression in patients with atherosclerotic renal artery stenosis. *Am J Hypertens* 1996;9:1055–1061.

CHAPTER 11 ■ Carotid Artery Disease Management

Debabrata Mukherjee and Aamer Abbas

In western countries, stroke affects approximately 0.2% of the population annually. In the United States alone, around 500,000 people experience a new stroke and 200,000 have a recurrence of a previous cerebrovascular event each year. About 90% of the strokes are ischemic and 10% are hemorrhagic (intracerebral hemorrhage or subarachnoid hemorrhage). The major cause of stroke is large-vessel atherosclerosis, with the highest risk occurring in patients with stenosis of the internal carotid arteries. Among patients who have suffered a stroke, one third may die within 1 year, one third may have permanent disability, and the remainder recovers. Stroke is the third leading cause of death in Western countries, accounting for 12% of all deaths. According to the data from Health Care Financing, in 1996, $3.8 billion ($5,945 per discharge) was paid in the United States to Medicare beneficiaries for stroke. The total stroke-related burden for the American economy is estimated to be $20 billion yearly due to health care costs and lost productivity. Stroke thus remains a major public health problem.

The classical risk factors of coronary atherosclerosis also apply to carotid atherosclerosis. Accordingly, presence and severity of carotid atherosclerosis correlate with the presence and severity of coronary atherosclerosis and peripheral vascular disease. Half of the men over 75 years of age have carotid atherosclerosis by ultrasonography, with a stenosis greater than 50% detected in 5% of cases. Important risk factors for carotid stenosis include smoking, diabetes, male gender, hypertension, and dyslipidemia. In patients with carotid atherosclerosis on ultrasound but no neurologic symptoms, the risk of subsequent stroke is best predicted by the percent carotid stenosis, the presence of disease progression on sequential ultrasound examinations, and the presence of carotid ulceration. Recent data demonstrated a risk of 1.6% per year on aspirin among asymptomatic patients with carotid stenosis less than 60% and of 3.2% per year among those with stenosis greater than 60%. Among patients with symptomatic [i.e., with previous stroke or transient ischemic attack (TIA)] carotid disease, the risk of recurrence may be as high as 10% in the first year and 30 to 35% at 5 years. High-risk features for recurrence include hemispheric TIA, recent TIA, increasing frequency of TIA, or high-grade carotid stenosis.

The most common site of cerebrovascular atherosclerotic disease is the carotid bifurcation, characteristically affecting the outer wall of the carotid sinus and extending into the distal common carotid artery. Atherosclerotic plaque rupture with subsequent total thrombotic occlusion of the carotid is a rare phenomenon. More commonly, atherosclerotic ulceration leads to luminal thrombus apposition and distal embolization. Both in asymptomatic and in symptomatic patients, the more severe the carotid lesion, the higher the risk of subsequent stroke. The presence of ulcerated lesions, seen in up to one third of the endarterectomy specimen but underappreciated with angiography, also increases the risk of ischemic events. In the medical arm of the North American Symptomatic Carotid Endarterectomy Trial (NASCET), the 2-year stroke incidence among symptomatic patients with evidence of carotid ulcers on angiography ranged from 26.3 to 73.2% as the degree of stenosis increased from 75 to 95%.

CLINICAL FEATURES

The majority of patients with carotid stenosis are asymptomatic, and diagnosis is made following auscultation of a carotid bruit or routine ultrasound screening. TIA is the leading symptom, and in the absence of neurologic deficits, the diagnosis is based on careful history taking. If no therapy is instituted, as many as 30 to 40% of these patients may subsequently develop stroke. Dysphasia, ipsilateral amaurosis fugax, contralateral visual field, and motor and sensory loss may be all manifestations of carotid disease. These findings must be differentiated from vertebrobasilar disease. While neurologic findings associated with carotid disease usually involve the contralateral face and body, posterior circulation events often cause bilateral or crossed deficits such as ataxia, dysarthria, diplopia, or bilateral visual field loss. Headache is an uncommon finding associated with cerebral embolic events. Hemicranial headache may occur with TIA originating from carotid stenosis, and occipital headaches may be reported in vertebrobasilar insufficiency. In patients with neurologic deficits associated with neck or retro-orbital pain, carotid or vertebral artery dissection should be excluded, particularly in the presence of trauma. The clinical triad of neck, head, or retro-orbital pain; new-onset Horner's syndrome; and contralateral sensory, motor, or cognitive deficits is pathognomonic for internal carotid artery (ICA) dissection.

DIAGNOSIS

Ultrasonography

Duplex ultrasonography, a combination of Doppler ultrasonography and B-mode imaging generated by a single transducer, is the diagnostic tool of choice for the initial assessment of carotid disease. This widely available technique allows morphological and functional assessment of the carotid lesion. When performed by trained sonographers using a standard protocol and with ongoing quality assurance, this method approaches 90% sensitivity and specificity compared with angiography for detection of severe carotid stenosis. Percent stenosis is determined by systolic and diastolic velocities with peak end-diastolic velocity greater than 135 cm/s and peak end-systolic velocity greater than 240 cm/s suggestive of stenosis greater than 80%. Duplex carotid scans may yield inadequate images in the following conditions: carotids that bifurcate high, long (greater than 3 cm) ICA plaque, calcific shadows, or near-complete occlusions. In these cases, magnetic resonance imaging is of value in differentiating between the two.

Magnetic Resonance Angiography

Magnetic resonance angiography (MRA) is a useful tool in carotid disease, allowing reliable imaging from the aortic arch to the intracranial branches. MR techniques for the diagnosis of carotid disease include gadolinium-based (contrast enhanced—CE) and time-of-flight (TOF-flow sensitive) approaches. CE-MRA techniques have been shown to have high sensitivity (greater than 90%), high negative predictive value (greater than 90%), and high specificity (greater than 90%) for detecting severe carotid stenosis. On the other hand, TOF (2D and 3D) techniques may be compromised by artifacts generated by vessel tortuosity, blood flow turbulence, and in-plane flow, and it is precisely in these situations that CE-MRA methodology may be superior. TOF is also time-consuming and subject to movement artifact. The specificity of CE-MRA is at least equal to and may even exceed that of duplex ultrasound in the diagnosis of 70 to 99% lesions and in the diagnosis of subtotaled arteries versus complete occlusions. In situations where duplex ultrasound yields suboptimal results, MRA may help resolve the issue and reduce the need for an invasive assessment [high bifurcation, long (greater than 3 cm) ICA plaque, calcific shadows]. MRA also provides the advantage that concomitant brain imaging may be performed to assess the extent of ischemic events and to exclude intracranial pathologies (e.g., tumors or vascular malformations) prior to endovascular therapy.

CT Angiography

MDCT angiography is an important diagnostic modality to assess the carotid circulation. The intracranial as well as extracranial circulation can be evaluated in the same sitting with this modality. In a study of 37 patients and 73 vessels, the reported sensitivity and specificity for high-grade stenosis were 75 and 96, respectively, and for moderate stenosis 88 and 82, respectively, as compared to contrast angiography. Furthermore, MDCT may assess the composition of the atherosclerotic plaque and the hemodynamics of the brain circulation by using the CT brain perfusion technology.

Angiography

Angiography remains the gold standard for diagnosis of carotid stenosis. It allows accurate measurement of luminal stenosis of the entire vessel from its origin to the intracranial branches, as well as proper assessment of plaque morphology, lesion length, and reference vessel diameter. In patients with symptomatic carotid disease, angiography may identify additional intracranial stenosis. However, it is an invasive procedure with a potential for embolization or vessel trauma. Currently, angiography is used in patients where noninvasive tests yield inconclusive or conflicting results and/or when percutaneous therapy is considered. Two different

NASCET   ECST

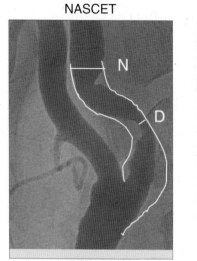
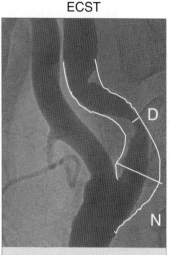

Percent stenosis = [(N–D/N) X 100]
NASCET = 67% stenosis   ECST = 84% stenosis

FIGURE 11-1.   Carotid stenosis severity measurements according to the NASCET and the ECST methods. For any given stenosis, the ECST method gives a higher percentage diameter stenosis. (N, presumed normal segment; D, diseased segment) (Adapted from Mukherjee D, Yadav SJ. Cerebrovascular diseases: pathophysiology and management. In: Fuster V, ed. Assessing and modifying the vulnerable atherosclerotic plaque. Armonk, NY: Futura Publishing, 2002:29–55.)

methods for calculating the degree of angiographic stenosis have been used in the major clinical trials (Fig. 11.1). Both the NASCET and the European Carotid Surgery Trial (ECST) define the stenotic segment the same way but differ in how they define the reference segment or the normal diameter. The NASCET method defines normal as the diameter just distal to the carotid bulb (neither the bulb itself nor a region of poststenotic dilatation), whereas the ECST method defines normal as the estimated diameter of the carotid bulb as it was prior to atherosclerotic narrowing. For any given stenosis, the ECST method gives a higher percentage diameter stenosis as illustrated in Figure 11.1. It is important to know which method was used to determine reference segment in order to interpret and apply trial results appropriately. Importantly, angiography remains the only scientifically validated method of defining ICA stenosis requiring endarterectomy, as in the large-scale randomized trials (i.e., NASCET, ECST) the degree of stenosis was assessed by angiography. However, in centers where MRA and duplex ultrasound imaging have been demonstrated to be concordant with angiography, angiography is usually not considered to be necessary in the clinical assessment of carotid disease prior to endarterectomy.

MANAGEMENT OF CAROTID DISEASE

Risk Factor Modification and Antiplatelet Therapy

Hypertension Control

Hypertension has a strong correlation with stroke, with both systolic and diastolic blood pressures being independently associated with primary and recurrent stroke risk. Diastolic pressures are correlated strongly with risk in younger individuals, and a reduction in diastolic blood pressure of 1 mm Hg has been shown to decrease the incidence of stroke by 7 to 10% over 5 years. In older individuals, a reduction in systolic pressure of 2 mm translates into a reduction of stroke incidence of 5 to 10%.

Smoking Cessation

Cigarette smoking increases the risk of stroke two- to threefold, especially in conjunction with hypertension. Smoking cessation is an essential part of stroke management.

Diabetes

Diabetes increases the risk of stroke 3- to 10-fold depending on the age of presentation. Diabetes doubles the rate of recurrent stroke, trebles the frequency of stroke-related dementia, and also increases stroke-related mortality. However, there are as yet no good data showing that tight glycemic control reduces stroke rates in diabetic individuals. Preliminary studies suggest that insulin sensitizers may have beneficial effects in reducing carotid atherosclerosis and intimal-medial thickening and may translate into reduction in strokes.

Lipid Lowering

The Stroke Prevention by Aggressive Reduction in Cholesterol Levels (SPARCL) trial was a randomized, double-blind study designed to determine whether atorvastatin 80 mg/d or placebo would reduce the risk of fatal or nonfatal stroke in patients with no known coronary disease who had experienced a stroke or TIA within the previous 6 months. During a median follow-up of approximately 5 years, 11.2% receiving atorvastatin and 13.1% receiving placebo reached the primary end point of fatal or nonfatal stroke (5-year absolute reduction in risk, 2.2%; adjusted HR, 0.84; 95% confidence interval, 0.71, 0.99; $P = 0.03$). The AHA/ASA recommendations state that on the basis of the SPARCL trial, administration of statin therapy with intensive lipid-lowering effects is recommended for patients with atherosclerotic ischemic stroke or TIA and without known CHD to reduce the risk of stroke and cardiovascular events.

Antiplatelet Therapy

Table 11.1 summarizes the data on antiplatelet therapy in high-risk individuals with a focus on stroke as a primary or a secondary end point. In the ASA in Carotid Endarterectomy (ACE) trial, low-dose ASA (75 to

TABLE 11.1

AGENTS EFFECTIVE IN VASCULAR RISK REDUCTION INCLUDING ONGOING CLINICAL TRIALS

Agent	Trials	Trial Specifics	N	1° End point (Reduction in Vascular Death/MI/Death)	Reduction in Nonfatal Stroke
Aspirin					
I° Prevention	Physicians Health Study British Physicians Health Study	DBPC trials, ASA 325 mg vs. placebo	22,071 5,139	41% RR ↓ in MI (limited to >50 y)	NS ↑ in hemorrhagic stroke
II° Prevention	Meta-analysis	Antithrombotic Trialist's Collaboration	>110,000	19%	25% RR ↓ with ASA compared to placebo in nonfatal stroke
II° Prevention, patients scheduled for endarterectomy	ACE	DBPC, Aspirin 81 mg vs. 325 mg vs. 650 mg or 1,300 mg for 3 mo	2,849	Rate of stroke, MI, and death was lower in the low-dose groups than the high-dose groups at 30 d (5.4 vs. 7.0%) and at 3 mo (6.2 vs. 8.4%)	Strokes occurred in 3–2% patients on low-dose ASA and 6–9% patients on high-dose acetylsalicylic acid
Clopidogrel					
II° Prevention High-risk patients with prior MI, stroke, or PAD	CAPRIE	DBPC, Clopidogrel 75 mg vs. ASA 325 mg	19,185	Statistically significant 8.7% RR ↓ in stroke, MI, or vascular death	Trend in reduction of stroke in subgroup with prior stroke
II° Prevention Patients with acute coronary syndrome	CURE	DBPC, Aspirin 75–325 mg vs. ASA + clopidogrel 75 mg	12,562	20% RR ↓ in (11.4% in placebo vs. 9.3% in clopidogrel arm) stroke, MI, or vascular death	14% RR ↓ in stroke with clopidogrel
II° Prevention Patients with acute coronary syndrome	CREDO	DBPC, Clopidogrel 75 mg for 4 wk vs. clopidogrel 75 mg for up to 9 mo	2,116	26.9% RR ↓ in (11.5 vs. 8.5% in long-term clopidogrel arm) of death, MI, and stroke	No ↑ in hemorrhagic strokes

(Continued)

TABLE 11.1

AGENTS EFFECTIVE IN VASCULAR RISK REDUCTION INCLUDING ONGOING CLINICAL TRIALS (*Continued*)

Agent	Trials	Trial Specifics	N	1° End point (Reduction in Vascular Death/MI/Death)	Reduction in Nonfatal Stroke
II° Prevention Patients with recent TIA or stroke	MATCH	DBPC, Clopidogrel 75 mg vs. ASA + clopidogrel 75 mg	7,600	15.7% reached the primary end point in the group receiving aspirin + clopidogrel vs. 16.7% in the clopidogrel alone group [relative risk reduction 6.4%, (95% CI 4.6–16.3)]; Life-threatening bleedings were higher in the group receiving aspirin + clopidogrel vs. clopidogrel alone [96 (2.6%) vs. 49 (1.3%); absolute risk increase 1.3% (95% CI 0.6–1.9)]	No benefit with dual therapy but ↑ bleed
II° Prevention Patients with small-vessel disease and lacunar infarcts	SPS3	DBPC, Aspirin 325 mg vs. aspirin 325 mg + clopidogrel 75 mg	2,500	Phase III trial ongoing	Trial ongoing
II° Prevention Patients who have recently recovered from a TIA	PRoFESS	DBPC, aspirin + extended-release dipyridamole vs. clopidogrel monotherapy	20,332	Recurrent stroke 1.01 (0.92–1.11); the secondary outcome, a composite of stroke, MI, and vascular death, was identical between groups	Neither aspirin plus extended-release dipyridamole or clopidogrel is superior to the other in the prevention of stroke

Dipyridamole

II° Prevention Patients with TIA or stroke within 3 mo	ESPS-2	DBPC, 2 × 2 factorial design, ASA 25 b.i.d. dipyridamole (ER-DP) 200 b.i.d.; placebo and ASA + ER–DP	6,602	No effect on MI or mortality; stroke rate at 24 mo – 9.5% with aspirin + dipyridamole vs. 12.5% with aspirin alone	37% reduction in stroke with aspirin + dipyridamole vs. aspirin alone 19% reduction with aspirin alone Dose of aspirin used was only 50 mg
II° Prevention Patients with TIA or stroke within 3 mo	ESPRIT	DBPC, aspirin (30–325 mg daily) vs. aspirin + dipyridamole (200 mg twice daily)	2,739	Hazard ratio with combination 0.80, (95% CI 0.66–0.98); absolute risk reduction 1.0% per year. (95% CI 0.1–1.8)	Combination regimen of aspirin plus dipyridamole is preferred over aspirin alone as antithrombotic therapy after cerebral ischemia of arterial origin

HMG CoA Reductase Inhibitors (Statins)

Patients with average cholesterol levels with prior MI	CARE	DBPC, randomized to pravastatin or placebo	4,159	24% reduction in heart attack or death	31% reduction in stroke
Patients with a history of heart attack or hospitalization for unstable angina pectoris	LIPID	DBPC, randomized to pravastatin or placebo	9,014	24% reduction in heart attacks, and a 22% decrease in deaths from any cause	19% reduction in stroke
Patients with acute coronary syndrome	MIRACL	DBPC, randomized to atorvastatin or placebo		16% RR ↓ in 14.8% in the atorvastatin group and 17.4% in the placebo group	50% reduction in stroke
People who have a high risk of coronary artery disease—even if their cholesterol levels are normal or low	HPS	DBPC, randomized to simvastatin or placebo	20,000		25% reduction in stroke

(Continued)

TABLE 11.1

AGENTS EFFECTIVE IN VASCULAR RISK REDUCTION INCLUDING ONGOING CLINICAL TRIALS (*Continued*)

Agent	Trials	Trial Specifics	N	1° End point (Reduction in Vascular Death/MI/Death)	Reduction in Nonfatal Stroke
2 secondary prevention studies, 5 mixed primary–secondary prevention population studies, and 10 regression trials	Meta-analysis of 17 trials	Meta-analysis of all randomized controlled trials published as of April 1997	21,303	24% RR ↓ in all-cause mortality	31% reduction in stroke
Patients who had had a stroke or TIA within 1–6 mo before study entry	SPARCL	DBPC, randomized to atorvastatin or placebo	4,731	During a median follow-up of 4.9 y, 11.2% receiving atorvastatin and 13.1% receiving placebo had a fatal or nonfatal stroke [5-y absolute reduction in risk, 2.2%; adjusted hazard ratio, 0.84; (95% CI 0.71–0.99; $P = 0.03$); unadjusted $P = 0.05$]	Atorvastatin reduced the overall incidence of strokes and of cardiovascular events by 16%

DBPC, double-blind placebo controlled trial; RR, relative risk; PAD, peripheral arterial disease; TIA, transient ischemic attack; ACE, ASA and carotid endarterectomy; CAPRIE, clopidogrel vs. aspirin in patients at risk of ischemic events; CURE, clopidogrel in unstable angina to prevent recurrent events; CREDO, clopidogrel for the reduction of events during observation; MATCH, management of atherothrombosis with clopidogrel in high-risk patients with recent TIA or ischemic stroke; SPS3, secondary prevention of small subcortical stroke; PRoFESS, prevention regimen for effectively avoiding second strokes; ESPRIT, European/Australian stroke prevention in reversible ischemia trial; ESPS, European stroke prevention study; CARE, cholesterol and recurrent events; LIPID, long-term intervention with pravastatin in ischemic disease; MIRACL, myocardial ischemia reduction with aggressive cholesterol lowering; HPS, Heart protection study; SPARCL, stroke prevention by aggressive reduction in cholesterol levels.

325 mg) was superior to high-dose ASA (650 to 1,300 mg) in preventing stroke, myocardial infarction (MI), or death both at 30 days (5.4 vs. 7.0%, $P = 0.07$) and at 3 months (6.2 vs. 8.4%, $P = 0.03$) in patients undergoing carotid endarterectomy. The Antiplatelet Trialists' Collaboration analyzed the results of 195 trials of greater than 135,000 patients and found that platelet antagonists lowered the risk of stroke, MI, and vascular death. On the basis of this, individuals at risk for vascular events should receive antiplatelet agents for the primary prophylaxis of stroke.

The efficacy of dual antiplatelet therapy with aspirin and clopidogrel was tested in the Management of Atherothrombosis with Clopidogrel in High-Risk Patients with Recent TIA or Ischemic Stroke (MATCH) trail. The MATCH trial did not show additional clinical value of adding aspirin to clopidogrel in high-risk patients with TIA or ischemic stroke. The European/Australian Stroke Prevention in Reversible Ischemia Trial (ESPRIT) was a randomized, open-label study comparing aspirin 30 to 325 mg with or without dipyridamole 200 mg b.i.d. in 2,763 subjects with TIA, transient monocular blindness, or minor stroke within 6 months of enrollment. The risk for the primary outcome of death from all vascular causes, nonfatal stroke, nonfatal MI, or major bleeding complication was significantly lower in the dipyridamole plus aspirin arm (HR, 0.80; 95% confidence interval, 0.66 to 0.98). The Prevention Regimen for Effectively Avoiding Second Strokes (PRoFESS) trial demonstrated that the risks of recurrent stroke or the composite of stroke, MI, or vascular death are similar with aspirin + extended-release dipyridamole combination and clopidogrel monotherapy. The update to the AHA/ASA recommendations for the prevention of stroke in patients with stroke and TIA recommends that aspirin (50 to 325 mg/d) monotherapy, the combination of aspirin and extended-release dipyridamole, and clopidogrel monotherapy are all acceptable options for initial therapy (Class I, Level of Evidence A). Based on ESPRIT trial, the combination of aspirin and extended-release dipyridamole is recommended over aspirin alone (Class I, Level of Evidence B).

Surgical Revascularization

Symptomatic Carotid Disease

The main findings of randomized trials comparing carotid endarterectomy with medical management are summarized in Table 11.2. Three pivotal studies in patients with symptomatic carotid disease have been completed and have documented improved outcomes with endarterectomy in patients with symptomatic severe carotid stenosis. The ECST trial was a multicenter, randomized trial in which patients with nondisabling stroke, TIA, or retinal infarction within the preceding 6 months were randomly assigned to carotid endarterectomy or medical therapy. The rate of perioperative major stroke or death was 7.0%. Patients with severe stenosis (greater than 70%) allocated to surgery had significant reduction in death or any stroke at 3-year follow-up (12.3 vs. 21.9%; $P < 0.01$). The risk of surgical death or ipsilateral stroke by 3 years was 10.3% in patients assigned to surgical intervention compared with 16.8% in patients assigned to medical therapy. Patients with mild and moderate carotid stenosis did not benefit with

TABLE 11.2

RESULTS OF MAJOR RANDOMIZED CAROTID ENDARTERECTOMY TRIALS

Study	Degree of Stenosis	NNT[a]	Event Prevented	Time Period
Symptomatic Patients				
NASCET	70–99%	6	Ipsilateral stroke	2 y
		10	Major stroke or death	
ECST	70–99%	15	Ipsilateral stroke	3 y
		20	Major stroke or death	
NASCET	50–69%	12 (men)	Ipsilateral stroke	5 y
		67 (women)	Ipsilateral stroke	
		16 (men)	Major stroke	
		125 (women)	Major stroke	
ECST	<70%	No benefit	Ipsilateral stroke	>4 y
NASCET	<50%	No benefit	Ipsilateral stroke	5 y
VA	>50%	No benefit	Stroke or death	Terminated
	>70%	26 (men)	Crescendo TIA or stroke	
Asymptomatic Patients				
CASANOVA	50–90%	No benefit	Any stroke or death	3 y
VA	>50%	No benefit	Any stroke or death	4 y
ACAS	>60%	17	Ipsilateral stroke or any stroke or death	5 y
ACST		Ongoing		

[a]NNT, number needed to treat; number of patients needed to be treated to prevent one event. NASCET, North American Symptomatic Carotid Endarterectomy Trial; ECST, European Carotid Surgery Trial; VA, Veteran Affairs study; CASANOVA, Carotid Artery Stenosis with Asymptomatic Narrowing: Operation Versus Aspirin; ACAS, Asymptomatic Carotid (Atherosclerosis Study; ACST, Asymptomatic Carotid Surgery Trial.
Adapted from Sila CA. Carotid stenosis: current strategies for choosing between medical and surgical management. Cleve Clin J Med 2000;67:851–861., with permission.)

surgery. The NASCET trial randomized patients with symptomatic 30 to 99% carotid artery stenosis to endarterectomy or medical management. Among 662 patients with 70 to 99% stenosis, at 2 years, those randomized to surgery had benefit in terms of ipsilateral stroke (9 vs. 26%; absolute risk reduction 17%; $P < 0.001$), any stroke (12.6 vs. 27.6%; $P < 0.001$), and major stroke or death (8.0 vs. 18.1%; $P < 0.01$). The perioperative (i.e., within 30 days) stroke or death rate in the trial was 5.8%. A total of 2,267 patients had stenosis less than 70% and were divided in post hoc analyses into groups with 50 to 69% stenosis and those with less than 50% stenosis. In patients with 50 to 69% stenosis, a 6.5% reduction in the primary end point of any ipsilateral stroke was observed by 5-year follow-up (15.7 vs. 22.2%; $P = 0.045$). In the group with less than 50% stenosis, a nonsignificant absolute reduction of 3.8% was observed (14.9 vs. 18.7%; $P = 0.16$). The risk for any stroke or death was significantly reduced in the surgical group at 5-year follow-up for patients with 50 to 69% stenosis (33.2 vs. 43.3%; $P = 0.005$), but no reduction was observed with surgery in patients with less than 50% stenosis (36.2 vs. 37%; $P = 0.97$). The Veterans Affairs Cooperative Studies Program Trialist Group randomly assigned 189 men with symptomatic carotid stenosis greater than 50% to medical therapy or carotid endarterectomy. At 1 year, a significant reduction in stroke or crescendo TIA in patients allocated to surgery was observed (7.7 vs. 19.4%; absolute risk reduction, 11.7%; $P = 0.011$). The benefit of surgery was more profound in patients with carotid stenosis greater than 70% (absolute risk reduction, 17.7%; $P = 0.004$). Perioperative (i.e., within 30 days) stroke or death rate was 6.6%.

Asymptomatic Carotid Disease

The benefit of carotid endarterectomy over medical management has been less impressive in patients with asymptomatic than in those with symptomatic carotid disease (Table 11.2). The Asymptomatic Carotid Atherosclerosis Study (ACAS) enrolled 1,659 patients with asymptomatic carotid stenosis ≥60% and followed these patients over 2.7 years (median). The perioperative stroke or death rate was exceedingly low (2.3%). The estimated aggregate risk at 5 years for ipsilateral stroke or any perioperative stroke or death was 5.1% for surgical patients and 11.0% for patients treated medically ($P = 0.004$). The Veteran Affairs Asymptomatic Carotid Stenosis study allocated 444 patients with asymptomatic carotid stenosis ≥50% to surgery or medical management. The combined incidence of ipsilateral neurologic events was 8.0% in the surgical group and 20.6% in the medical group ($P = 0.001$). However, due to high (mainly cardiac) mortality, no difference was observed in stroke or death rate at follow-up (41.2 and 44.2%, respectively).

Variables Impacting on Carotid Surgery Results

The "Randomized Trial" Effect. It is important to put the results achieved within the endarterectomy trials in perspective. Although randomized clinical trials remain the gold standard of clinical investigation in medicine, they have inherent limitations that may make difficult an extrapolation of the results to everyday clinical practice or its application to new therapies. The excellent results associated with endarterectomy in the randomized trials were achieved with accurate patient and operator selection. In NASCET, surgical centers had to demonstrate a perioperative stroke or death rate less than 6%. Multiple patient exclusions led to enrollment of only one third of patients operated at trial sites. In ACAS, both the hospital and the surgeon had to document a death or stroke rate less than 3%. Again, multiple exclusion criteria led to inclusion of 1 patient per 25 individuals screened. Another fact to keep in mind is that, cardiac complications such as MI have not been well tracked within the randomized trials. The importance of exacerbation of coronary disease following endarterectomy can be derived from the Mayo Asymptomatic Carotid Endarterectomy Study, a study that did not require and even discouraged the use of aspirin or any other anti-platelet drug in the surgical cohort. After randomizing only 71 patients, the trial was prematurely terminated due to 22% incidence of MI in the surgical arm.

Surgical Risk of Patients. The spectrum of perioperative endarterectomy mortality may range from as low as 0.1% in asymptomatic patients (ACAS) and 0.6% for symptomatic patients (NASCET) to 2.5% in Medicare (asymptomatic and symptomatic) patients operated in low-volume hospital. The Cleveland Clinic series including over 3,000 endarterectomies demonstrated that the 30-day mortality may be 15 times higher (4.4 vs. 0.3%) in patients at high risk for surgery (defined as coronary bypass surgery within 6 months, history of congestive heart failure, severe chronic obstructive pulmonary disease, or creatinine greater than 3 mg/dL) compared to those without such characteristics.

Importance of Center Endarterectomy Volumes. There is a direct correlation between center volume and risk from carotid endarterectomy. Complication rates at a hospital performing such surgeries should be less than 3% for individuals undergoing surgery for asymptomatic lesions and less than 6% for symptomatic individuals.

Predictors of Perioperative Risk

Sundt et al. graded patient risk for carotid endarterectomy based on the criteria listed in Table 11.3. Based on this, patients could belong to 4 grades of risk. Grade 1 (0.9% risk): No angiographic or medical predictors and stable neurologically. Grade 2 (1.7% risk): No medical but angiographic risk predictors. Stable neurologically. Grade 3 (3.1% risk): Major medical and/or angiographic predictors. Stable neurologically. Grade 4 (9.1% risk): Neurologically unstable.

Operative Complications

Table 11.4 lists complications with carotid endarterectomy other than stroke, MI, and death. Cranial nerve complications need to be watched for. Any individual with prior history of neck surgery of hoarseness should undergo laryngoscopy prior to carotid endarterectomy.

Technical Considerations in Carotid Surgery

General Versus Regional Anesthesia. With regional anesthesia, a local anesthetic is given to block levels C2 through C4. Because of the ease of intraoperative assessment of alterations in neurologic exam compared to baseline as assessed by speech, orientation, and contralateral strength, which can readily prompt maneuvers to improve cerebral perfusion, this approach has gained popularity. Potential complications with regional anesthesia include hypotension, seizure, anesthetic toxicity, hoarseness,

TABLE 11.3

RISK FACTORS FOR PERIOPERATIVE COMPLICATIONS FROM CAROTID ENDARTERECTOMY

Neurologic
   Deficit within past 24 h
   Stroke within the past 7 d
   Crescendo TIA
   Global cerebral ischemia
   CT evidence of stroke
Angiographic
   Ulcerated plaque on angiography
   >3 cm distal carotid stenosis
   >5 cm proximal carotid stenosis
   High bifurcation (at C2)
   Intraluminal thrombus
Medical
   Age > 50 y
   Hypertension
   Chronic obstructive pulmonary disease
   Severe obesity
   Diabetes mellitus

dysphagia, phrenic nerve palsy, and hematoma formation. This is currently the standard approach for CEA. Proponents of general anesthesia argue that intraoperative evaluation techniques such as carotid stump pressure measurement, EEG, transcranial Doppler, and evoked potential monitoring may help predict need for a shunt to augment cerebral flow. These techniques however correlate poorly with cerebral blood flow and do not translate into better outcomes.

Determination of Cerebral Tolerance to Ischemia. With local anesthesia, the common internal and external carotid arteries are occluded for 3 minutes, during this time the patient is asked to talk and lift his or her arms and legs. In 90% of patients, the collateral circulation is adequate to withstand this insult. In 10%, a shunt may need to be placed (see below). In individuals undergoing general anesthesia, the following modalities are used to determine adequacy of collateral flow in response to transient cerebral ischemia: (i) visual back bleeding from the ICA and (ii) ICA stump pressure of less than 25 mm Hg (except in those who have had prior strokes and may require routine placement of shunts)

Intraoperative Shunting. The selection of patients for shunt use has been controversial. Some advocate the use of shunts in all patients, while most cite that this is not universally required (shunting increases carotid clamp time and may damage the distal ICA). Prophylactic shunting is recommended

TABLE 11.4

COMPLICATIONS OF CAROTID ENDARTERECTOMY RELATED TO SURGERY

Complications	Incidence %	Clinical Features	Recovery/Management
Postoperative hypertension	19	Associated with hypovolemia (unsuspected)	Volume
Postoperative hypertension	28	Preoperative hypertension predicts development	Both complications related to carotid sinus mechanisms
Cervical hematoma	0.5–1.5	Often detected on removal of ET tube with patient valsalva. Prophylactic placement of drain may pick up continued bleeding	Reoperation; protamine if excessive bleeding perioperatively
Cranial Nerve Palsies[a]			
Recurrent laryngeal	7	Arises through vagal injury within carotid sheath; hoarseness postoperatively	PTFE (teflon) injection to vocal cord to return it to midline
Hypoglossal	6	Injured by excessive retraction; ipsilateral deviation of tongue, inarticulate speech, and clumsy mastication	80% resolve by 8 wk
Marginal mandibular	2	Injured by excessive retraction; drooping of angle of mouth (lower motor neuron type facial paralysis)	85% resolve spontaneously
Superior laryngeal	2	Carotid clamp may injure the main trunk (near carotid sinus) or the motor or sensory branches. Voice fatigue and loss of high-pitch phonation (may not be apparent in nonmusicians)	85% resolve spontaneously. Only 50% resolve
Glossopharyngeal	<0.5%	Rare; paralysis of the middle constrictor muscle with difficulty swallowing; most recover	Occurs only with mandibular subluxation for high carotid bifurcation; nutritional support
Recurrent restenosis	10–20%	Asymptomatic presentation Higher rates in women than in men	Only 1–2% require reoperation; vein patch angioplasty may reduce incidence

[a]Rates are for presentation in the immediate postoperative period.

in (i) contralateral carotid occlusion: The incidence of ipsilateral ischemia during carotid cross-clamping appears to be related to the patency of the contralateral carotid artery (50% incidence of ipsilateral cerebral ischemia during carotid cross-clamping when the contralateral artery is occluded) and (ii) ipsilateral CVA (recent). In patients who demonstrate signs of cerebral ischemia with carotid cross-clamping who do not fall under the two criteria mentioned above, a carotid shunt (most commonly used shunt is the Javid shunt) should be placed.

Primary Repair Versus Patch Closure. The debate over primary repair and patch closure is an ongoing one with proponents of each technique arguing their case. Proponents of primary repair argue that patching increases carotid occlusion time by 5 to 10 minutes and creates changes in shear stress along the wall of the carotid artery, which may result in thrombosis, atherosclerosis, and accelerated intimal hyperplasia. Saphenous vein harvesting to create a patch lengthens operating time, introduces a leg wound, and may prohibit the future use of the saphenous vein for other procedures besides being associated with a tangible risk of patch rupture (0.5 to 4%). The use of synthetic material to create the patch is not risk free either, with a definite risk for infection and rendering follow-up carotid duplex studies difficult owing to acoustic shadowing of the prosthetic material. Advocates for patch closure argue that primary closure results in narrowing of the artery by as much as 15%. Multiple randomized studies have been performed with mixed results. Several studies did not show any difference between patch closure and primary repair, while others showed some benefit with patch closure. In a meta-analysis of these studies, however, there appears to be a benefit to patch closure. The incidence of perioperative stroke decreased from 3.9% with primary closure to 1.2% with patch closure ($P = 0.008$). Similarly, the incidence of restenosis of at least 50% at 1 year was significant between primary and patch closure (7.4 vs. 2.1%, $P < 0.001$).

Carotid Stenting

Virtually all endovascular carotid interventions currently performed are stent based (Fig. 11.2). This trend appears appropriate based on the modest results in terms of residual stenosis or restenosis on follow-up achieved with angioplasty observed in the Carotid and Vertebral Artery Transluminal Angioplasty Study (CAVATAS) trial. Percutaneous intervention of the carotid arteries may have several advantages over surgical treatment (Table 11.5). In addition, the procedure is performed at lower costs, requires shorter hospital stay, and is less influenced by comorbidities. Therefore, it is particularly suited for patients at high risk for surgery (Table 11.6).

Technique and Complications

Procedural details are reported in Table 11.7. Appropriate patient selection is crucial in ensuring success of endovascular carotid intervention. Gaining access to the common carotid with the guiding catheter or sheath is a step associated with distal embolization and rarely vessel

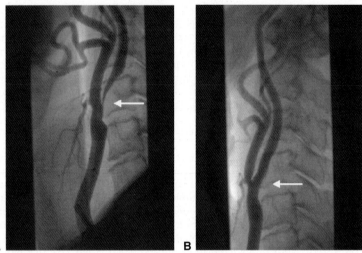

FIGURE 11-2. A: Severe stenosis of the proximal ICA. **B:** The results after stenting.

wall dissection. Hypotension and bradycardia are common at the time of angioplasty or stenting of the internal carotid bulb. These conditions are usually transient and mild and respond well to atropine and volume, only rarely requiring vasopressor support. Complications of endovascular procedures not specific to cerebral interventions include access-site hematomas, allergic reactions to contrast, heart failure, and contrast-induced nephropathy. Patients with severe peripheral vascular disease; severely calcified, tortuous or steep aortic arch; and/or severe calcification or tortuosity of cervicocranial vessels represent a high-risk subset for percutaneous intervention. Similarly, patients with severe renal insufficiency or a history of anaphylactic reaction to angiographic contrast may not be appropriate candidates, although alternatives to conventional contrast do exist.

Cerebral ischemia remains the most feared complication of carotid stenting (and of endarterectomy). The underlying mechanism is distal embolization, while acute vessel closure due to dissection, vasospasm, or thrombosis is rare. Transcranial Doppler monitoring, a noninvasive method to detect echogenic microemboli, has demonstrated frequent embolization during both carotid endarterectomy and stenting. The use of mechanical emboli protection devices may significantly reduce the risk of cerebral ischemia, as described below. Intracranial hemorrhage is another devastating complication, occurring in less than 1% of carotid revascularization cases (endarterectomy and stenting). Putative mechanisms include embolization and hemorrhagic conversion of an infracted region, the use of heparin and potent antiplatelet agents, and the hyperperfusion syndrome. High-risk features associated with the development of hyperperfusion syndrome

TABLE 11.5

PRO AND CONS OF CAROTID ENDARTERECTOMY AND STENTING

Carotid endarterectomy
- **Pros**
- Widely available
- Established technique
- Excellent results with the right surgeon (i.e., high volume) and the right patient (i.e., nonhigh risk)
- **Cons**
- General anesthesia (in the vast majority of cases)
- More frequent use of vasopressors
- Neck complications, cranial nerve palsies
- Not suitable for high (above C2) or low (below C7) lesions
- Outcome influenced by comorbidities
- Longer hospital stay, higher costs
- Carotid stenting
- **Pros**
- Local anesthesia
- No neck incision/scar/complications
- No violation of the body integrity
- Next day discharge, lower costs
- Outcome less influenced by comorbidities
- Randomized data available (in high-risk patients)
- **Cons**
- Require expertise, not widely available
- May be suboptimal for patients with
  - Severe peripheral vascular disease
  - Severely calcified, tortuous, or steep aortic arch
  - Severe calcification or tortuosity of cervicocranial vessels

include perioperative hypertension, revascularization of a severe stenosis with poor collateral blood flow, and the presence of bilateral severe stenoses or contralateral occlusion.

Adjuvant Antiplatelet Therapy and Anticoagulation Considerations

Carotid stenting is safely performed in the presence of aspirin and an ADP antagonist. Clopidogrel may be superior to ticlopidine in the setting of carotid stenting. The use of adjunctive glycoprotein IIb/IIIa receptor inhibitors (GP IIb/IIIa inhibitors) remains controversial. Currently, GP IIb/IIIa inhibitors should be considered only in selected patients and cannot be currently recommended as routine adjunctive treatment of carotid stenting. Periprocedural unfractionated heparin should be given to achieve activated clotting time (ACT) of 275 to 300 seconds. No postprocedural anticoagulation is needed. Dual antiplatelet therapy with aspirin and

TABLE 11.6

SAPPHIRE TRIAL HIGH-RISK CHARACTERISTICS

- Congestive heart failure (New York Heart Association class III/IV) and/or known severe left ventricular dysfunction (ejection fraction < 30%)
- Open heart surgery needed within 6 wk
- Recent MI (>24 h and <4 wk)
- Unstable angina (Canadian Cardiovascular Society class III/IV)
- Severe pulmonary disease
- Contralateral carotid occlusion
- Contralateral laryngeal nerve palsy
- Radiation therapy to neck
- Previous carotid endarterectomy with recurrent stenosis
- High cervical internal carotid/below the clavicle common carotid lesions
- Severe tandem lesions
- Age > 80 y

clopidogrel should be continued for at least a month, preferably longer, and lifelong aspirin is recommended.

Results of Carotid Stenting

Several reports have shown encouraging outcomes following carotid stenting. Importantly, the patients included were high-risk patients who were not candidates for surgery. Therefore, the results of carotid stenting should be put in perspective and not immediately compared with the results of the large-scale randomized endarterectomy trials, generated by highly selected surgeons performing surgery on a highly selected patient population. The largest series of carotid stenting with prospective assessment and rigorous long-term follow-up of the preemboli protection era has been reported by Roubin et al. The 30-day fatal stroke rate in this series was 0.6%, and the nonstroke death rate was 1%. The corresponding major stroke rate was 1%, the minor stroke rate was 4.8%, and the overall stroke and death rate was 7.4%. Over the 5-year study period, the stroke rate occurring after day 30 was 3.2%. Restenosis was rare (5%) despite consequent follow-up assessment with either angiography or ultrasound imaging.

Mechanical Emboli Protection

Several mechanical approaches to prevent distal embolization and thus to increase safety of carotid stenting have been investigated and include filter devices, distal balloon occlusion, and proximal balloon occlusion with flow reversal (Fig. 11.3). In the largest series investigating distal balloon occlusion (PercuSurge GuardWire, Medtronic, Santa Rosa, CA) in carotid stenting, Henry et al. reported excellent technical success with an intolerance to balloon occlusion in a minority of patients (4%) and 30-day stroke and death rate of 2.7%. Importantly, microscopic analysis of the aspirated

TABLE 11.7

PROTOCOL FOR CAROTID STENTING

- Arterial sheath inserted in the femoral artery; short-acting intravenous sedation if needed
- An aortic arch angiographic study (LAO 30° projection) is performed to determine the origin of the great vessels to choose an appropriate catheter for selective angiography
- Baseline angiography performed of the bilateral vertebral and carotid arteries to determine the extent of vascular disease and presence of collateral circulation
- Unfractionated heparin 60 U/kg administered with target ACT 275–300 s
- A 125-cm 5F JR4 diagnostic catheter (Cordis Corporation, Miami, FL) placed inside a 90-cm 7F Cook Shuttle Sheath (Cook Corporation, Bloomington, IN) or a 100-cm 8F H1 guiding catheter (Cordis Corporation, Miami, FL)
- The origin of the common carotid artery is intubated with the JR4 catheter and a 0.035 Magic-Torque (Boston Scientific, Miami, FL) guidewire advanced into the external carotid artery
- The 6F Cook Shuttle Sheath/8F H1 guiding catheter is advanced into the common carotid artery over the JR4 catheter
- The JR4 catheter is withdrawn at this time and diagnostic angiograms performed in the ipsilateral 30° oblique and left lateral projection for vessel sizing
- The lesion in the carotid artery is traversed with a 0.014-in Angioguard XP filter device (Cordis Corporation, Miami, FL)
- 0.5–1 mg of atropine IV usually administered
- 4.0 × 20-mm rapid exchange angioplasty balloon catheter used to predilate
- Stenting performed with a nitinol self-expanding stent (PRECISE stent, Cordis Corporation, Miami, FL)
- Stent postdilation with a 5.5 × 20-mm balloon catheter
- Final angiographic shots of the carotid bifurcation and intracranial angiogram
- All patients receive 325–500 mg of aspirin and 300 mg of clopidogrel prior to the procedure and are discharged home the following day on clopidogrel (75 mg PO q.d.) for 4 wk and on aspirin (100–325 mg PO q.d.) indefinitely

blood confirmed debris in all cases (particle mean diameter, 250 μm). The ACCULINK for Revascularization of Carotids (ARCHER) registry was a single-arm, prospective study addressing the use of the Accunet filter (Guidant, Indianapolis, IN) in 437 patients with symptomatic stenosis of ≥50% or asymptomatic stenosis ≥80% but with high-risk features for surgery (similar to the SAPPHIRE criteria, Table 11.6). The primary end point (composite of stroke, death, or MI) at 30 days was reached in 7.8%. Of particular clinical importance were the results among 141 patients treated for restenosis following carotid endarterectomy showing combined end point rate as low as 1.4% at 30 days. Similarly, the stroke, death, or MI rate of 7.6% among 66 patients with contralateral carotid occlusion compared favorably with the stroke and death rate of 14.3% reported in NASCET.

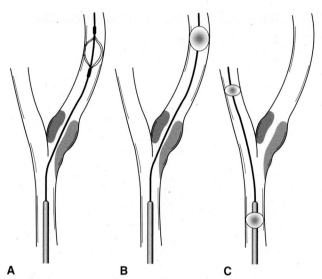

FIGURE 11-3. A number of distal protection devices that aim to reduce or elimi- nate distal embolization during percutaneous carotid interventions are being used. **A** demonstrates the Angioguard (Cordis Corporation, Miami Lakes, FL) device that incorporates an angioplasty guidewire with a filter that expands and is placed distal to the target lesion to capture and retrieve embolic debris. At the end of the proce- dure, the filter is collapsed, trapping the embolic debris, and removed from the artery. The AngioGuard filter has multiple, 100 μm, laser-drilled holes that allow perfusion during device deployment. This is a major advantage of filter devices since perfu- sion is maintained during the procedure. In contrast, the balloon occlusion device **B** results in complete occlusion of antegrade flow while the device is deployed. The PercuSurge GuardWire (Medtronic, Santa Rosa, CA) is an occlusion thrombectomy device that consists of a wire containing a central lumen that communicates with a low-pressure distal occlusion balloon incorporated into the tip. The wire serves as both the angioplasty guidewire and provides protection from distal embolization. An inflation device allows controlled expansion of the balloon in the treated vessel. An aspiration catheter is used to remove the debris from the treated vessel before the balloon is deflated and antegrade flow in the treated vessel is restored. The Parodi Anti-Emboli System (PAES; ArteriA Medical Science, Inc., San Francisco, CA) is a guiding catheter with an occlusion balloon attached at its distal end (**C**). The PAES establishes protection by reversing blood flow in the target vessel. The system works by occluding the common carotid, which creates a negative pressure gradient distal to the balloon occlusion and establishes retrograde flow in the ICA. The external carotid is also occluded to avoid flow traveling from the external one back up the internal one. Since there is no antegrade flow, embolization is prevented.

Surgery Versus Percutaneous Intervention

Several large clinical trials have compared endarterectomy with endovas- cular therapy (Table 11.8). The CAVATAS trial randomized 504 patients with symptomatic carotid stenosis to surgery or angioplasty. Stents were used in 26% of the patients in the endovascular arm. The 30-day

TABLE 11.8

CAROTID STENT STUDIES

Study	Year	N	30-day Death + Stroke (CEA) N (%)	30-day Death + Stroke (CAS) N (%)
Leicester	1998	23	0 (0%)	5 (45.5%)
Wallstent	2001	219	5 (4.5%)	13 (12.1%)
Kentucky-Sympt	2001	104	1 (2%)	0 (0%)
CAVATAS	2001	504	25 (9.9%)	25 (10%)
Kentucky-Asympt	2004	85	0 (0%)	0 (0%)
SAPPHIRE	2004	334	9 (5.4%)	8 (4.8%)
EVA-3S	2006	527	10 (3.9%)	25 (9.6%)
SPACE	2006	1183	38 (6.5%)	46 (7.7%)
BACASS	2008	20	1 (10%)	0 (0%)
ICSS	2009	1649	28 (3.4%)	61 (7.4%)
CREST[a]	2010	2502	56 (4.5%)	66 (5.2%)

[a]For CREST, the primary end point was any periprocedural stroke, myocardial infarction, or death or postprocedural ipsilateral stroke.
CAVATAS, Carotid And Vertebral Artery Transluminal Angioplasty Study; SAPPHIRE, Stenting and Angioplasty with Protection in Patients at High Risk for Endarterectomy; EVA 3S, Endarterectomy Versus Stenting in severe carotid stenosis; SPACE, Stent-protected Angioplasty versus Carotid Endarterectomy in symptomatic patients; BACASS, Basel Carotid Artery Stenting Study; CREST, Carotid Revascularization Endarterectomy versus Stenting Trial.

incidence of death or any stroke was 10% in both groups. The event-free survival remained identical in the 2 groups up to 3 years. Yadav et al reported the 30-day results of the Stenting and Angioplasty with Protection in Patients at High Risk for Endarterectomy (SAPPHIRE) trial, a multicenter randomized trial comparing carotid endarterectomy and carotid stenting with filter-based emboli protection (Angioguard, Cordis Corporation, Miami, FL) in patients deemed to be at high risk for surgery (Table 11.6). The required degree of stenosis was ≥50% in symptomatic patients and ≥80% in asymptomatic patients. A neurologist, a surgeon, and an interventionalist assessed all patients. The trial was stopped early after enrollment of 723 patients (307 patients were randomized, 409 were followed in the stent registry, and 7 were followed in a surgical registry) because, although the study was designed to assess noninferiority among the two strategies, carotid stenting with emboli protection turned out to be superior to surgery. Accordingly, the primary end point of 30-day death, stroke, or MI rate occurred in 5.8% among patients randomized to carotid stenting and in 12.6% among those who underwent surgery ($P = 0.047$). A nonstatistically significant benefit was observed across the individual end points. Importantly, patients who were considered to be at too high risk for surgery and therefore entered a carotid stent registry had a favorable death, stroke, or MI rate of 7.8%.

The Endarterectomy Versus Stenting in Severe Carotid Stenosis trial was a randomized noninferiority trial comparing CEA to carotid stenting in symptomatic patients with a 60 to 99% stenosis. This trial was terminated prematurely due to an increase in primary end points (any stroke or death within 30 days) in the stent arm (3.9 vs. 9.6%, respectively). The Stent-Protected Angioplasty Versus Carotid Endarterectomy in Symptomatic Patients trial was a noninferiority trial that enrolled 1,200 patients to either carotid stenting with or without cerebral protection versus CEA. The primary end point of stroke or death was achieved in 6.84% in the stent arm versus 6.34% in the CEA arm. The recently reported International Carotid Stenting Study (ICSS) showed superior results with surgery, at least at 30 days' postprocedure. The incidence of death, MI, and stroke was 5.1 in the surgical arm and 8.5% with stenting. The Carotid Revascularization Endarterectomy versus Stenting Trial (CREST) was a rigorous trial, using a single device and optimal medical management and showed similar net outcomes with CAS and CEA for the treatment of carotid stenosis. The composite primary end point of any stroke, MI, or death during the periprocedural period or ipsilateral stroke on follow-up was 7.2% with stenting versus 6.8% with surgery (P = NS). The CREST data provides evidence that there is clinical equipoise between CEA and CAS for patients who are at average surgical risk. It is also important to note that EVA, ICSS, and SPACE help us understand that operator experience influences the outcome of CAS, as it has likewise been shown to influence the outcome of CEA. Overall, the totality of the data suggests that carotid revascularization performed by highly qualified surgeons and interventionists is effective and safe.

Concomitant Carotid and Coronary Artery Disease

Carotid disease and coronary disease are often concomitant as atherosclerosis is a systemic disease. The overall perioperative stroke rate with routine coronary artery bypass grafting (CABG) is 1 to 3%. Patients with greater than 50% ICA stenosis carry a 9.2% risk of perioperative neurologic event, while individuals with greater than 75% stenosis carry a 14.3% of perioperative stroke rate. In this difficult patient population, controversy exists regarding in what order to perform the two operations: CEA followed by CABG (staged), CABG followed by CEA (reverse-staged), or a combined approach at one setting (Table 11.9). The majority of the reported literature is retrospective in nature. In the combined group, there was a 2.8 to 3.3% stroke rate and a 3.4 to 4.2% mortality rate. Reverse-staged is reported to have a 14% stroke rate and a 5.3% mortality rate. The staged approach resulted in a 3 to 4% stroke rate and a 3 to 4% mortality rate. In summary, retrospective reports show little difference between staged and combined approaches; however, reverse-staged appears to confer higher stroke and mortality rates. In general, the more severe and symptomatic problem should be addressed initially. In the setting of severe carotid disease with normal to moderate coronary disease, a combined or staged procedure (CEA prior to CABG) should be undertaken. With severe, unstable coronary

TABLE 11.9

STROKE AND MORTALITY RATES FOR CONCOMITANT CAROTID ENDARTERECTOMY [CEA] AND BYPASS SURGERY [CABG]

Order of Procedure	Stroke Rates	Mortality Rates
Staged (CEA prior to CABG)	3–4%	3–4%
Reverse-Staged (CABG prior to CEA)	14%	5.3%
Combined (Simultaneous CEA and CABG)	2.8–3.3%	3.4–4.2%

disease and asymptomatic unilateral carotid disease without contralateral disease, combined or reverse-staged approaches should be considered. In the setting of severe coronary and carotid disease, any of the three approaches should be considered depending on individual surgeons' experience and morbidity rates. One large observational study has reported that patients who underwent carotid stenting followed by heart surgery had significantly fewer adverse events than those undergoing CEA + CABG, despite a worse baseline risk profile. Carotid stenting may be a safer carotid revascularization option for this challenging patient population but needs to be validated further.

CONCLUSIONS

- Stroke is the leading cause of long-term serious disability and the third leading cause of death in Western countries.
- Carotid artery disease is the underlying etiology in up to two thirds of patients with stroke.
- In symptomatic carotid disease, medical management with antiplatelet agents does not provide adequate protection against stroke recurrence, and carotid revascularization has been shown to be superior in this setting.
- In asymptomatic patients, the value of revascularization is less well established. Patients with severe carotid stenosis may benefit from revascularization if this can be performed at a low periprocedural risk.
- In recent years, carotid stenting has gained widespread attention.
- Although mainly performed in patients at high risk for surgery, the results have been encouraging with acceptable periprocedural stroke rates.
- A major breakthrough has been the use of emboli protection devices.
- Available evidence from CREST and SAPPHIRE suggests that there is clinical equipoise between CEA and CAS for patients who are at average or high surgical risk.
- Currently, CAS is approved for symptomatic patients at high surgical risk.

PRACTICAL POINTS

■ Aspirin (50 to 325 mg/d) monotherapy, the combination of aspirin and extended-release dipyridamole, and clopidogrel monotherapy are all acceptable options for initial therapy for stroke prevention.

■ Lipid lowering with statins are effective in preventing stroke.

■ Carotid endarterectomy remains the gold standard for revascularization of carotid artery stenosis.

■ Carotid stenting is currently approved for patients at high risk for CEA who have symptomatic carotid artery stenosis greater than 70%, as long as stenting is performed using FDA-approved systems with embolic protection devices.

■ Clopidogrel appears superior to ticlopidine as an ADP receptor antagonist in the setting of carotid stenting.

■ An emboli protection device should be used during carotid stenting and potentially during carotid endarterectomy.

■ Carotid revascularization performed by highly qualified surgeons and interventionists is effective and safe.

RECOMMENDED READING

Adams RJ, Albers G, Alberts MJ, et al. Update to the AHA/ASA recommendations for the prevention of stroke in patients with stroke and transient ischemic attack. *Stroke* 2008;39: 1647–1652.

Amarenco P, Bogousslavsky J, Callahan A III, et al. High-dose atorvastatin after stroke or transient ischemic attack. *N Engl J Med* 2006;355(6):549–559.

American Heart Association. *Heart disease and stroke statistics - 2010 update.* Dallas, TX: American Heart Association, 2009.

Autret A, Pourcelot L, Saudeau D, et al. Stroke risk in patients with carotid stenosis. *Lancet* 1987;1:888–890.

Beneficial effect of carotid endarterectomy in symptomatic patients with high-grade carotid stenosis. North American Symptomatic Carotid Endarterectomy Trial Collaborators [see comments]. *N Engl J Med* 1991;325:445–453.

Bhatt DL, Kapadia SR, Bajzer CT, et al. Dual antiplatelet therapy with clopidogrel and aspirin after carotid artery stenting. *J Invasive Cardiol* 2001;13:767–771.

Brott TG, Hobson RW II, Howard G, et al for the CREST Investigators. Stenting versus endarterectomy for treatment of carotid-artery stenosis. *N Engl J Med* 2010;363(1):11–23.

Bucher HC, Griffith LE, Guyatt GH. Effect of HMGcoA reductase inhibitors on stroke. A meta-analysis of randomized, controlled trials. *Ann Intern Med* 1998;128:89–95.

Endarterectomy for asymptomatic carotid artery stenosis. Executive Committee for the Asymptomatic Carotid Atherosclerosis Study [see comments]. *JAMA* 1995;273:1421–1428.

Endovascular versus surgical treatment in patients with carotid stenosis in the Carotid and Vertebral Artery Transluminal Angioplasty Study (CAVATAS): a randomised trial. *Lancet* 2001;357:1729–1737.

Hebert PR, Gaziano JM, Chan KS, et al. Cholesterol lowering with statin drugs, risk of stroke, and total mortality. An overview of randomized trials. *JAMA* 1997;278:313–321.

Hobson RW, II, Krupski WC, Weiss DG. Influence of aspirin in the management of asymptomatic carotid artery stenosis. VA Cooperative Study Group on Asymptomatic Carotid Stenosis. *J Vasc Surg* 1993;17:257–263; discussion 263–265.

Mukherjee D, Yadav SJ. Cerebrovascular diseases: pathophysiology and management. In: Fuster V, ed. *Assessing and modifying the vulnerable atherosclerotic plaque.* Armonk, NY: Futura Publishing, 2002:29–55.

Ouriel K, Hertzer NR, Beven EG, et al. Preprocedural risk stratification: identifying an appropriate population for carotid stenting. *J Vasc Surg* 2001;33:728–732.

Randomised trial of endarterectomy for recently symptomatic carotid stenosis: final results of the MRC European Carotid Surgery Trial (ECST). *Lancet* 1998;351:1379–1387.

Roffi M, Mukherjee D, Clair DG. Carotid artery stenting versus endarterectomy. *Eur Heart J* 2009;30(22):2693–2704.

Sila CA. Carotid stenosis: current strategies for choosing between medical and surgical management. *Cleve Clin J Med* 2000;67:851–861.

Silvennoinen HM, Ikonen S, Soinne L, et al. CT angiographic analysis of carotid artery stenosis: comparison of manual assessment, semiautomatic vessel analysis, and digital subtraction angiography. *Am J Neuroradiol* 2007;28:97–103.

Sudlow CL, Warlow CP. Comparable studies of the incidence of stroke and its pathological types: results from an international collaboration. International Stroke Incidence Collaboration. *Stroke* 1997;28:491–499.

Sundt TM Jr, Meyer, FB, Piepgras, DG, et al. Risk factors and operative results. In: Weber FB, ed. *Sundt's occlusive cerebrovascular disease*, 2nd ed. Philadelphia, PA: WB Saunders Co, 1994:241–247.

Aneurysms: Diagnosis and Management
Sean J. English, Jonathan L. Eliason, and Gilbert R. Upchurch Jr

INTRODUCTION

Abdominal aortic aneurysms (AAAs) primarily affect the elderly and have a high mortality rate if left untreated. Encounters with this disease will become more frequent as society ages during the 21st century, as evidenced by the observation that AAA accounts for approximately 150,000 inpatient hospital admissions per year in the United States. Data from the CDC National Vital Statistics on deaths from the year 2006 demonstrated that aortic aneurysm constituted the 16th leading cause of death in all patients aged 65 to 85 years. Aortic disease represented the 15th leading cause of death for Caucasian males of the same age group. The year 2000 National Hospital Discharge Summary reports more than 30,000 open operations for the repair of AAA were performed in the United States. Dimick et al. using Medicare data from all hospitals in the United States from 2001 to 2003 that performed AAA surgery documented 54,302 open repairs that were performed during that time period, while 26,750 endovascular repairs were performed during that same time period. Better defining those patients who are most at risk for AAA development is therefore an important undertaking.

Risk Factors

Atherosclerosis, a common finding in patients with AAAs, is believed to be a secondary rather than a primary etiologic factor in AAA development and may potentiate its development by further compromising the structure of the aortic wall. Age, male gender, smoking, hypertension, and the presence of chronic obstructive pulmonary disease (COPD) place patients at increased risk for the development of AAAs. Genetic factors also appear important in AAA development, with 15% of patients having a first-degree relative with an AAA (Table 12.1). For example, a decrease in aortic wall type III collagen has been noted in individuals with a first-degree relative with an AAA, compared to those without a family history of AAAs. Increases in the frequency of the Hp-2-1 haptoglobin phenotype, as well as the Kell positive and MN blood groups, have been noted in patients with AAAs. By contrast, there is a decrease in the incidence of AAAs in patients with type A Rh-negative blood group. A number of genetic polymorphisms have been associated with AAAs. However, since most AAAs are degenerative in nature, a polygenic inheritance pattern is likely. Rarer causes of AAAs include trauma, dissections, vasculitis, and infection (Table 12.1).

TABLE 12.1

VARIOUS ETIOLOGIES OF AAAs

Degenerative
Atherosclerosis
Connective tissue disorder
Cystic medial necrosis
Marfan's syndrome
Ehlers-Danlos' syndrome
Trauma
Dissection
Vasculitis
Takayasu's arteritis
Mycotic
Bacterial (*Staph* sp.)

Pathogenesis

AAAs are characterized by marked inflammation and an imbalance between the production and the degradation of structural extracellular matrix proteins. Disruption and degradation of medial elastin and collagen is a particularly prominent feature of AAA formation. In this regard, increased local production of enzymes that degrade elastin and collagen, namely the matrix metalloproteinases, has been proposed as being pivotal in vessel wall initiation and clinical progression of aneurysmal disease.

Clinical Features

Most AAAs are asymptomatic and over 80% are located in the infrarenal aorta. Normal aortic pulsation is roughly the width of the patient's thumb. An aortic aneurysm may be suspected when the aortic pulse is expansile and larger than two centimeters. Extension of the pulsations to the xiphoid or costal margins should make one suspect a thoracoabdominal or suprarenal aortic aneurysm. Presence of tenderness over an aneurysm is an ominous sign and may indicate impending rupture. Palpation of the lateral borders of the aorta between one's fingertips on abdominal examination may suggest the presence of a large pulsatile mass. However, prominent anterior pulsations alone are more likely to be due to an ectatic, nonaneurysmal aorta than an AAA. It is often difficult to palpate the infrarenal aorta in the epigastrium because the aortic bifurcation is at the level of the umbilicus. Thus, physical examination alone is unreliable in most patients, especially if obese. In one series of patients with known AAAs, experienced clinicians were unable to make the diagnosis in close to half the patients with the disease.

Concomitant Aneurysmal Disease

Patients with AAAs may also have aneurysms of the femoral or popliteal arteries. A study in patients with AAAs from the University of Michigan documented a 14% incidence of aneurysms of the femoral and popliteal arteries, all occurring in hypertensive male patients. The presence of these extremity aneurysms may serve as a clue to the existence of an AAA. In addition, it is important to recognize that patients with femoral and popliteal artery aneurysms have approximately an 80 and 60% chance of having an AAA, respectively.

Clinical Features of a Ruptured Abdominal Aortic Aneurysm

The classic triad of acute hypotension, back or abdominal pain, and a palpable abdominal mass is rarely seen. The patient with an unsuspected AAA may present with a clinical picture that suggests exacerbation of chronic back pain. A more acute presentation with the acute onset of abdominal, flank, or back pain radiating to the groin may be secondary to AAA expansion or rupture. Without imaging studies or a high index of suspicion, this pain may be confused with diverticulitis, renal colic, irritable bowel syndrome, inflammatory bowel disease, ovarian torsion, or appendicitis. In the hemodynamically stable patient with symptoms consistent with the diagnosis of an AAA, the use of abdominal ultrasonography (US) may be performed expeditiously as it confirms the suspected diagnosis of a ruptured AAA (rAAA), requires no transport time, and is quite sensitive. CT angiography in a stable patient when the diagnosis is uncertain is also now routinely performed, with the advent of endovascular aortic repair (EVAR). Patients with severe hypotension, unrelenting abdominal or back pain, and a suspected rAAA should be transported urgently to the endovascular suite where an open or an endovascular approach may be used.

DIAGNOSIS

Once an AAA is suspected, a logical diagnostic algorithm should be followed (Fig. 12.1). Plain abdominal or lumbosacral radiographs performed in either the anterior-posterior (AP) or the lateral projections done for other reasons, such as to examine the lumbar spine, may suggest the presence of an AAA by demonstrating a rim of calcification in the outer aortic wall (Fig. 12.2).

Ultrasound

The most useful means to establish the diagnosis of an AAA is duplex US. US is a noninvasive, inexpensive test that provides reliable and reproducible measurements of the aortic diameter (Fig. 12.3). US correlates closely with operative measurements of AAA, and interobserver variability of less than 5 mm has been demonstrated in 80% of AP measurements. Errors and limitations with US are most often attributed to inexperienced technicians, lack of interpretive skills, or excessive bowel gas.

Computed Tomography Angiography

Computed tomography angiography (CTA) should be ordered if intervention is planned, as CT is highly predictive of AAA size, with interobserver variability of less than 5 mm existing in 91% of AP measurements. Importantly, CT is superior to US in assessing AAA wall integrity, the

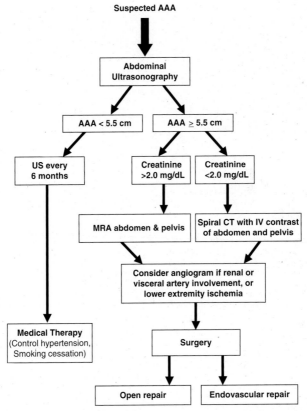

FIGURE 12-1. Algorithm for patient suspected of having an AAA. (*US*, ultrasound; *MRA*, magnetic resonance angiography; *CTA*, computed tomography angiography.)

location and amount of calcification within vessel walls, venous anomalies, retroperitoneal blood, aortic dissection, and infection or inflammation, as well as the proximal and distal extent of the aneurysm. CT may also demonstrate other intra-abdominal pathology (presence of various renal, adrenal, and gastrointestinal abnormalities) that may be important during planning for either an open or an endovascular approach. Limitations of CT include (a) need for nephrotoxic iodinated contrast administration, (b) increased radiation exposure, and (c) increased cost. Spiral or helical CTA provides excellent resolution and coronal reconstructions (Fig. 12.4). In addition to providing an anatomical roadmap prior to repair of AAAs, CT is the study of choice for assessing for postoperative endoleak following endovascular AAA repair (Fig. 12.5). Several recent studies have also suggested that US with power Doppler or various nonionic contrast agents (i.e., microbubbles) may also be used to follow AAA size and the presence of an endoleak (Fig. 12.6). This approach appears to be most useful in the setting of decreasing AAA size with prior CT evidence of no endoleak.

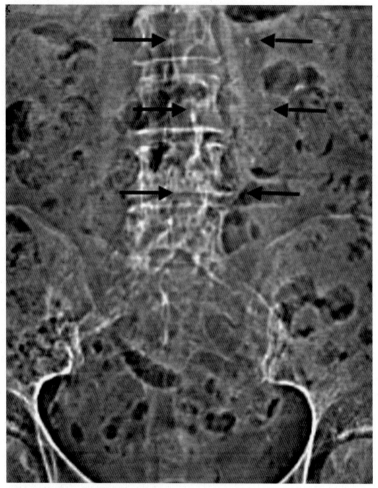

FIGURE 12-2. AP plain abdominal radiograph demonstrating calcification (*arrows*) in the aortic wall.

Magnetic Resonance Angiography

Magnetic resonance angiography (MRA) using nonnephrotoxic gadolinium with a breath-hold technique is comparable to CT scanning for AAA measurements. Images are based on T1 relaxation rather than blood flow, which means that slow flow in AAAs does not adversely affect the image. An earlier reported experience with 43 AAAs revealed that MRA correctly identified maximum AAA diameter and carried 94 and 98% sensitivity and specificity, respectively, for identifying significant stenoses of the splanchnic, renal, or iliac arteries. MRA limitations include the inability to scan

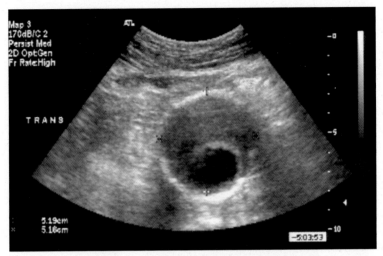

FIGURE 12-3. Duplex US documenting the AP (5.19 cm) and transverse diameter (5.16 cm) of an AAA. Note also the presence of a significant aortic thrombus.

patients who have pacemakers, defibrillators, or claustrophobia, and the fact that images may be obscured by artifacts caused by metallic objects including certain vascular stents. Disadvantages of MRA also include its inability to image calcified plaque, a finding important in endovascular interventions. However, MRA may be more sensitive than CTA for the detection of endoleaks after endovascular aortic aneurysm repair (EVAR).

Catheter-based Angiography

Catheter-based angiography with digital subtraction techniques is usually obtained when concomitant atherosclerotic vascular involvement is suspected, and treatment is planned prior to operative repair. Intravascular US (IVUS) may also be used concurrently when performing angiography. IVUS may be especially useful in assessing the size of the aortic neck, as most believe that CT tends to oversize aortic neck diameter. Angiography and IVUS may be useful in identifying the cephalad extent of the AAA, the number and location of renal arteries, the state of the splanchnic arteries, and the status of the iliac arteries, as well as the presence of occlusive disease in the lower-extremity arteries. Complications of angiography include bleeding or arterial occlusion at the catheterization site, atheroembolism, and impairment of renal function due to iodine-induced contrast nephrotoxicity.

Management of the Patient with Abdominal Aortic Aneurysm

The most serious complication of an AAA is continued expansion until aneurysm rupture occurs. Therefore, it is important to recognize factors contributing to AAA rupture. In accordance with the law of Laplace, a

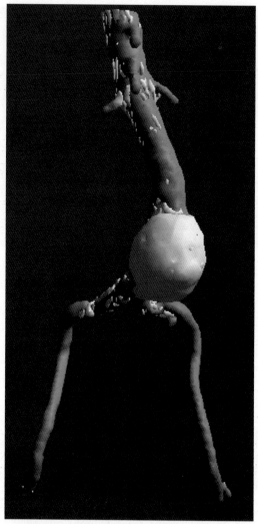

FIGURE 12-4. CTA scan of an AAA that would be considered a standard endovascular case, with an adequate infrarenal aortic neck length (>1.5 cm) and diameter (<3.2 cm), with minimal thrombus in the aortic neck, and with iliac arteries that are >6 mm in diameter, noncalcified, and nontortuous.

geometric increase in aortic wall pressure occurs with linear increases in AAA size. Thus, an increase in aortic diameter from 2 to 4 cm induces, not a twofold, but a fourfold increase in the pressure/cm^2 on the aortic wall. Rupture is directly proportional to aortic wall pressure. It is also known

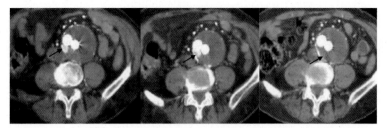

FIGURE 12-5.   CT scan demonstrating the presence of an endoleak after endovascular repair that resolved following coil embolization of a type 2 endoleak from a patent lumbar artery. *Arrows* marks endoleak.

that aortic elastic tissue loses its integrity with age. Acquired (smoking, hypertension), genetic factors, and patient characteristics (increasing age, male gender) hasten this process and add to the risk of accelerated AAA expansion. Aneurysm expansion greater than 6 mm over a 12-month time period suggests an unstable AAA and is a soft indication for early intervention in AAAs approaching 5 cm in diameter. An intact asymptomatic AAA with a diameter of 5 cm is generally recognized to carry a risk or rupture of 10% or less over 2 to 3 years. The risk of rupture for smaller aneurysms, 3 to 5 cm in size, is less well defined. However, greater anterior to posterior diameter, COPD, and diastolic hypertension all independently increase the

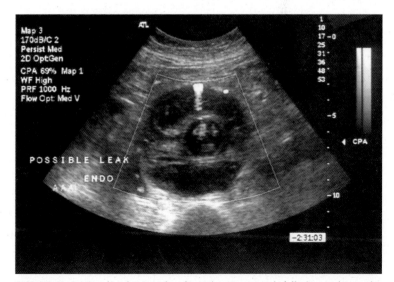

FIGURE 12-6.   Duplex ultrasound performed postoperatively following endovascular AAA repair showing a type 2 (branch vessel) endoleak.

chance of AAA rupture. Thus, the presence of a 5-cm AAA in a patient with diastolic hypertension and COPD is a cause for concern, with a predicted rupture rate of more than 30% in a year, compared to a 3-cm AAA in a normotensive patient without COPD, which has a rupture rate of only a few percentages over 5 years.

The risk of death following AAA rupture depends on performing an emergent and expeditious intervention. Attention to repairing the rAAA is paramount, and wasted time repairing small iliac artery aneurysms should be discouraged. Unfortunately, nearly 60% of patients with rAAAs die before reaching a hospital, and only 50% of the remainder survive an emergent operation. Thus, AAA rupture carries an 80% mortality rate.

Surgical Therapy

Elective operative intervention by open aortic repair (OAR) or an EVAR lessens the likelihood of death due to a rAAA. Conventional open repair in elective circumstances in a large population-based study from the state of Michigan carried a 5.6% mortality rate. Surprisingly, women fared worse than men following aneurysmectomy with operations for both intact and ruptured aneurysms. The elective mortality rate over an 11-year time period in women was 10.7% compared to 6.8% in men in this experience. Risk factors found to be predictive of a poor outcome and an increased in-hospital mortality following elective OAR include female gender, increased age (over 65 years), aneurysm rupture, and low volumes of aortic surgery. In fact, based only on age, gender, and hospital volume, up to an eightfold increase in mortality has been predicted.

Conventional Surgical Treatment of Intact Abdominal Aortic Aneurysms

A rapid operation is important for successful OAR, as an operation lasting longer than 5 hours is independently associated with an increase in mortality and significant cardiopulmonary complications. Other factors associated with poor surgical outcome include operative hypothermia, excessive blood loss, coagulopathy, and the need for supraceliac aortic cross clamping. Surgical approaches are individualized for each patient, with transperitoneal or retroperitoneal aortic exposure based on both the surgeon's preference and the aortic pathology. A transperitoneal approach is preferred when there is a need to revascularize the right kidney or if aneurysmal disease extends into the right iliac artery. Certain anatomic and clinical circumstances where a retroperitoneal approach is preferable include obese patients and those with multiple prior laparotomies and a "hostile" abdomen. Although the retroperitoneal approach does not significantly decrease mortality or major cardiopulmonary morbidity, multiple randomized trials suggest it expedites return of postoperative bowel function.

In the past, thrombotic and bleeding complications due to clamping and unclamping the aorta were the major complications following OAR. To address these issues, prior to occluding, the aorta patients are systemically anticoagulated with intravenous heparin, and the aorta is clamped distally prior to clamping proximally. The aneurysm is then incised, intraluminal clot is removed, and back-bleeding lumbar arteries are oversewn, before the aortic graft is sewn in place. The prosthetic grafts currently used are either woven or knitted Dacron or extruded polytetrafluoroethylene. After the graft is in place and blood flow is restored to the pelvis and the lower extremities, it is important that the graft be covered with the aneurysm sac and the retroperitoneum, so as to prevent contact with the intestines. Such contact may lead to later graft-enteric erosion, which is considered a life-threatening complication requiring graft removal.

Endovascular Surgical Treatment of Intact Abdominal Aortic Aneurysms

In 1999, two endovascular grafts were approved by the Food and Drug Administration for the treatment of infrarenal AAAs. Currently, there are four FDA-approved grafts including the AneuRx (Medtronic Inc., Minneapolis, MN, USA), the Excluder (WL Gore and Assoc., Flagstaff, AZ, USA), the Zenith (Cook Inc., Bloomington, IN, USA), and the Powerlink system (Endologix, Irvine, CA, USA) (Fig. 12.7). The Aorfix, Anaconda, Endurant, *LeMaitre* and Lifepath endografts have investigational device exemption and are undergoing trials in the United States. These endografts differ in design and deployment, although most of the devices are modular covered stent grafts and are deployed as a main aortic prosthesis with an ipsilateral iliac artery limb, followed by docking of a contralateral iliac

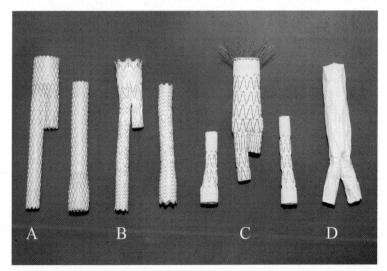

FIGURE 12-7. Current FDA-approved endografts for EVAR: **A:** AneuRx **B:** Excluder **C:** Zenith **D:** Powerlink system. Please note- Talent endograft not shown.

artery graft limb. Tubular endovascular stent grafts, for the most part, have been abandoned for infrarenal AAA repair due to increased endoleaks distally. Endografts are typically oversized 10 to 20% compared to the native aorta and iliac arteries in order to exclude flow and require surgical exposure of the access arteries, usually the proximal common femoral or distal external iliac arteries. Careful preoperative planning is necessary for selecting the length, diameter, and taper of the stent graft to match the aorta and iliac arteries. Many current devices and delivery sheaths are relatively rigid. Therefore, it is important to envision the position of the prosthesis in the target vessel. Angulation of the proximal and distal infrarenal aortic segments, as well as the iliac arteries, may make endograft deployment and fixation impossible. Sizing an artery by angiography alone can be difficult, even with specially constructed calibration catheters or intravascular ultrasound. Finally, covering the lumbar and the inferior mesenteric arteries with the device may lead to graft failure due to continued perfusion of the aneurysm by retrograde blood flow or an endoleak from a branch artery (Table 12.4).

Conventional Surgical Treatment of Ruptured Abdominal Aortic Aneurysms

The surgical approach to the patient with a rAAA must be focused on saving life. Nearly half these patients subjected to emergent surgery die from complications within the first 30 days of operation. Attention to controlling hemorrhage, restoring aortic blood flow, and avoidance of attempts to reconstruct less diseased vessels, such as asymptomatic stenosis of renal arteries or marginally aneurysmal iliac arteries, is mandatory. Supraceliac aortic cross clamp is often initially utilized to control continued bleeding, especially in patients with large retroperitoneal hematomas. The proximal aortic cross clamp may then be moved to below the renal arteries once the infrarenal aortic neck has been isolated and occluded. Adequate blood replacement and maintenance of normothermia are critical elements of these emergent procedures. Following aortic reconstruction, the adequacy of the blood flow to the colon and lower extremities should be assessed before leaving the operating room. One should consider delayed abdominal closure following rAAA repair. Massive fluid resuscitation and a large retroperitoneal hematoma in these patients may cause the usual abdominal closure to result in a compartment syndrome with decreased perfusion of the splanchnic and renal circulations. Delayed abdominal closure, using an open vacuum pack dressing, appears to confer survival benefits in select patients with rAAAs.

Endovascular Surgical Treatment of Ruptured Abdominal Aortic Aneurysms

Poor outcomes associated with OAR have driven the use of EVAR for rAAA treatment. Operative mortality associated with OAR is largely associated with the physiologic changes associated with the repair itself. The use of general anesthesia decreases sympathetic tone, resulting in hemodynamic instability, and entering the abdomen may cause an acute drop in blood pressure, with subsequent hypothermia and associated coagulopathy. EVAR allows for a minimally invasive approach, without the need for general anesthetic. Conversion from local anesthetic to general anesthesia may be indicated with loss of consciousness, hemodynamic decompensation, and respiratory distress. Patients who present with a rAAA often have a contained rupture or a controlled hemorrhage due to tamponade from periaortic tissue. Permissive hypotension is acceptable prior to obtaining a CT scan and/or transferring the patient to the endovascular suite. The use of an endovascular aortic occlusion balloon has been described for obtaining proximal hemorrhagic control. Use of FDA-approved endografts previously mentioned is dictated by the specifications of the graft and the AAA morphology, particularly that of the infrarenal aortic neck. The use of aorto-uni-iliac endografts allows for rapid exclusion of the aneurysm from aortic blood flow.

Prognosis and Follow-up Following Intact Abdominal Aortic Aneurysm Repair

When considering recent studies evaluating Medicare, NIS, and NSQIP databases, OAR and EVAR are associated with 30-day mortality rate of less than 5 and 3%, respectively (Table 12.2). Improved preoperative preparation and postoperative care have decreased the mortality rate following elective AAA repair over the past few decades. Most mortality following modern aortic surgery is secondary to myocardial ischemia. Guidelines that establish the need for preoperative cardiac assessment have been formulated. Common risk factors predicting postoperative cardiac events include advanced age, male gender, history of diabetes requiring medication, previous myocardial infarction (MI), and congestive heart failure. Patients undergoing elective surgery for intact AAAs have fewer postoperative complications and a lower mortality than do patients treated emergently for rAAAs. Coronary artery disease, COPD, and renal insufficiency all increase the hazards of surgery. Increasing complexity of the operation

TABLE 12.2
RESULTS AFTER OAR AND EVAR FOR INTACT AAAs

	Population	Study Period	N	30-D Mortality(%)
OAR				
Hua (2005)	NSQIP-PS	2000–2003	582	4.0
Schermerhorn (2008)	Medicare	2001–2004	22,830	4.8
Schwarze (2009)	NIS	2001–2006	75,222	3.6[a]
EVAR				
Hua (2005)	NSQUP-PS	2000–2003	460	2.8
Schermerhorn (2008)	Medicare	2001–2004	22,830	1.2
Schwarze (2009)	NIS	2001–2006	90,925	0.9[a]

[a]Average mortality, considering in-hospital mortality for each year of the study period.
NSQIP-PS, National Surgical Quality Improvement Program-Private Sector, NIS × Nationwide Inpatient Sample.

with involvement of the renal and the visceral vessels also increases the operative morbidity and mortality.

Different trials to date have determined the feasibility of EVAR for the treatment of AAAs. EVAR 1 was a randomized, controlled trial of 1,082 patients, age 60 years or older, who had aneurysms of at least 5.5 cm in diameter, and who were referred to 1 of 34 hospitals that performed the EVAR. This trial evaluated the use of EVAR and OAR for intact AAA disease, and the study demonstrated that aneurysm-related death is approximately 3% less likely to occur with EVAR compared to open repair; however, overall survival was comparable for the two groups in long-term follow-up. The Dutch Randomized Endovascular Aneurysm Management trial was a multicenter randomized trial comparing OAR with EVAR in 351 patients, who had an AAA of at least 5 cm in diameter and were considered candidates for both techniques. This trial demonstrated lower perioperative mortality after EVAR compared to OAR; however, no difference in overall mortality was observed after 2 years. EVAR 2 was a randomized, controlled trial of 338 patients, age 60 years or older, who had aneurysms of at least 5.5 cm in diameter, and who were referred to 1 of 31 hospitals in the United Kingdom. The trial considered patients who were determined to be unfit for open repair and received EVAR, compared to those patients who were determined to be unfit for open repair and received no treatment. The EVAR group demonstrated a 30-day mortality of 9%. No difference in mortality was found between the EVAR and the no-treatment group after 4 years. Studies considering patients in the NSQIP databases have demonstrated no difference in 30-day mortality rates for patients treated with EVAR compared to those treated by OAR; however, EVAR has been associated with significantly lower morbidity compared to that for OAR. Hua et al. demonstrated a significantly lower rate of pulmonary complications associated with EVAR at 6% compared to OAR at 18% ($P < 0.0001$), and this difference has been attributed to the differences in anesthetic and transfusion requirements associated with the two techniques. No significant differences in postoperative cardiac, renal, neurologic, or wound complication rates have been noted when comparing EVAR and OAR (Table 12.3). Longer-term follow-up is necessary to determine the ultimate superiority of one treatment modality over the other.

The most common complication following EVAR of an AAA is an endoleak (Fig. 12.8). An *endoleak* is defined as persistent blood flow in the aneurysm after the placement of the endovascular graft. Endoleaks are classified as: (a) graft-related, due to failure of the hemostatic seal at one end of the endovascular graft or within the fabric of the graft, or (b) graft-unrelated, with filling of the aneurysmal sac by back-bleeding from a branch artery (Table 12.4). Plain film of the abdomen may be used to follow graft migration, which is predictive of a type 1 endoleak (Fig. 12.9). In a large European registry of AAA endovascular grafts, the early endoleak rate was approximately 15%. In these cases, the endoleaks sealed spontaneously in 35% of patients, sealed following a second endovascular procedure in 18%, and were converted to OAR in 3%. In this same series, 7% of patients died within 30 days of unrelated causes, 12% had a persistent endoleak at late follow-up, and 27% were lost to follow-up. An additional

TABLE 12.3

COMPARISON OF COMPLICATIONS (%) AFTER OAR AND EVAR FOR INTACT AND rAAAs

Population	Study Period	N	30-D Mortality	Cardio-vascular	Pulmonary	Renal	Neuro-logic	Infectious	Shock	Bleeding	Wound	Graft Failure
Intact												
OAR												
Hua (2005) NSQIP-PS	2000–2003	582	4.0	3.1	18.2	4.5	2.6	8.6	NR	9.6	5.5	0.3
EVAR												
Hua (2005) NSQIP-PS	2000–2003	460	2.8	1.3	6.3	2.4	2.0	4.8	NR	5.0	5.7	2.0
Ruptured												
OAR												
Davenport (2010) NSQIP	2005–2007	328	37.2	8.2	50.0	20.4	5.2	8.5	29.9	NR	NR	NR
Giles (2009) ACS NSQIP	2005–2007	446	36.0	8.0	29.0	23.0	2.0	11.0	18.0	11.0	4.0	1.0
EVAN												
Davenport (2010) NSQIP	2005–2007	99	22.2	4.0	34.3	18.2	2.0	5.1	19.2	NR	NR	NR
Giles (2009) ACS NSQIP	2005–2007	121	24.0	7.0	19.0	20.0	2.0	6.0	14.0	7.0	7.0	4.0

NSQIP-PS, National Surgical Quality Improvement Program–Private Sector; Acs NSQIP, American College of Surgeons National Quality Improvement Program; NR, not reported.

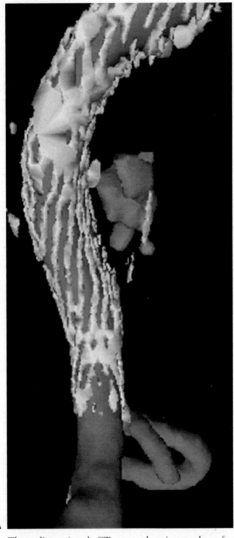

FIGURE 12-8. Three-dimensional CT scan showing endograft in place with evidence of a posterior endoleak. **A:** Image as only 3D reconstruction. (*Continued*)

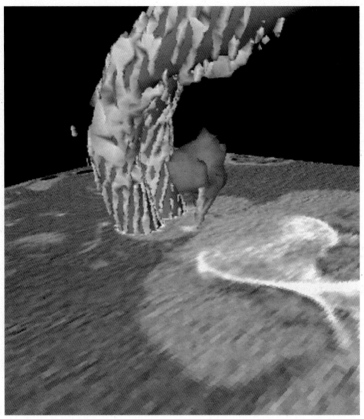

B

FIGURE 12-8. (*Continued*)   **B:** Image with 3D reconstruction and sagittal image.

18% of patients developed a late endoleak within the first year of follow-up. Unfortunately, it is clear that endoleaks may develop years after placement of the endovascular graft. Therefore, their resolution becomes crucial to the success of EVAR.

Prognosis and Follow-up Following Ruptured Abdominal Aortic Aneurysm Repair

In contrast to the relatively low mortality rates associated with elective AAA repair, the operative mortality rate following rAAA OAR is nearly 50%, and this rate has not changed significantly over recent decades, despite improved preoperative and postoperative care. Prospective trials have demonstrated significantly decreased 30-day mortality of EVAR for rAAA compared to that for OAR (Table 12.3). Survival analysis of patients matched by propensity score has shown a persistent benefit for EVAR over OAR over a four-year follow-up period. Despite improvements in AAA

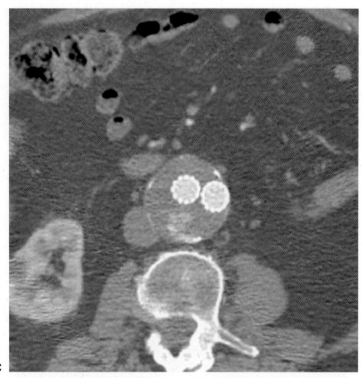

C

FIGURE 12-8. (*Continued*)   C: Example of a single slice of a sagittal image from which 3D reconstruction was created.

management, rupture mortality has not changed, and women continue to have a consistently higher risk of postoperative complications and mortality. Interestingly, with steadily decreasing postoperative mortality for the treatment of rAAA with EVAR, outcomes in nonteaching centers are substantially worse than those in teaching hospitals. The open versus endovascular repair of AAAs (IMPROVE) trial will prospectively determine whether a policy of endovascular repair improves the survival of patients with rAAA in a randomized, controlled fashion.

Early complications associated with EVAR for rAAA are as variable as those for elective repair. Failure to deploy a graft occurs in less than 2% of cases. Acute Type I and III endoleaks have been reported at rates of 2.2 to 25.5% and 2.7 to 4.0%, respectively, with the majority of these endoleaks subsequently treated endovascularly. Acute conversion to open repair has been reported at rates of 1.0 to 21.4%, with a perioperative mortality as high as 40%. Bilateral renal artery coverage, aortoiliac tortuosity preventing proper delivery of the endograft, persistent Type I endoleak, and aortic dissection from the proximal seal zone have been reported as possible causes for acute conversion to open repair. Rates of bowel ischemia after

TABLE 12.4

REVISED CLASSIFICATION OF ENDOLEAKS

Type of Endoleak

I. Leak at attachment site
   A. Proximal end of graft
   B. Distal end of graft
   C. Iliac occluder
II. Branch leaks
   A. Simple or to and fro (from only one patent branch)
   B. Complex or flow through (with two or more patent branches)
III. Graft defect
   A. Junctional leak or modular disconnect
   B. Fabric disruption (midgraft hole)
     • Minor (<2 mm; e.g., suture hole)
     • Major (≥2 mm)
IV. Graft wall (fabric) porosity (<30 d after graft placement)

(Adapted from Pearce WH. What's new in vascular surgery. *J Am Coll Surg* 2003;196:253–266.)

EVAR for rAAA have been reported at rates of 3.0 to 25.6%; however, EVAR has been associated with lower rates of colonic ischemia and subsequent bowel resection than those for OAR. Abdominal compartment syndrome (ACS) following EVAR for rAAA has been reported at rates of 2.2 to 20.0%. Severe coagulopathy, with significant transfusion requirements, use of an aortic occlusion balloon, and emergency conversion of a modular bifurcated graft to an aorto-uni-iliac graft have been associated with the development of ACS. Review of recent NSQIP data has demonstrated renal failure following EVAR for rAAA at rates of 18.2 to 20.0%, while previous studies have described patients subsequently requiring hemodialysis at rates of 2.2 to 18.8%. Hypotension, shock, atheroembolic or thromboembolic events, contrast nephropathy and endograft coverage of a renal artery have all been described as possible causes. Data from the NSQIP have demonstrated that cardiac events after EVAR for rAAA occurred at rates of 4.0 to 7.0%, and as high as 46% when evaluated by previous studies. Other studies have also described postoperative MI at rates of 2.0 to 14.0%. Poor preoperative cardiac functional status, increased intraoperative bleeding, lower intraoperative diastolic blood pressure, and increased intraoperative use of blood products were associated with higher rates of perioperative MI and cardiac death. It has been shown that aortic surgery patients who experienced perioperative MI had significantly higher bleeding rates during surgery, while those patients who subsequently died received more blood transfusions than matched survivors. In addition, pulmonary complications following EVAR have been reported at rates of 19.0 to 34.3%. COPD and home oxygen use have also been associated with poor outcomes following major surgery. COPD is associated with an increased prevalence of AAA, and it is an independent risk factor for AAA rupture (Table 12.3).

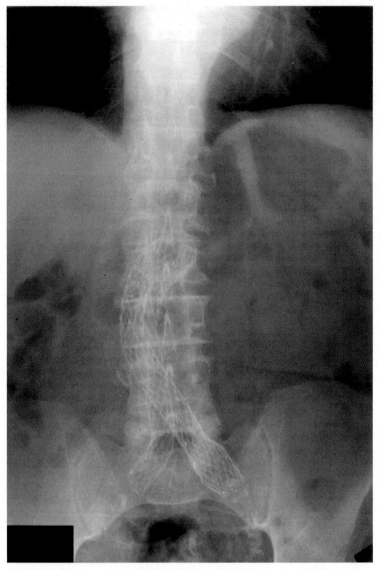

FIGURE 12-9. Plain film of the abdomen used to document correct placement of endograft and subsequently used serially to determine if graft migration is occurring.

CONCLUSION

AAAs are increasingly detected as the population ages. Physical examination alone is often unreliable in establishing the presence of an AAA. Diagnosis of AAA by US is efficient and cost effective and may be considered as part of screening for high-risk patients. CTA is the modality of choice when intervention is being considered for an aneurysm. The standard for AAA treatment has been replacement of the aneurysm with a prosthetic graft by conventional surgical means; however, EVAR is associated with lower morbidity and related complications. Studies are showing that EVAR is associated with a lower mortality rate compared to that for OAR, and ongoing trials will address this in a randomized control fashion.

PRACTICAL POINTS

- Incidence of aortic disease is increasing.

- The classic triad of acute hypotension, back or abdominal pain, and a palpable abdominal mass is rarely seen in patients with rAAAs.

- AAAs greater than 5.5 cm in diameter are life threatening and should be repaired in low-to-moderate risk patients.

- Three to five centimeter AAAs rupture with unpredictable frequency. Diastolic hypertension and COPD are independent variables contributing to a greater risk of rupture for smaller AAAs.

- While US is a good for screening, CTA should be performed if intervention is planned.

- Elective repair of AAA carries an overall 3 to 5% mortality rate for EVAR and OAR, respectively, with women faring worse than men.

- Emergent repair of rAAAs carries a near 50% operative mortality rate, with the overall mortality from AAA rupture approaching 80%, if those who succumb before reaching a hospital are included.

- The use of EVAR for the treatment of rAAA appears to be associated with a lower 30-day mortality rate than that for OAR.

RECOMMENDED READING

Beebe HG, Cronenwett JL, Katzen BT, et al. Results of an aortic endograft trial: impact of device failure beyond 12 months. *J Vasc Surg* 2001;33:55–63.

Bertges DJ, Rhee RY, Muluk SC, et al. Is routine use of the intensive care unit after elective infrarenal abdominal aortic aneurysm repair necessary? *J Vasc Surg* 2000;32:634–642.

Blum U, Voshage G, Lammer J, et al. Endoluminal stent-grafts for infrarenal abdominal aortic aneurysms. *N Engl J Med* 1997;336:13–20.

Carpenter JP, Baum RA, Barker CF, et al. Durability of benefits of endovascular versus conventional abdominal aortic aneurysm repair. *J Vasc Surg* 2002;35:222–228.

Chervu A, Clagett GP, Valentine RJ, et al. Role of physical examination in detection of abdominal aortic aneurysms. *Surgery* 1995;117:454–457.

Cronenwett JK, Murphy TF, Zelenock GB, et al. Actuarial analysis of variables associated with rupture of small abdominal aortic aneurysms. *Surgery* 1985;98:472–483.

D'Angelo AJ, Puppala D, Farber A, et al. Is preoperative cardiac evaluation for abdominal aortic aneurysm repair necessary? *J Vasc Surg* 1997;25:152–156.

Davenport DL, O'Keeffe SD, Minion DJ, et al. Thirty-day NSQIP database outcomes of open versus endoluminal repair of ruptured abdominal aortic aneurysms. *J Vasc Surg* 2010;51(2):305–309.

Desai M, Eaton-Evans J, Hillery C, et al. AAA stent-grafts: past problems and future prospects. *Ann Biomed Eng* 2010;38(4):1259–1275.

Dillavou ED, Muluk SC, Makaroun MS. A decade of change in abdominal aortic aneurysm repair in the United States: have we improved outcomes equally between men and women? *J Vasc Surg* 2006;43(2):230–238.

Dimick JB, Stanley JC, Axelrod DA, et al. Variation in mortality after abdominal aortic aneurysmectomy in the United States: impact of hospital volume, gender, and age. *Ann Surg* 2002;235:579–585.

Diwan A, Sarkar R, Stanley JC, et al. Incidence of femoral and popliteal artery aneurysms in patients with abdominal aortic aneurysms. *J Vasc Surg* 2000;31:863–869.

English SJ, Eliason JL, Rectenwald JE, et al. Complications after endovascular repair for ruptured abdominal aortic aneurysm. *J Vasc Endovasc Surg* 2009;16:133–144.

Ernst CB. Abdominal aortic aneurysm. *N Engl J Med* 1993;328:1167–1173.

Giles KA, Pomposelli FB, Hamdan AD, et al. Comparison of open and endovascular repair of ruptured abdominal aortic aneurysms from the ACS-NSQIP 2005–07. *J Endovasc Ther* 2009;16(3):365–372.

Gloviczki P, Pairolero PC, Mucha P, et al. Ruptured abdominal aortic aneurysms: repair should not be denied. *J Vasc Surg* 1992;15:851–859.

Hertzer NR, Mascha EJ, Karafa MT, et al. Open infrarenal abdominal aortic aneurysm repair: The Cleveland Clinic experience from 1989 to 1998. *J Vasc Surg* 2002;35:1145–1154.

Hua HT, Cambria RP, Chuang SK, et al. Early outcomes of endovascular versus open abdominal aortic aneurysm repair in the National Surgical Quality Improvement Program-Private Sector (NSQIP-PS). *J Vasc Surg* 2005;41(3):382–389.

Jaakkola P, Hippelainen M, Farin P, et al. Interobserver variability in measuring the dimensions of the abdominal aorta: comparison of ultrasound and computed tomography. *Eur J Vasc Endovasc Surg* 1996;12:230–237.

Johnston KW. Multicenter prospective study of non-ruptured abdominal aortic aneurysms. Part II. Variables predicting morbidity and mortality. *J Vasc Surg* 1989;9:437–447.

Katz DL, Stanley JC, Zelenock GB. Operative mortality rates for intact and ruptured abdominal aortic aneurysms in Michigan: an eleven-year statewide experience. *J Vasc Surg* 1993;19:804–817.

Katz DL, Stanley JC, Zelenock GB. Gender differences in abdominal aortic aneurysm prevalence, treatment, and outcome. *J Vasc Surg* 1997;25:561–568.

Lederle FA, Wilson SE, Johnson GR, et al. Aneurysm Detection and Management Veterans Affairs Cooperative Study Group. Immediate repair compared with surveillance of small abdominal aortic aneurysms. *N Engl J Med* 2002;346(19):1437–1444.

Lederle FA, Johnson GR, Wilson SE, et al. Rupture rate of large abdominal aortic aneurysms in patients refusing or unfit for elective repair. *JAMA* 2002;287(22):2968–2972.

Lesperance K, Andersen C, Singh N, et al. Expanding use of emergency endovascular repair for ruptured abdominal aortic aneurysms: disparities in outcomes from a nationwide perspective. *J Vasc Surg* 2008;47(6):1165–1170.

Matsumura JS, Brewster DC, Makaroun MS, et al. A multicenter controlled clinical trial of open versus endovascular treatment of abdominal aortic aneurysm. *J Vasc Surg* 2003;37:262–271.

May J, White GH, Waugh R, et al. Improved survival after endoluminal repair with second-generation prostheses compared with open repair in the treatment of abdominal aortic aneurysms: a 5-year concurrent comparison using life table method. *J Vasc Surg* 2001;33:21–26.

Menard MT, Chew DKW, Chan RK, et al. Outcome in patients at high risk after open surgical repair of abdominal aortic aneurysm. *J Vasc Surg* 2003;37:285–292.

Moore WS, Rutherford RB. Transfemoral endovascular repair of abdominal aortic aneurysm: result of the North American EVT Phase I Trial. *J Vasc Surg* 1996;23:543–553.

Mureebe L, Egorova N, Giacovelli JK, et al. National trends in the repair of ruptured abdominal aortic aneurysms. *J Vasc Surg* 2008;48(5):1101–1107.

National Center for Health Statistics (NHCS), National Vital Statistics System, WISQARS Query: 20 Leading Causes of Death, United States, 2006, All Races, Both Sexes, & Caucasian Males. Available at: http://webappa.cdc.gov/sasweb/ncipc/leadcaus10.html. Accessed 13 April 2010.

Ohki T, Veith FJ. Endovascular grafts and other image-guided catheter-based adjuncts to improve the treatment of ruptured aortoiliac aneurysms. *Ann Surg* 2000;232:466–479.

Parodi JC, Palmaz JC, Barone HD. Transfemoral intraluminal graft implantation for abdominal aortic aneurysms. *Ann Vasc Surg* 1991;5:491–499.

Pearce WH. What's new in vascular surgery. *J Am Coll Surg* 2003;196:253–266.

Powell JT, Thompson SG, Thompson, et al. The immediate management of the patient with rupture: open versus endovascular repair (IMPROVE) aneurysm trial–ISRCTN 48334791 IMPROVE trialists. *Acta Chir Belg* 2009;109:678–680.

Quinones-Baldrich WJ, Garner C, Caswell D, et al. Endovascular, transperitoneal, and retroperitoneal abdominal aortic aneurysm repair: results and costs. *J Vasc Surg* 1999;30:59–67.

Schermerhorn ML, O'Malley AJ, Jhaveri A, et al. Endovascular vs. open repair of abdominal aortic aneurysms in the Medicare population. *N Engl J Med* 2008;358:464–474.

Sicard GA, Reilly JM, Rubin BBG, et al. Transabdominal versus retroperitoneal incision for abdominal aortic surgery: report of a prospective randomized trial. *J Vasc Surg* 1995;21:174–183.

Schwarze ML, Shen Y, Hemmerich J, et al. Age-related trends in utilization and outcome of open and endovascular repair for abdominal aortic aneurysm in the United States, 2001–2006. *J Vasc Surg* 2009;50:722–729.

United Kingdom Small Aneurysm Trial Participants. Long-term outcomes of immediate repair compared with surveillance of small abdominal aortic aneurysms. *N Engl J Med* 2002;346:1445–1452.

van der Laan MJ, Bartels LW, Viergever MA, et al. Computed tomography versus magnetic resonance imaging of endoleaks after EVAR. *Eur J Vasc Endovasc Surg* 2006;32:361–365.

Wakefield TW, Whitehouse WM Jr, Wu SC, et al. Abdominal aortic aneurysm rupture: statistical analysis of factors affecting the outcome of surgical treatment. *Surgery* 1982;91:586–596.

Webster MW. Genetics of abdominal aortic aneurysm disease. In: Ernst CB, Stanley JC, eds. *Current therapy in vascular surgery*, 4th ed. St. Louis, MO: Mosby, 2001:206–208.

Williamson WK, Nicoloff AD, Taylor LM Jr, et al. Functional outcome after open repair of abdominal aortic aneurysm. *J Vasc Surg* 2001;33:913–920.

Zarins C, White RA, Schwarter S, et al. AneuRx stent-graft versus open repair of abdominal aortic aneurysms. Multicenter prospective clinical trial. *J Vasc Surg* 1999;29:292–305.

CHAPTER 13 ■ Approach to the Management of Thoracic and Thoracoabdominal Aneurysms

Shadi Abu-Halimah and Mark A. Farber

An aneurysm is currently defined as a localized dilatation of the aorta, 50% over the normal diameter, which includes all three layers of the vessel, intima, media, and adventitia. Thoracic aortic aneurysms are less common than aneurysms of the abdominal aorta.

The normal size for the thoracic and thoracoabdominal aorta is larger than that of the infrarenal aorta. The average diameter of the mid-descending thoracic aorta is 26 to 28 mm, compared with 20 to 23 mm at the level of the celiac axis.

Diagnosing and treating thoracic aneurysms (TAs) or thoracoabdominal aneurysms (TAAAs) have evolved in last few decades, but recent advances in endovascular surgery and adjuncts of open surgery potentially alter the prognosis of these aneurysms. However, TAAA repair is still associated with significant mortality and morbidity.

CLASSIFICATION

There are two major subtypes of aneurysm morphology: fusiform, which is uniform in shape with symmetrical dilatation that involves the entire circumference of the aortic wall, and saccular, which is more localized and appears as an out pouching of only a portion of the aortic wall. A pseudoaneurysm or false aneurysm is a collection of blood and connective tissue outside the aortic wall, usually the result of a contained rupture.

Aneurysms of the thoracic aorta can be classified into four general anatomic categories, although some aneurysms involve more than one segment:

Ascending aortic aneurysms arise anywhere from the aortic valve to the innominate artery—60%

Aortic arch aneurysms include any TA that involves the brachiocephalic vessels—10%

Descending aortic aneurysms distal to the left subclavian artery—40%

Thoracoabdominal aneurysms—10%

TAAAs can also be divided according to the Crawford classification, which was originally designed to help stratify patients into risk categories based upon the extent of disease:

I. Proximal descending thoracic to proximal abdominal aorta
II. Proximal descending to infrarenal aorta
III. Distal descending with abdominal aorta
IV. Primarily abdominal aorta

EPIDEMIOLOGY

The incidence of thoracic aortic aneurysm is estimated to be six to ten cases per 100,000 patient-years.

TAs occur most commonly in the sixth and seventh decade of life.

Males are affected approximately two to four times more commonly than females.

Hypertension is an important risk factor, being present in over 60% of patients.

Associated aneurysms can be detected in approximately 13% of patients with TAs. Approximately one forth of patients with a large thoracic aortic aneurysm also has an abdominal aortic aneurysm (AAA).

The Crawford classification (Fig. 13.1) is based on the extent of aortic involvement. Extent I aneurysms begin above the sixth intercostal space, usually near the left subclavian artery, and extend down to encompass the aorta at the origins of the celiac axis and superior mesenteric arteries; although the renal arteries may also be involved, the aneurysm does not extend into the infrarenal segment. Extent II aneurysms also arise above the sixth intercostal space but extend distally into the infrarenal aorta, often to the level of the aortic bifurcation. In some cases, they may also involve the ascending aorta. Extent III aneurysms begin in the distal half of the descending thoracic aorta, below the sixth intercostal space, and extend into the abdominal aorta. Extent IV aneurysms generally involve the entire abdominal aorta from the level of the diaphragm to the bifurcation.

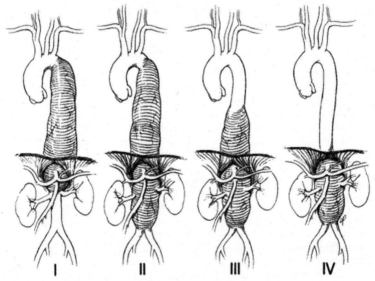

FIGURE 13-1.   Crawford classification of TAAAs.

ETIOLOGY AND PATHOGENESIS

The true etiology of aortic aneurysms is probably multifactorial, and the condition occurs in individuals with multiple risk factors. Risk factors include smoking, chronic obstructive pulmonary disease (COPD), hypertension, atherosclerosis, male gender, older age, high BMI, bicuspid or unicuspid aortic valves, genetic disorders, and family history. Aortic aneurysms are more common in men than in women and are more common in persons with COPD than in those without lung disease. TA most often results from cystic medial degeneration that leads to weakening of the aortic wall, which is highly associated with atherosclerosis in almost 80% of the cases. Cystic medial degeneration occurs normally with aging and is increased with hypertension.

In patients younger than 60 years of age, the discovery of a TA implies a genetic disorder. This may be the result of Ehlers-Danlos, Marfan's syndrome, and LD syndrome. Other causes may include inflammatory/infective cases.

Matrix metalloproteinases (MMPs) constitute a family of zinc-dependent proteases (endopeptidases) whose catalytic action is the degradation of the extracellular matrix components. In addition, they play the major role in the degradation of collagen and in the process of tissue remodeling. Multiple investigators have looked specifically at the profiles of proteolytic enzymes in the aortic wall of aneurysm patients and compared these profiles to those of normal individuals. These have implicated the MMP enzymes in the wall of the aorta as a prime agent of deleterious change in aneurysm and dissection disease. They found a marked elevation of the proteolytic enzymes (MMPs) and a marked depression of the inhibitory enzymes (TIMPs). Thus, in aneurysm patients, the balance is shifted strongly toward increased proteolysis—indicating an enzymatic attack on the fibrillin and collagen that form the structural basis of the aortic wall.

Association with Atherosclerosis

More than 80% of the descending TAs are associated with atherosclerosis sharing the same risk factors (e.g., hypertension, hypercholesterolemia, and smoking). It seems likely that there is a multifactorial, systemic, nonatherosclerotic causal process, such as a defect in vascular structural proteins, with atherosclerosis occurring secondarily.

Most theories emphasize the primary role of breakdown of the extracellular matrix proteins, elastin, and collagen by proteases such as collagenase, elastase, various MMPs, and plasmin. These proteolytic factors are derived from endothelial and smooth muscle cells and from inflammatory cells infiltrating the media and adventitia.

The combination of protein degradation and mechanical factors are thought to cause cystic medial necrosis, which has the appearance of smooth muscle cell necrosis and elastic fiber degeneration with cystic spaces in the media filled with mucoid material. These changes result in vessel dilatation and subsequent aneurysm formation and possible rupture.

The following observations in animal models are consistent with the importance of plasmin and metalloproteinases in aortic aneurysm formation.

Blockade of plasmin formation by overexpression of plasminogen activator inhibitor-1 prevents the formation of aneurysms and rupture by inhibiting metalloproteinase activation.

Aneurysm rupture correlates with an increase in metalloproteinase (gelatinases A and B) levels; local overexpression of tissue inhibitor of MMPs, produced by retrovirally infected smooth muscle cells, can prevent aneurysmal degeneration and rupture.

Genetic Factors

Connective tissue disorders such as the Marfan's or Ehlers-Danlos syndromes are associated with TA and TAAA. But familial associations with TAs have been reported in some patients without these disorders in 19% of TAs and thoracic dissection cases. Mutations in FBN1 have been identified in some patients with ascending thoracic aortic aneurysms who do not have Marfan's syndrome. Mutations in the transforming growth factor beta receptor 2 gene are responsible for about 5% of familial cases.

Marfan's Syndrome

Marfan's syndrome is associated with aortic root dilatation (normal ≤ 35 mm) due to cystic medial degeneration prior to aneurysm formation. This disorder is due to mutations in the fibrillin-1 (FBN1) gene.

Aortic root disease, which leads to the formation of aneurysmal dilatation, aortic regurgitation, and dissection, is the main cause of morbidity and mortality in Marfan's syndrome. Involvement of other segments of the thoracic aorta, the abdominal aorta, or even the carotid and intracranial arteries is reported.

Dilatation of the aorta is found in 50% of children and will progress with time. Echocardiography demonstrates that 60 to 80% of adult patients have dilatation of the aortic root (normal diameter ≤ 35 mm), often with aortic regurgitation. Marfan's syndrome is also frequently associated with aortic dissection, which typically begins just above the coronary ostia, that is, type A dissection, but can extend distally.

Ehlers-Danlos Syndrome Type IV

Etiology of this syndrome is due to defects in type III collagen that causes hyperelasticity and fragility of the skin and hypermobility of the joints. Although aortic root dilatation is uncommon, spontaneous rupture of large and medium-sized arteries, usually without dissection, is reported and is the most serious complication.

Loey-Dietz Syndrome

Loey-Dietz syndrome is a recently discovered autosomal dominant genetic syndrome, which has many features similar to Marfan's syndrome, but which is caused by mutations in the genes encoding transforming growth factor beta receptor 1 (TGFBR1) or 2 (TGFBR2).

Bicuspid Aortic Valve and Aortic Coarctation

There is an association between bicuspid aortic valve and ascending thoracic aortic aneurysms. In a study of young men with normally functioning bicuspid aortic valves, enlargement of the aortic root and/or ascending aorta was noted in 52%; this finding was independent of hemodynamic abnormalities, age, or body size. The tendency to aneurysm formation is associated with cystic medial degeneration and with decreased expression of FBN1, the gene for which is mutated in Marfan's syndrome.

In addition, a bicuspid aortic valve is an independent predictor of ascending aortic aneurysm formation after surgical correction of aortic coarctation and is associated with aortic root dilatation in patients with Turner's syndrome.

Inflammatory/Infectious Disorders

Aortitis has been associated with variety of inflammatory and infectious diseases, which can lead to aortic aneurysm. These diseases include giant cell arteritis, syphilitic aortitis, mycotic aneurysm often due to bacterial endocarditis, Takayasu arteritis, rheumatoid arthritis, psoriatic arthritis, ankylosing spondylitis, reactive arthritis, Wegener's granulomatosis, and reactive arthritis. TA formation is a particular problem in patients with giant cell arteritis that occurs in as many as 11% of patients and may be associated with aortic dissection. Chest x-ray is a recommended screening even for asymptomatic patients.

CLINICAL PRESENTATION

Patients with TAs are often asymptomatic at the time of presentation. Pain can be the presenting symptom according to the location of the aneurysm. This is usually attributed to compression or distortion of adjacent structures or vessels. Aortic regurgitation and thromboembolic disease can be the primary manifestation but is less common.

Ascending aneurysms are more prone to present with heart failure due to aortic regurgitation from aortic root dilatation and annular distortion. Compression of a coronary artery can result in myocardial ischemia or infarction, while a sinus of Valsalva aneurysm can rupture into the right side of the heart, producing a continuous murmur and sometimes heart failure.

Ascending and arch aneurysms can erode into the mediastinum compressing its structures: hoarseness due to compression of left vagus or left recurrent laryngeal nerve; hemidiaphragmatic paralysis due to compression of the phrenic nerve; wheezing, cough, hemoptysis, dyspnea, or pneumonitis if there is compression of the tracheobronchial tree; dysphagia due to esophageal compression; or the superior vena cava syndrome. Aneurysmal compression or erosion into adjacent bone may cause chest or back pain.

Aneurysmal compression of branch vessels or the occurrence of embolism to various peripheral arteries due to thrombus within the aneurysm can cause coronary, cerebral, renal, mesenteric, lower extremity and rarely, spinal cord ischemia (SCI) and resultant symptoms.

The most serious complications of thoracic aortic aneurysm are dissection or rupture. A descending thoracic aortic aneurysm can rupture into the adjacent esophagus, producing an aortoesophageal fistula and presenting with hematemesis. Rupture is often catastrophic, being associated with severe pain and hypotension or shock.

DIAGNOSIS

Chest x-ray

Most (75%) of TAs are asymptomatic. As such their detection is usually an incidental finding on CXR or axial imaging study done for other reasons. On CXR the aneurysm produces a widening of the mediastinal silhouette, enlargement of the aortic knob, or displacement of the trachea from midline. Other reported features include displaced calcification, aortic kinking, and opacification of the aorticopulmonary window.

However, chest x-ray cannot distinguish an aneurysm from a tortuous aorta and many aneurysms are not apparent on the chest x-ray, so it is not the initial diagnostic modality of choice for TAs or TAAAs.

Echocardiography

Echocardiography is a useful tool for the diagnosis of thoracic aortic aneurysm according to ACC/AHA 2003 guidelines. Transthoracic echocardiography (TTE) is the preferred procedure, with transesophageal echocardiography (TEE) usually being performed only if the examination is incomplete or additional information is needed. There are, however, two settings in which TEE is preferred: for examination of the entire aorta, especially in emergency situations, and for imaging when coexistent dissection is suspected.

Among patients with known bicuspid aortic valves, the 2006 ACC/AHA guidelines on valvular heart disease recommend an initial TTE to assess the diameters of the aortic root and ascending aorta. Patients with aortic root or ascending aorta diameter greater than 4.0 cm should undergo serial evaluation of aortic root/ascending aortic size and morphology by echocardiography, computed tomography (CT), or magnetic resonance on a yearly basis. A lower threshold for ascending aorta diameter should be considered in patients of small stature.

CT and MRI

CT with intravenous contrast and magnetic resonance imaging (MRI) are the preferred tests to detect a thoracic aortic aneurysm, determine its size, and define aortic and branch vessel anatomy. MRI is preferred for aneurysms involving the aortic root.

CT scans with contrast have become the most widely used diagnostic tool. They rapidly and precisely evaluate the thoracic and abdominal aorta to determine the location and extent of the aneurysm and the relationship of the aneurysm to major branch vessels and surrounding structures. They can help accurately determine the size of the aneurysm and assess dissection, mural thrombus, intramural hematoma, free rupture, and contained rupture with hematoma.

Sagittal, coronary, and axial images may be obtained with three-dimensional reconstruction. Stent graft planning for endovascular descending TA repairs requires fine-cut images from the neck through the pelvis to the level of the femoral heads. The takeoff of the arch vessels is critical to determine the adequacy of the proximal landing zone, as is assessing the patency of the vertebral arteries, if the left subclavian artery should be covered by the stent graft. Assessment of the common femoral artery access is essential to determine the feasibility of large-bore sheath access. A spiral CT scan with 1-mm cuts and three-dimensional reconstruction with the ability to make centerline measurements is crucial to stent graft planning.

Among patients with known bicuspid aortic valves, the 2006 ACC/AHA guidelines recommend MRI or CT when morphology of the aortic root or ascending aorta cannot be accurately assessed by echocardiography. MRI or CT is reasonable in patients with bicuspid aortic valves and aortic root dilatation on echocardiography to further quantify severity of dilatation and involvement of the ascending aorta.

Contrast Angiography

Contrast angiography is the best method for evaluating branch vessel pathology. However, this procedure is invasive with potential nephrotoxicity from contrast medium and is unable to discern extraluminal aneurysmal size. It is being replaced with 3D CT scan reconstructed images.

NATURAL HISTORY

It is not well studied but risk of rupture has been reported between 32 and 68% for large aneurysms. Most of the patients with TAs have associated cardiovascular disease, which accounts for the most common cause of death along with rupture in these patients. One- and five-year survival rate reported 65 and 20%, respectively.

The size of the aneurysm is the most important determinant of rupture. Reported incidence of rupture is around 16% for 40 to 59 mm aneurysms and more than 30% for 60 mm and above. Very low risk in cases of size below 40 mm. Aneurysms may rupture at smaller sizes in patients with Marfan's syndrome or other connective tissue disorders.

Reported rate of dissection or rupture ranged from 2 to 3 to 7%/y for aneurysms less than 50, 50 to 59, and ≥60 mm, respectively. Among patients with aneurysms ≥60 mm, the combined end point of rupture, dissection, or death occurred at a rate of 15.6%/y. The 5-year rate of survival was 56% in patients with aneurysms ≥60 mm.

Growth rates average 0.07 cm/y in the ascending aorta and 0.19 cm/y in the descending aorta. The rate of growth is related to the initial diameter with larger aneurysms growing more quickly. The rate of expansion was much greater for aneurysms more than 50 mm in diameter (7.9 vs. 1.7 mm/y in smaller aneurysms). The anatomic location of the aneurysm is another factor associated with the rate of expansion. Aneurysms located within the midportion of the descending aorta have the most rapid growth, while those in the ascending aorta have the slowest expansion rate, despite having the greatest initial diameter.

Elefteriades et al. published the natural history of thoracic aortic aneurysms and recommends elective repair of ascending aneurysms at 5.5 cm and descending aneurysms at 6.5 cm for patients without any familial disorders such as Marfan's syndrome. These recommendations are based on the finding that the incidence of complications (rupture and dissection) exponentially increased when the size of the ascending aorta reached 6.0 cm (31% risk of complications) or when the size of the descending aorta reached 7.0 cm (43% risk). Patients with Marfan's syndrome or familial aneurysms should undergo earlier repair, when the ascending aorta grows to 5.0 cm or the descending aorta grows to 6.0 cm.

MEDICAL MANAGEMENT OF ASYMPTOMATIC ANEURYSMS

Asymptomatic patients with an aneurysm are initially managed medically, while surgery is indicated for symptomatic patients and for asymptomatic patients with rapid aneurysm expansion or a diameter greater than 50 to 60 mm in diameter, depending on body size, cause of aortic dilation, and other clinical factors.

For smaller patients, including many women, we recommend elective repair for aneurysms greater than twice the size of the nonaneurysmal aorta (normal segment) or for those with rapid expansion, defined as growth of more than 0.5 cm during a 6-month interval.

In the asymptomatic patient, medical management includes

Aggressive blood pressure control, including beta-blockers being part of the regimen, in an attempt to slow aneurysm growth.

Patient education about signs and symptoms of the TAs through patient education.

Serial imaging of the aneurysm to evaluate growth and structure. The preferred imaging technique is CT scanning. Imaging should be repeated at 6 months after the initial study then yearly after that if there is no significant change in size.

There has been a real proven benefit of beta-blockers on the rate of aneurysms expansion except in adults with Marfan's syndrome. Beta-blockers are thought to act by decreasing left ventricular contractility (dp/dt) and shear stress. The goal systolic pressure is 105 to 120 mm Hg if tolerated. Beta-blockers are recommended for patients with bicuspid aortic valves and dilated aortic roots (diameter greater than 40 mm) who are not candidates for surgical correction and who do not have moderate or severe aortic regurgitation.

Beta-blocker therapy is recommended in patients with thoracic aortic aneurysm who are being followed nonoperatively and they are the preferred drug for the treatment of hypertension or angina.

Doxycycline effect has been investigated as a direct MMP inhibitor with some inhibitory effect on aneurysms expansion.

Smoking cessation, aspirin, and statins should be considered in all patients including preoperative workup.

SURGICAL THERAPY

The optimal timing of surgery for a thoracic aortic aneurysm is uncertain since the natural history is variable, particularly for aneurysms less than 50 mm in size, and the majority of patients have concomitant cardiovascular disease that increases the risks associated with surgery.

Indications

The indications for surgery include:

The presence of symptoms.

An end-diastolic aortic diameter of 50 to 60 mm for an ascending aortic aneurysm and 60 to 70 mm for a descending aortic aneurysm; often ≥70 mm in high-risk patients.

Aortic size index (aortic diameter [cm] divided by body surface area [m^2]) for the ascending aorta, patients are stratified into three groups: ASI < 2.75 cm/m^2 are at low risk for rupture (4%/y), ASI 2.75 to 4.25 cm/m^2 are at moderate risk (8%/y), and ASI > 4.25cm/m^2 are at high risk (20 to 25%/y). Relative aortic aneurysm size in relation to body surface area may be more important than absolute aortic size in predicting complications.

Accelerated growth rate (≥10 mm/y) in aneurysms less than 50 mm in diameter or greater than 5 mm in 6 months.

Evidence of dissection with diameter > 45 mm.

An aortic aneurysm >45 mm in diameter at the time of aortic valve surgery.

Pseudoaneurysm, saccular aneurysm, and mycotic aneurysms.

In patients with aortic regurgitation of any severity and primary disease of the aortic root or ascending aorta (such as Marfan's syndrome), the 2006 ACC/AHA valvular disease guidelines recommend aortic valve replacement and aortic root reconstruction when the degree of dilatation is ≥50 mm. The guidelines note that some have recommended surgery for this group at a lower level of dilatation (4.5 cm) or based on a rate of increase of 0.5 cm/y or greater in surgical centers with established expertise in repair of the aortic root and ascending aorta.

Preoperative Evaluation

Prior to surgical intervention, the patient should undergo evaluation for risk assessment and the presence of atherosclerotic disease of other vessels.

Preoperative assessment should include evaluation of left ventricular function and potential concomitant coronary artery disease.

Patients with ascending aortic and particularly arch disease should undergo carotid artery duplex ultrasound examination.

Patients with descending thoracic aortic disease require left thoracotomy and should undergo pulmonary function testing if clinical symptoms of pulmonary disease are present and a resting arterial blood gas on room air.

Patients with TAAA extension require delineation of any claudication history and a thorough arterial pulse examination. If the history or physical findings suggest peripheral arterial disease (PAD), then noninvasive lower extremity pulse-volume recordings and pressures are indicated to determine the level and severity of disease.

Perioperative Monitoring

Standard vascular surgery anesthetic techniques are applied in the perioperative setting. These include monitoring of arterial, central venous, and pulmonary arterial pressures; establishing vascular access appropriate for high volumes and vasoactive agent infusion; intubation with a single or double lumen endotracheal tube as indicated; and active blood product management including recycling systems. Continuous TEE to monitor both cardiac function and vascular flows is used routinely. Some surgeons routinely use somatosensory evoked potential monitoring during and after surgery for early detection of abnormal signals indicating SCI.

Surgical Technique

The location of the surgical incision depends upon the location of the aneurysm.

The standard incision for ascending and arch aneurysm repair is a median sternotomy.

The standard incision for descending aneurysms is a left thoracotomy.

For TAAAs, a left thoracotomy incision is extended across the costal margin for a retroperitoneal approach.

Operative repair of TAs involves tradition vascular principles with proximal and distal vascular control, minimal aneurysm manipulation, and prosthetic graft repair. Most aneurysm repairs involve aortic replacement with a Dacron tube graft. Dacron grafts allow ingrowth in the interstices to form a pseudoendothelial layer to minimize the risk of embolization. They may be knitted or woven. Knitted grafts are more porous and incorporate tissue well; however, they are prone to more bleeding unless collagen impregnated. Woven grafts are more impervious and therefore are the most commonly used for aortic replacement. Grafts are typically impregnated with collagen to avoid preclotting the graft and to promote optimal healing. End-organ revascularization is achieved with the distal anastomosis, native arterial reimplantation with or without endarterectomy, or bypass grafting with saphenous venous or prosthetic conduit.

Aortic root involvement generally necessitates coronary artery reimplantation and may or may not require aortic valve replacement or repair.

Vascular Control

One important difference between thoracic and abdominal aneurysm repair is the means for obtaining proximal vascular control during TA repair. TA repair often requires cardiopulmonary bypass with a cardioplegia-arrested heart, in ascending aneurysms, and specific circulatory measures to address end-organ protection of the brain, spinal cord, kidneys, liver, bowel, or lower extremities with left heart bypass in descending aneurysms.

In ascending aneurysm repair, protection against end-organ damage is accomplished with cardiopulmonary bypass and antegrade aortic perfusion distal to the aneurysm.

In arch aneurysm repair, the need for open vascular access to the brachiocephalic orifices mandates interruption of cerebral blood flow and the need for cerebral protection.

In descending aortic aneurysm repair, the utility of adjunctive end-organ protective measures is unclear. Reported risk of paraparesis or paraplegia developed in 16%, while acute renal failure severe enough to require dialysis occurred in 7%.

Initial reports found that a quick operation without adjunctive measures was sufficient for TAAA repair. However, newer studies suggest that measures such as distal aortic perfusion via bypass circuitry; selective perfusion of renal, segmental, and visceral arteries; cerebrospinal fluid (CSF) drainage combined with intrathecal papaverine in high-risk patients; intercostal reimplantation; and profound hypothermia, markedly decrease the likelihood of renal, mesenteric and spinal ischemia, which can result in paraplegia. As an example, one retrospective study of 132 patients found that reimplantation of the vessels between the eight thoracic intercostal and the second lumbar arteries reduced operative mortality (4.9 vs. 13.2% for no reimplantation) and the incidence of postoperative paraplegia (0 vs. 8.8%) or the overall rate of spinal cord dysfunction (2.4 vs. 9.9%).

Perioperative monitoring of spinal pressure and active management of spinal perfusion (mean arterial pressure—spinal pressure of greater than 80 mm Hg) have been shown to dramatically reduce and even reverse spinal cord injury in both open surgical as well as closed (endovascular) surgery, especially in higher risk patients including those with renal dysfunction, PAD, long segments surgery, and prior AAA.

Selective renal perfusion, intrathecal papaverine, and hypothermia are being used.

Cerebral Protection

Methods used for brain protection during deep hypothermic circulatory arrest (DHCA) include intraoperative EEG monitoring, evoked somatosensory potential monitoring, hypothermia (to temperatures less than 18°C), packing the patient's head in ice, Trendelenburg positioning (i.e., head down), mannitol, CO_2 flooding, thiopental, steroids, and antegrade and retrograde cerebral perfusion (RCP).

Hypothermia decreases oxygen consumption. For each drop in temperature by 1°C, the oxygen consumption by the tissues is reduced by 10%.

Air (i.e., nitrogen) is poorly soluble in blood. The risk of air embolism is reduced by flooding the surgical field with carbon dioxide. Carbon dioxide is denser than air and displaces air. It is rapidly soluble in blood and causes less risk of embolization. Any carbon dioxide absorbed in the blood is removed by increasing the sweep speed of cardiopulmonary bypass.

There are three common methods of providing cerebral protection:

With selective cerebral perfusion (SCP), antegrade cerebral blood flow is reestablished via a graft anastomosed to the brachiocephalic vessels. Although SCP is metabolically optimal, it is technically cumbersome and risks cerebral embolism and carotid dissection. A variation of SCP with a trifurcated graft and initial perfusion via the right axillary artery has also been described. This approach may reduce embolic complications.

Hypothermic circulatory arrest (HCA) involves the use of cardiopulmonary bypass with the establishment of profound systemic hypothermia, followed by controlled exsanguination and total body circulatory standstill. HCA provides the best operative field visualization; however, stroke rates increase significantly after 45 minutes of arrest.

RCP in which HCA is used in conjunction with retrograde jugular venous perfusion with cold oxygenated blood. Deoxygenated blood containing cellular metabolic by-products returns via the carotid orifices. There is a significantly reduced risk of stroke with RCP compared to HCA. Controversy exists over whether RCP functions by providing neuronal metabolic support, by preserving cerebral autoregulation, or by enhancing cerebral cooling and permitting retrograde evacuation of air and debris from the intracranial circulation.

Bicuspid Aortic Valve

Bicuspid aortic valves are often associated with ascending aortic aneurysms even in the absence of significant valve disease. In addition, the bicuspid valve usually becomes sclerotic, with progressive aortic stenosis and/or regurgitation that ultimately require valve replacement in over 75% of patients.

In some patients, repair of the aortic aneurysm becomes necessary before aortic valve repair is indicated. In such cases, the bicuspid valve is often replaced at the time of aortic surgery. However, preservation of the native valve has been attempted in some cases with a low percent need for valve repair later on.

The 2006 ACC/AHA guidelines recommend that among patients with bicuspid aortic valves undergoing aortic valve replacement because of severe aortic stenosis or severe aortic regurgitation, repair of the aortic root or replacement of the ascending aorta is indicated if the diameter of the aortic root or ascending aorta is greater than 45 mm. A threshold lower than 45 mm is suggested for patients of small stature.

Ascending Aortic Aneurysms

Surgical treatment of ascending aortic aneurysms depends on the extent of the aneurysm both proximally (e.g., involvement of the aortic valve, annulus, sinuses of Valsalva, sinotubular junction, coronary orifices) and distally (e.g., involvement to the level of the innominate artery). The choice of operation also depends on the underlying pathology of the disease, the patient's life expectancy, the desired anticoagulation status, and the surgeon's experience and preference.

Ascending aortic aneurysms with normal aortic valve leaflets, annulus, and sinuses of Valsalva are typically replaced with a simple supracoronary Dacron tube graft from the sinotubular junction to the origin of the innominate artery, with the patient under cardiopulmonary bypass.

If the aortic valve is diseased but the aortic sinuses and annulus are normal, the aortic valve is replaced separately and the ascending aortic aneurysm is replaced with a supracoronary synthetic graft, leaving the coronary arteries intact (i.e., Wheat procedure).

Sinus of Valsalva aneurysms with normal aortic valve leaflets and aortic insufficiency due to dilated sinuses may be repaired with a valve-sparing aortic root replacement (ARR). Two valve-sparing procedures have been developed: the remodeling method and the reimplantation method. The remodeling method involves resecting the aneurysmal sinus tissue while maintaining the tissue along the valve leaflets and scalloping the Dacron graft to form new sinuses to remodel the root. The reimplantation method involves reimplanting the scalloped native valve into the Dacron graft. Both require reimplantation of the coronary ostia into the Dacron graft.

Patients with an abnormal aortic valve and aortic root require ARR. In nonelderly patients who can undergo anticoagulation with reasonable safety, the aortic root may be replaced with a composite valve-graft consisting of a mechanical valve inserted into a Dacron graft coronary artery reimplantation (e.g., classic or modified Bentall procedure, Cabrol procedure).

For elderly patients, young active patients who do not desire anticoagulation, women of childbearing age, and patients with contraindications to warfarin, the options include stentless porcine roots, aortic homografts, and pulmonary autografts (i.e., Ross procedure). For elderly patients who cannot undergo a complex operation, another option is reduction aortoplasty (i.e., wrapping of the ascending aorta with a prosthetic graft).

Patients with Marfan's syndrome have abnormal aortas and cannot undergo tube graft replacement alone. They must have either a valve-sparing ARR or a complete ARR.

ARR with a homograft is ideal in the setting of aortic root abscess from endocarditis.

Aortic Arch Aneurysms

Arch aneurysms pose a formidable technical challenge. DHCA with or without antegrade or RCP is usually used to facilitate reanastomosis of the arch vessels. Aortic arch reconstruction techniques vary depending on the arch pathology.

In patients with proximal arch involvement extending from the ascending aorta, a hemiarch replacement may be performed. The ascending aorta is replaced with a Dacron graft beveled as a tongue along the undersurface of the arch. In patients whose conditions mandate replacement of the entire arch, the distal anastomosis is the Dacron graft to the descending thoracic aorta. The head vessels are reimplanted individually or as an island. Grafts have been developed with a trifurcated head-vessel attachment and with a fourth attachment for the cannula. In this case, the head vessels are attached individually to the trifurcated branches.

For patients in whom the arch replacement is part of a staged procedure, preceding the delayed repair of a concomitant descending TA, an "elephant trunk" is used. That is, the Dacron graft used to reconstruct the transverse arch ends distally in an extended sleeve that is telescoped into the descending thoracic aorta, facilitating later replacement of the descending thoracic/abdominal aneurysm (two-stage procedure).

In the operating room, steroids are often given at the onset of the procedure if HCA is anticipated. Evidence suggests that steroids given preoperatively several hours before the operation may have benefit. Some institutions monitor electroencephalogram silence to assess for adequate duration and temperature of cerebral cooling for HCA.

Descending Thoracic Aortic Aneurysms and Thoracoabdominal Aneurysms

Descending TAs may be repaired with open surgery or, if appropriate, with endovascular stent grafting techniques. Stent graft repair of descending thoracic aortic aneurysms should be performed if the predicted operative risk is lower than that of medical therapy. Patient age, comorbidities, symptoms, life expectancy, aortic diameter, characteristics and extent of the aneurysm, and landing zones should also be taken into consideration.

Surgically, descending TAs may be repaired with or without the use of a bypass circuit from the left atrium to the femoral artery or femoral vein–femoral artery cardiopulmonary bypass, depending on the length of the anticipated ischemic cross-clamping and the experience of the surgeon. Discrete aneurysms with an anticipated clamp time of less than 30 minutes may be repaired without left heart or cardiopulmonary bypass (i.e., "clamp and sew" technique). More complex or larger aneurysms are probably safer to repair with the aid of either left heart, partial, or full cardiopulmonary bypass with HCA. The use of left heart or cardiopulmonary bypass is favored to reduce hemodynamic instability and the risk of spinal cord paraplegia.

TAAAs, comprising approximately 10% of TAs, may be repaired with the use of a partial bypass of the left atrium to the femoral artery. Crawford type I TAAAs involve Dacron graft replacement of the aorta from the left subclavian artery to the visceral and renal arteries as a beveled distal anastomosis, using sequential cross-clamping of the aorta. Crawford type II TAAA repair requires a Dacron graft from the left subclavian to the aortic bifurcation with reattachment of the intercostal arteries, visceral arteries, and renal arteries. Crawford type III or IV TAAA repairs, which begin lower along the thoracic aorta or upper abdominal aorta, may use either the partial bypass of the left atrial artery to the femoral artery or a modified atriovisceral and/or renal bypass. Prevention of paraplegia is one of the principal concerns in the repair of descending and TAAAs.

A devastating complication of descending TA and TAAA repair is spinal cord injury with paraparesis or paraplegia. Preoperatively, some groups perform spinal arteriograms to attempt to localize the artery of Adamkiewicz for reimplantation during surgery. Neurologic monitoring with somatosensory evoked potentials or motor evoked potentials is used by some to assess SCI and identify critical segmental arteries for spinal cord perfusion. Lastly, preoperative placement of catheters for CSF drainage is performed to increase spinal cord perfusion pressure during aortic cross-clamping.

Spinal cord injury is less prevalent with endovascular stent grafting than with open repair but exists with both types of surgical treatment. For endovascular stent grafting, CSF drainage and avoidance of hypotension are the primary mechanisms used to prevent paraplegia. The use of CSF drainage is selective among most centers. For some discrete aneurysms, stent graft coverage may allow for preservation of spinal arteries. Others require coverage of the entire descending thoracic aorta. Indications for use of CSF drains include anticipated endograft coverage of T9-T12, coverage of the long segment of the thoracic aorta, compromised collateral pathways from prior infrarenal AAA repair, and symptomatic spinal ischemia.

Atrial femoral bypass is established with a Bio-Medicus circuit, and the patient is cooled to 32 to 34°C (89.6 to 93.2°F). Distal cross-clamping is performed at T4-T7 to allow continued spinal cord, visceral, and renal perfusion. The proximal anastomosis is performed, when complete, the proximal clamp is released and reapplied more distally on the tube graft. The distal cross clamp is moved sequentially down, if feasible, to allow visceral and renal perfusion. The intercostal arteries may be reimplanted, if desired, or oversewn. If sequential cross-clamping is not feasible, direct catheters may be placed in the visceral and renal vessels to allow continuous perfusion.

If the distal aneurysm extends to the renals, then the distal anastomosis may be beveled to incorporate the visceral and renal vessels and distal aorta. If the distal aneurysm extends to the bifurcation, the visceral and renal vessels are reattached to the tube graft. The left renal artery typically requires a separate anastomosis, but the celiac, superior mesenteric, and right renal arteries are often incorporated as a single island. The patient is rewarmed, and the partial bypass is discontinued as the tube graft perfuses the intercostals and abdominal vessels. The distal anastomosis at the bifurcation is performed as an open distal procedure.

Ross Procedure (Pulmonary Autograft)

The aortic root and proximal ascending aorta are replaced with a pulmonary autograft. The pulmonary valve is then replaced with a pulmonary homograft. Most commonly performed in children with congenital disease, the Ross operation may be used for active young adults with aneurysmal disease (excluding those with connective tissue disorders), women of childbearing age who desire pregnancy, or patients with contraindications to anticoagulation.

POSTOPERATIVE DETAILS

Patients who have undergone ascending aneurysm repairs are observed for signs of coronary ischemia, particularly if the coronary ostia were reimplanted, and for signs of aortic insufficiency when the aortic valve is repaired. Following the repair of arch aneurysms, particular attention must be given to neurological status, and patients who have had the elephant trunk repair must be observed for signs of paraplegia because the telescoped sleeve in the descending aorta may obstruct critical spinal vessels.

Paraplegia is most feared in patients who have had repair of the descending and thoracoabdominal aorta. Cerebrospinal fluid drainage may be continued for up to 72 hours postoperatively if necessary, along with motor evoked potential monitoring. Paraplegia and paraparesis may be acute or delayed postoperatively. If paraparesis or paraplegia is delayed, increased mean arterial pressure with pressors and reinstitution of CSF drainage may augment spinal cord perfusion to reverse this complication. Paraplegia due to occlusion of critical spinal arteries that were not reimplanted cannot be reversed by these maneuvers. Acute postoperative renal dysfunction may be due to extended periods of ischemic cross-clamping or to HCA.

FOLLOW-UP

Development of another aneurysm postoperatively is not uncommon in these patients. For this reason, serial evaluations (i.e., CT scans or MRI for ascending, arch, or descending aneurysms; echocardiography for ascending aneurysms) may be performed every 3 to 6 months during the first postoperative year and every 6 months thereafter.

COMPLICATIONS

Morbidity and mortality in TA repair are higher than most elective surgical procedures given the anatomic constraints and operative complexity. The subsets of aortic arch and Crawford type II (proximal descending to infrarenal aorta) aneurysms have the highest morbidity and mortality rates.

Early morbidity and mortality are related to bleeding, neurologic injury (e.g., stroke), cardiac failure, pulmonary failure (e.g., acute respiratory distress syndrome [ARDS]), and renal failure. The long-term mortality and morbidity were related to aneurysm in other areas, MI, and stroke.

In earlier studies, the overall 30-day postoperative mortality rates were 4 to 10% and stroke rates of 2 to 5% in patients undergoing ascending and arch aneurysm repair. Spinal injury was seen in 10 to 20% and renal injury rates around 10 to 15% with repair of a descending aneurysm, with around 7% severe acute renal failure requiring dialysis.

Bleeding is a potential complication for all aneurysm repairs. It is minimized by the use of antifibrinolytics, felt strips, and factors, including fresh frozen plasma and platelets. For patients who undergo HCA, the use of aprotinin, an antifibrinolytic agent used to reduce operative blood loss in patients undergoing open heart surgery, is controversial, but most groups routinely use aminocaproic acid (Amicar). Coagulopathy and bleeding in severe cases may warrant the use of recombinant factor VII.

Stroke is a major cause of morbidity and mortality and typically results from embolization of atherosclerotic debris or clot. TEE and epiaortic ultrasound may be beneficial in localizing appropriate areas to clamp. Patients undergoing arch repairs are at the highest risk of permanent and transient neurologic injury. RCP is beneficial for flushing out embolic debris, but it may be detrimental, with increased intracranial pressure and cerebral edema. Antegrade cerebral perfusion is beneficial for reducing neurologic injury during HCA. Stroke incidence for open surgical repair versus endovascular repair of descending TAs is equivalent.

Myocardial infarction may occur with technical problems with coronary ostia implantation during root replacement for ascending aortic aneurysms and may require reoperation. Pulmonary dysfunction and renal dysfunction are other potentially morbid complications.

Paraparesis and paraplegia, either acute or delayed, are the most devastating complications of descending TA and TAAA repairs. Despite cerebrospinal drainage, reimplantation of intercostal arteries, evoked potential monitoring, mild hypothermia, and atrial femoral bypass, spinal cord injury still occurs. Endovascular stent grafting has not eliminated spinal cord paraplegia; however, it appears to have reduced its incidence compared to open repair. Whether this is related to the technique or limiting risk factors associated with the development of SCI is difficult to determine.

Complications specific to endovascular stenting include endoleaks, stent fractures, stent graft migration or thrombosis, iliac artery rupture, retrograde dissection, microembolization, aortoesophageal fistula, and complications at the site of delivery (e.g., groin infection, lymphocele, seroma).

The early hospital mortality rate following repair of ascending aneurysms is 4 to 10%. Stroke occurs in 2 to 5% of patients. As would be expected, the early mortality rate after repair of arch aneurysms is considerably higher of 6 to 12% with some reports up to 25% with stroke rate varying from 3 to 22%. Renal failure that required dialysis occurred in 7% of patients. The mortality rate after repair of descending TAs is lower, approximately 5 to 15%.

The results of a phase II multicenter trial for the GORE-TAG thoracic endovascular stent demonstrated 30-day mortality of 1.5%. Temporary or permanent spinal cord paraplegia occurred in 3% of patients and stroke in 4% of patients. At 2 years, aneurysm survival was 97% and overall survival 75%. For the Medtronic Talent device, the incidence of in hospital paraplegia in the stent group was 1.75%, stroke 3.7%, mortality 4 to 7.9%, and procedural success greater than 95%.

When endovascular stent grafting was compared to open surgery for the GORE-TAG device, the rate of paraplegia was 3% in the stent group versus 14% in the open group; operative mortality was 1 versus 6%, and early death was 2 versus 10%. The patients in the stent group had a shorter ICU and hospital stay, a quicker recovery time, and a lower incidence of major adverse events (except for vascular complications). Complications at 2 years included 4% proximal stent migration, 6% migration of the graft components, and 15% of patients had an endoleak. Survival rates were the same (80% in both the open and stent groups).

Midterm results comparing open descending TA repair with endovascular stent grafting demonstrated lower early operative mortality with endovascular repair (10% for stent grafting vs. 15% for open repair) but similar late survival (actuarial survival rate at 48 months of 54% for stent grafting vs. 64% for open repair).

Predictors of Outcome with Thoracoabdominal Aneurysm

The main adverse predictors of outcomes after repair include preoperative renal insufficiency, increasing age, symptomatic aneurysms, and Crawford type II aneurysms (proximal descending to infrarenal aorta).

Other risk factors include emergent operation, dissection, congestive heart failure (CHF), prolonged cardiopulmonary bypass time, arch replacement, previous cardiac surgery, need for concomitant coronary revascularization, and reoperation for bleeding.

Emergency Surgery

Emergency surgery for TAAA that has ruptured or dissected is associated with a substantial morbidity and mortality with reported 30 days mortality of 42%, renal failure of 36%, respiratory failure of 36%, and paraplegia/paraparesis of 27%.

Thoracic Endovascular Aortic Repair

Thoracic endovascular aortic repair (TEVAR) was initially developed to treat patients who were considered to not be surgical candidates but is now considered a suitable alternative to OS in most cases. Potential benefits of TEVAR relative to OS include avoidance of long incisions in the thorax or abdomen, no cross-clamping of the aorta, less blood loss, lower incidence of visceral, renal, and SCI, fewer episodes of respiratory dependency, and quicker recovery.

Computed tomography angiography (CTA) of the chest, abdomen, and pelvis with 3D reformatting is performed preoperatively. It provides accurate information regarding the external and luminal diameter of the aorta to be used for the proximal and distal seal zones, the length of coverage required, the degree of angulation and tortuosity of the aorta, identification of important side branches, as well as characteristics of the lumen and wall of the aorta, including thrombus burden and calcification. From this information, the diameter and length of the graft(s) needed for successful repair can be chosen.

The procedure is typically done under general endotracheal anesthesia. A lumbar drain is placed in the L3-L4 disc space for drainage of CSF in cases where extensive coverage of the thoracic aorta is anticipated, where interruptions of contributing blood supply to the artery of Adamkiewicz (T8-L1) is high, and in cases where the patient has had prior AAA repair. Other risk factors included aortoiliac occlusive disease, use of a conduit, and procedural hypotension. Some institutions have taken the approach of routine use of lumbar drainage in all cases; however, this must be balanced with the risks of the additional procedure and the ability to promptly insert a lumbar drain if symptoms develop after the implantation.

Performance of the procedure requires the delivery of a large-bore sheath into the aorta as well as angiographic access. This is typically accomplished transfemorally, although patients presenting with disadvantaged femoral access sites may require delivery of the sheath through the common iliac artery, an iliac conduit, or an endovascular stent graft in the external iliac artery.

The high force of blood flow in the thoracic aorta may be one of the reasons why longer seal zone (20 mm) is recommended, defined as to either the proximal or distal ends of the thoracic stent graft where it is opposed to relatively normal aorta, on either end (compared with the abdominal aorta) to prevent displacement. Other suggests the sealing length should be proportional to the diameter of the vessel being treated. The curve of the thoracic aorta at the arch presents special challenges in attempting to achieve adequate proximal fixation and seal. With advanced age, atherosclerotic changes lead to lengthening and increased tortuosity, adding to the difficulty of accurate device deployment and adequate proximal landing. When device deployment is performed close to or within the arch, the graft must closely appose the "inner curve" of the arch. If the proximal end of the graft is oriented toward the apex of such a curve, "bird-beaking" where the graft is not apposed to the aortic wall will occur, increasing the risk of graft collapse, migration, and failure of aneurysm exclusion. With adequate preoperative planning, landing more proximally and debranching the arch as needed can usually circumvent these issues.

Placement of the proximal or distal end of the device to obtain adequate aneurysm exclusion may require covering important side branches. "Hybrid" procedures which combine open vascular bypass to important vessels followed by thoracic stent grafting have been developed. The proximal seal zone may abut or involve branch vessels of the arch. Debranching procedures using "hybrid" techniques can be performed, allowing coverage of the origins of these vessels.

When coverage of the left subclavian artery is required, preoperative planning consists of carotid and vertebral artery duplex, with a CTA or MRA of the head and neck. Planned coverage of the left subclavian in a patient with a dominant left vertebral, hypoplastic right vertebral, inferior mammary bypass graft, left handed individual, or incomplete circle of Willis should be preceded by left carotid-subclavian arteries bypass or left subclavian transposition. Some authorities suggest it be done routinely to decrease the risk of SCI; however, Level I evidence is lacking in this regard.

For more proximal landing zones involving the left common carotid artery or brachiocephalic trunk, antegrade bypass from the ascending aorta/transposition of the great vessels can be performed or, alternatively, extra-anatomic bypass can be performed to avoid sternotomy.

The distal seal zone must also be at least 20 mm in length. Typically, the celiac axis is spared. Reports of covering the celiac artery in patients with a documented patent pancreaticoduodenal arcade have been successful in achieving up to an additional 25 mm in seal length with nominal incidence of mesenteric ischemia. Once the device is deployed, the stent graft is typically ballooned at the seal zones and graft junctions. This however is not without risks. Perioperative complications leading to hypotension or vasoconstrictive agent and hinder collateral perfusion and result in detrimental hepatic ischemia.

On occasion, the distal end of a TAAA may extend below the level of the renal artery blood flow, and intercostal, visceral, and renal arteries may be compromised. Surgical and stenting techniques have been developed to decrease the likelihood of this complication with debranching or fenestrations.

DEVICES

The Gore-TAG device is made of e-PTFE and a nitinol stents exoskeleton.

The Medtronic Talent thoracic stent graft system was studied in the VALOR I trial. It is made of two components, a proximal straight tubular stent graft with a proximal bare stent configuration and a distal tapered tubular stent graft with an open web proximal configuration and closed web distal configuration. It consists of a woven polyester graft with a nitinol endoskeleton.

The Medtronic Valiant endograft has a modified proximal bare stent configuration with eight bare peak wires compared with the five bare peak wires found in the Talent stent graft. The long connecting bar of the Talent device was removed in the Valiant device to afford better flexibility of the device.

The Cook TX2 stent graft is a two-piece modular endograft system made of proximal and distal tubular endografts with and without tapering. The proximal endograft is covered and has stainless steel barbs, allowing for active fixation to the aortic wall. The distal component has at its distal end a bare metal stent. This allows active fixation of the device over the origins of the visceral vessels. The TX2 is made of Dacron fabric covered by stainless steel Z-stents.

The Bolton Relay stent graft is an investigational device. It is composed of self-expanding nitinol stents sutured to a polyester fabric graft with a curved longitudinal nitinol wire intended to provide columnar strength. It has a proximal bare stent, which remains constrained until the endograft is fully deployed and maintains a sinusoidal connecting bar to provide device longitudinal stability as well as flexibility.

COMPLICATIONS

Stroke

Risk factors for embolic stroke include the need for proximal deployment of the graft, presence of mobile atheroma in the arch, and prior stroke. The vertebral arteries arising from the subclavian may be the source for posterior circulation strokes. Perioperative stroke has ranged from 4 to 8%, comparable to open surgery.

Ischemia

Left upper extremity symptoms may occur in up to 15.8% of patients but only required intervention in a minority of patients around 5.3%.

Spinal Cord Ischemia

Extensive coverage of the thoracic aorta as well as prior history of AAA repair places the patient at increased risk for SCI with the potential for paraplegia. The risk of SCI has been reported to be between 3 and 11%, comparable to the rate of open surgery. Some studies have demonstrated a lower rate of SCI with TEVAR than with open surgery. The extent of aortic disease was the strongest predictor of SCI.

Visceral Ischemia

Visceral ischemia can occur with coverage of the celiac axis. Although, reports have suggested that collateralization through an intact pancreati-coduodenal arcade allows for extension of the distal seal zone to the level of the superior mesenteric artery (SMA) without physiologic consequence. Similarly, stenting below the SMA or renal artery levels requires revascularization of these vessels, or use of specialized fenestrated grafts.

Postimplantation Syndrome

This syndrome occurs during the early postoperative period and is characterized by leukocytosis, fever, and elevation of inflammatory mediators such as C-reactive protein, IL-6, and TNF-alpha. It is thought to be due to endothelial activation by the endoprosthesis. For thoracic aortic stent grafts, development of either unilateral or bilateral reactive pleural effusions is not uncommon, with a reported incidence 30 to 70%.

Thirty-day Mortality

Perioperative mortality with second generation stent grafts is low around 2%.
   Late stent graft complications occurred in 38% of patients and included stent graft misdeployment or removal, endoleak, aortic dissection, distal embolization, gut ischemia, and infection. Fatal complications occurred in 4%, including rupture of the treated aneurysm, stent graft erosion into the esophagus (aortoesophageal fistula), arterial injury, and excessive bleeding.

Device Migration

Migration of the graft (greater than 10 mm) cranially or caudally can occur, with a published incidence of 1 to 2.8% over a 6- to 12-month period. Factors predisposing to migration include excessive oversizing usually more than 30% and tortuous seal zone anatomy.
   The rate of secondary intervention required following stent grafting due to either endoleak or device migration is around 4%.

Long-term Surveillance

CTA is usually obtained within a month of the procedure, followed by an imaging study at 6 months and annually thereafter. Evidence of attachment site endoleak is intervened upon promptly. Type II endoleaks can be observed if the sac does not enlarge. Magnetic resonance angiography can also be used, although it is of limited applicability in patients with ESRD or CRI. Noncontrast CT allows for measurement of the sac diameter and is sufficient in most circumstances to document effective aneurysm exclusion.

PRACTICAL POINTS

■ Males are affected two to four times more than females.

■ Hypertension is the strongest risk factor for aortic aneurysm.

■ Aortitis associated with inflammatory and infectious disorders can lead to aortic aneurysm.

■ Aggressive blood pressure control, with beta-blockers being part of the regimen in an attempt to slow aneurysm growth.

■ Indication for surgery include, among others, an end-diastolic aortic diameter of 50 to 60 mm for an ascending aortic aneurysm and 60 to 70 mm for a descending aortic aneurysm.

■ Surgery is indicated for a thoracic aorta of greater than 45 mm if patient is undergoing aortic valve replacement or has an aortic dissection.

■ Patients with ascending aortic and particularly arch disease should undergo detailed imaging of the arch vessels.

■ The main adverse predictors of outcomes after repair include preoperative renal insufficiency, increasing age, symptomatic aneurysms, and Crawford type II aneurysms (proximal descending to infrarenal aorta).

■ The proximal and distal "seal zone" for TEVAR must be at least 20 mm in length

■ Potential complications from TEVAR include stroke, spinal cord or visceral ischemia, postimplantation syndrome, and graft migration.

RECOMMENDED READING

Hiratzka LF, Bakris GL, Beckman JA, et al. ACCF/AHA/AATS/ACR/ASA/SCA/SCAI/SIR/STS/SVM guidelines for the diagnosis and management of patients with thoracic aortic disease: a report of the American College of Cardiology Foundation/American Heart Association Task Force on Practice Guidelines, American Association for Thoracic Surgery, American College of Radiology, American Stroke Association, Society of Cardiovascular Anesthesiologists, Society for Cardiovascular Angiography and Interventions, Society of Interventional Radiology, Society of Thoracic Surgeons, and Society for Vascular Medicine. *Circulation* 2010;121(13):e266–e369.

Adams JN, Trent RJ. Aortic complications of Marfan's syndrome. *Lancet* 1998;352:1722.

Allaire E, Forough R, Clowes M, et al. Local overexpression of TIMP-1 prevents aortic aneurysm degeneration and rupture in a rat model. *J Clin Invest* 1998;102:1413.

Amabile P, Grisoli D, Giorgi R, et al. Incidence and determinants of spinal cord ischaemia in stent-graft repair of the thoracic aorta. *Eur J Vasc Endovasc Surg* 2008;35:455.

Bavaria JE, Appoo JJ, Makaroun MS, et al. Endovascular stent grafting versus open surgical repair of descending thoracic aortic aneurysms in low-risk patients: a multicenter comparative trial. *J Thorac Cardiovasc Surg* 2007;133:369.

Baxter BT, Pearce WH, Waltke EA, et al. Prolonged administration of doxycycline in patients with small asymptomatic abdominal aortic aneurysms: report of a prospective (phase II) multicenter study. *J Vasc Surg* 2002;36:1–12.

Bonow RO, Carabello BA, Chatterjee K, et al. 2008 Focused update incorporated into the ACC/AHA 2006 guidelines for the management of patients with valvular heart disease: a report of the American College of Cardiology/American Heart Association Task Force on Practice Guidelines (Writing Committee to Revise the 1998 Guidelines for the Management of Patients With Valvular Heart Disease): endorsed by the Society of Cardiovascular Anesthesiologists, Society for Cardiovascular Angiography and Interventions, and Society of Thoracic Surgeons. *Circulation* 2008;118:e523.

Davies RR, Gallo A, Coady MA, et al. Novel measurement of relative aortic size predicts rupture of thoracic aortic aneurysms. *Ann Thorac Surg* 2006;81:169.

Davies RR, Goldstein LJ, Coady MA, et al. Yearly rupture or dissection rates for thoracic aortic aneurysms: simple prediction based on size. *Ann Thorac Surg* 2002;73:17.

Demers P, Miller DC, Mitchell RS, et al. Midterm results of endovascular repair of descending thoracic aortic aneurysms with first-generation stent grafts. *J Thorac Cardiovasc Surg* 2004;127:664.

Elefteriades JA. Natural history of thoracic aortic aneurysms: indications for surgery, and surgical versus nonsurgical risks. *Ann Thorac Surg* 2002;74:S1877.

Elefteriades JA. Indications for aortic replacement. *J Thorac Cardiovasc Surg* 2010; 140(6 Suppl):S5–S9; discussion S45–S51.

Elefteriades JA, Farkas EA. Thoracic aortic aneurysm clinically pertinent controversies and uncertainties. *J Am Coll Cardiol* 2010;55(9):841–857.

Greenberg RK, Lytle B. Endovascular repair of thoracoabdominal aneurysms. *Circulation* 2008;117:2288.

Kouchoukos NT, Masetti P, Rokkas CK, et al. Safety and efficacy of hypothermic cardiopulmonary bypass and circulatory arrest for operations on the descending thoracic and thoracoabdominal aorta. *Ann Thorac Surg* 2001;72:699.

Svensson LG, Crawford ES, Hess KR, et al. Experience with 1509 patients undergoing thoracoabdominal aortic operations. *J Vasc Surg* 1993;17:357.

Makaroun MS, Dillavou ED, Wheatley GH, et al.; Gore TAG Investigators. Five-year results of endovascular treatment with the Gore TAG device compared with open repair of thoracic aortic aneurysms. *J Vasc Surg* 2008;47:912.

Makaroun MS, Dillavou ED, Kee ST. Endovascular treatment of thoracic aortic aneurysms: results of the phase II multicenter trial of the GORE TAG thoracic endoprosthesis. *J Vasc Surg* 2005;41(1):1–9.

Matsumura JS, Cambria RP, Dake MD, et al. International controlled clinical trial of thoracic endovascular aneurysm repair with the Zenith TX2 endovascular graft: 1-year results. *J Vasc Surg* 2008;47:247.

Pannu H, Fadulu VT, Chang J, et al. Mutations in transforming growth factor-beta receptor type II cause familial thoracic aortic aneurysms and dissections. *Circulation* 2005;112:513.

Riesenman PJ, Farber MA, Mendes RR, et al. Coverage of the left subclavian artery during thoracic endovascular aortic repair. *J Vasc Surg* 2007;45:90.

Ross D. Replacement of the aortic valve with a pulmonary autograft: the "switch" operation. *Ann Thorac Surg* 1991;52(6):1346–1350.

Shores J, Berger KR, Murphy EA, et al. Progression of aortic dilatation and the benefit of long-term beta-adrenergic blockade in Marfan's syndrome. *N Engl J Med* 1994;330:1335.

Szeto WY, Bavaria JE, Bowen FW, et al. The hybrid total arch repair: brachiocephalic bypass and concomitant endovascular aortic arch stent graft placement. *J Card Surg* 2007;22:97.

CHAPTER 14 ■ Thoracic Aortic Aneurysm and Dissection

Mark A. Farber, Matthew A. Mauro, Debabrata Mukherjee, and Walter A. Tan

Diseases of the thoracic aorta, although relatively uncommon, remain among the most lethal and difficult to treat problems in all of medicine. There are two general categories of aortic disease: aortic dissection and aortic aneurysms.

Acute aortic dissection is the most common aortic emergency, and more than one in four patients die in hospital. Thoracic aortic aneurysms (TAAs) are much less common than abdominal aortic aneurysms (AAAs), but rupture is typically catastrophic and results in sudden death. The overall goal for these entities is aggressive blood pressure management and elective repair, where indicated, to avoid acute events.

ETIOLOGY

TAAs are principally caused by medial degeneration related to atherosclerosis. This accounts for up to three fourths of cases. Additionally, secondary dilatation of aortic dissections accounts for approximately a fifth of cases. The remaining etiologies include inherited abnormality of collagen, spondyloarthropathies, infection, aortitis, and trauma. Two well-described inherited connective tissue disorders that can cause thoracic aortic pathology are Marfan's syndrome and Ehlers-Danlos' syndrome. The presence of a bicuspid aortic valve increases the risk of developing an ascending thoracic aneurysm.

Pathophysiology

Aortic aneurysm histopathology, which is more accurately termed *medial degeneration*, is characterized by disruption and loss of elastic fibers and increased deposition of proteoglycans. Typically, there are areas of loss of smooth muscle cells in the aortic media and the presence of inflammatory cell infiltration in this disease. Aortic pathology associated with myosin heavy chain 11, smooth muscle (*MYH11*) and actin, alpha 2, and smooth muscle aorta (*ACTA2*) mutations leading to ascending aortic aneurysms demonstrates a hyperplastic response by smooth muscle cells in the aortic media. Although accumulation of proteoglycans in the aortic media is a consistent finding in TAAs, studies have not determined why this accumulation occurs or whether these are causal in nature.

Clinical Presentation

TAAs are usually asymptomatic but can present as chest, back, abdominal, or flank pain depending on which adjacent structure is compressed, stretched, or eroded into. These include the recurrent laryngeal nerve (hoarseness), bronchus (coughing or stridor), esophagus (dysphagia), or rarely even superior vena cava (upper-extremity edema) or the vertebrae and spinal cord (paralysis). Congestive heart failure due to aortic regurgitation or myocardial ischemia due to coronary compression is common. In many patients, identification of thoracic aneurysm disease occurs only incidentally when they undergo x-rays or tomographic scans for other indications.

Classification

The Crawford classification is important for surgical and endovascular intervention planning. The classification scheme is based on the location and extent of involvement of the descending aorta (Fig. 14.1). This allows patients to be stratified into different risk categories for cardiac, renal, and spinal cord complications. Aneurysms proximal to the left subclavian

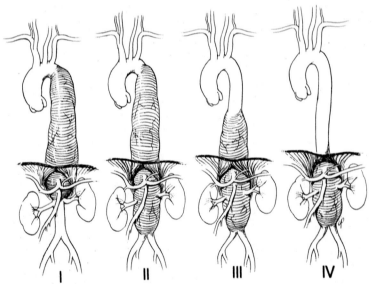

FIGURE 14-1. Crawford classification of thoracoabdominal aneurysms of the descending aorta. Type I involves most of the descending aorta above the renal arteries; type II involves virtually the entire descending aorta; type III involves the distal segment of the thoracic aorta and varying lengths of the abdominal aorta; and type IV involves most or all of the abdominal aorta including the visceral vessels. (From Morrisey NJ, Hamilton IN, Hollier LH. Thoracoabdominal aortic aneurysms. In: Moore WS, ed. *Vascular surgery*. Philadelphia, PA: WB Saunders, 2002:438.)

artery are described on the basis of whether the aortic root or any brachio-cephalic branch (arch aneurysms) is involved.

Diagnosis

Definitive diagnosis of thoracic aortic disease requires aortic imaging. Selection of the most appropriate imaging study depends on several patient-related factors (i.e., hemodynamic stability, renal function, and contrast allergy) and institutional capabilities (i.e., availability of individual imaging modalities, technology, and imaging specialist expertise). Consideration should also be given to patients with borderline abnormal renal function (serum creatinine greater than 1.8 to 2.0 mg/dL) by assessing the tradeoffs between the use of iodinated intravenous contrast for computerized tomography (CT) and the risk of contrast-induced nephropathy and between gadolinium agents used with MR and the risk of nephrogenic systemic fibrosis. It is recommended that external aortic diameter be reported for CT- or MR-derived size measurements. This is important because lumen size may not accurately reflect the external aortic diameter in the setting of intraluminal clot, aortic wall inflammation, or dissection.

Chest X-Ray

Chest x-ray is often a part of the evaluation of patients with aortic diseases. However, chest x-ray is inadequately sensitive to definitively exclude the presence of aortic aneurysm or dissection and therefore rarely excludes the disease.

Computerized Tomography

CT has been shown to have 92% accuracy for diagnosing abnormalities of the thoracic aorta, in a series of examinations that included 33 thoracic aneurysms, 3 ruptured TAAs, 6 PAUs, 5 aortic dissections, and 2 pseudoaneurysms. The sequence for CT performed in the potential setting of acute aortic dissection generally would include a noncontrast study to detect subtle changes of intramural hematoma followed by a contrast study to delineate the presence and extent of the dissection flap, identify regions of potential malperfusion, and demonstrate contrast leak indicating rupture. Technical parameters recommended for image reconstruction are slices of 3-mm or less thickness with a reconstruction interval of 50% or less than the slice thickness at 50% or greater overlap, tube rotation of 1 second or less, and 120 to 140 kVp.

Magnetic Resonance Imaging

MR has been shown to be very accurate in the diagnosis of thoracic aortic disease, with sensitivities and specificities that are equivalent to or may exceed those for CT and transesophageal echocardiography (TEE). Black blood imaging, using spin-echo sequences, is used to evaluate aortic anatomy and morphology (such as aortic size and shape) and the aortic wall for hematoma or other causes of thickening, such as vasculitis. Noncontrast white blood imaging is performed using either basic gradient echo sequences or the more advanced balanced steady-state free precession T2-weighted techniques that generate images with subsecond temporal resolution. Signal is generated from blood, making it appear white in the absence of contrast.

Contrast Angiography

Angiography provides accurate information about the site of dissection, branch artery involvement, and communication of the true and false lumens. Additionally, angiographic and catheter-based techniques allow for evaluation and treatment of coronary artery and aortic branch disease, as well as assessment of aortic valve and left ventricular function if indicated. Several disadvantages such as timely availability, exposure to iodinated contrast, and potential false-negative results with a thrombosed false lumen have replaced catheter-based angiography with CT, MR, and TEE as the first-line diagnostic tests to establish the presence of the acute aortic syndrome.

Transesophageal Echocardiography

TEE is safe and can be performed at the bedside, with a low risk of complications (less than 1% overall, less than 0.03% for esophageal perforation). The echocardiographic diagnosis of TAAs is determined on demonstration of aortic enlargement relative to the expected aortic diameter, based on age-adjusted and body size–adjusted nomograms. Overall, the sensitivity for proximal aortic dissection is 88 to 98% with a specificity of 90 to 95%. Advantages of TEE include its portability, rapid imaging time, and lack of intravenous contrast or ionizing radiation. Additionally, dissection-related cardiac complications can be evaluated including aortic regurgitation, proximal coronary artery involvement, and the presence of tamponade physiology. Disadvantages include a potential lack of availability at small centers and during off hours and sedation requirements that may include endotracheal intubation. Furthermore, the accuracy of TEE can be quite operator dependent. The recommendations for aortic imaging techniques to determine the presence and progression of thoracic aortic diseases are outlined in Table 14.1.

MANAGEMENT

Clinicians should routinely evaluate any patient presenting with complaints that may represent acute thoracic aortic dissection to establish a pretest risk of disease that can then be used to guide diagnostic decisions. This process should include specific questions about medical history, family history, and pain features as well as a focused examination to identify findings that are associated with aortic dissection. Meticulous control of hypertension, lipid profile, smoking cessation, and other atherosclerosis risk–reduction measures should be instituted for patients with small aneurysms not requiring surgery as well as for patients who are not considered to be surgical or stent-graft candidates. The optimal diameter at which a TAA should be repaired is not completely defined. Repair is indicated in

TABLE 14.1

RECOMMENDATIONS FOR AORTIC IMAGING TECHNIQUES TO DETERMINE THE PRESENCE AND PROGRESSION OF THORACIC AORTIC DISEASE

- Measurements of aortic diameter should be taken at reproducible anatomic landmarks, perpendicular to the axis of blood flow, and reported in a clear and consistent format.
- For measurements taken by computed tomographic imaging or MRI, the external diameter should be measured perpendicular to the axis of blood flow. For aortic root measurements, the widest diameter, typically at the midsinus level, should be used.
- For measurements taken by echocardiography, the internal diameter should be measured perpendicular to the axis of blood flow. For aortic root measurements, the widest diameter, typically at the midsinus level, should be used.
- Abnormalities of aortic morphology should be recognized and reported separately even when aortic diameters are within normal limits.
- The finding of aortic dissection, aneurysm, traumatic injury, and/or aortic rupture should be immediately communicated to the referring physician.
- Techniques to minimize episodic and cumulative radiation exposure should be utilized whenever possible.

asymptomatic patients with degenerative thoracic aneurysm, chronic aortic dissection, intramural hematoma, penetrating atherosclerotic ulcer, mycotic aneurysm, or pseudoaneurysm, who are otherwise suitable candidates and for whom the ascending aorta or aortic sinus diameter is 5.5 cm or greater. Patients with Marfan's syndrome or other genetically mediated disorders (vascular Ehlers-Danlos' syndrome, Turner's syndrome, bicuspid aortic valve, or familial TAA and dissection) should undergo elective operation at smaller diameters (4.0 to 5.0 cm depending on the condition; see Chapter 13 also) to avoid acute dissection or rupture. Similarly, patients with a growth rate of more than 0.5 cm/y in an aorta that is less than 5.5 cm in diameter should be considered for operation. Patients undergoing aortic valve repair or replacement and who have an ascending aorta or aortic root of greater than 4.5 cm should also be considered for concomitant repair of the aortic root or replacement of the ascending aorta (Fig. 14.2).

Contemporary management of TAAs has changed substantially with the evolution of endovascular stents (Fig. 14.3). The choice of surgical or endovascular intervention is influenced by aneurysm anatomy, involvement of the arch, and distal extent of the aneurysm. The specifics of operative strategy will vary based on the aneurysm morphology and preference of the surgeon. The most commonly applied surgical techniques include the clamp-and-sew technique. This is supplemented by protective adjuncts, and distal aortic perfusion is often provided as an atriofemoral bypass. An "elephant trunk" procedure has been used to reconstruct the arch and then provide a Dacron graft landing zone for endovascular stent-graft treatment of descending TAAs (Fig. 14.4).

Postoperative paraplegia related to spinal cord ischemia is the most feared nonfatal complication of TAA repair. In an effort to minimize this risk, a variety of adjunctive techniques have been developed. These include

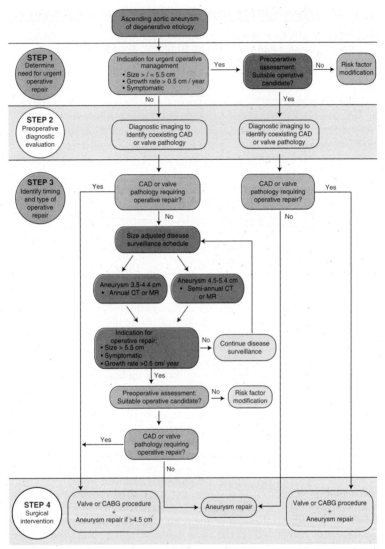

FIGURE 14-2. Ascending aortic aneurysm management strategy. (CABG, coronary artery bypass graft surgery; CAD, coronary artery disease; CT, computed tomographic imaging; MR, magnetic resonance imaging.) (Adapted from 2010 ACCF/AHA/AATS/ACR/ASA/SCA/SCAI/SIR/STS/SVM guidelines for the diagnosis and management of patients with thoracic aortic disease. *Circulation* 2010;121;1544–1579.)

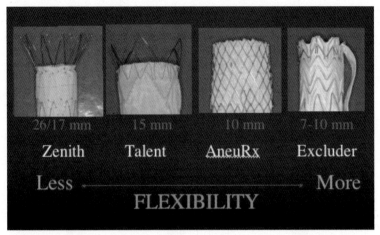

FIGURE 14-3.   Types of thoracic stent grafts: proximal fixation segments.

cerebrospinal fluid drainage, regional hypothermic protection using ice saline epidural infusion, reimplantation of critical intercostals arteries, evoked-potential monitoring, and distal aortic perfusion via atriofemoral bypass.

The feasibility of endoluminal stent grafting for TAAs has resulted in renewed evaluation and approach to thoracic aortic treatments. While now firmly established and having three FDA-approved devices, there remains controversy as to optimal indications, technical feasibility, and follow-up. Stent grafts have been applied to a broad range of clinical settings and indications. As a result, the risks of stent grafting the thoracic aorta have been more clearly defined. There is, however, a lack of long-term follow-up data and ongoing controversy as to a complete understanding of the risk-benefit ratio of stent grafting versus either medical management or open surgical repair.

Recently reported literature has reported a wide variation in operative mortality between 2 and 26%. This variation has largely been related to the urgency of the procedure, the extent of comorbid disease, and the experience of the operator. Analysis of midterm results demonstrates a 3- to 8-year survival of 25 to 90% over a broad range of clinical indications. Despite low operative mortality, thoracic stent grafting has been associated with a variety of late complications. These complications include endoleaks, graft migration, stent fractures, and aneurysm-related deaths. The late complications are reported much more commonly than what has been reported with open surgical repair.

The indication for stent grafting of descending TAAs needs to be based on the predictive operative risk that is lower than the risk of either conventional open repair or medical management. Consideration of a patient's age, comorbidity, life expectancy, and quality of life is significant. Aneurysm morphology and adequacy for stent grafting along with operator experience are also relevant considerations. It is also important to remember that postprocedure surveillance involves routine CT scans, and aortic reintervention is commonly required.

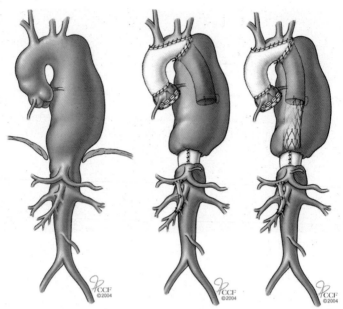

FIGURE 14-4.   Elephant trunk procedure. **Left:** Preoperative disease. **Middle:** Stage I with replacement of the ascending aorta and arch with a Dacron graft with the distal graft sutured circumferentially to the aorta distal to the left subclavian artery and the free end of the graft ("elephant trunk") within the descending aneurysm. **Right:** Completion of the procedure using an endovascular stent graft attached proximally to the "elephant trunk" and the distal end secured to a Dacron graft cuff. (Adapted from 2010 ACCF/ AHA/AATS/ACR/ASA/SCA/SCAI/SIR/STS/SVM guidelines for the diagnosis and management of patients with thoracic aortic disease. *Circulation* 2010;121;1544–1579.) (See color insert.)

The Gore TAG phase II study provides the best currently available comparison of open versus surgical treatment of descending TAAs. In this nonrandomized trial, TAG devices were placed in 137 patients, and compared to an open surgical control of 94 patients, 44 were concurrent and 50 historical. Perioperative mortality was 2.1% with endografting and 11.7% with open surgery. A 30-day analysis of complications demonstrated a significantly lower incidence of spinal cord ischemia, 3% versus 14%; reduced respiratory failure, 4% versus 20%; and reduction of renal failure, 1% versus 13%. Peripheral vascular complications were higher in the endograft cohort, that is, 14% versus 4%. Follow-up at 1 and 2 years demonstrated an endoleak rate of 6 and 9%, respectively, and reintervention in three endograft patients at 2 years. No reintervention was required in the surgical group. No difference in overall mortality was observed at 2 years by Kaplan-Meier analysis. Additional data have been forthcoming from a number of industry-sponsored trials. The VALOR trial using Medtronics Talent device completed enrollment in 2005. The PIVITOL group consisted of patients with degenerative thoracic aneurysms who were considered to be at low-to-moderate risk for surgical repair. Thirty-day mortality was 2.1% with a paraplegia rate of 1.5% and a stroke rate of 3.6%. All-cause mortality was reported at 1 year of 16.1% with aneurysm-related death of 3.1%. The STARZ trial was sponsored by Cook and used the Zenith TX2 endograft device. Enrollment was completed in 2006. Thirty-day mortality was 1.9% compared to 5.7% in the surgical control. Major preoperative events were also lower in the endograft group, 2.5% versus 7.1%. The incidence of paraplegia was 1.3% in the stent-graft group compared to 5.7% in the control group.

The most common morphology of descending TAAs is bursiform. These aneurysms appear to behave relatively predictably and assessment of aortic dimensions can be used to determine suitability for endografting as well as prognosticate about risk of rupture. Aneurysms that are secular or eccentric may be associated with increased risk of leak or disruption. Our understanding of other variant etiologies such as mycotic, penetrating aortic ulceration, and aneurysms associated with connective tissue disorders such as Marfan's syndrome remains incomplete. Management of saccular aneurysms and penetrating ulcers that may be associated with pseudoaneurysms lend themselves to endovascular treatment. These localized pathologies are often ideally suited for stent-graft repair because the aorta both proximally and distally is often relatively normal and a good landing zone for endografts. The role for endograft repair for managing patients with mycotic aneurysms is unknown. Successful endograft treatment has been reported in a small number of patients. Since the infected tissue remains, the likelihood of longer-term success is doubtful. Endovascular repair of mycotic aneurysm is not recommended and should be reserved for patients who are at prohibitive risk of open surgical repair. Patients with Marfan's syndrome or other connective tissue disorders require special consideration. While there are reported successful endograft interventions in this group of patients, there remains significant controversy and limited information about longer-term durability. Specifically, concerns have been raised about the effects of persistent radial force from the stent graft on an abnormal aorta. Stent-graft repair of aneurysms in patients with Marfan's syndrome or other connective tissue disorders is not recommended. In the event a patient is deemed to be at prohibitive open surgical risk, it should be considered but only as a last resort. Patients with Ehlers-Danlos' syndrome or polycystic kidney disease appear to have an increased risk of dissection following stent-graft placement.

Hybrid Procedures

The anatomical limitations for successful endovascular repair include inadequate seal zones, branch vessel involvement, and aneurysmal disease that extends into the thoracoabdominal area. With increasing extent of surgery, the risks of paraplegia, renal failure, and death increase. The extension of stent-graft repair to patients with thoracic aneurysms involving the arch or the visceral abdominal aortic segment with a hybrid operation has the ability to afford benefit in these high-risk patients. In some cases, the proximal or distal seal zone can be extended by surgical bypass of branch vessels commonly referred to as *debranching*. This technique has been performed on relatively small numbers of patients. While a number of small reported series have suggested successful outcomes with low paraplegia rates, no comparative trial data are available. The expected evolution of these hybrid procedures is the development of branch-graft technology and fenestrated grafts that will likely replace these hybrid procedures in high-risk patients.

AORTIC DISSECTION

The pathogenesis of aortic dissection is classically the result of an intimal tear. Following exposure of the intima to pulsating blood under high pressure, mural separation occurs and propagates distally. The propagated flap or septum results in the formation of a dual lumen that can cause obstruction or malperfusion. Most cases of aortic dissection are due to degenerative atherosclerotic changes in the aorta wall. Aortic dissection is also seen in younger patients with Marfan's syndrome, Ehlers-Danlos' syndrome, Turner's syndrome, and Noonan's syndrome. Crack cocaine use and trauma are thought to be predisposing risk factors that can also lead to aortic dissection.

Clinical Presentation

Based on the largest contemporary consecutive series, the International Registry of Acute Aortic Dissection (IRAD), the abrupt onset of severe chest or back pain is the single most common presenting complaint for patients with aortic dissection. Dissection can be unsuspected in patients and may be entirely missed in up to a third of patients prior to autopsy. The "classic" presentation is lacking in many patients: almost half of patients do not have sharp or ripping pain, and more than three fourths do not have radiating or migratory pain or peripheral pulse deficits (Table 14.2). Even more disconcerting is that no abnormalities were noted in the initial chest radiograph or electrocardiogram in upward of 70% of these patients, giving a false sense of security. A high degree of suspicion must therefore be maintained. Other manifestations include cardiac tamponade, acute myocardial infarction (usually due to right coronary artery compromise), acute aortic regurgitation, syncope, and hemothorax due to hemorrhage into the pleural space.

Classification

There are two primary classification schemes that have been developed to define aortic dissection (Fig. 14.5). The Stanford system classifies dissection as type A when the ascending aorta is involved and type B involving the descending aorta. This system is useful because of its inherent prognostic value and because this classification is fundamental to making management decisions. The most clinically important distinction is whether the ascending aorta or arch is involved (type A dissection), or just the segments beyond the left subclavian artery (type B dissection). Type A dissection comprises about 60 to 70% of all aortic dissections and is the most common aortic emergency. Type A dissections have a high mortality. The mortality rate averages up to 1% per hour within the initial 24 hours of presentation. As a result, urgent surgical consultation and repair are indi-

TABLE 14.2

CLINICAL PRESENTATION OF ACUTE AORTIC DISSECTION IN THE IRAD

Presenting Symptoms and Physical Examination of Patients with Acute Aortic Dissection (N = 464)[a]

Category	Present, No. Reported (%)	Type A, No. (%)	Type B, No. (%)	P Value, Type A vs. B
Presenting Symptoms				
Any pain reported	443/464 (95.5)	271 (93.8)	172 (98.3)	0.02
Abrupt onset	379/447 (84.8)	234 (85.4)	145 (63.8)	0.65
Chest pain	331/455 (72.7)	221 (78.9)	110 (62.9)	<0.001
Anterior chest pain	262/430 (60.9)	191 (71.0)	71 (44.1)	<0.001
Posterior chest pain	149/415 (35.9)	86 (32.8)	64 (41)	0.09
Back pain	240/451 (53.2)	129 (46.6)	111 (63.8)	<0.001
Abdominal pain	133/449 (29.6)	60 (21.6)	73 (42.7)	<0.001
Severity of pain: severe or worst ever	346/382 (90.6)	211 (90.1)	135 (90)	NA
Quality of pain: sharp	174/270 (64.4)	103 (62)	71 (68.3)	NA
Quality of pain: tearing or ripping	135/267 (50.6)	78 (49.4)	57 (52.3)	NA
Radiating	127/449 (28.3)	75 (27.2)	52 (30.1)	0.51
Migrating	74/446 (16.6)	41 (14.9)	33 (19.3)	0.22
Syncope	42/447 (9.4)	35 (12.7)	7 (4.1)	0.002
Physical examination findings				
Hemodynamics (n = 451)[b]				
Hypertensive (SBP ≥ 150 mm Hg)	221 (49.0)	99 (36.7)	122 (70.1)	
Normotensive (SBP 100–149 mm Hg)	156 (34.6)	110 (39.7)	46 (26.4)	<0.001
Hypotensive (SBP < 100 mm Hg)	36 (8.0)	32 (11.6)	4 (2.3)	
Shock or tamponade (SBP ≤ 80 mm Hg)	38 (8.4)	36 (13.0)	2 (1.5)	
Auscultated murmur of aortic insufficiency	137/434 (31.6)	117 (44)	20 (12)	<0.001
Pulse deficit	69/457 (15.1)	53 (18.7)	16 (9.2)	0.006
Cerebrovascular accident	21/447 (4.7)	17 (6.1)	4 (2.3)	0.07
Congestive heart failure	29/440 (6.6)	24 (8.8)	5 (3.0)	0.02

[a]SBP, systolic blood pressure; NA, not applicable.
[b]Systolic blood pressure is reported for 277 patients with type A and 174 patients with type B acute aortic dissection, respectively.

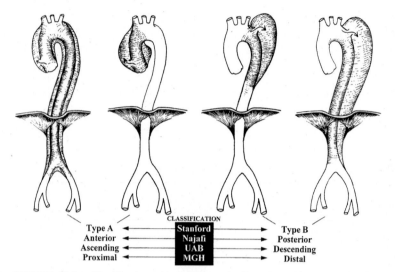

FIGURE 14-5. Classification schemes for aortic dissections. (From Morrisey NJ, Hamilton IN, Hollier LH. Thoracoabdominal aortic aneurysms. In: Moore WS, ed. *Vascular surgery*. Philadelphia, PA: WB Saunders, 2002:440.)

cated for these patients. By contrast, type B dissections are associated with a relatively low initial mortality. This allows for medical treatment in many cases surgical or endovascular intervention is not required. Intervention is reserved for those patients with evidence of malperfusion to the viscera, limb ischemia, or refractory pain.

IMAGING

The initial diagnostic modality employed (CT, MR, or TEE) for a patient suspected of having an aortic dissection is less important than expeditious assessment of the ascending aorta, the aortic valve, and the pericardium at the time of presentation.

The involvement of the ascending aorta or the transverse arch often signifies the need for urgent surgery under full cardiopulmonary bypass or circulatory arrest. Some of these patients may not have the luxury of time for detailed CT or MR and may go directly to the operating room where TEE is performed. In general, coronary catheterization is not recommended and, in cases of suspected tamponade pericardiocentesis, may worsen outcomes.

For type B dissections in which emergent intervention is not required, a thorough evaluation is necessary to define the extent of aortic pathology and evaluate other contributing comorbidities in an effort to reduce potential complications. It is critical to define the extent of aortic pathology, particularly on the basis of the proximal and distal extent, and whether branch vessels are involved. Concomitant AAA can be seen in up to 10%

of patients with thoracic aortic disease. Lack of adventitial integrity (e.g., contained rupture) should be meticulously examined for. For patients requiring surgical intervention, this anatomical information is helpful and allows planning for the proximal and distal suture lines. For poor surgical candidates, determination of adequate "landing zone" for proximal and distal device attachment may allow for endovascular intervention. Aortic dissections that can be effectively treated with endovascular stent grafts must have a seal zone that allows for both proximal and distal exclusion. The aortic morphologies that best suit this typically are those that spare the transverse arch and are relatively discrete. Any prior pathology such as chronic or repaired aortic dissection or aortic aneurysm should be delineated. Sagittal views or reconstructions from aortography, CT, or MR can be helpful and may reveal aortic tortuosity or overt buckling that may significantly alter diameter and length estimates taken from nontangential cuts. The presence of thrombus in the involved aortic region may signify early aneurysmal changes and can influence the selection of the specific site of anastomosis. Aortic calcification and atherosclerotic disease may also be present. Extensive atherosclerotic plaque and or dense calcification can contribute significantly to the difficulty of any surgical or endovascular procedure. Furthermore, it is advisable to define any associated chronic dissection since the anticipated increased complexity of repair or cross-clamp time may prompt some surgeons to alter their intraoperative strategy. Intercostal artery reconstructions are frequently attempted if they are deemed important for spinal cord perfusion either preoperatively or intraoperatively.

There are some special considerations for optimal imaging of aortic dissections. The ascending aorta is almost twice as frequently involved as the descending aorta, and there is a mortality gradient depending on the site of tear. More proximal tears such as those involving the aortic root are associated with approximately 37% mortality compared to those starting from the arch (~23%) and less than 15% beyond the left subclavian artery (type B). The region of the right lateral wall is frequently the proximal entry site, and consequent compromise of the right coronary artery is seen. The entire course of the true and false lumens should be clearly delineated and followed; therefore, scanning should include the iliofemoral arteries. Whether the false lumen is patent, or incompletely or completely thrombosed, is critical for choosing the optimal treatment strategy.

In addition, the thoracic aorta should also be carefully studied for other pathology (Fig. 14.6). *Intramural hematomas*, or noncommunicating static blood in the aortic wall that is not associated with intimal tear, have been detected in 3 to 13% of autopsy series. Those that do not involve the ascending aorta have a more favorable long-term prognosis. Older patients or those who develop ulceration, enlargement, or direct flow communication between the aortic wall and the lumen are at high risk for adverse events. Surgery is considered when these affect the ascending aorta, whereas lesions in the descending aorta tend to resorb or remain stable with expectant medical management. Conversely, *localized dissection*, or intimal tears without hematoma, has been discovered at surgery in up to 5% of a consecutive series of 181 consecutive aortic and arch repairs. These are worrisome as they were not detected preoperatively despite multiple

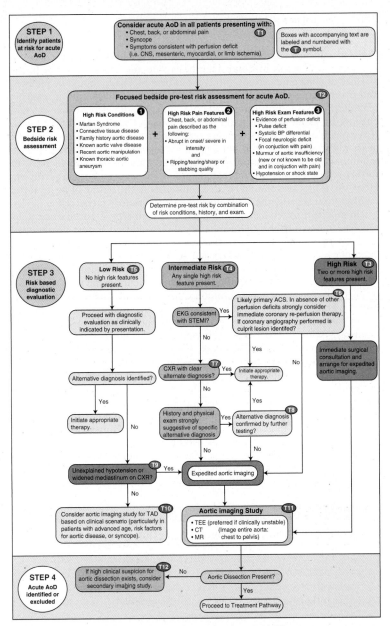

FIGURE 14-7. Aortic dissection evaluation pathway. (ACS, acute coronary syndrome; AoD, aortic dissection; BP, blood pressure; CNS, central nervous system; CT, computed tomographic imaging; CXR, chest x-ray; EKG, electrocardiogram; MR, magnetic resonance imaging; STEMI, ST-elevation myocardial infarction; TAD; thoracic aortic disease; TEE, transesophageal echocardiogram.) (Adapted from 2010 ACCF/AHA/AATS/ACR/ASA/SCA/SCAI/SIR/STS/SVM guidelines for the diagnosis and management of patients with thoracic aortic disease. *Circulation* 2010;121;1544–1579.)

Initial management of thoracic aortic dissection should be directed at decreasing aortic wall stress by controlling heart rate and blood pressure. In the absence of contraindications, intravenous beta blockade should be initiated and titrated to a target heart rate of 60 beats/min or less, and in patients with clear contraindications to beta blockade, nondihydropyridine calcium channel–blocking agents should be used as an alternative for rate control. If systolic blood pressures remain greater than 120 mm Hg after adequate heart rate control has been obtained, then angiotensin-converting enzyme inhibitors and/or other vasodilators should be administered intravenously to further reduce blood pressure that maintains adequate end-organ perfusion. However, β-blockers should be used cautiously in the setting of acute aortic regurgitation because they will block the compensatory tachycardia.

In an effort to reduce mortality, patients with type A aortic dissections require emergent surgery. Urgent surgical consultation should be obtained for all patients diagnosed with thoracic aortic dissection regardless of the anatomic location (ascending versus descending) as soon as the diagnosis is made or highly suspected. It is estimated that without surgical intervention, the mortality rate is at least 50%. Surgical intervention can reduce mortality to 10 to 30%. The most common causes of death include cardiac tamponade, aortic rupture, stroke, visceral ischemia, and circulatory failure.

In patients with type B aortic dissections, medical therapy has been the mainstay. Acute thoracic aortic dissection involving the descending aorta should be managed medically unless life-threatening complications develop (e.g., malperfusion syndrome, progression of dissection, enlarging aneurysm, inability to control blood pressure or symptoms). In patients without evidence of visceral ischemia, uncontrolled hypertension, progression of the dissection, inadequate pain control, or Marfan's syndrome medical management results in 30-day mortality of approximately 10%. Surgical and endovascular intervention is reserved for type B dissections that are complicated and have evidence of hemodynamic instability or malperfusion syndromes. Endovascular treatment has emerged and now exceeds open surgical intervention as the primary modality for treating acute complicated type B aortic dissections. Table 14.3 discusses endovascular

TABLE 14.3

ENDOVASCULAR OPTIONS FOR AORTIC DISSECTION

1. Stent grafting for the thoracic or abdominal aorta or iliac arteries to reestablish true lumen or seal entry site(s)
2. Stenting of the aortic true lumen for dynamic obstruction
3. Stenting of obstructed branch origin for static obstruction
4. Balloon or wire fenestration of dissection flap or septum
5. Fenestration to provide a reentry tear for a dead-end false lumen to prevent thrombotic occlusion or promote blood flow to branch vessels
6. Stenting to scaffold open a fenestration

(Adapted from Erbel R, Alfonso F, Boileau C, et al. Diagnosis and management of aortic dissection: Task Force on Aortic Dissection, European Society of Cardiology. *Eur Heart J* 2001;22:1642.)

TABLE 14.4

ELIGIBLE PATHOLOGIES FOR STENT-GRAFT THERAPY IN CURRENT CLINICAL TRIALS

Valor Trial (Medtronic)
Aneurysms
Dissections (acute and chronic)
Penetrating ulcer
Pseudoaneurysm
Traumatic injury
Aortic transection
Contained rupture
TX2 (Cook)
Aneurysms
Penetrating ulcer
TAG Confirmatory Arm (WL Gore)
Aneurysms
No ruptures or dissections

options for aortic dissection, and Table 14.4 lists eligible pathologies for stent-graft therapy in current clinical trials.

In an IRAD propensity analysis of type B aortic dissections, open surgical repair was associated with an independent increased risk of in-hospital mortality. In-hospital complications with endovascular management occurred in 20% of patients and 40% in patients managed with open surgery. In-hospital mortality was 33.9% with surgery and 10.6% with endovascular treatment. Figure 14.8 demonstrates management pathway for aortic dissections.

FENESTRATION IN AORTIC DISSECTION

Aside from aortic rupture and exsanguination, a common cause of death is ischemia and infarction of visceral organs that are supplied by arterial branches from the aorta. The kidneys, the gut, and the lower extremities can be compromised, and may result in gangrene, shock, and intractable systemic inflammatory response. In particular, patients with aortic dissection with branch vessel compromise have greater than 50% mortality. Unfortunately, these can be occult in as many as one in four patients, becoming apparent only when irreversible organ damage is established. There are numerous reasons for this poor detection rate, not the least of which are lack of diagnostic sensitivity even with contrast CTA, interpretation error in these complex cases, and the time lag between organ death and biochemical markers.

Perfusion to these compromised vital organs can be reestablished either with surgical or with endovascular techniques. An initial EVAR strategy that includes bare stents, stent grafts, fenestration, or combination therapy

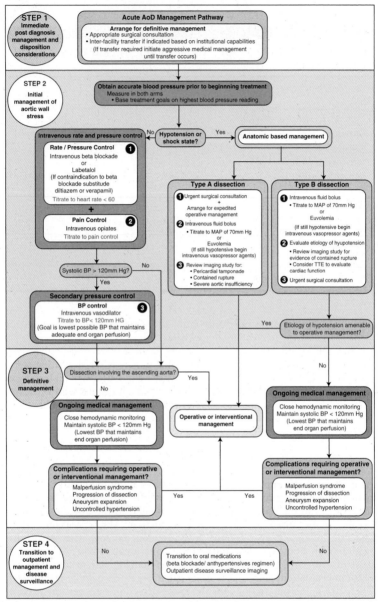

FIGURE 14-8. Acute aortic dissection management pathway. (AoD, aortic dissection; BP, blood pressure; MAP, mean arterial pressure; TTE, transthoracic echocardiogram.) (Adapted from 2010 ACCF/AHA/AATS/ACR/ASA/SCA/SCAI/SIR/STS/SVM guidelines for the diagnosis and management of patients with thoracic aortic disease. *Circulation* 2010;121;1544–1579.)

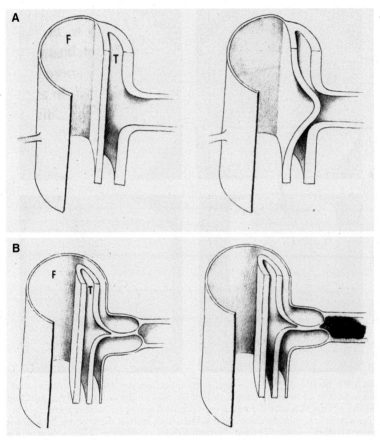

FIGURE 14-9.   Mechanisms of arterial obstruction in dissection: **A:** Dynamic, where the intimal flap can intermittently occlude a branch artery depending on the relative pressures and flows across the true and false lumens. **B:** Static or fixed impediment to flow (e.g., dissection extending into the aorto-ostial segment of splanchnic arteries).

may be applicable to cases of aortic dissections beyond the left subclavian artery, and some instances of retrograde dissection from the descending thoracic aorta. In the series from Stanford, successful endovascular reperfusion was accomplished in 22 of 22 patients with dynamic obstruction compared to only 6 of 15 (40%) for those who had a concomitant static obstruction (Fig. 14.9). In view of this and promising outcomes from other centers, many experts now believe that this is the therapy of choice for dynamic visceral artery obstruction, and that surgery be attempted only when this fails. An initial surgery still has a role for patients with acute or early visceral ischemia who require definitive aortic repair.

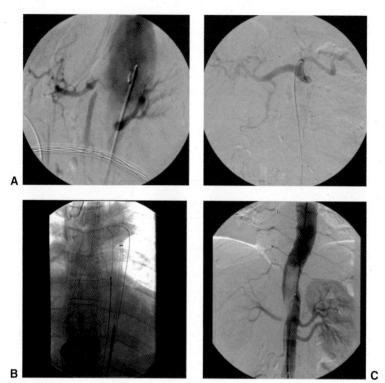

FIGURE 14-10.   Fenestration and its complication. **A:** "Floating" visceral arteries indicative of poor communication of blood with the aorta. **B:** After puncture of the intimal flap (not shown), a wire is pulled across this fenestration from the true lumen into the false lumen and snared. Both ends of the wire are then pulled taut across the aortic flap, and then caudally in an effort to create a rend across the septum to allow freely communicating blood flow to perfuse the mesenteric arteries. **C:** Extension of separation of the intimal flap from the aortic wall with partial aortic obstruction due to bunching up of intimal tissue (rectangular-shaped lucency).

It must be kept in mind that there are already natural fenestrations along the flap, since a branch orifice is divided into two pieces: the "button" of ostium that is pulled off with the intimal flap, and the corresponding ostial button on the aortic adventitial wall that remains connected to the main arteries. The orificial slits in the flap may serve as reentry sites for continued pressurization of the false lumen, preventing it from thrombosing. On the other hand, these may be beneficial in cases where visceral perfusion is predominantly derived from the false lumen.

Fenestration of the intimal flap can be done to reestablish flow into the lumen that subserves the compromised visceral branch. This technique has also been used in patients with embolization arising from thrombus in an aortic lumen to remedy flow stasis and further clot formation. This can be accomplished either by puncturing or ballooning the aortic septum, or additionally using a wire to slice across this flap, in essence intentionally tearing through the septum to create free communication of blood flow (Fig. 14.10). Stenting may be required to scaffold open the orifice of a visceral artery where a dissection flap may have extended into the vessel. Occasionally, embolization may be necessary to address endoleaks or retrograde branch perfusion that maintains patency of an aortic false lumen.

SUBACUTE AND CHRONIC AORTIC DISSECTION

The perioperative morbidity and mortality associated with open surgical repair of aortic dissection has resulted in the consensus that for chronic type B dissections, medical therapy is the treatment of choice. Despite adequate medical management, the longer-term prognosis of patients with type B dissections is suboptimal. Conceptually, the idea is that stent grafting the proximal primary intimal tear and scaffolding the true lumen would facilitate aortic remodeling and avoid complications of dissection extension or secondary aneurysmal dilatation. In a small series reported by Nienaber and associates, successful stent grafting was performed in a small number of patients. No mortality or significant morbidity was observed. Subsequently, a randomized study was organized. The INSTEAD study is the only randomized study comparing stent grafting with optimal medical management in patients with uncomplicated subacute or chronic dissection. The data were published in *Circulation* in 2009. The data demonstrated that thoracic stent grafting failed to improve the rates of 2-year survival and adverse events compared to optimal medical therapy. In the recent Talent Thoracic Registry, patients were treated with the Medtronic Talent device. In the cohort of treated patients, 38% had an aortic dissection and 8% had an acute or subacute type B dissection. In-hospital mortality was low, and paraplegia events were reported as 1.7%. These data suggest that stent grafting has a relatively low mortality and morbidity risk. The available observational data suggest that endografting of patients with chronic or subacute dissections can be performed with a high degree of technical success and the prevalence of complications may be lower than in those patients undergoing stent-graft placement for acute dissection. Despite the lack of efficacy data, stent grafting remains a therapeutic option for a patient who is deemed to be at high surgical risk and who has suitable anatomical morphology that allows covering of the proximal entry tear. The role of stent grafting for patients with chronic dissections in which the septum has begun to form scar tissue and is no longer pliable remains uncertain.

Acute Traumatic Aortic Transection

Emergency surgical intervention for traumatic disruptions or ruptures of the thoracic aorta is associated with significant morbidity and mortality. Many of these patients die in the field before ever reaching medical attention. The reported 30-day mortality for patients who survive and undergo emergent or nonemergent surgical repair is reported to vary from 6 to 23%. Pioneering work by Kato et al. demonstrated that an endovascular approach may have advantages and reduce the mortality and morbidity of conventional surgical repair. In a multicenter study, 30 patients with chest trauma and multiple injuries underwent endovascular stent grafting. Initial technical success was reported as 100%. Complications included late death in 6.7%, stroke in 3.3%, and partial stent collapse in 3.3%. Limited follow-up did not demonstrate endoleaks, migrations, or late pseudoaneurysm formation. Technical difficulties with this approach include the necessity to cover the left subclavian artery to achieve adequate seal. Problems with oversizing leading to infolding and obstruction have been noted. Additionally, many of these patients are younger and the aorta has not enlarged and unfolded as is typically seen in older patients. The resulting acute angulation of the aortic arch does not allow the stent graft to accommodate to the aortic anatomy. This failure of apposition can lead to a "bird beak" deformity and result in compression of the proximal lip of the graft resulting in a type1 endoleak or frank collapse of the device.

The long-term durability of the current stent-graft technology in these types of patients is unknown. It is hoped that with newer devices that are smaller and have improved angulation capability, some of these obstacles can be overcome.

CONCLUSION

■ Thoracic aortic diseases are usually asymptomatic and not easily detectable until an acute and often catastrophic complication occurs.

■ Imaging of the thoracic aorta with CT, MRI, or in some cases, echocardiographic examination is the only method to detect thoracic aortic diseases and determine risk for future complications.

■ Repair of TAA is indicated in asymptomatic patients with degenerative thoracic aneurysm, chronic aortic dissection, intramural hematoma, penetrating atherosclerotic ulcer, mycotic aneurysm, or pseudoaneurysm, who are otherwise suitable candidates and for whom the ascending aorta or aortic sinus diameter is 5.5 cm or greater.

■ Patients with Marfan's syndrome or other genetically mediated disorders (vascular Ehlers-Danlos' syndrome, Turner's syndrome, bicuspid aortic valve, or familial TAA and dissection) should undergo elective operation at smaller diameters (4.0 to 5.0 cm depending on the condition; see Section 5) to avoid acute dissection or rupture.

■ Initial management of thoracic aortic dissection should be directed at decreasing aortic wall stress by controlling heart rate and blood pressure.

■ Urgent surgical consultation should be obtained for all patients diagnosed with thoracic aortic dissection regardless of the anatomic location (ascending versus descending) as soon as the diagnosis is made or highly suspected.

■ Stringent control of hypertension, lipid profile optimization, smoking cessation, and other atherosclerosis risk–reduction measures should be instituted for patients with small aneurysms not requiring surgery as well as for patients who are not considered to be surgical or stent-graft candidates.

■ CT or MRI of the aorta is reasonable at 1, 3, 6, and 12 months post-dissection and, if stable, annually thereafter so that any threatening enlargement can be detected in a timely fashion.

PRACTICAL POINTS

■ For many thoracic aortic diseases, results of treatment for stable, often asymptomatic, but high-risk conditions are far better than the results of treatment required for acute and often catastrophic disease presentations.

■ An echocardiogram is recommended at the time of diagnosis of Marfan's syndrome to determine the aortic root and the ascending aortic diameters and 6 months thereafter to determine the rate of enlargement of the aorta.

■ For patients with a current TAA or dissection, or previously repaired aortic dissection, employment and lifestyle restrictions are reasonable, including the avoidance of strenuous lifting, pushing, or straining that would require a Valsalva maneuver.

■ A brain protection strategy to prevent stroke and preserve cognitive function should be a key element of the surgical, anesthetic, and perfusion techniques used to accomplish repairs of the ascending aorta and transverse aortic arch.

■ Women with Marfan's syndrome and aortic dilatation, as well as patients without Marfan's syndrome who have known aortic disease, should be counseled about the risk of aortic dissection as well as the heritable nature of the disease prior to pregnancy.

RECOMMENDED READING

2010 ACCF/AHA/AATS/ACR/ASA/SCA/SCAI/SIR/STS/SVM guidelines for the diagnosis and management of patients with thoracic aortic disease. *Circulation* 2010;121;1544–1579.

Bavaria JE, Appoo JJ, Makaroun MS, et al. Endovascular stent grafting versus open surgical repair of descending thoracic aortic aneurysms in low risk patients: a multicenter comparative trial. *J Thorac Cardiovasc Surg* 2007;133:369–377.

Conrad MF, Cambria RP. Contemporary management of descending thoracic and thoracoabdominal aortic aneurysms: endovascular versus open. *Circulation* 2008;117:841–852.

Dake MD, Kato N, Mitchell RS, et al. Endovascular stent-graft placement for the treatment of acute aortic dissection. *N Engl J Med* 1999;340:1546–1552.

Hagan PG, Nienaber CA, Isselbacher EM, et al. The International Registry of Acute Aortic Dissection (IRAD): new insights into an old disease. *JAMA* 2000;283(7):897–903.

Kato N, Hirano T, Kawaguchi T, et al. Aneurysmal degeneration of the aorta after stent-graft repair of acute aortic dissection. *J Vasc Surg* 2001;34:513–518.

Kaya A, Heijmen RH, Rousseau H, et al. Emergency treatment of the thoracic aorta:results in 113 consecutive acute patients (the Talent Thoracic retrospective registry). *Eur J Cardiothoracic Surg* 2009;35:276–281.

Morrisey NJ, Hamilton IN, Hollier LH. Thoracoabdominal aortic aneurysms. In: Moore WS, ed. *Vascular surgery*, 6th ed. Philadelphia, PA: WB Saunders, 2002:437–480.

Nienaber CA, Eagle KA. Aortic dissection: new frontiers in diagnosis and management: Parts I and II. *Circulation* 2003;108(5):628–635 and 108(6):772–778.

Nienaber CA, Fattori R, Lund G, et al. Nonsurgical reconstruction of thoracic aortic dissection by stent-graft placement. *N Engl J Med* 1999;340:1539.

Shimono T, Kato N, Yasuda F, et al. Transluminal stent-graft placements for the treatments of acute onset and chronic aortic dissections. *Circulation* 2002;106(Suppl I):I-241–I-247.

Svensson LG, Kouchoukos NT, Miller DC, et al. Expert consensus document on the treatment of descending thoracic aortic disease using endovascular stent grafts. *Ann Thorac Surg* 2008;85:S1–S41.

Tan WA. Endovascular treatment of aortic dissections. *Catheterization Cardiovasc Intervent* 2003;58:101–102.

Task Force on Aortic Dissection, European Society of Cardiology. Diagnosis and management of aortic dissection. *Eur Heart J* 2001;22:1642–1681.

Tsai TT, Trimarchi S, Nienaber CA. Acute aortic dissection: perspectives from the international registry of acute aortic dissection (IRAD). *Eur J Vas Endovasc Surg* 2009;37:149–159.

Williams DM, Lee DY, Hamilton BH, et al. The dissected aorta: percutaneous treatment of ischemic complications—principles and results. *J Vasc Intervent Radiol* 1997;8:605–625.

CHAPTER 15

■ Approach to and Management of Mesenteric Vascular Disease

Leslie Cho and Jeffrey A. Skiles

INTRODUCTION

Acute mesenteric ischemia may be caused by embolic/thrombotic arterial occlusion, nonocclusive mesenteric arterial insufficiency, or mesenteric venous occlusion. Chronic mesenteric ischemia is usually related to progressive atherosclerotic narrowing of the mesenteric arteries. Because of the wide range of causes, mesenteric ischemia often goes undiagnosed and untreated, leading to high morbidity and mortality. This chapter reviews the clinical features, diagnosis, and management of patients with acute and chronic mesenteric ischemia. Acute mesenteric ischemia may be due to embolic mesenteric artery occlusion, thrombotic mesenteric artery occlusion, mesenteric venous occlusion, and nonocclusive mesenteric occlusion. A thorough understanding of mesenteric arterial anatomy is crucial to understanding and managing these patients.

Clinical Anatomy

The gastrointestinal tract is supplied by the celiac trunk, the superior mesenteric artery (SMA), and the inferior mesenteric artery (IMA). The celiac trunk originates from the anterior aorta just below the diaphragm at the level of the thoracic vertebrae 12 (T12) or the first lumbar vertebra (Fig. 15.1). It branches into the common hepatic, splenic, and the left gastric arteries. The left gastric artery supplies the lesser curvature of the stomach and collateralizes with the right gastric artery branch of the hepatic artery. The common hepatic artery gives off the hepatic and gastroduodenal artery, which supplies the distal stomach and duodenum. In a minority of patients (15%), the gastroduodenal artery branches off from the SMA. The gastroduodenal artery supplies the greater curvature of the stomach via the right gastroepiploic artery.

The SMA is located few centimeters below the celiac artery usually around the first lumbar vertebra at 20- to 30-degree caudal angulation and supplies the pancreas, duodenum, jejunum, and the right half of the colon. The branches of the SMA are the inferior pancreaticoduodenal artery, the jejunal and ileal branches, the ileocolic artery, the right colic artery, and the middle colic artery (Fig. 15.2).

The IMA originates from the mid to distal infrarenal aorta around the third lumbar vertebra, which is usually 5 cm or more below the origin of the SMA. It supplies the distal transverse, left, and sigmoid portions of the colon and the rectum. Its branches are the left colic artery, the sigmoid (inferior left colic) arteries, and the superior rectal artery (Fig. 15.3). The SMA and IMA collateralize via the marginal artery of Drummond and the meandering mesenteric artery.

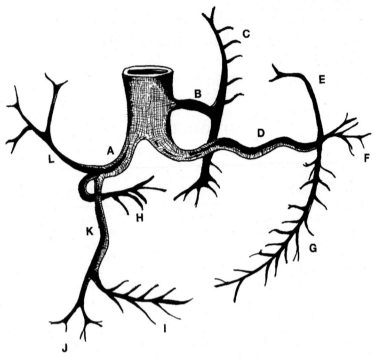

FIGURE 15-1. Normal anatomy of the celiac trunk and its major branches. (*A*, Common hepatic artery; *B*, left gastric artery; *C*, esophageal branches; *D*, splenic artery; *E*, short gastric branches; *F*, splenic branches; *G*, left gastroepiploic artery; *H*, right gastric artery, *I*, right gastroepiploic artery; *J*, superior pancreaticoduodenal artery; *K*, gastroduodenal artery; *L*, hepatic artery.)

The venous drainage follows a similar pattern as the arterial circulation, with the vena recta forming a venous arcade that drains the small bowel and proximal colon through the ileocolic, middle colic, and right colic veins to form the superior mesenteric vein (Fig. 15.4). The superior mesenteric vein and the splenic vein join and continue to the liver as the portal vein. There are three areas especially vulnerable to ischemia during low-flow states because of their more remote position between the major arteries. These are the hepatic flexure of the colon between the ileocolic and the middle colic branches of the SMA, the splenic flexure between the middle colic and the left colic arteries, and the distal sigmoid and rectum.

CLINICAL FEATURES AND DIAGNOSIS

Acute Mesenteric Ischemia

Acute mesenteric ischemia (Table 15.1) most commonly occurs as a result of embolism, acute thrombosis on preexisting atherosclerotic disease, or a low-flow state caused by systemic illness. Prompt diagnosis requires a

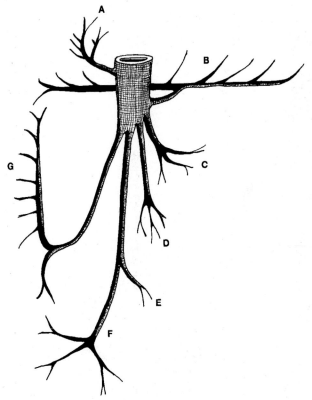

FIGURE 15-2.   Normal anatomy of the SMA and its major branches. (*A*, Inferior pancreaticoduodenal (anterior and posterior branches); *B*, middle colic artery; *C*, jejunal artery; *D*, ileal artery; *E*, ileal artery; *F*, ileocolic artery; *G*, right colic.)

high index of suspicion since even with aggressive treatment, a patient with acute mesenteric ischemia has 40 to 50% mortality. Table 15.1 summarizes clinical features for acute mesenteric ischemia based on etiology.

Acute Embolic Mesenteric Artery Occlusion

Acute ischemia may be caused by mesenteric arteries becoming occluded by emboli. The SMA receives 3 to 4% of all arterio-arterial emboli. Atrial fibrillation with left atrial thrombus, mitral stenosis with left atrial thrombus, and transmural myocardial infarction with mural thrombus are the most frequent sources of emboli. Other causes are proximal aortic atheroma, left atrial myxoma, and paradoxical emboli from venous circulation.

Clinical Features.   Embolic mesenteric occlusion occurs in patients with one or more of the cardiac risk factors described above and usually without antecedent history of weight loss or intestinal angina. One third of patients may

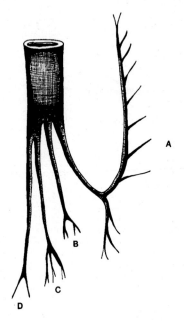

FIGURE 15-3. Normal anatomy of the IMA and its major branches. (*A*, Left colic artery (superior and inferior branches); *B*, lower left colic artery; *C*, sigmoid artery; *D*, superior rectal artery.)

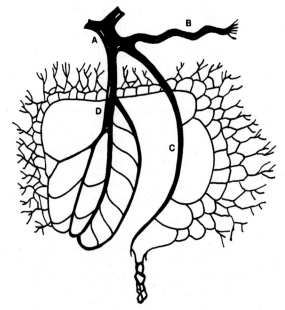

FIGURE 15-4. Normal anatomy of the mesenteric venous system. (*A*, Portal vein; *B*, splenic vein; *C*, inferior mesenteric vein; *D*, superior mesenteric vein.)

TABLE 15.1

ACUTE MESENTERIC ISCHEMIC CONDITIONS

	Acute Embolic Occlusion	Acute Thrombotic Occlusion	Nonocclusive Mesenteric Ischemia
Clinical features	Sudden abdominal pain	Gradual and progressive postprandial pain	Several days of vague abdominal pain and distension
Gender (M:F)	2:1	1:2	1.5:1
Diagnostic study	Operative diagnosis	Angiography	Angiography
Pathology	Embolic occlusion of SMA	Atherosclerosis	Low cardiac output Vasospasm from medications
Treatment	Embolectomy	Bypass or endarterectomy	Improve cardiac output, vasodilators, and IV fluids

SMA, Superior mesenteric artery.

have had a prior history of peripheral embolic episodes. Usually, patients describe sudden onset of severe abdominal pain. The nature of the pain has been described as initially crampy and then constant. Abdominal pain is the most common manifestation of ischemia and is often described as severe and "pain out of proportion to the exam." Rapid evacuation of the bowel sometimes occurs. Leukocytosis, hemoconcentration, and systemic acidosis are often seen. Elevated serum amylase, alkaline phosphatase, and creatinine phosphokinase may indicate bowel infarction. There are few physical examination signs of early acute mesenteric ischemia. If the ischemia progresses without intervention, patients can have abdominal distention, signs of peritoneal irritation, and gastrointestinal bleeding.

Diagnosis. There are no abdominal x-ray signs for the early diagnosis of mesenteric artery occlusion. Radiographs are helpful in discerning free air resulting from perforation. Plain x-ray may rule out other causes of an acute abdomen such as the presence of small bowel obstruction, renal or biliary stone, chronic calcific pancreatitis, or a perforated viscus. Late findings range from "thumbprinting," which signifies intramural edema or hemorrhage, to pneumatosis or portal vein gas, which represents bowel infarction. Frequently, mesenteric artery occlusion from embolism occurs in patients in the intensive care setting who are intubated, and laboratory abnormalities such as significant uncorrected metabolic acidosis from increasing lactic acid or unexplained persistent leukocytosis may be the first sign. Unfortunately, these signs occur when ischemic bowel has progressed to infarction.

Duplex scanning has been advocated in patients with acute mesenteric ischemia. However, the inability to obtain accurate B-mode images, difficulty in obtaining a good image in patients with truncal obesity, visualization difficulties depending on bowel gas pattern, tortuosity of the vessel, and technician inexperience make duplex scanning still a questionable modality.

Angiography with delayed filming to demonstrate the venous phase is the gold standard in the setting of suspected mesenteric ischemia when no signs of peritoneal irritation exist. Lateral aortography should be performed as the initial study to identify the origin of the mesenteric vessels. Selective cannulations of the celiac, SMA, and IMA can usually be performed using a JR4 catheter in the lateral projection. In some cases, catheters with longer tips, such as SOS or the Cobra catheter, may be needed for selective injections. For good quality mesenteric angiograms without streaming, the rate of injection should match the flow rate of the vessel being studied. The typical flow rates are 10 mL/s for the celiac trunk, 8 mL/s for the SMA, and 3 mL/s for the IMA. Digital subtraction angiography acquisition may be less helpful for mesenteric angiography because of the presence of bowel gas. In individuals who are being evaluated for GI bleeding, the clinically suspected vessel should be injected first. Arteriography may help in distinguishing the different causes of acute mesenteric ischemia. A "meniscus" sign located 4 to 6 cm from the origin of the SMA is the classic angiographic finding in mesenteric artery occlusion from an embolus. Emboli typically lodge distal to the origin of either the middle colic artery or the first jejunal branch of the SMA. Therefore, the proximal jejunal branches fill rapidly on the angiogram, while the distal jejunal and ileal branches fill slowly.

Acute Thrombotic Mesenteric Artery Occlusion

Clinical Features. Acute SMA thrombosis with the development of intestinal ischemia commonly afflicts women in their 60s and 70s. It often occurs in patients with preexisting chronic mesenteric ischemic symptoms such as weight loss, altered bowel habits, and chronic abdominal pain. Acute SMA thrombotic occlusion is typically associated with preexisting SMA atherosclerosis, although it has been associated with fibromuscular dysplasia, hypercoagulable states, inflammatory arteritis, and aortic dissection.

Diagnosis. As with acute mesenteric ischemia from embolism, radiographs are not helpful. Angiography is the gold standard for the diagnosis of acute mesenteric artery occlusion from thrombus. Atherosclerosis of the SMA most commonly affects the origin and proximal few centimeters of the artery. Unlike SMA embolus, there is a sharp cutoff in the proximal 3 cm of the SMA without jejunal branch sparing. Extensive collateral circulation from the celiac artery or IMA is often seen in patients with thrombotic mesenteric artery occlusion.

Acute Mesenteric Venous Thrombosis

Clinical Features. Mesenteric venous thrombosis encompasses a wide range of presentations from asymptomatic nonocclusive thrombus to portal venous occlusion with associated liver failure and extensive bowel necrosis. Mesenteric vein occlusion accounts for approximately 10% of acute mesenteric ischemia. There are multiple causes of mesenteric vein occlusion, including hypercoagulable state, abdominal malignancies, prior abdominal operations, oral contraceptive use, and inflammatory abdominal disease (Table 15.2). When mesenteric vein occlusion occurs, fluid begins to accumulate in the wall and lumen of the affected intestine. If diagnosis is not made early, thrombosis may extend into the vasa recti and intramural venous collaterals. When this occurs, the arterial circulation is compromised from the decrease in effective perfusion pressure resulting from the increase in capillary pressure.

Acute mesenteric venous occlusion with sudden abdominal pain has been associated with bowel infarction and peritonitis. In patients with subacute mesenteric vein occlusion, abdominal pain may have been present for several days to weeks without bowel infarction or variceal hemorrhage. Chronic mesenteric venous occlusion usually presents with complications of portal or splanchnic vein thrombosis such as variceal bleeding. Patients with chronic occlusion do not complain of pain because of their extensive collateral formation.

Diagnosis. Physical exam and routine blood test are not helpful in the diagnosis of mesenteric vein occlusion. Abdominal radiographs may show "thumbprinting," which is a blunt, semiopaque indentation of the bowel

TABLE 15.2

CAUSES OF MESENTERIC VENOUS THROMBOSIS

Prothrombotic State	Hematologic Disease	Inflammatory Disease	Post-op State	Others
Antithrombin III deficiency	Polycythemia vera	Pancreatitis	Abdominal operation	Cirrhosis
Protein C deficiency	Paroxysmal nocturnal hemoglobinuria	Peritonitis	Splenectomy	Portal hypertension
Protein S deficiency	Essential thrombocythemia	Ulcerative colitis	Sclerotherapy	Abdominal trauma
Factor V Leiden		Crohn's disease		Decompression sickness
Antiphospholipid antibody		Diverticulitis		
Hyperhomocysteinemia				
Oral contraceptives				
Pregnancy				
Neoplasms				

lumen indicative of mucosal edema. Bowel infarction as a result of mesenteric vein occlusion may show gas in the wall of the bowel or in the portal vein and free peritoneal air. Therefore, barium contrast studies should be avoided. Abdominal ultrasound can diagnose portal vein thrombosis and show ascites and intestinal edema; however, superior mesenteric and splenic venous thromboses are difficult to diagnose on ultrasound. Therefore, computed tomography (CT) is the test of choice. An acute thrombosis will show central lucency in the mesenteric vein. However, a small mesenteric vein may be difficult to visualize even with a CT scan. Other CT findings are enlargement of the superior mesenteric vein and a sharply defined vein wall with a rim of increased density. Persistent enhancement of bowel wall, pneumatosis intestinalis, and portal vein gas are late findings. Extensive collateral system in the mesentery and retroperitoneum indicates mesenteric venous thrombosis of more than a few weeks' duration. Angiography may show distal arterial spasm, stretching of the peripheral vessels due to bowel wall edema, and prolongation of the capillary phase of the study. A venous phase may or may not be present depending on the extent of the thrombosis.

Nonocclusive Mesenteric Ischemia

Clinical Features. Nonobstructive mesenteric ischemia is the most common cause of acute mesenteric ischemia. Elderly males and females are equally affected. It generally occurs in patients with low cardiac output or those with sustained mesenteric vasoconstriction (Table 15.3). Nonocclusive mesenteric ischemia occurs as a direct result of the effects of systemic processes on the mesenteric circulation. For ischemia to occur without focal occlusive disease, low-flow state, vasoconstriction, or a combination of both must be severe enough to overwhelm the compensatory mechanism found in the normal intestinal state. However, low cardiac output alone can result in intestinal ischemia. This may be aggravated by the treatment of heart failure with vasopressors and/or digitalis, which can cause mesenteric vasoconstriction. The initial splanchnic response to decreased blood flow is vasodilation, but if there is no increase in blood flow, vasoconstriction occurs. Prolonged vasoconstriction can injure the

TABLE 15.3
CAUSES OF NONOCCLUSIVE MESENTERIC ISCHEMIA

Low Output State	Mesenteric Vasoconstriction
CHF	Medications
	Digitalis, vasopressors
Cardiac arrhythmia	Hypovolemia
Post cardiac surgery	Septic shock
Cardiomyopathy	Hemoconcentration
	Post abdominal surgery

CHF, Congestive heart failure.

intestinal wall, and the progression to ischemic injury is inevitable unless the vasoconstriction can be reduced and splanchnic perfusion improves. The colon's splenic flexure is the most vulnerable area of low-flow state due to the watershed blood supply.

Diagnosis. Patients may present with abdominal signs and symptoms associated with systemic and/or mesenteric hypoperfusion. A gradual onset of lower abdominal pain is usually the norm and is accompanied by minimal physical findings. Unfortunately, the diagnosis is often delayed due to focus on the treatment of the underlying problems. As with other types of mesenteric ischemia, routine labs and abdominal radiographs are nonspecific and unhelpful. Barium enema studies may reveal "thumbprinting" pattern in the colon due to hemorrhage or edema. A high index of suspicion is required for diagnosis. Arteriography is the gold standard for diagnosis. A normal proximal SMA with smooth tapering of the distal artery and poor or absent opacification of distal branches suggests severe vasospasm. Although proximal SMA disease may be seen, it is unusual. Diagnosis at the time of operation may be difficult since decreased pulse from a proximal to distal portion may also be found in mesenteric artery occlusion due to embolization or thrombosis.

Chronic Mesenteric Ischemia

Clinical Features. This is a rare disease involving insufficient blood flow to the small intestine, resulting in intestinal ischemia. Chronic mesenteric ischemia is usually due to atherosclerosis but rarely may be caused by extensive fibromuscular disease or trauma. Celiac artery, SMA, and IMA usually have ostial disease, and occlusions are typically found in the proximal few centimeters of these arteries. Chronic mesenteric ischemia results when two of the three major splanchnic arteries have severe stenosis. At rest, patients have sufficient intestinal blood flow to maintain gut viability and prevent symptom development. However, the increased demand in mesenteric circulation after eating may overwhelm the compensatory ability of the collateral circulation, thereby causing intestinal angina.

Diagnosis. Patients with chronic mesenteric ischemia present in their fifth or sixth decade of life. They typically have atherosclerotic disease elsewhere, such as peripheral vascular disease, coronary artery disease, and/or cerebrovascular disease. Females are more likely to be affected than males. Most patients complain of postprandial abdominal pain. The classic description is crampy or colicky pain located in the epigastric area that begins 15 to 30 minutes following eating, which lasts for 2 to 3 hours and gradually subsides. Patients may compensate by eating smaller portions. Most patients with chronic mesenteric ischemia have marked weight loss. Physical exam reveals weight loss and generalized signs of atherosclerosis. Rarely, some patients may have abdominal bruit. Most often, patients receive a malignancy workup. Plain abdominal x-ray, CT, and endoscopy are insensitive in diagnosing chronic mesenteric ischemia but can rule out other diseases such as malignancy. Duplex ultrasound requires excellent technical skills and a well-prepared patient. Vessel tortuosity, respiratory motion, and the presence of bowel gas impede good visualization. Velocity parameters used to determine the presence of 70% or greater stenosis (peak systolic velocity above 275 cm/s for the SMA and above 200 cm/s for the celiac artery) have been reported with sensitivities and specificities around 90% compared to angiography. Therefore, duplex ultrasound can be used reliably to exclude the diagnosis of chronic mesenteric ischemia. Gadolinium-enhanced MRA has also been used and is increasingly becoming the preferred diagnostic modality. Biplanar angiography including selective engagement of celiac artery, SMA, and IMA remains the diagnostic test of choice. In addition to defining the extent of the disease, angiography determines collateral flow. Chronic mesenteric ischemia requires flow-limiting stenosis or occlusion of at least two of the three mesenteric arteries. In general, large collaterals are present and help confirm the presence of lesions that are suspected to be flow limiting.

Chronic Mesenteric Venous Thrombosis

Clinical Features. Unlike acute mesenteric venous thrombosis, patients with chronic mesenteric venous thrombosis are usually asymptomatic. Diagnosis is often made during CT scan of the abdomen for some unrelated reasons. On CT, superior mesenteric vein is not visualized, and there are extensive venous collaterals. Angiography is not needed for diagnosis. Patients with chronic mesenteric venous thrombosis involving portal or splenic vein may have portal hypertension with esophageal varices, splenomegaly, or hypersplenism. Of note, isolated splenic vein thrombosis may be due to pancreatic neoplasm or pancreatitis, and these should be ruled out.

MANAGEMENT

Acute Mesenteric Ischemia

Acute embolic mesenteric ischemia is a surgical emergency. Arteriography should be obtained only if there is a question of diagnosis. If there is a strong suspicion of acute mesenteric occlusion from embolism, the patient should proceed to the operating room. The treatment of choice is embolectomy. Following adequate reperfusion time, bowel viability is assessed using Doppler ultrasound, intravenous fluorescein with Wood's lamp illumination, and clinical assessment. If questionable regions remain, a second-look operation should be planned in 12 to 24 hours. SMA embolectomy is technically successful in the majority of patients. However, because of their comorbid conditions, mortality rates are high. Mortality appears to be directly related to the length of time from onset of symptoms to treatment and the extent of bowel necrosis. An overall mortality rate of 70% was reported from a pooled analysis. Recently, mortality rates of 50% have been reported.

There have been reports of thrombolytic agents for the lysis of SMA thromboemboli. A late complication of thrombolysis is the development of ischemic intestinal strictures within 2 months following successful thrombolysis. These may represent persistent areas of ischemia due to peripheral emboli or reperfusion injury. Even though thrombolysis may seem more convenient and less invasive, the advantage of open abdomen evaluation cannot be underestimated. At the current state, thrombolysis may be considered only in patients with early SMA embolism when no signs of peritoneal irritation exist and there is a prohibitive surgical risk.

For thrombotic mesenteric artery occlusion, surgery is also the treatment of choice. When a significant portion of small intestine appears potentially salvageable, SMA reconstruction should be performed with subsequent assessment of bowel viability and resection as indicated. If extensive necrosis has occurred, mortality rates are high. Mortality rates for acute mesenteric thrombosis approach 90% and can be correlated with the amount of bowel infarction. Therefore, it is urgent that a rapid diagnosis be made. Lysis and angioplasty have been associated with unacceptably high rates of hemorrhage.

Surgical exploration is not mandatory in all patients with acute mesenteric vein occlusion. Only patients with peritonitis require emergency surgery. For these patients, resection is performed on necrotic bowel with or without perforation. Thrombectomy may be performed on fresh thrombus and is restricted to the superior mesenteric vein only. The more diffuse venous thrombosis seen in the acute form of the condition is not optimal for thrombectomy. Arterial spasm, which accompanies acute venous occlusion, may be treated with intra-arterial papaverine and anticoagulation. Early anticoagulation, even intraoperatively, has been associated with increased survival and decreased recurrence rates. Acute abdominal findings mandate broad-spectrum antibiotic coverage. If there is no evidence of bowel infarction, mesenteric vein occlusion can be managed medically. Immediate anticoagulation should be started. Systemic anticoagulation should be started with bolus of heparin and adjusted so that the activated partial thromboplastin time is more than twice the normal level. Anticoagulation may be started even in the presence of gastrointestinal bleeding, if the risk of bleed is outweighed by the benefit of preventing bowel necrosis. Oral anticoagulation with warfarin should be started if there is no longer a threat of bowel ischemia. Although varices and variceal bleeding may occur, the benefits of long-term anticoagulation cannot be disputed. The duration of anticoagulation is dependent on the cause of mesenteric vein occlusion. In the absence of an ongoing thrombotic disorder, anticoagulation may be limited to 6 months to 1 year. During systemic anticoagulation, it is important to provide supportive measures such as rapid intravascular fluid volume resuscitation, nasogastric tube intestinal decompression, and bowel rest. The treatment for chronic mesenteric venous thrombosis is aimed at controlling and preventing variceal bleeding. Long-term anticoagulation is recommended for patients with a prothrombotic state.

The management of nonocclusive mesenteric ischemia is focused toward treating the underlying cause. Inotropic support to increase cardiac output or aggressive diuresis in congestive heart failure and fluid resuscitation in hypovolemia should be the initial goal. Digitalis and alpha agonists should be avoided. A pulmonary artery catheter should be considered for optimal fluid management. All patients should also receive bowel rest and bowel decompression.

While underlying problems are being addressed, mesenteric vasodilators can be initiated. Selective catheter-directed pharmacotherapy is the treatment of choice. Bolus injection of tolazoline (Priscoline) 25 mg followed by continued infusion of papaverine at 30 to 60 mg/h or papaverine alone at 30 to 60 mg/h may be instituted to reduce mesenteric vasoconstriction. Therapy is terminated after the resolution of vasoconstriction is documented on angiography or when symptoms resolve. Some have advocated continuous epidural infusion of papaverine in cases of refractory vasoconstriction. Systemic glucagon treatment has also been used; however, to date, efficacy of these agents has not been proven in clinical studies. Surgery is recommended when symptoms do not resolve after pharmacotherapy. Because of the underlying severe medical problems in these patients, mortality rates are as high as 60%.

Chronic Mesenteric Ischemia

Surgical revascularization is the traditional treatment in patients with chronic mesenteric ischemia. Overall, the operative mortality remains high and is 7.5%. There are several surgical revascularization strategies including visceral endarterectomy, antegrade supraceliac aorta to visceral bypass, and retrograde infrarenal aorta to visceral bypass. Before surgical revascularization, patients may benefit from total parenteral nutrition (TPN). Although there is controversy regarding the length and benefit of TPN, improving the nutritional status of the patient prior to surgery seems rational. Transaortic visceral endarterectomy is a technically challenging procedure that requires extensive retroperitoneal vascular exposure. This technique also has a greater risk of paraplegia because of supraceliac aortic cross-clamping. Endarterectomy may be particularly beneficial in cases where the patient has both visceral and renal artery stenoses. Endarterectomy is very difficult in patients with extensive aortic atherosclerosis, and an alternative technique must be considered.

Retrograde SMA bypass is the most commonly performed visceral bypass procedure. The simplicity of the approach to the infrarenal aorta and infrapancreatic SMA makes this surgery attractive to the surgeon. With retrograde bypass, care must be taken to configure a graft that will not kink. Antegrade bypass is the procedure of choice when there is marked infrarenal aortic atherosclerosis. Endarterectomy appears to have the lowest rates of recurrence followed by antegrade bypass reconstruction and then retrograde reconstruction. Endovascular treatment for chronic mesenteric ischemia is evolving as a first-line therapy at many experienced centers. Earlier studies had found high restenosis rates; however, stenting has significantly improved outcomes. Visceral surgical revascularization in a malnourished patient, even in particularly specialized centers, leads to significant morbidity and mortality, in contrast with endovascular treatment. The endovascular approach is less invasive and compares favorably with surgery in terms of clinical success, complications, and long-term outcomes (Table 15.4).

TABLE 15.4

SUMMARY OF STUDIES OF ENDOVASCULAR THERAPY FOR CHRONIC MESENTERIC ISCHEMIA

	No.	Vessels Revascularized[a]	Technical Success	Complications (Perioperative Deaths)	Clinical Success	Primary Patency [n/N(%)]	Long-term Pain Relief (%)	Mean Follow-up [Months (Range)]
Sniderman et al.	14	NA	12/14	0	12/14	7/14 (50)	71	NA (1–96)
Matsumoto et al.	19	20 (1.05)	15/19	3 (0)	12/19	10/19 (53)	52	25 (4–73)
Hallisey et al.	15	25 (1.67)	13/15	1 (1)	14/15	9/12 (75)	75	28 (4–60)
Allen et al.	19	24 (1.26)	18/19	2 (1)	15/18	12/18 (67)	79	39 (4–101)
Maspes et al.	23	41 (1.78)	21/23	2 (0)	18/23	13/15 (87)	75	27 (2–36)
Nyman et al.	5	6 (1.2)	5/5	2 (0)	3/5	2/5 (40)	80	21 (8–42)
Sheeran et al.	12	13 (1.08)	11/12	1 (1)	11/12	74	75	22 (13–38)
Kasirajan et al.	28	32 (1.14)	28/28	5 (3)	NA	73	66	36
Steinmetz et al.	19	19 (1)	19/19	3 (0)	19/19	12/16 (75)	85	31 (1–69)

NA, Not applicable.

[a]Rate of vessels revascularized per patient.

Data from Steinmetz E, Tatou E, Favier-Blavoux C, et al. Endovascular treatment as first choice in chronic intestinal ischemia. *Ann Vasc Surg* 2002;16: 693–699, with permission; From Sniderman KW. Transluminal angioplasty in the management of chronic intestinal ischemia. In: Strandness DE, van Breda A. eds. *Vascular diseases: Surgical and interventional therapy.* New York: Churchill Livingstone. 1994:803–809; Matsumoto AH, et al. *J Vasc Interv Radiology* 1995;6: 165–174; Hallisey et al. *J Vasc Interv Radiology* 1995;6:785–791; Allen RC, et al. *J Vasc Surg* 1996;24:415–421; Maspes F, et al. *Abdominal Imaging* 1998;23:358–363; Nyman U, et al. *Cardiovasc Interv Radiol* 1998;21:305–313; Sheeran SR, et al. *J Vasc Interv Radiol* 1999;10:861–867; Kasirajan K, et al. *J Vasc Surg* 2001;33:63–71.

SPECIAL ISSUES

Median Arcuate Ligament Syndrome

Median arcuate ligament syndrome is caused by the compression of celiac trunk by the median arcuate ligament of the diaphragm. It is found in middle-aged, female patients. They complain of abdominal pain with eating and have marked weight loss. The pain is usually less severe than intestinal ischemic pain. On physical exam, bruit is heard on the upper abdomen. On angiography with camera in lateral position, compression of the celiac axis by the median arcuate ligament is seen during deep expiration. Surgical division of the median arcuate ligament is the treatment of choice.

Mesenteric Aneurysms

Splenic Artery Aneurysm

Clinical Features. The splenic artery is the most common visceral artery to become aneurysmal. The pathophysiology is degeneration of artery media and occurs most likely in women of childbearing age. Women outnumber men by 4 to 1. These women tend to have multiple pregnancies. In one study, 40% of the patients had more than six pregnancies. Fibromuscular dysplasia accounts for about 15% of splenic artery aneurysms, and almost 5% of the patients with fibromuscular dysplasia (FMD) of the renal artery have splenic artery aneurysms. About 10% of patients with splenic artery aneurysm have portal hypertension as the etiology. Usually, patients are asymptomatic; however, a quarter of the patients will complain of vague upper abdominal pain.

Diagnosis. Abdominal x-ray may show "signet ring" calcification. The usual angiographic appearance is concentric calcification. Splenic artery aneurysms are usually saccular and occur at bifurcations. The usual location for aneurysm is the distal third of the splenic artery.

Treatment. The rupture rate in nonpregnant patients is 2% with a mortality rate of 25%. In pregnant women, the risk of rupture is greatly increased, and the maternal and fetal mortality rates are 70 and 75%, respectively. Therefore, repair of these aneurysms in pregnant women is indicated. Otherwise, aneurysms larger than 2.5 cm, symptomatic aneurysms, and aneurysms in women of childbearing age should be repaired. The treatment is aneurysmectomy or ligation and exclusion of the aneurysm. Splenectomy is required if the aneurysm is hilar or in the distal artery. If pseudoaneurysm is found in patients with pancreatitis, distal pancreatectomy and splenectomy are required. Percutaneous catheter embolization may be an attractive option in high-risk surgical patients; however, it is not recommended for patients with previous surgery.

Hepatic Artery Aneurysm

Clinical Features. The hepatic artery aneurysm accounts for 20% of visceral aneurysms. The causes are most likely atherosclerosis, degeneration of the artery media, trauma, or infection. Polyarteritis nodosa, cystic medial necrosis, and other arteriopathies may also cause hepatic artery aneurysms. Most aneurysms are extrahepatic with the common hepatic artery accounting for majority of cases. Typically, intrahepatic aneurysms result from trauma. Patients tend to be men over the age of 60. Most patients are asymptomatic. Patients complain of right upper abdominal pain radiating to the back of the right shoulder. Jaundice from bile duct compression may also occur with large aneurysms.

Diagnosis. Angiography is the gold standard for locating and confirming the diagnosis. Hepatic artery rupture occurs in 20% of the patients with mortality rates of 35%.

Treatment. Repair is advocated regardless of size in majority of cases. An intrahepatic aneurysm may be treated with catheter-based embolization, although it has been associated with hepatic and biliary necroses. For an extrahepatic aneurysm, it may be excised or excluded. Common hepatic artery aneurysms may be treated with proximal and distal ligation. A proper hepatic artery aneurysm requires arterial reconstruction. Flow restoration with vein graft is recommended to avoid hepatic necrosis.

Celiac Trunk Aneurysm

Celiac artery aneurysms are uncommon and may result from atherosclerosis, medial degeneration, trauma, aortic dissection, or infection. Patients are middle-aged with equal numbers of males and females. The patient typically complains of significant abdominal pain. Angiography is the gold standard. Because of the high rates of rupture, repair with arterial reconstruction is recommended for all patients regardless of symptoms.

Superior Mesenteric Artery Aneurysm

SMA aneurysms affect men and women equally. Infection from nonhemolytic streptococci from a left-sided endocarditis accounts for the majority of cases. Infection from illicit drug use, medical degeneration, atherosclerosis, or trauma may also cause superior mesenteric aneurysms. Aneurysms tend to be mycotic in patients younger than 50 years of age. Epigastric pain is common. Vascular calcification on abdominal radiograph or angiogram leads to the diagnosis. Although the rupture rates are low, thrombosis rates are high. Therefore, most of these lesions should be repaired. Aneurysmectomy with arterial reconstruction is the treatment of choice. The operative mortality is less than 15%. The mortality rate with rupture is 50%.

CONCLUSIONS

- Mesenteric vascular diseases encompass a wide spectrum of conditions that have high mortality rates if left untreated.
- These diseases require physicians to have a high index of suspicion.
- Only early diagnosis and aggressive treatment can decrease the high mortality rates found with mesenteric vascular diseases.

- Angiography is the gold standard to diagnose acute mesenteric ischemia from embolism, thrombosis, or nonobstructive mesenteric occlusion.
- CT scan has a sensitivity of 90% in the diagnosis of mesenteric venous thrombosis. Operative findings include gradual transition from ischemic to normal bowel in venous thrombosis.
- Mesenteric venous thrombosis can be managed with medications alone if there is no evidence of bowel infarction. Anticoagulation should be started immediately, even intraoperatively.
- Visceral aneurysms should be repaired in most cases.

PRACTICAL POINTS

- There are three watershed areas in the colon circulation. These are (i) the hepatic flexure of the colon between the ileocolic and the middle colic branches of the SMA, (ii) the splenic flexure between the middle colic and the left colic arteries, and (iii) the distal sigmoid and rectum.

- Do *not* wait for angiography if you suspect acute mesenteric ischemia from embolism or thrombosis. Emergent surgery is needed!

- Operative findings show abrupt transition from ischemic to normal bowel in arterial thromboembolism.

- Involvement of inferior mesenteric vessels is common in arterial thromboembolism and uncommon in venous thrombosis.

- Thrombolysis may be useful in arterial thromboembolism but rarely useful in venous thrombosis.

- Infection from nonhemolytic streptococci from a left-sided endocarditis accounts for the majority of superior mesenteric artery aneurysms.

- The splenic artery is the most common visceral artery to become aneurysmal.

- Three conditions are associated with splenic artery aneurysms: (i) fibrodysplasias, (ii) portal hypertension with splenomegaly, and (iii) multiparity.

RECOMMENDED READING

Barkhordarian S, Gusberg RJ. Mesenteric ischemia: identification and treatment. *ACC Curr J Rev* 2003;12:19–21.

Bergan JJ. Visceral ischemic syndromes. In: Moore W, ed. *Vascular surgery: a comprehensive review*, 4th ed. Philadelphia, PA: WB Saunders, 1993:523–531.

Bradbury MS, Kavanagh PV, Bechtold RE, et al. Mesenteric venous thrombosis: diagnosis and noninvasive imaging. *Radiographic* 2002;22:527–541.

Brandt LJ, Boley SJ. AGA technical review on intestinal ischemia. *Gastroenterology* 2000;118:954–968.

Chang JB, Stein TA. Mesenteric ischemia: acute and chronic. *Ann Vasc Surg* 2003;17(3): 323–328.

Chitwood RW, Ernst CB. Visceral ischemic syndromes. In: Young JR, Olin JW, Bartholomew JR, eds. *Peripheral vascular disease*, 2nd ed. St. Louis, MO: Mosby, 1996:305–320.

Eton D. Mesenteric vascular disease. In: Eton D, ed. *Vascular disease*, 2nd ed. Landes Bioscience, 1999:298–307.

Graham LM, Mesh CL. Celiac, hepatic, and splenic artery aneurysms. In: Ernst CB, Stanley JC, eds. *Current therapy of vascular surgery*, 3rd ed. St. Louis, MO: Mosby 1995:714–718.

Greenwald DA, Brandt LJ, Reinus JF. Ischemic bowel disease in the elderly. *Gastroenterol Clin North Am* 2001;30:445–473.

Kumar S, Sarr MG, Kamath PS. Mesenteric venous thrombosis. *N Engl J Med* 2001;345: 1683–1688.

McKinsey JF, Gewertz BL. Acute mesenteric ischemia. *Surg Clin North Am* 1997;77:307–318.

Moawad J, Gewertz BL. Chronic mesenteric ischemia: clinical presentation and diagnosis. *Surg Clin North Am* 1997;77:357–369.

Mukherjee D, Cho L. Renal and mesenteric artery stenosis. In: Bhatt DL, ed. *Handbook of peripheral and cerebrovascular intervention*. London, UK: Remedica, 2004.

Rosenblum JD, Boyle CM, Schwartz LB. The mesenteric circulation: anatomy and physiology. *Surg Clin North Am* 1997;77:289–306.

Stanley JC. Mesenteric arterial occlusive and aneurysmal disease. *Cardiol Clin North Am* 2002;20:611–622, vii.

Steinmetz E, Tatou E, Favier-Blavoux C, et al. Endovascular treatment as first choice in chronic intestinal ischemia. *Ann Vasc Surg* 2002;16:693–699.

Sreenarasimhaiah J. Diagnosis and management of intestinal ischaemic disorders. *Br Med J* 2003;326(7403):1372–1376.

Vicente DC, Kazmers A. Acute mesenteric ischemia. *Curr Opin Cardiol* 1999;14:453–458.

CHAPTER 16 ■ Overview of Upper Extremity Artery Disease

Steven M. Dean

Although significantly less common than typical atherosclerotic peripheral artery disease (PAD) of the lower extremities, upper extremity artery disease (UEAD) is an important and often challenging cause of arm ischemia and/or distal vasospasm. Hemodynamically significant atherosclerosis is approximately 20 times less common in the arms than in the legs and is usually limited to the proximal or "inflow" arteries. However, vasospastic disorders are more likely to affect the upper than the lower extremities. A variety of unique nonatherosclerotic etiologies can provoke UEAD. Some of these causes are exclusive to the upper limb and include thoracic outlet syndrome (TOS) and occupation-related occlusive disease.

Pathophysiologically, UEAD can be divided into large-artery (proximal to the wrist) and small-artery (distal to the wrist) diseases. A classification scheme for UEAD is outlined in Table 16.1. During the initial patient assessment, the clinician attempts to assign the affected patient into one of these three broad categories. However, prompt and definitive differentiation of these etiologies based on an isolated history and physical is not always possible. Consequently, adjunctive serology testing and noninvasive and/or invasive vascular studies are frequently required to explicitly define the locus and etiology of a patient's UEAD. Classification overlap may occur between categories. For instance, a patient with thromboangiitis obliterans can be categorized as having both large- and small-artery occlusive disease as well as secondary Raynaud's syndrome.

ANATOMY AND PHYSIOLOGY OF UPPER EXTREMITY CIRCULATION

Anatomy

The inflow arteries of the upper extremities comprise the innominate and subclavian arteries. Figure 16.1 illustrates the remaining intrinsic vessels of the upper extremity including the axillary, brachial, radial, ulnar, palmar, and digital arteries. Upon traversing the wrist, the radial and ulnar arteries form the deep and superficial palmar arches, respectively (Fig. 16.2). The deep palmar arch yields three palmar metacarpal arteries that anastomose with four common palmar digital branches of the superficial palmar arch. At the level of the finger webs, the common digital arteries bifurcate into paired medial- and lateral-based proper digital arteries that ultimately fuse at the distal tuft (Fig. 16.3).

The radial, ulnar, and proper digital arteries form a parallel arterial system that can preserve normal resting perfusion despite underlying obstructive disease. Consequently, one must remain cognizant that these

TABLE 16.1

CLASSIFICATION SCHEME FOR UPPER EXTREMITY ARTERIAL DISEASE

I. Thromboembolic Diseases

A. Embolism
- Proximal primary aneurysm
- Post-stenotic aneurysm
- Cardiogenic (including patent foramen ovale)
- Ulcerated aortic arch and/or innominate, subclavian, axillary arteries

B. Thrombosis
- Thrombophilia
  - Antiphospholipid antibody syndrome
  - Heparin-induced thrombocytopenia
  - Proteins S and C, and antithrombin deficiencies; homocysteinemia, factor V Leiden mutation, prothrombin gene mutation (these causes are rare)
- Hematologic disorders
  - Myeloproliferative syndromes, leukemias, hypereosinophilic syndromes
  - Multiple myeloma, Waldenstrom's macroglobulinemia, cryoglobulinemia
  - Paroxysmal nocturnal hemoglobinuria
- Malignancy
- Vasculitis

II. Arterial Occlusive Diseases

A. Large Artery (proximal to wrist)
- Atherosclerosis
- Large vessel vasculitis (giant cell, Takayasu's)
- Medium vessel vasculitis (polyarteritis nodosa, Kawasaki's disease)
- Thromboangiitis obliterans
- Fibromuscular dysplasia
- Radiation fibrosis
- Entrapment (TOS, axillary artery crutch injury)
- Aneurysms (subclavian through radioulnar level)

B. Small Artery (distal to wrist)
- Autoimmune diseases
- Small- and medium-sized vasculitis
- Thromboangiitis obliterans
- Hypothenar hammer syndrome, thenar hammer syndrome, hand-arm vibration syndrome
- Hematologic disorders (as above)
- Thrombophilia (as above)
- Malignancy
- Frostbite
- Calciphylaxis/calcific azotemic arteriopathy

(Continued)

TABLE 16.1

CLASSIFICATION SCHEME FOR UPPER EXTREMITY ARTERIAL DISEASE *(Continued)*

III. Vasospastic Diseases
A. Large Artery
- Ergotamines
- Methamphetamine and related medications
- Cocaine

B. Small Artery
- Primary Raynaud's syndrome
- Secondary Raynaud's syndrome

duplicate arteries can potentially decrease the sensitivity of noninvasive testing (pressure measurements and plethysmographic waveforms) in identifying UEAD. For example, normal forearm and digital pressures as well as pulsed volume recording (PVR) waveforms may be obtained in the setting of an occluded ulnar artery.

Anomalous Circulation

In order to avoid a false-positive diagnosis of UEAD, a clinician should be aware that a variety of arterial anomalies may occur in the upper extremity. Arterial variants of the upper extremity are listed in Table 16.2.

Collateral Pathways

In addition to the previously described dual arterial system, the upper extremity possesses an abundance of complementary arterial tributaries that can function as collaterals in the presence of significant UEAD. This highly redundant system can significantly delay the onset of ischemic symptoms despite underlying arterial occlusive disease. The prototypical upper extremity collateral pathway is exemplified by the vertebral artery functioning as a collateral conduit in the setting of a proximal subclavian (or innominate) artery severe stenosis or occlusion. Figure 16.1 illustrates several arterial branches that can function as collaterals in the event of a brachial artery occlusion (e.g., profunda brachii, radial recurrent, superior and inferior ulnar collaterals).

Physiologic and Pathophysiologic Vasospasm

The sympathetic nervous system regulates local perfusion via adrenergic receptors on the smooth muscle of cutaneous vessels. Typically, the cutaneous circulation assumes a predominant role in preserving a stable core body temperature by adjusting the surface blood flow contingent on the ambient temperature. For example, cold temperatures evoke shunting of blood away from the surface, consistent with physiological or "normal" vasospasm. Conversely, exposure to warm environments augments perfusion to the skin. Raynaud's syndrome arises when this normal or physiological response to ambient cold temperatures is exaggerated and

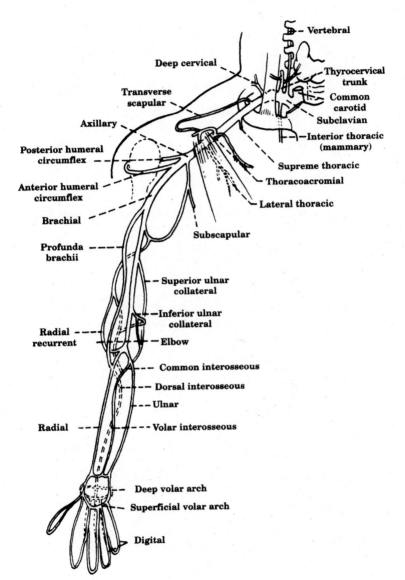

FIGURE 16-1.   Arterial supply of the upper extremity.

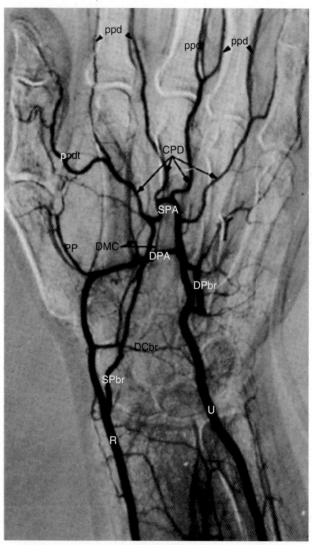

FIGURE 16-2.   Normal arteriogram of the hand showing the arches (superficial and deep). (CPD, common palmar digital; DCbr, dorsal carpal branch; DMC, dorsal metacarpal; DPA, deep palmar arch; DPbr, deep palmar branch of ulnar; PP, princeps pollicis (main artery to the thumb); ppd, palmar proper digital; ppdt, palmar proper digital thumb; R, radial; SPA, superficial palmar arch; SPbr, superficial palmar branch of radial; U, ulnar.) (Adapted from Kadir S. *Atlas of normal and variant angiographic anatomy.* W. B. Saunders Company, 1991.)

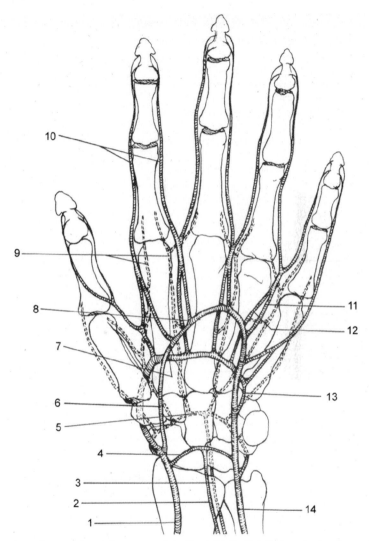

FIGURE 16-3.   Arterial anatomy of the hand. (*1*, Radial; *2*, Anterior interosseus; *3*, Posterior interosseus; *4*, Palmar carpal branch; *5*, Dorsal carpal branch forming the dorsal carpal rete; *6*, Superficial palmar branch of the radial artery; *7*, Deep palmar arch; *8*, Superficial palmar arch; *9*, Dorsal metacarpal arteries; *10*, Proper palmar digital arteries; *11*, Common palmar digital arteries; *12*, Palmar metacarpal; *13*, Deep palmar branch of the ulnar artery; *14*, Ulnar artery.) (Adapted from Kadir S. *Atlas of normal and variant angiographic anatomy.* W. B. Saunders Company, 1991.)

TABLE 16.2

ARTERIAL VARIANTS OF THE UPPER EXTREMITY

Variant	Frequency of Occurrence in the Population (%)
Aortic arch and great vessels	
Common origin of the right brachiocephalic and left common carotid arteries (bovine arch)	22
Left vertebral artery origin directly from the aorta	4–6
Brachial artery	
Radial artery origin from the brachial or axillary	15–20
Ulnar artery origin from the brachial or axillary	1–3
Accessory (duplicated) brachial artery (rejoin in the antecubital fossa)	0.1–0.2
Radial artery	
Radial artery origin from the brachial or axillary	15–20
Aplasia, hypoplasia, and duplication	<1
Ulnar artery	
High origin (axillary/brachial)	1–3
Low origin (5–7 cm below the elbow joint)	1
Persistent median artery	<0.1
Persistent interosseous branch	<0.1
Palmar arch variants	
Incomplete deep and superficial palmar arches	0.5–1.5

digital perfusion intermittently ceases. Physiological vasospasm is never associated with complete cessation of digital perfusion. Primary Raynaud's syndrome only involves functional alterations, whereas secondary Raynaud's syndrome also involves associated structural microvascular abnormalities. The pathogenesis of Raynaud's syndrome includes defects in one of more of these three systems: (a) vascular (endothelial dysfunction; structural defects), (b) neural (central dysfunction; impaired vasodilation; impaired vasoconstriction), and (c) intravascular abnormality (increased platelet activation and aggregation; impaired fibrinolysis).

HISTORY AND PHYSICAL EXAMINATION

History

Salient historical items to consider in the evaluation of the patient with UEAD are outlined in Table 16.3. Additionally, the reader is requested to review Chapter 1 as well. The examiner should remain cognizant of the frequent association of autoimmune and hematologic disease with UEAD when obtaining a review of systems. Both large- and small-artery disease may provoke digital vasospasm, distal rest pain, fixed digital

TABLE 16.3

HISTORICAL POINTS IN UPPER EXTREMITY ARTERIAL DISEASE

1. **Description of Symptoms**
   Unilateral vs. bilateral symptoms; intermittent vs. constant symptoms; presence of digital ulcerations; severity of symptoms
2. **Comorbid Disease**
   Autoimmune, hematologic/oncologic, atherosclerosis
3. **Tobacco Use**
   Pack year history
4. **Occupational**
   Chemical exposure—polyvinylchloride
   Thoracic outlet compression—weightlifting, baseball pitching, rowing, swimming
   Hypothenar hammer syndrome—auto repair or mechanical work, carpentry, karate, baseball catching, walker usage
   Vibration injury—chain saws, pneumatic tools, grinders, riveting machines
   Crutch use
5. **Medications**
   Ergotamines, beta blockers, interferon alpha and beta, bleomycin, vinblastine, cisplatin, amphetamine, methysergide, oral contraceptives
6. **Illicit Drug Use**
   Cocaine, cannabis, amphetamine
7. **Pertinent ROS**
   Especially rheumatologic and hematologic—myalgias, arthralgias, rashes, photosensitivity, xerostomia, xerophthalmia, GERD, fatigue, weight loss, venous thromboembolic disease, anemia, miscarriages, etc.

cyanosis, ulcerations, and/or gangrene. The presence of exertional aching (claudication) or rest pain within the arm or forearm connotes underlying large-artery disease. The following historical features can be potentially useful in elucidating the diagnosis of UEAD:

Unilateral Versus Bilateral Symptoms

A patient who presents with unilateral exertional arm aching and/or Raynaud's symptoms should be assessed for a proximal embolic source. The presence of bilateral symptoms generally reflects an underlying systemic process.

Intermittent Versus Constant Digital Symptoms

Persistent, fixed ischemia within the digits indicates a secondary pathological process is responsible (e.g., large- and/or small-artery occlusive disease), whereas primary Raynaud's syndrome is exemplified by intermittent, reversible symptoms. However, one must remain cognizant that patients with secondary Raynaud's syndrome can also present with transient, reversible symptomatology as well.

Hand and/or digital ulcerations: if identified, an underlying secondary process definitely exists (e.g., autoimmune disease, the antiphospholipid antibody syndrome, severe atherosclerosis). Primary Raynaud's syndrome does not provoke digital ulcerations.

Physical Examination

General Exam

When evaluating a patient with UEAD, a comprehensive physical examination should be performed that includes a detailed cardiovascular, dermatologic, and hematologic assessment. From a cardiovascular standpoint, observe for signs that could be associated with an embolus or endocarditis (atrial fibrillation, murmurs, Janeway's lesions, Roth's spots, and/or Osler's nodes). A dermatologic evaluation for evidence of autoimmune disease (heliotrope rash, butterfly rash, facial telangiectasias, perioral furrowing, diffuse livedo) and vasculitis (palpable purpura, diffuse ulcerations, diffuse livedo) is warranted. Last of all, assess for hepatosplenomegaly that can complicate solid and lymphoreticular malignancies as well as myeloproliferative syndromes.

Upper Extremity Exam

The upper extremity examination as summarized in Chapter 1 should be followed when assessing a patient. Table 16.4 provides an overview of physical examination findings and associated diagnoses.

TABLE 16.4

UPPER EXTREMITY EXAMINATION IN THE PATIENT WITH UEAD

Inspection:
    Telangiectasias—CREST syndrome, scleroderma
    Gottron's papules—dermatomyositis
    Janeway's lesions/Osler's nodes—bacterial endocarditis
    Sclerodactyly—scleroderma, CREST syndrome, MCTD, dermatomyositis
    Splinter hemorrhages—trauma, bacterial endocarditis, APAS, autoimmune disease
    Abnormal nail fold capillaroscopy—scleroderma, CREST syndrome, dermatomyositis
Palpation:
    Aneurysms:
        Subclavian—post-stenotic in association with TOS, atherosclerotic, traumatic
        Brachial—iatrogenic (postcatheterization), traumatic, fibromuscular dysplasia
        Ulnar artery—traumatic (hypothenar hammer syndrome)
        Radial artery—traumatic, iatrogenic
        Cervical rib—thoracic outlet syndrome
        Thrill—arteriovenous fistula/arteriovenous malformation
Auscultation:
    Systolic bruit—arterial stenosis or tortuosity
    Continuous murmur—arteriovenous fistula

Thoracic Outlet Syndrome Maneuvers and Allen's Test

A thorough UEAD assessment should include both TOS maneuvers and Allen's test. A detailed description of how to perform TOS maneuvers is included in Chapters 1 and 17. The examiner should remain cognizant that positive thoracic outlet maneuver testing including diminution of pulse can be achieved in up to 50% of the asymptomatic "normal" population. Conversely, a normal study does not exclude the diagnosis of TOS. Recall that TOS maneuvers assess for the presence of subclavian artery compression, yet 95% of TOS cases are due to neurogenic rather than arteriovenous compromise. Performing these maneuvers while contemporaneously auscultating for subclavian artery bruits and assessing for scalene tenderness increases their accuracy.

Palpable distal radial and ulnar pulses only signify arterial patency at the level of the wrist. Consequently, Allen's test must be performed to assess the arterial luminal integrity within the hand. For instance, in the hypothenar hammer syndrome, the ulnar artery usually occludes just distal to the wrist where the artery traverses the hook of the hamate bone. A positive Allen's test would be obtained in this scenario. A positive reverse Allen's test indicates a distal radial artery occlusion.

DIAGNOSTIC TESTING

Although a comprehensive history and physical examination will sometimes identify the etiology of UEAD, additional diagnostic testing is often required to substantiate the examiner's impression, assess disease severity, and monitor treatment response. Testing should be employed in a safe, logical, and cost-effective fashion.

Segmental Limb Pressures, Arterial Doppler Waveforms, and Pulse Volume Recordings

All patients who present for evaluation of UEAD should undergo initial noninvasive testing via segmental blood pressure measurements with contemporaneous arterial Doppler and/or PVR waveforms. Similar to lower extremity testing, pneumatic cuffs are placed at the brachium, forearm, and wrist and systolic blood pressure measurements are obtained at each level. Systolic pressures are compared with those at adjoining levels of the ipsilateral limb as well as to the same level of the contralateral limb. A pressure differential that exceeds 15 mm Hg suggests hemodynamically significant large-artery occlusive disease is present.

Multiphasic (triphasic or biphasic) arterial Doppler waveforms indicate normal resting arterial perfusion, whereas a monophasic waveform connotes significant large-artery stenosis. A normal PVR waveform exhibits a dicrotic notch that excludes the presence of significant arterial occlusive disease. In the setting of hemodynamically significant arterial occlusive disease, the PVR waveform upstroke is less steep, the peak becomes rounded and delayed, the downslope bows away from the baseline, and the reflected dicrotic wave disappears. With further progression of stenosis, the upslope and downslope of the waveform appear nearly equal, and the waveform amplitude diminishes (Fig. 16.4).

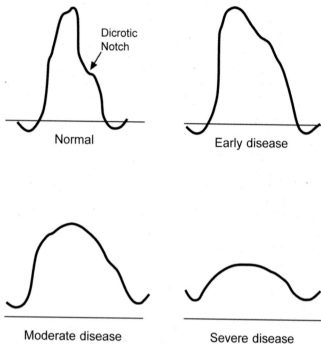

FIGURE 16-4. Segmental volume plethysmography in peripheral vascular disease. Variations in the contours of the pulse volume recording with segmental volume plethysmography reflect the severity of peripheral vascular disease. Mild disease is characterized by the absence of a dicrotic notch. With progressive obstruction, the upstroke and downstroke become equal, and with severe disease, the amplitude of the waveform is blunted.

Finger Systolic Blood Pressures

In order to eliminate potentially conflicting vasospasm, digital testing should be completed in a warm, draft-free environment and the patient should be relaxed. Digital cuffs are applied to the proximal phalanges of all ten digits in order to obtain systolic blood pressure measurements. The normal finger brachial index average is 1.0 with a range of 0.8 to 1.3. Abnormal readings include a finger brachial index of 0.7 or less, an absolute digital pressure of less than 70 mm Hg, or a difference of more than 15 mm Hg between fingers. On account of dual digital arterial perfusion, it is possible to obtain a normal digital pressure (false-negative study) in the presence of an isolated digital artery occlusion. Additionally, obtaining a normal pressure at the proximal phalangeal level does not exclude distal digital artery occlusive disease. Rarely, the digital arteries can be calcified and poorly compressible, which results in supraphysiological pressures.

Finger Pulse Contours

Pulse contours are easily obtained via distal digital photoplethysmographic studies. Similar to obtaining digital pressures, waveform testing should be performed in an environment where vasospastic stimuli have been eliminated. Waveforms should be compared between digits of the ipsilateral and contralateral hands. A normal waveform is marked by a systolic rise time of less than 0.2 seconds with associated brisk upstroke and high amplitude. In contrast, significant palmar and/or digital artery occlusive disease yields a delayed waveform upstroke (systolic rise time greater than 0.2 seconds) and blunted amplitude. Unique digital "peaked" pulse waves can be seen in the patient with primary, vasospastic, or secondary, yet nonobstructive, Raynaud's syndrome. Peaked pulse waves are reported to be 100% specific and 66% sensitive for diagnosis of primary, vasospastic Raynaud's syndrome. Figure 16.5 outlines these various digital pulse contours. A false-negative study can occur when only one digital artery is obstructed. Arterial Doppler waveforms of all paired digital arteries can be obtained, yet this testing modality is time-consuming and therefore rarely performed.

Duplex Arterial Ultrasound

Duplex scanning yields accurate anatomic and physiologic data in addition to identifying and distinguishing between arterial stenoses and occlusions. The duplex scan can also assess for peripheral aneurysms, dissections, and potentially distinguish between large-artery atherosclerotic plaque and vasculitis. All of the predominant upper extremity arteries can be insonated from the innominate-subclavian to the wrist level. A retroclavicular "blind spot" sometimes obviates focal subclavian imaging; however, assessing the juxtaposed proximal and distal subclavian artery Doppler flow patterns provides an indirect assessment of this suboptimally imaged region. Although technically demanding, even the palmar and digital arteries can be imaged via duplex ultrasonography with a high-frequency transducer.

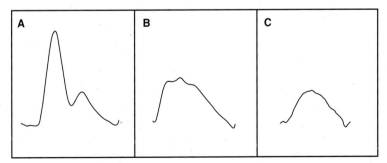

FIGURE 16-5. Plethysmographic pulse contours. A: Normal. B: Peaked. C: Obstructed. (From Sumner DS. Noninvasive Assessment of upper extremity ischemia. In: Bergan JJ, Yao JST, eds. *Evaluation and treatment of upper and lower extremity circulatory disorders*. Orland, FL: Grune & Stratton, 1984:75–95.)

Contrast Arteriography, Magnetic Resonance Angiography, and Computed Tomography Angiography

Contrast arteriography (CA), magnetic resonance angiography (MRA), and computed tomography angiography (CTA) are most useful when large-artery occlusive disease is suspected or clinically obvious in the evaluation of UEAD. These studies can precisely define the location of arterial stenosis and/or occlusions (thrombotic and/or embolic). Additionally, an anatomic display of the distal perfusion into the forearm and hand can be demonstrated. MRA and CTA can easily assess the thoracic aorta for associated pathology such as atheromatous plaque, dissection, or vasculitis. CA provides a superior assessment of the digital arteries. When any of these anatomic studies are performed, it is critical that the aortic arch and both upper extremities are imaged. Failure to visualize all arteries can potentially lead to a misdiagnosis. For instance, a patient presenting with unilateral digital ischemia should not be limited to unilateral imaging as a bilateral arteriogram may identify subclinical contralateral digital occlusive disease suggestive of a systemic vasculopathy or vasculitis; consequently, a proximal arterial embolic source is unlikely. Alternatively, if the innominate and/or proximal subclavian arteries are not imaged, a causative ulcerated plaque may be overlooked as the embolic nidus of digital artery occlusions.

Laboratory Assessment

Table 16.5 outlines various serological studies that may be useful when a systemic illness is suspected in a patient who presents with UEAD.

TABLE 16.5

LABORATORY EVALUATION IN UEAD

Primary Raynaud's Syndrome	Secondary Raynaud's Syndrome
Complete blood count	Identical testing as primary Raynaud's syndrome
ESR	Antiphospholipid antibodies (anticardiolipin antibodies, lupus anticoagulant, B2-glycoprotein 1 antibodies)
CRP	Double-stranded DNA
ANA	Homocysteine
Rheumatoid factor	SPEP and immunoelectrophoresis
	Extractable nuclear antibodies
	Anti-Scl 70 Ab, Anticentromere Ab
	Cryopathy serology (cold agglutinins, cryoglobulins, cryofibrinogen)
	Complement levels
	Hepatitis B and C assays
	Ergotamine blood levels
	Toxicology screen

Ancillary Studies

Echocardiography and electrocardiography should be employed when proximal emboli are entertained. Radiographs of the hand may uncover the soft-tissue calcifications of CREST syndrome or arterial calcification of uremic or diabetic medial calcinosis. When TOS is suspected, a radiograph for a cervical rib or an anomalous first rib should be obtained.

Nail Fold Capillaroscopy

The capillaries within the nail fold can be seen by placing a drop of high-resolution immersion oil on the cuticular region of the digit and subsequently imaging with an ophthalmoscope between 10 and 40 diopters. Normal capillaries appear as delicate, regularly spaced "hairpin" loops. In contradistinction, abnormal capillaries are enlarged, tortuous, and often interspersed with avascular regions or "capillary dropout." Capillary hemorrhages are another abnormal finding. Nail fold capillaroscopy provides useful diagnostic and prognostic information since observing normal capillaries implies primary Raynaud's syndrome exists, whereas identifying abnormal capillaries suggests a secondary cause for Raynaud's syndrome is present (or will eventuate in time). Nail fold abnormalities are most often found in systemic sclerosis and CREST syndrome yet can occur in systemic lupus erythematosus, Sjogren's syndrome, antiphospholipid antibody syndrome, and dermatomyositis as well.

Cold Immersion Testing

As the diagnosis of Raynaud's syndrome is historically and clinically based, this test is not and should not be routinely utilized. Sophisticated, cumbersome, and expensive vascular laboratory testing can be employed to measure digital blood flow and temperature after a painful cold challenge in an attempt to distinguish between simple cold sensitivity, primary Raynaud's syndrome, and secondary Raynaud's syndrome. Unfortunately, significant testing overlap can occur between these three patient groups as well as control groups. One must also remain aware that cold immersion testing may precipitate a digit-threatening ischemic crisis in the setting of secondary Raynaud's syndrome.

TABLE 16.6

CRITERIA FOR THE DIAGNOSIS OF PRIMARY RAYNAUD'S SYNDROME

Symmetric attacks
Absence of tissue necrosis or gangrene
No history or physical findings suggestive of a secondary cause
Normal nail fold capillaries
Normal erythrocyte sedimentation rate
Negative serological findings (especially negative ANA)

TABLE 16.7

CRITERIA SUGGESTIVE OF SECONDARY RAYNAUD'S SYNDROME

Age of onset >30 y
Male gender
Abnormal Allen's test/absent upper extremity pulses
Painful, intense vasospasm
Asymmetric vasospasm
Digital pits, ulcerations, necrosis
Abnormal nail fold capillaroscopy
Clinical features of autoimmune disease (e.g., arthritis, myositis)
Specific autoantibody positivity (e.g., anticentromere antibodies)

Primary Versus Secondary Raynaud's Syndrome

Primary Raynaud's syndrome is suggested by the clinical criteria outlined in Table 16.6. Additionally, a patient with primary vasospastic disease will have normal upper extremity segmental pressures and waveforms with either normal or "peaked" digital plethysmographic waveforms. Twelve to twenty percent of patients whose condition was initially classified as primary Raynaud's syndrome will evolve into secondary Raynaud's syndrome over 10 or more years. The frequency of secondary transformation is higher in males and the elderly. In contrast, patients with secondary Raynaud's syndrome exhibit one or more of the clinical features shown in Table 16.7. Such patients are more likely to have abnormal upper extremity noninvasive studies. Digital plethysmographic waveforms may be either normal or "peaked" in early secondary Raynaud's syndrome cases, but as the digital ischemia becomes more severe and fixed, a blunted or even flat waveform ensues. Nail fold capillary abnormalities, strongly positive ANA, elevated ESR, and additional specific autoantibodies are associated with a 30% incidence of developing secondary Raynaud's syndrome within 5 years.

CONCLUSIONS

Upper extremity arterial disease is relatively rare in comparison to lower extremity occlusive disease. It can be very disabling, sometimes affecting hand and finger function. When symptomatic, Raynaud-type symptoms are invariably present. Fortunately, major amputation is rare. In contrast to lower extremity PAD, atherosclerosis is not the predominant cause of UEAD; rather, a myriad of diverse etiologies exist that can affect either the large or the small arteries of the upper limb. Segmental limb pressures with Doppler and PVR waveforms in addition to digital pressures and plethysmographic waveforms are useful complementary studies after a thorough history and physical examination has been undertaken. Subsequent adjunctive testing may be required to further assist the examiner in ascertaining the etiology of UEAD and should be individualized in a cost-efficient fashion.

PRACTICAL POINTS

■ Patients who present with unilateral upper extremity ischemic symptoms should be assessed for a proximal embolic source.

■ Approximately two thirds of patients who present with significant hand and finger ischemia are afflicted with small-artery disease of the upper extremity (occlusive disease distal to the wrist).

■ Both duplicate and complementary tributary arteries form a highly redundant arterial cascade that can delay the onset of upper ischemic symptoms despite significant underlying arterial occlusive disease.

■ Persistent, severe upper extremity digital ischemia (including ulcerations) excludes the diagnosis of primary Raynaud's syndrome, which is only characterized by intermittent vasospasm.

■ Subjects can present with ischemic symptoms isolated to one digit, yet non-invasive testing may uncover subclinical involvement in the ipsilateral and contralateral digits.

■ Falsely negative digital plethysmography and pressure studies can occur when only one digital artery is obstructed.

■ The presence of an abnormal nail fold capillaroscopy examination in a patient with Raynaud's syndrome may be the most powerful predictor for the subsequent development of an autoimmune disease.

■ Twelve to twenty percent of patients whose condition was initially classified as primary Raynaud's syndrome will evolve into secondary Raynaud's syndrome over 10 or more years.

■ Nail fold capillary abnormalities, strongly positive ANA, elevated ESR, and autoantibodies are associated with a 30% incidence of developing secondary Raynaud's syndrome within 5 years.

RECOMMENDED READING

Blockmans D, Beyens G, Verhaeghe R. Predictive value of nailfold capillaroscopy in the diagnosis of connective tissue diseases. *Clin Rheumatol* 1996;15:148–153.

Cutolo M, Sulli A, Secchi ME, et al. Nailfold capillaroscopy is useful for the diagnosis and follow-up of autoimmune rheumatic diseases. A future tool for the analysis of microvascular heart involvement? *Rheumatology* 2006;45:43–46.

Edwards JM, Porter JM. Upper extremity arterial disease: etiologic considerations and differential diagnosis. *Semin Vasc Surg* 1998;11:60–66.

Greenfield LJ, Rajagopalan S, Olin JW. Upper extremity arterial disease. *Cardiol Clin* 2002;20: 623–631.

Herrick AL, Illingworth K, Blann A, et al. Von Willebrand factor, thrombomodulin, thromboxane, beta-thromboglobulin and markers of fibrinolysis in primary Raynaud's phenomenon and systemic sclerosis. *Ann Rheum Dis* 1996;55(2):122–127.

Mackinnon SE, Novak CB. Thoracic outlet syndrome. *Curr Probl Surg* 2002;9(11):1070–1145.

Ochoa VM, Yeghiazarians Y. Subclavian artery stenosis: a review for the vascular medicine practitioner. *Vasc Med* 2011; Feb;16(1):29-34. Epub 2010 Nov 15.

Ouriel K. Noninvasive diagnosis of upper extremity vascular disease. *Semin Vasc Surg* 1998; 11:54–59.

Palmer RA, Collin J. Vibration white finger. *Br J Surg* 1993;80:705–709.

Sumner DS. Noninvasive assessment of upper extremity and hand ischemia. *J Vasc Surg* 1986;3:560–564.

Sumner DS. Evaluation of acute and chronic ischemia of the upper extremity. In: Cronenwett J, Gloviczki P, Johnston K, et al., eds. *Vascular surgery*, 5th ed. Philadelphia, PA: Saunders, 2000.

Yao JS. Upper extremity ischemia in athletes. *Semin Vasc Surg* 1998;11(2):96–105.

CHAPTER 17 ■ Subclavian, Innominate, Axillary Artery Disease and Thoracic Outlet Syndrome

Debabrata Mukherjee

Upper extremity arterial disease is significantly less common than disease of the lower extremities. Large-vessel occlusive disease of the arm typically involves the subclavian arteries. The Joint Study of Extracranial Arterial Occlusion reported a 17% incidence of subclavian or innominate artery stenosis, but clinical symptoms or angiographic steal occurred in only 2.5% of cases. The most common site of disease is the left subclavian artery, and this vessel is involved three to four times more frequently than the right side. Significant proximal subclavian artery stenosis may result in subclavian steal syndrome (SSS) leading to vertebrobasilar insufficiency, upper extremity claudication, and myocardial ischemia due to hyperfusion of the internal mammary artery (IMA) in patients with an IMA bypass. The axillary artery is only rarely involved by atherosclerosis, and more commonly, axillary artery stenosis or aneurysm is related to long-term use of axillary crutches. Table 16.1 lists etiologies of large-artery involvement. For the most part, large-vessel disease has limited etiologies [embolic, aneurysm, vasculopathy (vasculitis and atherosclerosis), and entrapment]. Long-term use of crutches may cause axillary artery stenosis or aneurysms. Giant cell arteritis (typically Takayasu's) should be considered in young individuals presenting with upper extremity involvement, whereas atherosclerosis is a common etiology in older individuals. Thoracic outlet syndrome (TOS) should be considered in any individual with acute or chronic upper extremity symptoms.

CLINICAL FEATURES

Innominate Arterial Disease

Involvement of the innominate artery is uncommon, and the etiologies are limited to atherosclerosis and inflammatory vasculitis. Involvement of the innominate artery is seen in 5 to 17% of patients undergoing arteriography of the arch/cerebral vessels. While most cases are asymptomatic, other presentations include upper extremity–related symptoms (right-sided claudication or microembolization) or cerebrovascular ischemic symptoms related to the vertebrobasilar distribution.

Subclavian Artery Disease

Most individuals with subclavian artery stenosis are asymptomatic, and involvement is detected as an incidental finding during Doppler ultrasound examination of the carotid and vertebral arteries. Arm claudication may occur but is generally rare, owing to exuberant collateral formation

329

in most individuals but may be seen with very high-grade stenosis or subclavian occlusions. *Radiologic vertebral-subclavian steal* occurs in the setting of subclavian artery stenosis proximal to the origin of the vertebral artery, associated with flow reversal in the vertebral artery. This may be demonstrated by ultrasound, phase-contrast magnetic resonance angiography (MRA), or retrograde opacification of the vertebral artery on diagnostic angiography. Symptoms suggestive of vertebrobasilar or posterior cerebral circulation ischemia such as dizziness, unsteadiness, vertigo, or visual changes may occur in response to upper extremity arm exertion. The combination of retrograde vertebral flow and neurologic symptoms in response to upper extremity exertion has been labeled *SSS*. In this disorder, blood is shunted through the ipsilateral vertebral artery from the contralateral posterior circulation to ameliorate blood flow to the subclavian artery beyond a tight proximal stenosis. This is mostly encountered in the context of contralateral carotid or posterior circulation disease or hypoplastic posterior communicating arteries (common anomaly), resulting in inadequate blood flow to the ipsilateral vertebral artery and resultant posterior circulation ischemia. The Joint Study of Extracranial Arterial Occlusion found that 80% of patients with SSS had concomitant lesions in the contralateral carotid or vertebral circulation. The existence of this clinical entity has, however, been questioned, as there can be imprecise correlation between the presence of these symptoms and the existence of stenosis. Moreover, individuals with atherosclerosis of the subclavian artery also harbor concomitant cerebrovascular disease, making precise attribution of symptoms difficult. Individuals with left internal mammary artery (LIMA) coronary bypass grafts may develop angina with arm exercise related to coronary-subclavian steal where there is flow reversal in the LIMA and blood is diverted from the coronary circulation resulting in myocardial ischemia.

Giant Cell Arteritis (Takayasu's)

Takayasu's arteritis commonly involves the subclavian arteries. Typically, type I (arch vessels) and type II (arch and abdominal vessels) variants of the disease display subclavian artery involvement. In contrast to the involvement with atherosclerosis, the involvement with vasculitis tends to be diffuse (proximal and distal to the origin of the vertebral artery), andconsequently, patients do not present with SSS. The involvement is typically asymptomatic, presenting with evidence of a bruit over the subclavian artery, absent radial artery pulses, or a blood pressure differential between upper and lower extremities. A few patients may complain of upper extremity claudication. All patients with Takayasu's should have blood pressures measured in all four extremities.

Aneurysms of the Subclavian and Axillary Artery

Subclavian Artery Aneurysms

These result from atherosclerosis, trauma, TOS, and rarely collagen-vascular diseases. This is an unusual site, and the presence of an aneurysm at this location should prompt an investigation for arterial aneurysms in other sites.

Clinical features include embolization and pain in the neck/shoulder region due to impingement on the brachial plexus with or without Raynaud's symptoms. Uncommon manifestations include hoarseness due to compression of the recurrent laryngeal nerve and dyspnea (compression of the trachea) and transient ischemic attacks due to retrograde embolization in the vertebral and carotid arteries. Pulsatile masses in the supraclavicular region may represent tortuous rather than aneurysmal subclavian arteries. Aneurysms in the distal subclavian artery are usually secondary to TOS (almost always a cervical rib).

"Kommerell's Diverticulum" and Aneurysm of an Aberrant Right Subclavian Artery

An *aneurysm of an aberrant right subclavian artery* (ARSA) arising from a left aortic arch is a common abnormality of the aortic arch, occurring in 0.4 to 2% of the population. ARSA originates in the thoracic aorta, distal to the left subclavian artery, and crosses the midline between the spinal column and the esophagus to the right axilla. In 60% of cases, its origin in the thoracic aorta is saccular, as a diverticulum first described by Kommerell (hence referred to as *Kommerell's diverticulum*). This abnormality tends to be asymptomatic and discovered by chance when a chest radiograph is taken or endoscopic examination is performed. When symptomatic, it commonly causes intermittent dysphagia for solids because of its retroesophageal course, a condition known as *dysphagia lusoria*. These aneurysms display a marked propensity to rupture.

Axillary Artery Aneurysm

This is usually a result of repetitive trauma as is the case with "crutch aneurysm" or may be seen with blunt or penetrating trauma to the area (as occurs with motor vehicle accidents, humeral fractures, and anterior dislocation of the shoulder). In a crutch aneurysm, the presentation is often one of upper extremity ischemia and should always be suspected in anybody using a crutch who has an abnormal pulse exam. With trauma associated with brachial plexus injury or new neurologic findings (in the context of previously normal findings), the presence of an expanding axillary artery aneurysm should be considered as an etiology and an arteriogram or a carefully performed duplex exam ordered as part of the workup.

DIAGNOSTIC APPROACH FOR SUSPECTED ARTERIAL DISEASE

Physical examination may suggest significant subclavian or innominate stenosis through detection of weak or absent radial and ulnar pulse on the ipsilateral side and reduced blood pressure (difference greater than 15 mm Hg) when compared to the contralateral arm. Detection of a bruit over the subclavian artery (subclavian artery stenosis) or proximal (base of carotid) carotid and subclavian artery is a suggestive clue. Upper extremity embolization (unilateral) should prompt a workup for proximal disease in the innominate and subclavian arteries. In some individuals, bilateral involvement of subclavian or innominate artery as well as the subclavian vessels may result in blood pressures being low in both upper extremities. Thus, lower-than-expected blood pressures in the upper extremity should prompt measurement of lower extremity blood pressure. The evaluation of large-vessel disease of the upper extremity would not be complete without performing diagnostic maneuvers for TOS as described in detail in Chapter 1 and later in this chapter, including palpation for tenderness over the scalenus anticus. Every patient with suspected TOS should have a radiograph to rule out a thoracic rib. Figure 16.1 provides a general outline for testing in patients presenting with upper extremity symptoms. Also refer to the Diagnostic Testing section in that chapter for specific tests. Aspects specific to large-arterial involvement are outlined here.

Segmental Limb Pressures, Finger Pressures, and Doppler Pulse Contours

The normal pressure differential between adjacent levels of the same limb or compared to the same level of the contralateral limb is less than 7 mm Hg. A significant pressure drop (more than 10 mm Hg) or an index below 0.80 indicates disease at that level [ratio of brachial/brachial, forearm/ forearm, wrist/wrist, wrist/brachial (same arm) or forearm/brachial indices (same arm) is normally above 0.90, with ratios below 0.85 being considered abnormal]. The presence of monophasic or damped signals is adjunctive qualitative evidence of disease. Normally, the pulse contours in the upper extremity arteries (evaluated by Doppler or pulse volume recordings) are triphasic or biphasic (see Chapter 16). Monophasic or damped signals indicate disease at that level. Concomitant finger pressures should also be obtained in cases with evidence of Raynaud's or small-vessel disease (see Chapter 16).

Duplex Ultrasonography

Duplex evaluation of the arteries of the upper extremity is extremely helpful in suspected large-vessel involvement. The proximal left subclavian artery and segments of the subclavian system under the clavicle are one area that may be difficult to image. Duplex scanning facilitates an image-directed Doppler exam of specific upper extremity arteries and their branches. Normal systolic velocity in the subclavian and innominate arteries is 80 to 120 cm/s. A greater than twofold elevation in velocities in the stenotic zone versus the prestenotic zone indicates a more than 50% narrowing. Spectral characteristics that suggest turbulence are very helpful adjunctive findings. Arterial occlusion is diagnosed by diagnosing the absence of flow within the artery, taking care not to confuse various solid nonvascular structures with an occluded artery. In individuals with arm claudication and normal patterns at baseline, Doppler flow should be remeasured after 3 to 5 minutes of arm exercise.

Magnetic Resonance Angiography

3D contrast-enhanced magnetic resonance angiography may be used to evaluate the aortic arch vessels as well as the upper extremity arteries. The arch evaluation provides information on the proximal and middle portions of the subclavian artery that may be sufficient for the diagnosis of atherosclerotic involvement. Additional phase-contrast MRA (PC-MRA) measurements may be required to demonstrate retrograde flow in a vertebral artery in cases of subclavian artery steal (most commonly seen in the left side). Improvements in coil technology are enabling simultaneous demonstration of the arch vessels and the carotid bifurcations. Two artifacts that are particularly relevant to imaging arch and subclavian disease that may simulate a stenosis in an artery are (a) *Coil drop-out artifact:* In patients with low aortic arch or elevated shoulders, the coil sensitivity may drop out in the periphery resulting in loss of signal and simulation of a stenosis. (b) *Venous susceptibility artifact:* This may occur around the subclavian and innominate vessels because of the high concentration of contrast agent in the venous system (innominate or subclavian veins) that may obscure signal in the adjoining arteries. To avoid this artifact, right arm injections are preferred (as the region of the left innominate vein is more prone to obscure the arch vessels including the subclavian), and contrast should be chased with a saline bolus followed by arm elevation to clear contrast as rapidly as possible.

Computed Tomography Angiography

CT angiography uses iodinated contrast material and gives excellent anatomical detail concerning the location of subclavian arterial lesions. However, if endovascular treatment is considered, then conventional 4-vessel arteriography is more appropriate, since the diagnostic study as well as the treatment can be performed at the same time.

Catheter-based Angiography

Catheter-based angiography allows direct visualization of blood vessels in the body by the injection of iodinated contrast material via a catheter placed directly into the artery or vein. It remains the gold standard to determine the severity and extent of subclavian/innominate arterial disease. Digital subtraction angiographic technology allows high-quality images using small amounts of contrast material. A number of unique catheter shapes have been developed to facilitate intubation/cannulation of the ostium of the great vessels based on the architecture of the aortic arch (see Chapter 3 on "Diagnostic Angiography"). An aortic arch angiographic study (LAO 30-degree projection) is initially performed to determine the origin of the great vessels to choose an appropriate catheter for selective angiography (Fig. 17.1). The left subclavian artery is well visualized in the LAO 30-degree projection. Innominate artery bifurcation is best visualized in right anterior oblique (RAO) 20 to 30 degrees and caudal 10- to 20-degree view. Baseline angiography of the bilateral vertebral and carotid arteries should be performed to determine the extent of vascular disease and the presence of collateral circulation. Angiography should demonstrate the entire arterial circulation from the origin (subclavian/innominate) to the digital arteries.

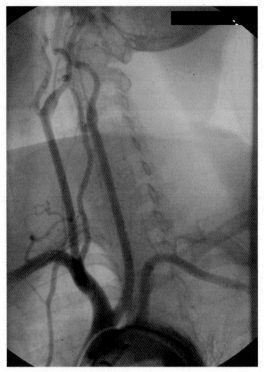

FIGURE 17-1. Aortic arch angiographic study (LAO 30-degree projection) to determine the origin of the great vessels. This angiogram shows a bovine arch where the left carotid artery arises from the innominate trunk. The LAO 30-degree projection is excellent for visualization of the left subclavian artery, but significant overlap is noted in the innominate system.

MANAGEMENT OF PATIENT
Medical Treatment

Most patients with asymptomatic subclavian artery stenosis can be managed medically (Fig. 17.2) in a manner akin to lower extremity peripheral arterial disease. Intensive risk factor modification is therefore indicated in these individuals to reduce the risk of cardiovascular morbidity and mortality. Antiplatelet agents reduce both the risk of limb loss and the need for revascularization in patients with peripheral arterial disease. All patients should be on aspirin unless contraindicated. The adenosine diphosphate antagonists clopidogrel or prasugrel may be considered in patients intolerant to aspirin. Based on ATP III guidelines and available data, all patients with peripheral arterial disease should be on lipid-lowering therapy with a target LDL of preferably less than 70 mg/dL.

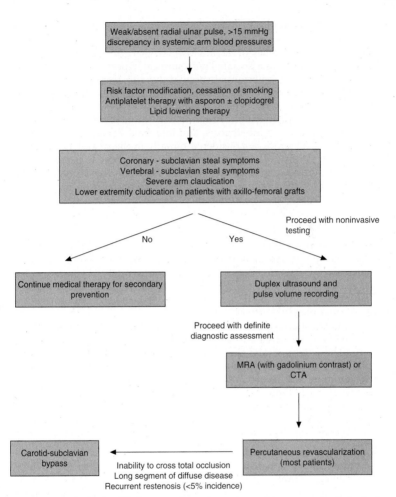

FIGURE 17-2. A simplified approach to the patient with suspected subclavian/innominate artery stenosis.

Surgical Treatment

Subclavian Disease

Surgical or percutaneous revascularization is indicated in individuals with symptoms of coronary or vertebral steal syndrome and severe arm claudication or rest pain. The surgical treatment for symptomatic subclavian stenosis is carotid-to-subclavian artery bypass if the ipsilateral carotid artery is free of disease. The use of extra-anatomic bypass of the carotid and subclavian arteries was first introduced by Diethrich et al. in 1967 to reduce the complication rate of transthoracic reconstruction.

In a review of carotid subclavian artery bypass with PTFE performed for symptomatic stenosis or occlusion, AbuRahma et al. reported an overall 10-year primary patency of 92%. However, there are significant periprocedural complications associated with surgical bypass in these individuals (who usually harbor substantial vascular disease) averaging 13% including stroke in 3% and death in 2%. The main complications associated with carotid subclavian bypass include injury to the thoracic duct with development of early lymph fistula or chylothorax, injury to cranial or sympathetic nerves, graft stenosis, and infection. Percutaneous interventions should therefore be considered initially in the treatment of subclavian artery stenosis. However, when this is not possible because of the inability to cross complete occlusions, the extent of disease in the subclavian artery, or stent failure, extra-anatomic reconstruction may provide an alternative treatment option.

Innominate Disease

Stenosis of the innominate artery can be approached percutaneously when feasible. In cases where this is not possible (for reasons mentioned under the subclavian artery stenosis section), surgical bypass or direct reconstruction are potential treatment options. Extra-anatomic bypasses that are commonly used include carotid-subclavian bypasses. Direct reconstruction of the artery may be feasible in select cases and includes innominate endarterectomy and aortic origin grafting (to the carotid and subclavian arteries as a bifurcated graft or a single limb graft with a side arm). The extent of and the numbers of bypasses depend on the concomitant vessels involved. In individuals with concomitant asymptomatic left common carotid artery stenosis, restoration of flow to the carotid lesions alone without subclavian bypass/reconstruction has resulted in improvement in symptoms.

Percutaneous Treatment of Subclavian and Innominate Disease

Recent data suggest that angioplasty and stenting may be preferable to surgery in most patients with symptomatic subclavian and innominate stenosis (Table 17.1). The advantages of percutaneous intervention include fewer surgical- and anesthesia-related complications, lower procedural morbidity, and a shorter hospital stay. Hadjipetrou et al. reported a 100% success rate in 18 patients undergoing aortic arch vessel stenosis who were treated with primary stent placement. There were no major complications. The follow-up at 17 months demonstrated no restenosis and all patients remained asymptomatic. Jain et al. reported a series of 245 patients undergoing subclavian artery intervention from six centers. The overall success rate was 98.5%, with a major complication rate of 1%. The mean gradient across the lesions was reduced from 52.5 mm Hg to 3.1 mm Hg ($P < 0.01$). Complications included distal embolization in three patients (1.2%), including one transient ischemic attack. After almost 2 years of follow-up, the primary patency rate was 89% and the secondary patency rate was 98.5% in this large series. The generally accepted consensus is that peripheral vascular stenting of aortic

TABLE 17.1

PROTOCOL FOR SUBCLAVIAN/INNOMINATE ARTERY STENTING

- Patients sedated with short-acting intravenous sedation, and arterial sheath inserted in the femoral artery.
- An aortic arch angiographic study (LAO 30° projection) is performed to determine the origin of the great vessels to choose an appropriate catheter for selective angiography.
- The left subclavian artery is well visualized in the LAO 30° projection.
- Innominate artery bifurcation is best visualized in right anterior oblique (RAO) 20–30° and caudal 10–20° view.
- Baseline angiography performed on the bilateral vertebral and carotid arteries to determine the extent of vascular disease and presence of collateral circulation. In patients with intracranial vertebral artery disease, successful treatment of subclavian artery stenosis may not improve symptoms of vertebrobasilar ischemia.
- Unfractionated heparin 60 U/kg with target activated clotting time >250 s is administered.
- A 125-cm 5F JR4 diagnostic catheter (Cordis Corporation, Miami, FL) placed inside a 90-cm 7F Brite-tip Sheath (Cordis Corporation, Miami, FL) is introduced.
- The origin of the left subclavian/innominate artery is intubated with the JR4 catheter and a 0.035 Wholey guidewire (Mallinckrodt, Inc., Hazelwood, MO) advanced into the distal subclavian artery.
- The 7F Brite-tip Sheath is advanced into the proximal subclavian artery over the JR4 catheter.
- The JR4 catheter is withdrawn at this time and diagnostic angiograms performed in the ipsilateral 30° oblique for vessel sizing.
- An undersized balloon (6.0-mm Opta-Pro, Cordis Corporation, Miami, FL) is used to predilate the lesion to allow subsequent passage of a stent.
- Stenting performed with a balloon expandable stent (GENESIS stent, Cordis Corporation, Miami, FL; EXPRESS LD stent, Boston Scientific) for ostial/proximal lesions.
- Stenting performed with a nitinol stent (SMART stent, Cordis Corporation, Miami, FL; DYNALINK, Abbott Vascular or SENTINOL, Boston Scientific) for distal subclavian stenosis.
- All patients receive 325 mg of aspirin and 300 mg of clopidogrel prior to the procedure and are discharged home the following day on clopidogrel (75 mg PO once a day.) for 4 wk and on aspirin (325 mg PO q.d.) indefinitely. Prasugrel 60-mg loading dose and 10 mg q.d. maintenance dose may also be used in place of clopidogrel.

arch vessel disease is equal in efficacy to surgical procedures with less morbidity and mortality than surgery. The long-term patency and symptomatic improvement appear to be excellent, which makes percutaneous stent therapy the treatment of choice in most centers with experienced interventionists (Fig. 17.3).

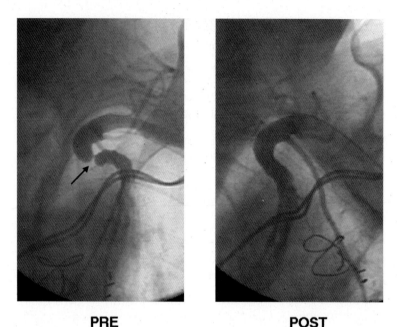

PRE   **POST**

FIGURE 17-3. Successful balloon angioplasty and stenting of a severe stenosis as depicted by the arrow in the proximal left subclavian artery of a 64-year-old male with anterior myocardial ischemia and class III angina. Angina completely resolved after revascularization.

Management of Subclavian and Axillary Aneurysmal Disease

The treatment of subclavian/axillary artery aneurysms is dependent on the etiology. In subclavian aneurysms that are associated with a cervical rib, the treatment should comprise thoracic outlet decompression, with cervical rib removal. Mild poststenotic arterial dilation alone (without other manifestations of upper extremity ischemia) due to compression may return to normal caliber with this intervention alone. When significant dilation is present, resection of the aneurysm or endoaneurysmography and placement of a short interposition graft (vein is preferred) is the operation of choice. Most authors would recommend resection of a symptomatic aneurysm or an asymptomatic aneurysm (subclavian and axillary) when the diameter of the aneurysms exceeds twice the normal arterial diameter. Aneurysms of an aberrant subclavian artery should be resected promptly on identification because of a propensity for these aneurysms to rupture. Operative mortality associated with the resection of extrathoracic subclavian and axillary aneurysms should be less than 5%, whereas that associated with repair of intrathoracic aneurysms is higher. This is related to complications associated with rupture related to emergency presentations. Another treatment option is the insertion of an endoprosthesis in the subclavian artery, excluding the aneurysm from its proximal neck until the distal neck. The endovascular treatment offers a minimally invasive alternative for this subgroup of patients. Patency rates between 80 and 100% have been reported in the literature with covered stents.

THORACIC OUTLET SYNDROME

This refers to compression of the neurovascular structures at the superior aperture of the thorax. The narrow space called the *scalene triangle* (Fig. 17.4) is bounded by the first rib, the clavicle, the scalenus medius muscle, and the costoclavicular ligament. TOS is used to describe a variety of symptoms resulting from the compression of the brachial plexus and/or subclavian vein and/or artery. Neurogenic TOS is by far more the most common form than venous or arterial TOS (95, 4, and 1% of all operations for TOS) due to the greater propensity for brachial plexus structures to be entrapped than vascular structures.

Clinical Features and Symptoms

Most patients with neurogenic TOS have a history of neck trauma preceding their symptoms, with accidents and repetitive stress being common. Repetitive physical exertion may result in venous TOS and thrombosis of the subclavian artery also referred to as *effort thrombosis* or *Paget-Schrotter disease*. Arterial TOS is almost always associated with a cervical rib or an anomalous first rib, and the absence of these may essentially exclude arterial TOS. The presence of these, however, in antecedent trauma may predispose to neurogenic TOS. Since ATOS is usually asymptomatic until arterial emboli occur, asymptomatic patients found to have one of these rib anomalies are followed with duplex scans every few years to detect silent arterial abnormalities.

Neurogenic Thoracic Outlet Syndrome

Pain, paresthesia, and weakness in the hand, arm, and shoulder, plus neck pain and occipital headaches, are the classical symptoms of neurogenic TOS. Raynaud's phenomenon, hand coldness and color changes, are also frequently seen, and the symptoms are typically confused as symptoms of arterial TOS. The brachial plexus, especially the lower elements, C8 and T1 spinal nerves and lower trunk, becomes compressed or irritated in the interscalenic triangle. Pain and sensory changes (numbness, tingling) in a brachial plexus distribution, aggravated with use of the upper extremity, especially on elevation are the main complaints.

Venous Thoracic Outlet Syndrome

Arm swelling is good evidence of subclavian vein obstruction/thrombosis in venous TOS and almost never occurs with arterial or neurogenic TOS. Pain or aching may sometimes occur but is frequently. Paresthesia in the fingers and hands is common in venous TOS and may be secondary to swelling in the hand rather than nerve compression in the thoracic outlet area.

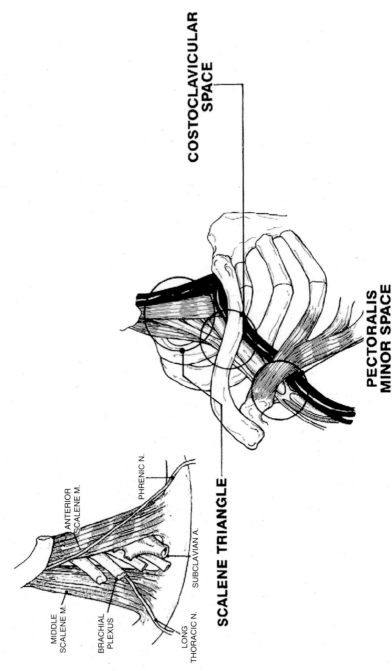

FIGURE 17-4. Anatomy of the thoracic outlet area demonstrating the three main spaces. (From Sanders RJ, Haug CE. *Thoracic outlet syndrome: a common sequela of neck injuries.* Philadelphia, PA: JB Lippincott, 1991:34.)

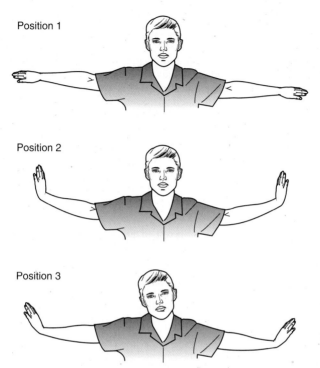

Position 1

Position 2

Position 3

FIGURE 17-5.   Upper limb tension test. Position 1: Arms abducted to 90 degrees with elbows extended. Position 2: Additional dorsiflexion of wrists. Position 3: Tilt head to side, ear to shoulder. Each maneuver progressively increases stretch on the brachial plexus. While positions 1 and 2 elicit symptoms on the ipsilateral side, position 3 elicits symptoms on the contralateral side. Pain down the arm, especially around the elbow, and/or paresthesia in the hand is a positive response. The strongest positive test is onset of symptoms in position 1 with increased symptoms in positions 2 and 3. The weakest response is onset of symptoms only in position 3. (Adapted from Sanders RJ, Hammond SL, Rao NM. Diagnosis of thoracic outlet syndrome. *Vasc Surg* 2007;46:601–604.)

Arterial Thoracic Outlet Syndrome

The symptoms of ATOS include digital ischemia, claudication, pallor, coldness, and pain in the hand but rarely in the shoulder or neck and occur secondary to embolization either from mural thrombus in the compressed subclavian artery or from an aneurysm and not secondary to Raynaud's phenomenon as is common with neurogenic TOS.

Clinical Evaluation of Thoracic Outlet Syndrome

The clinical evaluation of suspected TOS should include the measurement of the blood pressure in both arms and specific findings including on provocative maneuvers (see Chapter 1 for thoracic outlet maneuvers).

Arterial TOS is commonly associated with an absent radial pulse and seldom requires provocative tests such as Adson's and the EAST maneuver, which are often falsely positive even in normal individuals. These latter maneuvers are often more helpful in diagnosing neurogenic TOS.

Venous TOS is readily identified by the presence of arm swelling, cyanosis, and distended superficial veins over the shoulder and chest wall (almost ever occurs with arterial/neurogenic TOS).

NTOS usually demonstrates tenderness over the scalene muscles and duplication of symptoms by the following provocative maneuvers:

1. EAST Maneuver (External rotation and abduction stress test): Abducting the arms to 90 degrees in external rotation (90 degrees AER), which brings on symptoms within 60 seconds and often, in less than 30 seconds. An easy way to accomplish this is to ask the patient to adopt the "stick-up posture" with arms extended, externally rotated, and behind the head.

Modified upper limb tension test of Elvey: Figure 17.5 demonstrates the test in three incremental postures of increasing stress.

Diagnostic Studies

An x-ray is useful to assess for cervical rib or an anomalous first rib. The absence essentially rules out arterial TOS, while the presence (through sheer probability) especially with symptoms and appropriately positive provocative maneuvers makes the diagnosis of neurogenic TOS likely. The distinction between arterial and other forms of TOS should be based on history and physical exam alone and seldom requires arteriography including CTA or MRA. Arteriography should be employed only when a patient has signs and symptoms suggestive of ischemia and when surgery is under consideration. Noninvasive tests such as measurement of pulse volume in positions of provocation may be useful to detect arterial compression; however, this is rarely necessary if the symptoms are consistent with neurogenic TOS. Electromyography and nerve conduction velocity tests are normal in the large majority of patients with clinical signs of NTOS and are probably not indicated. A study from France seems to suggest that measurement of conduction velocities of the NCV of the medial antebrachial cutaneous nerve may reveal early abnormalities in neurogenic TOS. This could prove to be a helpful test to confirm diagnoses, but data from other centers on use of this modality are currently limited.

Treatment

Decompression of the subclavian artery is accomplished by releasing the scalene muscles and the removal of any abnormal bony structures such as a cervical rib or occasionally the first rib. Decompression of the artery and removal of the anomalous bony structures is also used to treat poststenotic dilatation or aneurysm.

CONCLUSIONS

The most common site of upper extremity arterial stenosis is origin of the left subclavian artery, and this vessel is involved three to four times as often as the right side. Physical examination may suggest significant subclavian stenosis by the detection of a bruit over the artery and/or a weak or absent radial and ulnar pulse and reduced blood pressure in the involved side, when compared to the contralateral arm. Duplex scanning, contrast-enhanced MRA, and CTA enable accurate depiction of subclavian artery stenosis. The high technical success, low restenosis rate, minimal complications, elimination of general anesthesia, and low cost make percutaneous revascularization for symptomatic subclavian artery stenosis the treatment modality of choice. If percutaneous revascularization is not possible because of inability to cross a complete occlusion, extent of disease in the subclavian artery, or stent failure, extra-anatomic reconstruction provides a reasonable alternative treatment option. The most common form of TOS is neurogenic, which may mimic arterial TOS due to the common occurrence of Raynaud-type symptoms. Provocative maneuvers such as Modified upper limb tension test and the EAST maneuver are often positive in neurogenic TOS and are often associated with scapen tenderness. Arterial TOS almost never occurs in the absence of a cervical rib/anomalous first rib.

PRACTICAL POINTS

■ Atherosclerosis commonly involves the subclavian arteries. Takayasu's arteritis commonly affects the subclavian arteries, especially in young individuals.

■ In patients with extensive atherosclerosis or Takayasu's arteritis, always measure BP in both extremities and lower extremity.

■ The evaluation of upper extremity symptoms must include consideration of TOS.

■ Radiologic subclavian steal is more common than clinical SSS.

■ Percutaneous intervention point:

■ Total occlusions of the subclavian arteries are easier to cross from the ipsilateral brachial approach.

■ Arterial TOS almost never occurs in the absence of a cervical rib/anomalous first rib.

■ Obliteration of the pulse in response to EAST/Adson's test often occurs in normal individuals and cannot be used to rule in arterial TOS.

RECOMMENDED READING

AbuRahma AF, Robinson PA, Jennings TG. Carotid-subclavian bypass grafting with polytetrafluoroethylene grafts for symptomatic subclavian artery stenosis or occlusion: a 20-year experience. *J Vasc Surg* 2000;32:411–419.

Diethrich EB, Garrett HB, Ameriso J. Occlusive disease of the common carotid and subclavian arteries treated by carotid-subclavian bypass. *Am J Surg* 1967;114:800–808.

Fields WS, Lemak NA. Joint study of extracranial arterial occlusion. VII. Subclavian steal—a review of 168 cases. *JAMA* 1972;222(9):1139–1143.

Hadjipetrou P, Cox S, Piemonte T, et al. Percutaneous revascularization of atherosclerotic obstruction of aortic arch vessels. *J Am Coll Cardiol* 1999;33:1238–1245.

Hilfiker PR, Razavi MK, Kee ST, et al. Stent-graft therapy for subclavian artery aneurysms and fistulas: single center mid-term results. *J Vasc Interv Radiol* 2000;11:578–584.

Jain SP, Zhang SY, Khosla S, et al. Subclavian and innominate stenting: acute and long-term results. *J Am Coll Cardiol* 1998;31:63A.

Mackinnon SE, Novak CB. Evaluation of the patient with thoracic outlet syndrome. *Semin Thorac Cardiovasc Surg* 1996;8(2):190–200.

Paty PS, Mehta M, Darling RC, et al. Surgical treatment of coronary subclavian steal syndrome with carotid subclavian bypass. *Ann Vasc Surg* 2003;17(1):22–26.

Plewa MC, Delinger M. The false-positive rate of thoracic outlet syndrome shoulder maneuvers in healthy subjects. *Acad Emerg Med* 1998;5:337–342.

Sanders RJ, Hammond SL, Rao, NM. Diagnosis of thoracic outlet syndrome. *Vasc Surg* 2007;46:601–604.

Seror O. Medial antebrachial cutaneous nerve conduction study, a new tool to demonstrate mild lower brachial plexus lesions. A report of 16 cases. *Clin Neurophysiol* 2004;115:2316–2322.

RAYNAUD'S PHENOMENON

Introduction

Raynaud's phenomenon (RP) (first described by Maurice Raynaud in 1862) is characterized by episodic vasospasm on exposure to cold. In its classic triphasic form, RP is typified by the development of digital blanching and cyanosis following cold exposure, and rubor with rewarming. In most cases, though, cyanosis may be absent and the episodes consist of pallor associated with pain followed by rubor. The most common site of occurrence is the fingers, and in initial stages, only a few fingers may be affected. Other sites of occurrence are the toes, nose, and ears. The diagnosis of RP is primarily made on an historical basis, but vascular laboratory testing and blood work may be required in ruling out secondary etiologies. The symptoms of RP may be lifestyle limiting, especially in the colder months, and significantly alter quality of life in severely afflicted patients. RP is an extremely common disorder (prevalence rates above 5% even in warm climates). The risk factors classically associated with its occurrence include cold weather, female sex, and a family history of the disorder. Some patients relate emotional stress as a precipitating factor of symptoms. Other components of the history that may be relevant in the evaluation of the patient include exposure to vibratory tools, palmar trauma, and chemotherapeutic agents.

Clinical Features

Signs and Symptoms

RP is a historical diagnosis. The physical examination in primary RP is typically negative as almost all patients do not present at the time of the episode. Table 18.1 lists the diagnostic criteria for primary RP. A useful historical clue in differentiating intermittent vasospasm (primary RP and early secondary RP) from spasm in conjunction with arterial obstruction (typical in severe secondary RP) is whether the symptoms are constant or intermittent. Constant, symptomatic ischemia evidenced by rest pain or ulceration is invariably caused by fixed obstruction that may occur with severe secondary forms of RP. Thus, findings of rest pain or ulcerations are not consistent with a diagnosis of primary RP. Table 18.2 lists other features that are helpful in the differentiation of primary from secondary RP. Nail fold capillaroscopy should be performed in all patients with manifestations of RP with "scleroderma pattern" representing the most specific finding associated with connective tissue disease. It is typified by dilated capillaries,

345

TABLE 18.1

CRITERIA FOR THE DIAGNOSIS OF PRIMARY RP

Vasospastic attacks precipitated by cold or emotional stress
Symmetric attacks (involving both hands)
Normal nail fold capillaries
No history/physical examination findings of diseases implicated in secondary RP
Normal ESR and negative ANA

hemorrhages, avascular areas, and neoangiogenesis and is found in about 90% of patients with clinically overt systemic sclerosis. Similar changes also occur in dermatomyositis, mixed connective tissue disease (MCTD), and overlap syndromes. The absence of abnormal capillaroscopic findings is one of the diagnostic criteria for primary RP. *Unilateral RP*: The presence of unilateral features again should warrant a careful investigation for secondary, especially embolic, causes. The most common embolic sources are the proximal large upper extremity arteries that may be involved as part of atherosclerosis, vasculitis, thoracic outlet syndrome (TOS), and Buerger's disease. Other potential causes of unilateral symptoms may originate distal to the wrist and include occupational and trauma-related conditions (see below under differential diagnosis).

Classification

RP is classified as primary (idiopathic) or secondary. The latter is associated with underlying disease states or conditions associated with vasospasm and is generally associated with more severe symptoms. Only 30% of primary RP patients suffer from severe attacks, whereas 75% of patients with secondary RP suffer from severe attacks. RP in the setting of tissue necrosis and advanced signs of ischemia or abnormal findings on noninvasive

TABLE 18.2

FEATURES THAT HELP DIFFERENTIATE PRIMARY AND SECONDARY RP

Features	Primary RP	Secondary RP
Age of onset	15–30	>40 y
Severity of symptoms	Mild	Severe
Tissue necrosis and gangrene	Absent	May be present
Risk of progression	Minimal	High
Autoantibodies[a]	Absent	Present
Endothelial dysfunction	+	+++
Circulating vasoconstrictors[b]	+	+++

[a]Autoantibodies: ANA, anticentomere, antiribonucleoprotein (RNP), anti-Smith (Sm), and antitopoisomerase (Scl-70).
[b]Vasoconstrictors: Endothelin-1, asymmetric dimethylarginine.

laboratory testing excludes primary RP. Collagen-vascular disease is by far the most common associated condition with secondary RP, and indeed, the latter may commonly precede more classic features of these diseases.

Pathophysiology

The etiology of RP is not clearly understood. The etiology of vasospasm in both primary and secondary RP is complex and reflects the complex interaction of the endothelium, smooth muscle, and neural and circulating or paracrine mediators that may all play a role in the regulation of cutaneous vascular tone. The normal neural regulation of cutaneous blood flow in response to stimuli such as cold (as opposed to other areas of circulation) is through sympathetic adrenergic vasoconstrictor fibers via the postjunctional $\alpha_2 c$ receptors in the vascular smooth muscle cells. Vasodilation is partially through the withdrawal of the sympathetic stimulus. Elevations in vasoconstrictors such as endothelin-1, asymmetric dimethylarginine (ADMA), and thromboxane A2 have all been demonstrated in RP. In addition, diminished fibrinolytic and potentiation of prothrombotic factors have also been noted. These factors have been suggested to represent consequences of disordered nitric oxide generation or may play a primary etiologic or potentiating role in the genesis of the abnormal responses that are typical of RP. Genetic and hormonal factors may also play a role in influencing propensity as indicated by the familial aggregation of this disorder and its tendency to affect females in excess of males. Recently, five candidate regions have been mapped out; some of which may contain genes that may play a role in the inheritance of this condition.

Differential Diagnosis

RP is a historical diagnosis. This implies that it may need to be distinguished from other physiologic symptoms and signs that may be encountered on exposure to cold or conditions such as acrocyanosis that may mimic RP. Rarely, even acrocyanosis patients may develop superimposed episodes of Raynaud's syndrome. A variety of neurologic conditions may result in nonspecific tingling or vasomotor symptoms and should be distinguished from true RP. To complicate matters, true RP may occur in 10% of patients with compressive neuropathies such as carpal tunnel syndrome (compression of the median nerve from etiologies such as localized tenosynovitis, trauma, hypothyroidism, amyloidosis, or activities associated with repetitive motion of the wrist). The diagnosis of carpal tunnel syndrome is entertained when tapping the volar surface of the wrist (Tinel's sign) or maintaining flexion of the wrist (Phalen's maneuver) elicits symptoms. Complex regional pain syndrome or CRPS [reflex sympathetic dystrophy (RSD)] should also be considered in the differential diagnosis (see below).

Once the diagnosis of RP is made, it is important to differentiate primary from secondary etiologies, as this has important prognostic and therapeutic ramifications. A complete list of causes of secondary RP is given in Table 18.3.

TABLE 18.3

CAUSES OF SECONDARY RP

Connective tissue diseases
  Systemic sclerosis spectrum (scleroderma, CREST)
  Systemic lupus erythematosus
  Dermatomyositis or polymyositis
  Rheumatoid arthritis
  Primary biliary cirrhosis
Thromboangiitis obliterans (Buerger's disease)
Mechanical injury
  Vibration (vibration-induced white finger) and recurrent trauma (hypothenar hammer
    syndrome)
  Frostbite
  Crutch pressure
  Thoracic outlet syndrome
Large-vessel diseases
  Atherosclerosis of brachiocephalic artery
  Vasculitis (Takayasu's and giant cell arteritis)
Vasospastic disorders
  Migraine or vascular headaches
  Prinzmetal angina
Altered blood rheology
  Paraproteinemia
  Polycythemia, chronic myeloid leukemia
  Cryoglobulins, cryofibrinogenemia, cold agglutinins
Infection
  Parvovirus B19
  Helicobacter pylori
  Hepatitis B
Chemicals or drugs
  Bleomycin and vinblastine
  Polyvinyl chloride
  β blockers
  Ergot and methysergide
  Interferon α and β
Endocrine disorders
  Carcinoid syndrome
  Pheochromocytoma
  Hypothyroidism

Connective Tissue Diseases. Connective tissue diseases account for fewer than 20% of all patients with RP but account for the majority of patients with secondary forms of RP. These patients tend to have the most severe form of the disease. RP can occur with PSS or the CREST variant (more than 90% suffer from RP), MCTD (more than 80%), SLE (more than 30%), dermatomyositis (more than 25%), and rheumatoid arthritis (more than 10%).

Buerger's Disease (Thromboangiitis Obliterans). Upper extremity involvement is frequently reported in Buerger's disease, with 20 to 50% of these patients demonstrating secondary RP with evidence of obstructive lesions in the digits.

Mechanical Injury. Trauma-induced RP can occur with frostbite or crush injury and with traumatic aneurysms of the radial and ulnar arteries. A vascular steal syndrome following dialysis shunting may also cause a severe form of RP, which leads to severe distal ischemic injury. The "hypothenar hammer syndrome" occurs with repetitive injury to the ulnar artery (pounding or twisting) at the level of the hypothenar prominence that results in injury to the ulnar artery and/or the development of aneurysms. Patients typically present with RP confined to a few digits of the dominant hand (fourth and fifth digits) and an abnormal Allen's test (owing to occlusion of the distal ulnar artery.

Thoracic Outlet Syndrome. TOS is a rare cause of RP and most often results in vasomotor symptoms that can be confused historically for RP. True vascular TOS is extremely rare, and more often, compression of the neurovascular bundle in the neck and shoulder region may result in neurovascular symptoms that may be mistaken for RP. Unilateral presentations should raise the possibility of this disorder. Diagnostic difficulties may arise with primary RP and a cervical rib that may be an incidental finding. See Chapters 16 and 17 for diagnosis and management of this disorder.

Arterial Disorders. RP may occur as a consequence of embolic phenomena from proximal large-vessel involvement due to atherosclerosis, aneurysmal disease, and vasculitis (Takayasu's and giant cell arteritis). A high index of suspicion for embolic disease must be maintained, particularly in the setting of unilateral symptoms. Patients with atherosclerosis are generally older, unless they have severe dyslipidemias or long-standing tobacco use.

Toxins. Heavy metal poisoning (arsenic, mercury, and lead) and exposure to vinyl chloride may cause secondary RP. Exposure to vinyl chloride causes acroosteolysis-a disorder associated with resorption of the distal phalangeal tufts, a finding similar to that seen with PSS. Angiography reveals multiple arterial stenosis and occlusions along with hypervascularity adjacent to areas of bony resorption.

Rheologic and Hematological Causes. Diseases that alter the macromolecular or cellular components of blood and increase blood viscosity may contribute to the development of RP. Polycythemia, thrombocythemia, and chronic myeloid leukemia may all be associated with RP. Cryoglobulinemia, cryofibrinogenemia, cold agglutinins, and paraproteinemia may also present with RP but are rarer causes.

Drugs. The ergot derivative bromocriptine mesylate, used to treat Parkinson's disease; drugs used to treat migraine headaches; and amphetamines are all reported to aggravate arterial vasospasm. RP may also occur with β blockers due to unopposed α-adrenergic vasoconstriction. Chemotherapeutic agents and interferon α/β may also precipitate RP.

Risk of Progression of Raynaud's Phenomenon and Prognosis

In patients with RP and no associated symptoms and normal serology (normal ESR and normal ANA), the risk of an eventual diagnosis of a rheumatologic disorder is 2 to 3% over 5 years, while the risk of progression of symptoms is 6% over a 10-year period. The risk of an eventual rheumatologic disorder being diagnosed at the time of initial evaluation or in the future in the presence of RP and a positive ANA is high (above 50%). The 2-year risk of a rheumatologic disease in patients with RP and/or an abnormal nail fold examination and positive autoantibodies is 15 to 20%. The risk for development of secondary etiologies with an initial diagnosis of primary RP and borderline elevations in ANA titers remains unknown. A number of specific autoantibodies are much more helpful in predicting risk of eventual diagnosis of a rheumatologic disease. The most useful tests include anti-Smith (anti-Sm), which is predictive for development of SLE; Scl-70 (predicts PSS); and anticentromere antibodies (predicts CREST). The presence of antibodies to antiribonucleoprotein (anti-RNP) (MCTD) is predictive of severe RP compared with those with other serologic markers.

Diagnosis

Figure 18.1 details a suggested approach for the workup of patients with RP. The initial diagnosis of RP is clinical. The three screening questions that are often very helpful in differentiating this condition from other disorders are (a) Are your fingers unusually sensitive to cold? (b) Do your fingers change color when they are exposed to cold temperatures? and (c) Do they turn white, blue, or both? The diagnosis of RP is excluded if the answers to questions 2 and 3 are negative. The history should include a detailed review of symptoms, comorbid illnesses, occupational/exposure history (vinyl chloride exposure), trauma history (hypothenar hammer syndrome or vibratory tool history), and complete drug history (medications that may provoke vasospasm, β blockers, etc.), including recreational drug and tobacco use. The differentiation of primary from secondary RP is through a process of exclusion and through careful physical examination in conjunction with vascular and blood testing. Physical examination should focus on signs of systemic disease as well as evidence of large-vessel disease (absent pulses and abnormal Allen's test [Chapter 16]). Patients with PSS and other rheumatologic diseases may demonstrate enlarged and deformed capillary loops, surrounded by relatively avascular areas

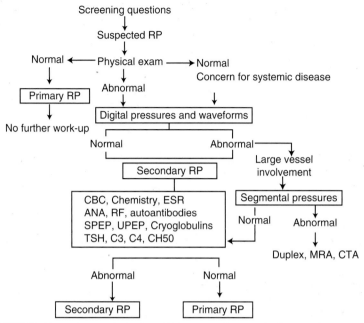

FIGURE 18-1. Approach to RP. ANA, antinuclear antibody; RF, rheumatoid factor; C3, C4 and CH50, complement 3, 4, and hemolytic complement 50; SPEP and UPEP, serum protein and urinary protein electrophoresis; MRA, magnetic resonance angiography; TSH, thyroid-stimulating hormone.

on capillary microscopy of the nail folds (scleroderma pattern). Digital ulcerations are most commonly caused by vasculitis (50 to 75% of all cases; half of the vasculitis cases are caused by PSS/CREST), Buerger's, and atherosclerosis-related complications (embolism). Segmental pressures are helpful in the assessment of proximal large-vessel disease (atherosclerosis) that may be associated with RP. Unilateral RP symptoms and signs of ischemia should raise the possibility of proximal large-vessel etiologies (atherosclerosis, vasculitis), TOS, and thromboangiitis obliterans (TAO). Digital pressures and waveforms are helpful in differentiating primary from secondary RP in patients presenting with a clinical diagnosis of RP. The finger to ipsilateral brachial index, measured at the proximal phalanx, averages 1.0 in normal subjects (range 0.8 to 1.3) with patients with obstructive lesions demonstrating an index below 0.7 or absolute finger pressures of less than 70 mm Hg. Since the presence of normal pressures at the proximal phalanx does not rule out more distal involvement, digital waveforms recorded by a photoplethysmograph are obtained at the same time. Normal contours are very specific for absence of obstructive lesions. Patients with primary RP usually have normal digital pressures and waveforms. In contrast, patients with secondary RP have concomitant digital obstructive disease and have abnormal finger pressures and/or waveforms. This could be symmetric and bilateral as in secondary RP due to rheumatologic or other systemic disease or asymmetric in cases associated with peripheral embolization, occupational causes, or trauma. Unilateral symptoms in a patient with bilateral abnormalities of digital waveforms and pressures suggest a systemic disorder associated with RP. RP symptoms with normal waveforms and pressures in conjunction with abnormal capillaroscopy and/or systemic symptoms may suggest a secondary etiology (nascent or undetected), and this may warrant additional testing. In general, invasive studies such as contrast arteriography should be reserved for situations when there is a high index of suspicion for a proximal arterial embolic source. The lab testing for secondary causes of RP is outlined in Figure 18.1. Cold immersion testing is rarely required for the diagnosis of RP. The test measures the time to recovery of skin temperature in the digits (the Porter method) or the digital artery pressure (the Nielsen method).

Treatment

The approach to the patient with RP depends on the underlying cause and severity of symptoms. In general, therapy can be categorized as (a) conservative, (b) pharmacological intervention, or (c) sympathectomy. In all cases of secondary RP, the underlying etiology should be treated and inciting stimuli (such as drugs) removed. Figure 18.2 provides treatment approach to RP.

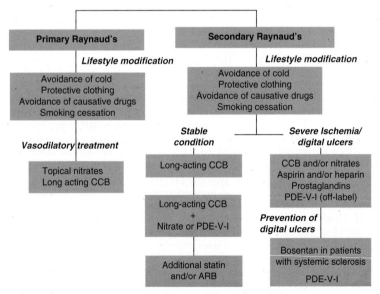

FIGURE 18-2.   Treatment approach in RP. (PG, prostaglandin)

Conservative Care

This approach is sufficient in treating cases with mild RP (mostly primary RP) and involves reassurance and an explanation that this disorder is a benign process and does not result in amputation. Patients should be advised to wear warm clothing in order to reduce risk of symptoms from cold exposure. Patients may benefit from moving to warmer climes. Cigarette smoking or even rooms filled with cigarette smoke may elicit symptoms and should be avoided. Electrically heated gloves and socks are often very helpful and may be used. Chemical hand warmers may be used with the appropriate precautions. Studies have been conducted evaluating whether behavioral therapy, such as biofeedback training, results in decreased vasospastic attacks. The current data are insufficient to recommend routine use in patients with RP. Treatment of the underlying condition is important such as the treatment of rheumatic disease. Although this may be associated with a reduction in the severity of attacks of RP, the frequency of attacks and severity may be difficult to predict.

Pharmacological Intervention

Table 18.4 lists pharmacological interventions to treat RP. A number of drugs have been used in this disorder. The benefits of therapy in general are modest and the results are better in primary RP compared to secondary RP.

Vasodilator Therapies. These are the most widely used and at the present time the most effective. Topical nitrates as transdermal patches or as different cream or gel formulations as well as in oral applications may be effective in RP. Sustained release patches with glycerol trinitrate have been shown to be effective and demonstrated to significantly reduce severity and number of Raynaud's attacks in patients with primary and also in patients with secondary RP. However, headache limits the use of topical nitrates.

Calcium channel blockers (CCB) may be of benefit with prior clinical trials demonstrating some effects in reducing frequency and severity in primary RP by dihydropyridine CCB. The typical starting dose of nifedipine is 30 mg/d, preferably administered as a sustained release preparation and gradually increased if no improvement to as much as 90 mg/d. Patients should be warned regarding possible side effects including hypotension, light-headedness, peripheral edema, and indigestion. Longer acting CCB such as amlodipine may be effective and are better tolerated but are not well studied in this condition. Of note, verapamil was not shown to be effective in a small series of patients with RP due to scleroderma. Overall, if dihydripyridines are ineffective, there is no role for alternate agents in the same class. In patients with a CREST syndrome, CCB can reduce sphincter tone in the lower esophagus and should be used with caution.

Phosphodiesterase V Inhibitors. PDE V inhibitors have been demonstrated to have beneficial effects in primary and secondary RP in several studies and case reports. In a single-center trial with 16 patients with secondary

TABLE 18.4

PHARMACOLOGIC THERAPIES IN RP

Agents	Mechanism of Action	Dosage	Side Effects
Calcium channel blockers			
Nifedipine SR	Vasodilator through	30–120 mg/d	Reflex tachycardia,
Amlodipine	blockade of L-type	5–20 mg/d	flushing, dizzi-
Felodipine	calcium channels	2.5–10 mg/d	ness, hypotension,
Isradipine		2.5–5.0 mg/d	constipation,
Diltiazem SR		120–300 mg/d	peripheral edema
Nitrates			
Topical nitroglycerin	Nitric oxide generation and smooth muscle relaxation	2% ointment applied locally to fingers	Headache, dizziness, and hypotension
Miscellaneous			
Prazosin	An $\alpha2$ agonist and vasodilator	1–5 mg/d	Dizziness, hypotension
Fluoxetine	Selective serotonin reuptake inhibitor	20–40 mg d	Sleep disturbances, impotence
Losartan	Angiotensin type 1 receptor antagonist	25–100 mg/d	Hypotension
Prostaglandins			
PDE V Inhibitors			
Sildenafil	Smooth muscle relaxation	50 mg b.i.d.	Dizziness, stuffy nose, priapism
Tadalafil		20 mg q.o.d.	Dizziness, stuffy nose, priapism, myalgias
Prostanoids			
Epoprostenol	Vasodilator prostanoids are used only in critical upper extremity ischemia associated with secondary RP	0.5–6 ng/kg/min IV for 2–7 d	Diarrhea, flushing, headache, hypotension, and rash
Alprostadil		0.1–0.4 µg/kg/ min IV, 6–24 h for 2–7 d	
Iloprost		0.5–2.0 ng/kg/min for 2–7 d	

RP resistant to vasodilatory treatment, 4-week treatment with 50 mg b.i.d. reduced number of attacks and mean Raynaud's condition score. Tadalafil at a dose of 20 mg q.o.d. may be beneficial in treatment-resistant secondary RP. In a randomized controlled crossover study, this dose on top of CCB resulted in a reduction in frequency and duration of attacks in conjunction with improvement in digital ulcers when administered over a duration of 6 weeks.

Statins and Rho-kinase Inhibitors. There is no role for these agents in primary RP. In cases of secondary RP with tissue necrosis or secondary RP with ongoing cardiovascular risk factors, these drugs may be considered on an individual basis. Statins display pleiotropic effects on endothelial function, which may be beneficial also in RP. In patients with secondary RP due to systemic sclerosis, 40 mg of atorvastatin reduced digital ulcers. More data are necessary to judge the definite role of this class of drugs. Rho-kinase inhibitors are not approved in the United States. Where available, Fasudil may be a potential consideration, in light of its known effects in alleviating vasospasm and increasing nitric oxide–dependent vasodilation.

Other Vasodilator Approaches. Adrenergic receptor blockers such as prazosin and doxazosin may decrease episodes of vasospasm in primary and secondary RP, but these drugs are only modestly effective. There are case reports suggesting benefit for the serotonin reuptake inhibitors such as fluoxetine and the phosphodiesterase 3 inhibitor cilostazol.

Prostaglandin Analogues. Intravenous iloprost, epoprostenol, and alprostadil may be beneficial in severe secondary RP associated with tissue necrosis and may aid in healing. These agents may also be used in the event of an acute ischemic crisis as may occur in cases of RP associated with rheumatologic disease.

Side effects of prostaglandins include headache, flush, and nausea and are dose dependent. Low-dose treatment (0.5 ng/kg/min of iloprost) may be equally effective to high-dose treatment (2.0 ng/kg/min iloprost).

Antiplatelet Agents

There is no role for these agents in primary RP, but aspirin may be considered in severe secondary RP with digital skin necrosis and ulcerations based on anecdotal data.

Sympathectomy

Sympathectomy has been a treatment of RP for a number of years with adoption of local and less invasive techniques over surgical approaches.

Chemical Sympathectomy. This can be achieved by the injection of an anesthetic locally or near the appropriate cervical or lumbar sympathetic ganglia. A local digital or wrist block with lidocaine or bupivacaine, without epinephrine, can reverse vasoconstriction. Although this procedure may be successful in reversing acute vasospasm, there is no sustained benefit.

Cervical Sympathectomy. This is rarely recommended for RP because of the risks of surgical complications and lack of sustained benefit. Although morbidity and complications are reduced with the less invasive endoscopic technique, the long-term symptom recurrence rate is not improved over the open technique.

Localized Digital Sympathectomy. Digital sympathectomy appears to be a reasonable treatment in patients with ischemia or severe RP but only after medical therapy has been exhausted. The effectiveness of this technique appears to depend on the expertise of the surgeon. The procedure involves stripping of the adventitial layer away from the affected arteries thereby, theoretically, irreversibly interrupting sympathetically mediated vasoconstriction. The extent of the surgery may vary from adventitial dissection of the digital arteries alone or that of the palmar common digital arteries, superficial palmar arch combined with denervation of the radial and ulnar arteries. Additional procedures, including vascular reconstruction, digital debridement, and amputation, can be performed at the time of the surgery, if indicated.

COMPLEX REGIONAL PAIN SYNDROME

Introduction

Complex regional pain syndrome (CRPS), formerly known as RSD or Sudeck's atrophy, is a regional, posttraumatic, neuropathic pain problem that most often affects one or more limbs. The term causalgia was previously used to describe the characteristic burning pain that is typical of this disorder, most commonly seen after limb injury that results in damage to a major peripheral nerve. The term CRPS was proposed in 1993 by a consensus conference to replace numerous, often misleading eponyms and to convey the complexity of this disorder (variable and dynamic presentation), its regional presentation (distribution pattern that is wider than the area of original injury), and pain that is characteristically disproportionate to the initiating event.

Clinical Features

Classification

CRPS is subdivided into type 1 and type 2 (Table 18.5). The clinical features of the two types are identical. The distinguishing feature is the presence of a major peripheral nerve injury in patients with type 2. Diagnostic criteria for CRPS types 1 and 2 are listed in Table 18.5.

Etiology

There are three precipitating causes for CRPS. These may be categorized as (a) traumatic, (b) nontraumatic, and (c) idiopathic. Most cases of CRPS are type 2 and result from clearly identifiable episodes of trauma such as burns, crush injury fractures, and dislocations. Nontraumatic causes

TABLE 18.5

CLASSIFICATION OF CRPS

Type 1
- Pain that develops after an initial painful event that may or may not have been traumatic
- Allodynia, hyperalgesia, or spontaneous pain is present and is not congruent with the distribution of a single peripheral nerve
- History of edema, skin blood flow, or sudomotor abnormalities in the painful region
- No other concomitant conditions account for the pain

Type 2
- Pain that develops after an identifiable trauma or nerve injury
- Allodynia, hyperalgesia, or spontaneous pain is present and is not congruent with the distribution of a single peripheral nerve
- History of edema, skin blood flow abnormalities, or sudomotor abnormalities in the painful region
- No other concomitant conditions account for the pain

---

include myocardial infarction, deep venous thrombosis, prolonged bed rest, and neoplasms. CRPS 1 following a heart attack was referred to as the shoulder-hand syndrome.

Clinical Symptoms and Signs

The clinical presentation of CRPS is variable and the syndrome may present with a combination of symptoms and signs in children and adults. The salient aspects of the disorder are as follows:

1. The pain is described as a burning or throbbing discomfort arnd is not in a neural distribution. It often extends beyond the distribution of the peripheral nerve.
2. Allodynia and hyperalgesia in response to normal sensory stimuli. Occasionally, hyperpathia is seen, characterized by disproportionately increased pain response to a stimulus.
3. Sudomotor and vasomotor instability. Sweating could be increased, decreased, or unchanged, while the extremity may be reported as being warm and red or alternately cold and blue.
4. Swelling that may be intermittent or constant.
5. Trophic changes that include atrophy of skin and nails.
6. Motor and joint symptoms including tremor, weakness, and joint stiffness.

Diagnosis

No specific test or feature is diagnostic for CRPS. Thus, identifying the constellation of historical features and clinical examination findings and ruling out other disorders by appropriate laboratory testing are important.

Vascular studies (when vasomotor signs and symptoms predominate), EEG (neuropathic symptoms and signs), radiographic studies to rule out bone or soft-tissue pathology, and blood tests to rule out infection or a rheumatologic condition are important.

Diagnostic testing in CRPS should include the following: (a) Sensory evaluation. (b) Sudomotor and vasomotor studies using infrared thermography to measure temperature and sweat studies on the affected area. The latter may employ subjective measures such as indicator-starch powder; the quantitative sudomotor axon reflex test is a provocative test that determines the sweat output in response to an iontophoresis cholinergic challenge, such as acetylcholine or methacholine. (c) Radiologic testing with technetium-99m bone scanning may reveal evidence of increased uptake, while bone films may reveal osteoporosis. These findings generally take months to develop. (d) Diagnostic sympathetic block. The analgesic response to a sympathetic nerve block is considered by some to be the most important diagnostic tool. However, based on the new system (CRPS), sympathetic dysfunction may or may not play a role in the etiopathogenesis since a positive response to a block is not essential to diagnose CRPS. A diagnostic sympathetic block should be considered for patients with clinical evidence of vasomotor or sudomotor dysfunction and severe pain. A lumbar paravertebral sympathetic block is performed for lower extremity symptoms, while a cervicothoracic block (often called stellate ganglion block) or upper thoracic sympathetic block is performed for upper extremity symptoms. It is important to obtain selective blockade of the sympathetic nerves and to avoid inadvertent blockade of the somatic nerves as the pain relief may then be erroneously ascribed to the sympathetic block, and this may lead to inappropriate diagnosis and treatment.

Treatment

Physical therapy is the cornerstone and first-line treatment for CRPS and is one of the few interventions shown to be effective in controlled studies. The goal of medications is to facilitate participation in physical therapy. The medications that have been found to be useful for treating CRPS include antidepressant agents such as doxepin or nortriptyline (both at 10 to 75 mg/d), gabapentin (100 mg/d initially and then 600 to 1,200 mg t.i.d.), opioids (oxycodone or hydrocodone), and corticosteroids. A recent small trial suggests that IVIG, 0.5 g/kg, can reduce pain in refractory CRPS. Studies are required to determine the best immunoglobulin dose, the duration of effect, and when repeated treatments are needed. Patients with moderate to severe pain that does not respond to medication who experience marked improvement after a diagnostic sympathetic block (sympathetically maintained pain) are candidates for regional anesthetic blocks. The two major types of regional techniques are sympathetic nerve blocks and combined somatic/sympathetic nerve blocks. A series of daily or every other day sympathetic ganglion blocks with use of local anesthetic for 1 to 3 weeks is the preferred approach. Cervical and lumbar sympathetic trunk blocks can be performed as a series of intermittent blocks, or a catheter can be placed next to the sympathetic trunk and local anesthetic boluses performed daily. To maximize advantage of the analgesic effects of the blocks, physical therapy should be initiated immediately after the block. If the benefit from blockade is limited, neurolysis with either neurolytic injections or radiofrequency ablation may be considered.

ERYTHERMALGIA

Introduction

Erythermalgia (EM) is a disorder of the extremities but may involve other body parts such as the face and is characterized by increased temperature, burning pain, and erythema. The original terminology for this disorder was "erythromelalgia" based on the Greek words *erythros* (red), *melos* (extremities), and *algos* (pain) that are characteristic for this disorder. Since the term eythromelalgia did not incorporate the increased skin temperature as an integral part of the condition, the term "erythermalgia" (*thermé* heat) was suggested. The term "erythroprosopalgia" (*prosopon*, face) describes "facial EM." Figure 18.3 illustrates the typical features of EM.

Clinical Features

Signs and Symptoms

The diagnosis of EM is historical and is based on an assessment of symptoms. Although no uniform diagnostic criteria exist, the following criteria proposed by Thompson are used for the diagnosis. The criteria are as follows: (a) burning extremity pain, (b) pain aggravated by warming, (c) pain relieved by cooling, (d) erythema of affected skin, and (e) increased temperature of affected skin during attacks and in association with pain and erythema. Symptoms are intermittent, usually involve the lower extremities, and are typically symmetric. Pruritus and "pins and needles" may precede

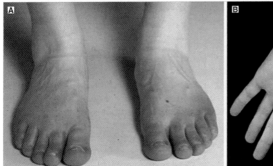
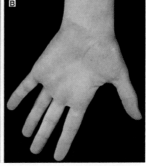

FIGURE 18-3. Erythermalgia affecting the feet (A) and the hand (B). (Reprinted from Sandroni P, Davis MDP et al. Combination gel of 1% Amitriptyline and 0.5% Ketamine To Treat Refractory Erythromelalgia: A New Treatment Option? *Arch Dermatol* 2006;142:283–286, with permission). (See color insert.)

the burning pain. The duration varies from minutes to several hours, or in severe cases, continuous symptoms and signs are seen. Symptoms may be precipitated by hot weather, dependency of lower extremities, exercise, excessive warmth (sleeping under bedcovers, wearing shoes and gloves), and alcohol ingestion. Relief is obtained by lowering skin temperature or by elevating the affected extremity. Relief with cooling is mandatory for the diagnosis.

Classification

EM may be primary or secondary to an identifiable disorder. Primary EM usually occurs in middle-aged individuals but may be seen at any age; men are affected more commonly than women. The most common causes of secondary EM are myeloproliferative disorders, especially polycythemia vera and essential thrombocythemia. EM may precede the diagnosis of a secondary disorder by several years. In all new cases, underlying causes should be sought and appropriate laboratory studies should be performed periodically. Table 18.6 lists conditions associated with EM.

Pathophysiology

The pathogenesis of primary EM is not entirely known. A localized defect in the vascular and neural function of the involved skin has been proposed. Arteriovenous shunting in the affected skin, with subsequent hypoxia and metabolic deficits, may play a significant role. A familial form (autosomal dominant) of primary EM exists called SCN9A-related EM and involves mutations in the SCN9A gene encoding the sodium channel protein $Na_v1.7$ subunit. $Na_v1.7$ is abundantly expressed in nociceptive neurons and their nerve endings, close to trigger zones where receptor potentials are generated, and plays an important role in pain. A role for $Na_v1.7$ in inflammatory pain has been demonstrated in a series of neuron class-specific knockout experiments in mice in which inflammatory pain responses were markedly attenuated after $Na_v1.7$ was deleted in dorsal root ganglion cells.

Differential Diagnosis

With a good history and classic findings, the diagnosis of EM is easily made. EM may be confused with CRPS and with neuropathic pain. The former is also associated with symptoms such as heat, erythema, and burning pain, and these patients may sometimes soak affected limbs in ice water. Although CRPS usually occurs after an injury, some cases may occur spontaneously. Conversely, although EM typically occurs spontaneously, it can occur following injury. EM generally is bilateral and is typically intermittent as opposed to CRPS, which may be continuous. EM may be confused with neuropathic syndromes, especially because the pain sometimes precedes erythema. To compound matters further, EM may occur with neuropathic syndromes such as sciatica and skin biopsies from patients with EM have revealed evidence of small- and large-fiber neuropathies in a high proportion of patients.

TABLE 18.6

CLASSIFICATION OF EM

Primary
Secondary
   Hematologic/malignancy
      Polycythemia, thrombocythemia
      Leukemia, particularly chronic myeloid leukemia
      Hereditary spherocytosis
      Pernicious anemia
      Thrombotic thrombocytopenic purpura
      Lymphoma
   Connective tissue disorders
      Rheumatoid arthritis
      Systemic lupus erythematosus
      Mixed connective tissue disorder
      Sjogren's syndrome
   Infectious diseases
      AIDS
      Recurrent bacterial infections
      Syphilis
   Musculoskeletal and neurologic disorders
      Neuropathies
      Multiple sclerosis
      Spinal cord disease
   Drug induced
      Iodide contrast
      Vaccines: influenza, hepatitis
      CCB, bromocriptine, norephedrine, pergolide, ticlopidine
   Vascular and systemic disorders
      Diabetes
      Atherosclerosis
      Cholesterol embolization
   Traumatic and cold exposure

Treatment

The treatment for EM includes conservative, pharmacologic, and surgical treatment approaches. The ideal therapeutic approach remains to be defined, but the majority of patients respond to conservative treatment in conjunction with pharmacologic approaches. Irritable nociceptors are likely involved in the maintenance of pain in erythromelalgia. The extreme sensitiveness of the skin (i.e., allodynia) in these patients clearly supports this concept. However, it does not explain the complexity of the pain, which most likely involves central sensitization. Since evidence indicates that altered hyperexcitable sodium channels are expressed in inherited painful neuropathies and inherited erythromelalgia, one approach is to block these channels locally with appropriate approaches.

Conservative approaches include counseling patients to avoid precipitating factors and treatment of underlying secondary causes (if any). Cold-water exposure may temporarily relieve symptoms but is not useful for long-term care as an immersion injury can ensue. Topical lidocaine patches may be helpful and work through blockade of sodium channels. Oral aspirin and misoprostol may be beneficial in patients with a secondary cause such as thrombocytosis or erythrocytosis but is not beneficial in the primary form. Recently a topical applied combination of 1% amitriptyline hydrochloride and 0.5% ketamine hydrochloride applied up to four or five times daily has been shown to be of benefit. Gabapentin may also provide benefit. Other options include sertraline, amitriptyline, imipramine, paroxetine, and fluoxetine, usually begun at low doses. Responses are quite variable but through trial and error, substantial benefit can be achieved. Invasive approaches are reserved for severe cases and are similar to treatment of CRPS.

ACROCYANOSIS

Introduction

Acrocyanosis is a disorder involving bluish discoloration of the digits of the hands and, less frequently, of the feet. Signs and symptoms of vasospasm may intensify during cold exposure and hyperemia with rubor may develop on warming. The resultant decrease in blood flow and an increase in oxygen extraction are thought to produce cyanosis. Acrocyanosis affects men and women equally and typically occurs between the ages of 20 and 45 years. The etiology of this condition is thought to be due to vasospasm in small cutaneous arteries and arterioles, causing compensatory dilation of the capillaries and postcapillary venules.

Clinical Features

This disorder is distinguished from RP as it occurs on a persistent basis, rather than being episodic, and is generally devoid of other features associated with RP including pain. Patients with this condition do not routinely have blanching, and there is proximal extension beyond the digits to involve the hands or feet. Other areas of the body such as the forehead, nose, cheeks, earlobes, elbows, and knees may be also affected. The prognosis is extremely good with this disorder, and the loss of digital tissue is extremely uncommon. Hyperhidrosis often complicates the disorder during the warmer months.

Treatment

The treatment involves dressing warmly and wearing gloves in order to avoid reflux sympathetic vasoconstriction during body cooling. Pharmacologic intervention is rarely necessary or beneficial.

LIVEDO

Introduction

Livedo is a dermopathy characterized by a violaceous reticular or "netlike" mottling that surrounds a pallorous central core of skin. Livedo most commonly involves the lower extremities yet the upper extremities can be affected as well. The term "livedo reticularis" is frequently used in an arbitrary fashion. It is very useful to think of livedo in terms of the anatomy and physiology of the cutaneous microvascular system. Arterial inflow consists of a series of ascending arterioles that rise perpendicularly to the skin surface. Each arteriole divides to form a capillary bed, which in turn drains into venous plexus at the periphery of the bed. Blood flows from the arteriole at the center of the bed to venules at the periphery of the bed. Anything that increases the visibility of the venous plexus can result in a livedo appearance. Venodilation and deoxygenation of blood in the venous plexus are the two main causes of increased visibility of the plexus. Examples of potential causes of venodilation include altered autonomic nervous system function, circulating venodilators, and local hypoxia. Deoxygenation is mainly caused by decreased arteriolar inflow or increased resistance to venous outflow. Examples of causes of decreased arteriolar inflow are vasospasm caused by cold or autonomic input, arterial thrombosis, and increased blood viscosity. Venous thrombosis and increased blood viscosity are causes of increasing venous outflow resistance.

Clinical Features

It is imperative that a clinician differentiates between the frequently benign, often reversible physiologic livedo reticularis and the pathologic, permanent form of livedo called livedo racemosa. In livedo reticularis, the discoloration is exemplified by symmetric, regular, "unbroken" rings, whereas livedo racemosa is marked by irregular "broken" rings. Livedo reticularis symmetrically affects the extremities, whereas livedo racemosa often involves the limbs in an asymmetric fashion. Additionally, livedo racemosa tends to be more generalized than livedo reticularis often involving the buttocks, trunk, and even the feet and hands. Figures 18.4 and 18.5 contrast the regular and irregular cones of both forms of livedo. Livedo reticularis and livedo racemosa are often associated with vasospastic digits and/or acrocyanosis. Whereas patients with livedo reticularis usually have an unremarkable dermatologic exam, subjects with livedo racemosa may manifest associated purpura, nodules, macules, ulcerations, and/or atrophie blanche–type scarring. Table 18.7 outlines various causes of livedo racemosa. In the majority of cases of livedo reticularis, laboratory testing is typically negative and is usually unwarranted. The need for additional serology in a patient with livedo racemosa (and rare cases of livedo reticularis) should be directed by the history and clinical assessment. A large punch or wedge biopsy of the deep reticular dermis and subcutaneous fat is sometimes helpful in identifying the secondary cause of livedo racemosa. Sneddon's syndrome is a rare entity characterized by livedo and

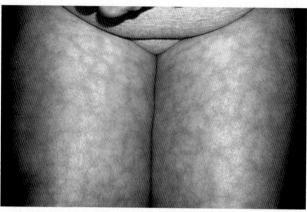

FIGURE 18-4.   Livedo reticularis. Note the symmetric, regular, "unbroken" rings. (See color insert.)

cerebrovascular events including stroke. Sneddon's syndrome typically affects women before or during middle age, with the first cerebrovascular event typically occurring before age 45.

Treatment

Other than cold avoidance, medical therapy for primary livedo reticularis is usually unwarranted. In rare instances, vasodilator therapy

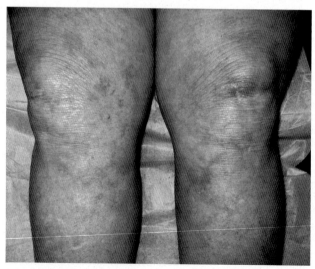

FIGURE 18-5.   Livedo racemosa. Note the asymmetric and irregular appearance of the cones. (See color insert.)

TABLE 18.7
CONDITIONS ASSOCIATED WITH LIVEDO RACEMOSA

Antiphospholipid antibody syndrome
Sneddon's syndrome
Autoimmune disease/vasculitis
Myeloproliferative syndromes (polycythemia vera, essential thrombocytosis)
Paraproteinemias
Cryopathies (cryoglobulinemia/cryofibrinogenemia/cold agglutinin disease)
Atheroembolic disease
Calciphylaxis
Hyperoxaluria
Atrial myxoma
Erythema ab igne
Livedoid vasculopathy
Infections/disseminated intravascular coagulation/septic emboli

may be tried in the patient who is socially inhibited by the cosmetic appearance of the disorder. Treatment of livedo racemosa should be directed toward the underlying disorder. Subjects with livedo racemosa and the antiphospholipid antibody syndrome with thrombosis require anticoagulant therapy.

PERNIO (CHILBLAINS)

Introduction

Patients with severe cold exposure may develop a vasculitic disorder called pernio. The acute form involves raised red to blue lesions on the lower parts of the leg, frequently the shins and the toes following cold exposure.

Clinical Features

The lesions are classically pruritic with an associated burning sensation that may blister and ulcerate. The lesions usually resolve in 7 to 10 days, frequently leaving a residual pigmented area. Women are more commonly affected than men, and occurrences are usually between the ages of 15 and 30 years. The chronic form of pernio, called "chilbains," typically involves the lower extremity in areas that are repeatedly exposed to cold. The lesions are usually composed of crops of raised erythematous patches ranging in size from 2 to 10 mm. Similar to the acute form, lesions gradually blister and ulcerate and are often very painful. The blister base may be blue, violet, or hemorrhagic. Upon healing, scarring and pigmentation may occur. Pathologic evaluation of these lesions reveals a vasculitis characterized by intimal proliferation and perivascular infiltration of mononuclear and polymorphonuclear leukocytes. Also, giant cells may be present in the subcutaneous tissue.

Treatment

The treatment of this condition mainly involves avoiding cold exposure, and patients are advised to dress warmly. The sympathetic nervous system is not thought to be involved in the pathology and, thus, sympathetic-blocking drugs and sympathectomy are not effective. CCB such as nifedipine may reduce the time to resolution of existing lesions and prevent development of new lesions.

CHOLESTEROL EMBOLISM

Introduction

Cholesterol embolism occurs secondary to showering of cholesterol crystals usually secondary to invasive procedures such as coronary or vascular catheterization, coronary artery bypass graft surgery, and percutaneous coronary intervention, measured after surgery or anticoagulation. Sometimes, the provocative stimulus may be absent or hard to recognize. The primary organ systems involved with cholesterol embolism include the kidneys, skin, and the gastrointestinal tract. Cholesterol embolism most commonly occurs in patients with significant vascular disease, diabetes, and history of tobacco use.

Clinical Features

The classic clinical presentation of cholesterol embolism includes livedo reticularis and acute renal failure, in the setting of normal peripheral pulses. However, the presentation may be atypical with symptoms such as fever or myalgias, gastrointestinal bleeding, and multiorgan involvement that may mimic necrotizing vasculitis, and dust may not be readily recognized.

Livedo reticularis is characterized by a bluish "lacelike" pattern that is most commonly seen in the lower legs and feet bilaterally. This may extend to the thighs, buttocks, trunk, and, rarely, the upper extremities. Purpuric skin eruptions, subcutaneous nodules, and, rarely, ulcerations may also be present. These manifestations are possibly secondary to an inflammatory reaction surrounding cholesterol crystals. Blue toe syndrome is a characteristic manifestation of cholesterol embolism characterized by blue-black or violaceous discoloration of the toes and feet. The lesions are painful as the changes are secondary to decreased blood supply with secondary tissue ischemia. Laboratory findings are often nonspecific and peripheral eosinophilia can occur but is not consistent. Skin muscle or renal biopsy demonstrating needle-shaped cholesterol clefts within intravascular microthrombi is the most specific finding but may not be possible.

Treatment

If the source of embolization can be definitively identified, surgery to remove the source may be a consideration. However, in most patients, medical therapy options are limited to traditional atherosclerosis risk reduction measures including statin therapy. In severe cases, progression to dialysis and gangrene necessitating amputation may occur.

PYODERMA GANGRENOSUM

Introduction

Pyoderma gangrenosum (PG) is a painful, noninfectious ulcerative cutaneous disorder that most commonly affects the lower extremities.

Clinical Features

The diagnosis is made by recognizing the characteristic clinical manifestations in the setting of a causative systemic disease yet excluding other causes of similar-appearing ulcerations. PG often evolves in the setting of systemic illnesses such as inflammatory bowel disease, rheumatologic disorders, and lymphoproliferative disease. PG often begins as isolated or multiple pustules (which can be mistaken for a spider bite) that evolve into painful large necrotic ulcerations with undermined erythrocyanotic margins (Fig. 18.6). The ulcerations of PG sometimes evolve after trauma to the skin, which connotes the process of pathergy.

An appropriate workup for PG should include routine blood work including a CBC with peripheral smear, comprehensive chemistry profile, hepatitis profile, serum and/or urine protein electrophoresis, and a urinalysis. An autoimmune/vasculitis and antiphospholipid antibody profile is typically needed as well. If indicated, a bone marrow biopsy should be obtained if a lymphoproliferative disorder is suspected. Cultures of the ulcer for not only bacteria but also fungi and atypical mycobacteria are needed. Finally, a skin biopsy should be obtained in all cases. Although the histopathologic findings in the disorder typically reveal marked yet nonspecific neutrophilic infiltration, a biopsy is useful to exclude other ulcerative etiologies.

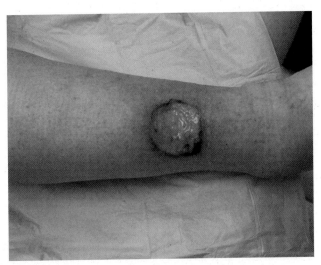

FIGURE 18-6. Pyoderma gangrenosum (See color insert.)

Treatment

There is no definitive therapy that is consistently effective in the setting of PG. Treating the associated systemic disease will sometimes mitigate PG ulcerations. Topical treatment includes topical/intralesional corticosteroids, cromolyn sodium 2% solution, tacrolimus/pimecrolimus, nitrogen mustard, and 5-aminosalicylic acid. Systemic therapies are diverse and include corticosteroids, dapsone, cyclosporine, cyclophosphamide, mycophenolate mofetil, azathioprine, tacrolimus, chlorambucil, thalidomide, and tumor necrosis factor-alpha inhibitors. In refractory cases, intravenous medications can be tried that include pulsed methylprednisolone, intravenous immune globulin, pulsed cyclophosphamide, and infliximab. The clinician should remain cognizant that surgical debridement and/or skin grafting should typically be avoided as these endeavors can provoke the pathergic phenomenon and subsequent wound deterioration.

PRACTICAL POINTS

- The presence of advanced ischemia (tissue necrosis and gangrene) rules out primary RP.

- The 2-year risk of a rheumatologic disease in patients with RP and/or an abnormal nail fold exam and positive autoantibodies is 15 to 20%.

- Unilateral RP should raise the possibility of embolic (proximal artery) or traumatic causes due to recreation or vocation (hypothenar hammer or vibrational white finger).

- Unilateral symptoms in a patient with bilateral abnormalities of digital waveforms and pressures suggest a systemic disorder associated with RP including Buerger's disease.

- Acrocyanosis is persistent while RP is intermittent. Hyperhidrosis often complicates the disorder during the warmer months.

- The lesions of pernio are classically pruritic with an associated burning sensation.

- A history of trauma or injury should be carefully sought in CRPS.

- Response to a diagnostic sympathetic block is often helpful in the diagnosis of CRPS.

- The relief of pain and symptoms with cold is typical of EM and is not seen with CRPS.

RECOMMENDED READING

Bakst R, Merola R, Franks AG, et al. Raynaud's phenomenon: pathogenesis and management. *J Am Acad Dermatol* 2008;59:633–653.

Bailey SR, Eid AH, Mitra S, et al. Rho kinase mediates cold-induced constriction of cutaneous arteries: role of alpha2C-adrenoceptor translocation. *Circ Res* 2004;94(10):1367–1374.

Balogh B, Mayer W, Vesely M, et al. Adventitial stripping of the radial and ulnar arteries in Raynaud's disease. *J Hand Surg* 2002;6:1073–1080.

Baumhakel M, Bohm M. Recent achievements in the management of Raynaud's phenomenon. *Vascul Health Risk Manage* 2010;6:207–214.

Block JA, Sequeira W. Raynaud's phenomenon. *Lancet* 2001;357(9273):2042–2048.

Cohen JS. Erythromelalgia: new theories and new therapies. *J Am Acad Dermatol* 2000;43: 841–847.

Dean SM, Satiani B. Three cases of digital ischemia successfully treated with cilostazol. *Vasc Med* 2001;6:245–248.

Dziadzio M, Denton CP, Smith R, et al. Losartan therapy for Raynaud's phenomenon and scleroderma: clinical and biochemical findings in a fifteen-week, randomized, parallel-group, controlled trial. *Arthritis Rheum* 1999;42:2646–2655.

Fries R, Shariat K, von Wilmowsky H, et al. Sildenafil in the treatment of Raynaud's phenomenon resistant to vasodilatory therapy. *Circulation* 2005;112(19):2980–2985.

Furspan PB, Chatterjee S, Freedman RR. Increased tyrosine phosphorylation mediates the cooling-induced contraction and increased vascular reactivity of Raynaud's disease. *Arthr Rheum* 2004;50(5):1578–1585.

Gibbs MB, English JC, Zirwas MJ. Livedo reticularis: an update. *J Am Acad Dermatol* 2005; 52:1009.

Herrero C, Guilabert A, Mascaro-Galy JM. Diagnosis and treatment of livedo reticularis on the legs. *Actas Dermosifiliogr* 2008;99:598–607.

Janig W, Baron R. Complex regional pain syndrome: mystery explained? *Lancet Neurol* 2003: 687–697.

Kawald A, Burmester GR, Huscher D, et al. Low versus high-dose iloprost therapy over 21 days in patients with secondary Raynaud's phenomenon and systemic sclerosis: a randomized, open, single-center study. *J Rheumatol* 2008;35(9):1830–1837.

Matsumoto Y, Ueyama T, Endo M, et al. Endoscopic thoracic sympathectomy for Raynaud's phenomenon. *J Vasc Surg* 2002;36:57–61.

Rajagopalan S, Pfenninger D, Kehrer C, et al. Increased asymmetric dimethylarginine and endothelin 1 levels in secondary Raynaud's phenomenon: implications for vascular dysfunction and progression of disease. *Arthritis Rheum* 2003;48(7):1992–2000.

Rho RH, Brewer RP, Lamer TJ, et al. Complex regional pain syndrome. *Mayo Clin Proc* 2002;77(2):174–180.

Shenoy PD, Kumar S, Jha LK. Efficacy of tadalafil in secondary Raynaud's phenomenon resistant to vasodilator therapy: a double-blind randomized cross-over trial. *Rheumatology* 2010; 49:2420–2428.

Spencer-Green G. Outcomes in primary Raynaud phenomenon: a meta-analysis of the frequency, rates, and predictors of transition to secondary diseases. *Arch Intern Med* 1998;158: 595–600.

Thompson AE, Pope JE. Calcium channel blockers for primary Raynaud's phenomenon: a meta-analysis. *Rheumatology (Oxford)* 2005;44(2):145–150.

Tucker AT, Pearson RM, Cooke ED, et al. Effect of nitric-oxide-generating system on blood flow in skin of patients with severe Raynaud's syndrome: a randomised trial. *Lancet* 1999; 354:1670–1675.

Wigley FM. Clinical practice. Raynaud's phenomenon. *N Engl J Med* 2002;347(13):1001–1008.

CHAPTER 19 ■ History, Physical Examination, and Diagnostic Approach to Venous Disorders

Teresa L. Carman

Venous disease includes a broad spectrum of clinical conditions from acute disease to chronic ailments. Both acute and chronic venous disorders are common, prompting many patients to seek medical attention. It is important to carefully define venous disorders in order to help differentiate them on history and physical examination.

It is estimated that 27% of the American population has a detectable form of chronic lower extremity venous disease (mainly varicose veins), and 1 to 3% may have ongoing symptoms of chronic venous insufficiency (CVI). *Varicose veins* are one of the most common chronic venous disorders encountered in clinical practice. The term *varicose veins* refers to any dilated tortuous elongated vein. This designation is without regard to the size of the vessel. Varicosities can be subdivided into three categories. *Trunk vein varicosities* are the enlargement of the great or small saphenous systems and their tributaries. *Reticular veins* are subcutaneous veins arising from the tributaries of trunk veins. These are usually one to three millimeters in size. *Telangiectasias* are also called *spider veins*. These are small intradermal varicosities that are rarely symptomatic.

Many chronic venous disorders are caused by venous reflux. Reflux is defined as the retrograde flow of blood in veins of the lower extremity due to incompetent valves. Some degree of venous reflux may be seen in up to 20% of asymptomatic individuals older than 20 years. Reflux can arise as a consequence of (i) perforator vein incompetence in the calf or thighs; (ii) incompetence of the saphenofemoral junction (SFJ), or the saphenopopliteal junction (SPJ); (iii) incompetence of deep venous valves, most commonly due to destruction by DVT (valve reflux is detected in ~50% of veins that are thrombosed); or (iv) ineffective calf muscle pump mechanism, as a result of which ejection of blood from the lower limb is inadequate, increasing residual venous volume (VV).

The functional consequence of communication of deep venous pressures to the low-pressure superficial system is venous hypertension. Venous hypertension is perceived as symptoms of lower extremity heaviness, aching, and fatigue. CVI is a consequence of venous hypertension and chronic venous reflux related to structural or functional abnormalities of veins. Chronic long-standing venous hypertension leads to cutaneous changes such as edema, dilated veins, skin hyperpigmentation or hemosiderin staining, lipodermatosclerosis, and ulceration.

Acute venous thromboembolism (VTE), a term that typically includes deep vein thrombosis (DVT), pulmonary embolism (PE), and may include superficial venous thrombosis (SVT), is the third most common vascular disorder in the United States exceeded by only cardiovascular disease and stroke syndromes. Acute SVT and DVT are characterized by the development of thrombus in the superficial and deep veins, respectively. While DVT is commonly recognized as a vascular urgency, it is important to note that superficial thrombophlebitis may propagate into the deep venous system and become a DVT in 10 to 15% of cases. Many medical and surgical conditions may contribute to the underlying risk for VTE. Common causes of DVT and SVT may include trauma or injury, inherited or acquired hypercoagulable states including cancer, drugs such as oral contraceptives (OCPs), infection, or immobility including surgery (Table 19.1). Postthrombotic syndrome (PTS) is the long-term sequelae of DVT. PTS is caused by a combination of venous valve injury as well as obstruction from persistent intraluminal fibrosis and webs. PTS may affect up to 70% of patients following DVT.

TABLE 19.1

CLINICAL RISK FACTORS FOR ACUTE VTE

Strong risk (OR > 10)
   Knee or hip replacement
   Major trauma
   Fracture hip or knee
   Spinal cord injury
Moderate risk (OR 2–9)
   Abdominal and thoracic surgery
   Arthroscopic surgery
   Congestive heart failure
   Stroke with paralysis
   Cancer/myeloproliferative disorders/chemotherapy
   Hormonal therapy including HRT, OCPs, and SERMs
   Previous venous thromboembolism
   Thrombophilia
Low risk (OR < 2)
   Age
   Bed rest > 3 d
   Obesity
   Varicose veins
   Laparoscopic surgery
   Prolonged car or airplane travel
   Pregnancy

OR, odds ratio; HRT, hormone replacement therapy; OCPs, oral contraceptives; SERMs, selective estrogen receptor modulators.

CLINICAL FEATURES

Medical History

Demographics

Age. Venous disease is typically a disease of an aging population. VTE occurs both in the young and in the old, although there is an age-dependent increase (30- to 40-fold higher incidence in 80-year-old compared to 30-year-old persons). It is estimated that VTE risk doubles with each decade of age. VTE in the young is almost always a consequence of a thrombotic diathesis. The incidence of varicose veins and CVI sequelae also increases with age, and age independently predicts the development of these complications.

Gender. The overall incidence of VTE in women and men is quite similar. However, men appear to have increased risk for VTE recurrence compared to women. Women have a three-fold to four-fold higher risk for varicose veins than men. Despite the strong link between varicosities and the eventual development of CVI, sequelae of CVI paradoxically tend to be more common in men than in women.

Race. The risk for VTE show racial differences, with whites at greater risk than Hispanics. Asians have the lowest risk for VTE. This may be due to differences in genetic factors that predispose to DVT.

Obesity. Obesity increases the risk for varicosities in women but not in men. Obesity is an independent predictor of development of CVI. Whether obesity increases the risk of VTE is debated. If obesity results in significant immobility, indeed the risk may increase.

History of Present Illness

While many patients with venous disease are asymptomatic, pain, swelling, and skin changes are the most common signs and symptoms of acute or chronic venous disease. Patients may present with any combination of these symptoms. The variability in presentation can be fairly remarkable. Some patients may present for the evaluation of asymptomatic skin abnormalities such as a telangiectasia, while at the other end of the spectrum, patients may present with fulminant manifestations of CVI including edema, hyperpigmentation, lipodermatosclerosis, and venous ulceration.

A careful history should be focused on defining the onset, progression, and exacerbating and relieving factors, and associated clinical signs and symptoms for the clinical complaint (Table 19.2). It may be helpful to know what diagnostic studies have been performed and whether the symptoms are improving or worsening with time. The history, examination, differential diagnosis, and testing will also be affected by unilateral vs. bilateral symptoms. The history should include cataloging whether the patient has had a recent surgical procedure, prolonged travel, immobility, history

TABLE 19.2

DIFFERENTIATING LOWER EXTREMITY SWELLING

Feature	Orthostatic	Chronic Venous Disease	Lymphatic
Laterality	Bilateral; symmetrical	Usually unilateral; occasionally bilateral but unequal; rarely symmetric	Usually unilateral; occasionally bilateral; rarely symmetric
Effect of elevation	Relieved completely	Partial or complete resolution	Mild or minimal relief
Distribution	Diffuse involvement with maximal edema in the ankles and feet	Ankles and legs (feet may be spared)	Diffuse, greatest distally
Pain	None/little	Fatigue, heaviness, aching; bursting discomfort (venous claudication)	Minimal pain
Skin changes	Shiny skin, no pigmentation or trophic changes	Medial aspect of lower legs (gaiter area); hyperpigmentation, thickening or fibrosis, lipodermatosclerosis, ulcers in advanced cases	Lichenification and thickening of skin

of cancer, trauma, medications, or illnesses that may predispose to acute VTE. A careful assessment of risk factors for DVT may be helpful in identifying factors that may have played a role. Table 19.1 lists various risk factors including surgical procedures and risk for developing a DVT. *Prolonged immobility* increases the risk of DVT. Hospitalization, air travel (greater than 8 hours), or long car trips are included in this assessment. The increase with air travel appears to be modest, and this does not appear to translate into an increase in the incidence of PE in the general population. Trauma is strongly associated with DVT, with more than 50% of individuals with trauma to the lower extremities and more than 40% of those with trauma elsewhere (chest and abdomen) demonstrating evidence of DVT with duplex evaluation. A history of *fracture* of the long bones of the lower extremity or the pelvic bones increases the risk of asymptomatic DVT. The use of indwelling devices such as central venous catheters, pacemakers, and infusion ports is strongly associated with the development of DVT at the site of insertion.

Pain Associated with Venous Disease. The majority of patients with DVTs are asymptomatic. Pain may however occur in the context of any acute or chronic venous disorder. In superficial thrombophlebitis and DVT, the clinical findings (see physical examination) that accompany the pain may suggest the need for further evaluation and intervention. Typically, the pain is of new or abrupt onset and associated with new or acute swelling, warmth, or erythema of the limb. In addition, the patient may report a cordlike structure that is painful, tender, and/or red. Individuals with extensive DVT (iliofemoral disease) may often experience a bursting discomfort in the lower extremities on exertion (venous claudication) that is relieved slowly with rest and elevation (see venous claudication in Table 19.2).

The pain of CVI is typically described as an ache toward the end of the day felt in the entire lower extremity or in a portion of the limb. This is also true in the setting of PTS. In acute exacerbations of CVI, including stasis dermatitis, patients may have fairly acute onset of symptoms; thus, imaging to exclude DVT is sometimes warranted. Pain is not a typical complaint in varicosities, and the presence of pain over a varix should raise the suspicion of associated thrombophlebitis. It is common for patients with varicosities to experience atypical symptoms such as pricking, tingling, prurutis, or burning discomfort over the site. Restless leg syndrome is an underappreciated disorder that can complicate both varicose veins and CVI.

Swelling. This is the second most common manifestation of venous disease and is a manifestation of venous hypertension. Venous hypertension is the pathophysiologic hallmark of CVI. Venous hypertension represents transmission of venous pressure to the deep and superficial veins. Obstruction and/or reflux aided by gravity and incompetent valves increases pressure within the deep and communicating veins. Other causes for venous hypertension that should be considered include (i) intrinsic venous thrombosis, (ii) extrinsic venous compression such as May-Thurner syndrome or Cockett's syndrome where the left iliac vein is compressed by the overlying right common iliac artery, and (iii) elevated right heart pressure due to various causes. The location, onset, duration, and aggravating or relieving factors for swelling should be carefully considered. Table 19.2 provides differentiating features of venous edema from other causes of lower extremity swelling.

Past Medical and Surgical History

A history of DVT makes recurrent DVT a strong consideration in a patient presenting with other suggestive signs and symptoms. Similarly, a history of DVT makes PTS and CVI a more likely cause of the lower extremity swelling. The risk of VTE is increased by concomitant associated influences (see Table 19.1). A personal or family history of venous thromboembolism, spontaneous abortion, or pregnancy morbidity should increase concern for an inherited or acquired form of thrombophilia.

A history of *malignancy* or *myeloproliferative syndrome* is associated with a higher incidence of DVT. In addition, DVT could be the first manifestation of a malignancy in 3 to 20% of individuals. Carcinoma of the lung is the most common tumor associated with a DVT by virtue of its higher prevalence compared to other malignancies. Gastrointestinal (pancreas and stomach)- and genitourinary-associated carcinomas and adenocarcinomas of unknown primary are more strongly linked to development of thrombosis. *Paralysis* due to spinal cord injury is also associated with an increased risk for VTE including PE. The risk of DVT after paralysis is greatest during the first 2 weeks after injury; deaths resulting from PE are relatively rare after 3 months. *Pregnancy* increases the risk of VTE with the highest risk in the immediate postpartum period (20 times higher than control nonpregnant women). *Inflammatory bowel disease* has also been associated with increased risk for DVT.

Medication History

Estrogen, hormone replacement, OCPs, and selective estrogen receptor modulators (SERMs) increase the risk for DVT. Newer OCPs have a significantly lower amount of estrogen than prescribed decades ago but nonetheless still increase risk of DVT. In addition, OCPs with third-generation progestins have increased risk for VTE compared to OCPs containing second-generation progestins. Still, a woman's risk of VTE-related death from estrogen-based contraceptive therapy is lower than her risk of dying from pregnancy. The risk (hazard ratio) for a postmenopausal woman on hormone replacement therapy developing a DVT is approximately 2.1 (based on HERS and the Women's Health Initiative studies). Combining hormonal therapy with other VTE triggers magnifies the VTE risk. For example, oral contraceptive use may be at increased risk for DVT or cerebral thrombosis. However, in individuals with inherited thrombophilia, OCP use dramatically increases the risk. In patients with the prothrombin 20210 mutation risk increases up to 120-fold and with Factor V Leiden mutation risk is increased 30- to 40-fold.

In cancer patients, the introduction of chemotherapy or radiation therapy may increase the risk for VTE. The use of medications such as hydralazine, procainamide, and phenothiazines should be considered since they are known to potentially induce antiphospholipid antibodies. Exposure to heparin or low-molecular-weight heparin predisposes patients to formation of heparin-induced platelet factor 4 antibodies and heparin-induced thrombocytosis that may increase the risk for VTE.

Family History

A first-degree relative with a history of DVT raises concern for the presence of a hereditary thrombophilic defect. Table 19.3 lists the inherited thrombophilias and their prevalence in the general population as well as in patients presenting with a DVT. In general, there is an inverse relationship between the prevalence of a disorder and the thrombophilic risk. The most common disorders (i.e., factor V Leiden and prothrombin gene mutation) seem to have a modest influence on VTE and likely do not increase the risk for future events, while the less common thrombophilias (antithrombin deficiency, protein C and protein S deficiency) typically present at an earlier age and may indeed increase the risk for additional life-time events.

TABLE 19.3

PREVALENCE OF GENETIC THROMBOPHILIAS IN THE GENERAL POPULATION AND PATIENTS WITH DVT

Syndrome	General Population (%)	Patients with DVT (%)
Factor V Leiden (APC resistance)	3–6	21
Prothrombin G20210A	1.5–3.0	6
Protein C deficiency	0.1–0.5	3
Protein S deficiency	—	2
Antithrombin deficiency	0.02–0.17	1

Physical Examination

The physical examination of the patient with suspected venous disease should not be limited to the legs and should include the entire individual. Up to 50% of patients with acute DVT may have a PE at presentation. Abnormalities in routine vital signs including heart rate, blood pressure, respiratory rate, and temperature may all accompany acute VTE. Cardiac examination may be normal or reveal findings of elevated right heart pressure including jugular venous distension, a loud second heart sound, or a new flow-related murmur. Similarly, examination of the lungs may be normal or reveal nonspecific findings of diminished breath sounds, crackles, or induced pleuritic chest pain that may suggest an underlying infiltrate or infarction. No examination of the venous system is complete without an evaluation of the abdominal organs for possible malignancies and masses.

Complete examination of the venous system requires adequate understanding of venous anatomy including the presence of perforating veins (PV). Figures 19.1 and 19.2 illustrate the location of the most clinically important veins in the lower extremity. Common clinical findings of venous disease include pain, swelling, and skin changes as previously noted. A number of patients with DVT may have a normal physical exam. Only phlegmasia and SVT can be reliably diagnosed with any degree of a certainty via a clinical examination. However, it is important to have a methodical approach to the patient with suspected venous disease.

Inspection and Palpation

Inspection and palpation should be done with the entire lower extremity exposed. Patients with acute DVT may present with erythema, pain/tenderness on palpation or ambulation, or swelling (either proximal or distal). Unfortunately, physical examination alone is insufficient to exclude or diagnose DVT, and additional imaging is required in patients with suspected VTE.

Patient with chronic venous disease presenting with varicose veins should be examined both supine and standing. Great saphenous varicosities start along the medial side of the leg in front of the medial malleolus and travel proximally to the saphenofemoral junction. Small saphenous varicosities are seen from behind the lateral malleolus. Since the small saphenous vein is embedded in fascia, it is much easier to see tributaries to this vein in conditions associated

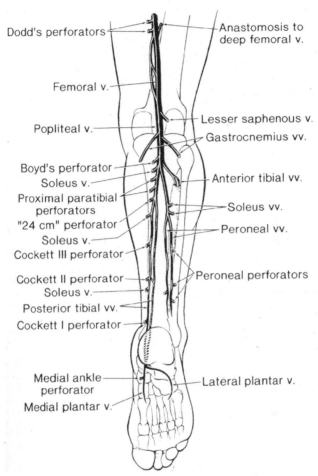

Dodd's perforators

Anastomosis to deep femoral v.

Femoral v.

Popliteal v.

Lesser saphenous v.

Gastrocnemius vv.

Boyd's perforator
Soleus v.
Proximal paratibial perforators
"24 cm" perforator
Soleus v.
Cockett III perforator

Anterior tibial vv.

Soleus vv.

Peroneal vv.

Cockett II perforator
Soleus v.
Posterior tibial vv.
Cockett I perforator

Peroneal perforators

Medial ankle perforator
Medial plantar v.

Lateral plantar v.

FIGURE 19-1.   Anatomy of the deep veins and perforators of the lower extremity (from the posterior aspect).

with high venous pressure. The calf and thigh perforators are relatively constant (Figs. 19.2 and 19.3). Incompetence of the Hunterian's perforator is a common cause of medial thigh (middle) varicosity, while Dodd's perforator incompetence results in varicosities in the lower thigh (medial aspect). The anteromedial calf perforator (Boyd's) connects the greater saphenous vein to the crural veins and is a common site for a primary varicosity. Figure 19.3 illustrates the current nomenclature of perforator veins.

Swelling and Skin Changes. Swelling is common manifestation associated with venous disease. It may be due to obstruction as in deep venous thrombosis but may also occur with inflammation or superficial

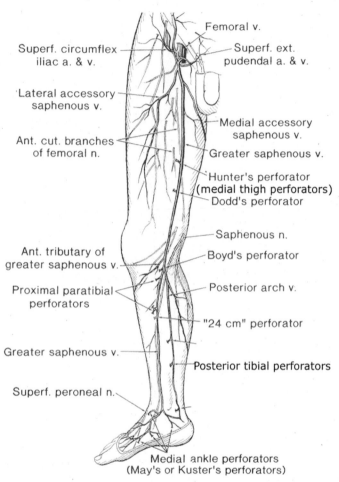

FIGURE 19-2.   Anatomy of the superficial and PV of the leg from the medial aspect.

thrombophlebitis. Localized redness and swelling may be due to thrombophlebitis; however, it may also be seen in patients with an exacerbation of CVI. Swelling related to venous thromboembolism typically
depends on the extent of the disease with proximal venous thrombosis
causing more severe symptoms compared to isolated distal DVT. Phlegmasia cerulea dolens may occur with extensive DVT that extends to the
iliofemoral veins. The limb appears diffusely swollen, turgid, and blue
(erythrocyanosis) due to concomitant arterial insufficiency.

With varicosities and in CVI, swelling is related to venous hypertension and usually occurs at the ankle and lower leg. Many practitioners
confuse the edema associated with venous disease and lymphedema. Lymphedema typically involves the toes (square toe sign), and there is usually

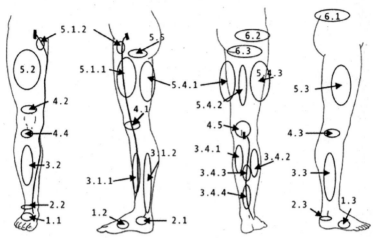

FIGURE 19-3. New nomenclature for PV. *1.1*, *1.2*, *1.3* are the dorsal, medial, and lateral foot PVs. *2.1*, *2.2*, and *2.3* are medial, anterior, and lateral PVs of the ankle. Leg PVs: *3.1.1* paratibial PV *3.1.2* posterior tibial PV *3.2* anterior leg PV *3.3* lateral leg PV *3.4.1* medial gastrocnemius PV *3.4.2* lateral gastrocnemius PV *3.4.3* intergemellar PV *3.4.4* para-achillean PV. Knee PVs: *4.1* medial knee PV *4.2* suprapatellar PV *4.3* lateral knee PV *4.4* infrapatellar PV *4.5* popliteal fossa PV. Thigh PVs: *5.1.1* PV of the femoral canal *5.1.2* inguinal PV *5.2* anterior thigh PV *5.3* lateral thigh PV *5.4.1* posteromedial thigh PV *5.4.2* sciatic PV *5.4.3* posterolateral thigh PV *5.5* pudendal PV. Gluteal PVs: *6.1* superior gluteal PV *6.2* midgluteal PV *6.3* lower gluteal PV. (From Caggiati A, Bergan JJ, Gloviczki P, et al. Nomenclature of the veins of the lower limbs: An international interdisciplinary consensus statement. *J Vasc Surg* 2002;36:416–422.)

a prominent hump on the dorsum of the foot (dorsal hump). Generally, venous edema does not involve the toes or the forefoot, providing a clinical clue that distinguishes these two problems (Table 19.2).

Few skin changes are typical of DVT. In some cases, there may be associated erythema or erythrocyanosis due to venous congestion and inflammation. However, the presence of pigmentation and eczematous changes in the medial aspect of the lower leg ("stasis dermatitis") is almost pathognomonic for CVI. In cases of long-standing stasis dermatitis, one may see a "venous" ulceration. These are typically seen above the medial malleolus with the surrounding skin displaying signs of CVI. The ulcer is shallow (never penetrates the deep fascia), and the floor of the ulcer is usually covered with a moist granulating base while edge is sloping and pale blue in color. Table 19.4 details clinical considerations associated with different vascular-related ulcers.

Clinical Signs. The majority of patients with DVT may have a relatively normal physical exam. While there are historical clinical signs espoused to indicate DVT, these signs are neither sensitive nor specific for the diagnosis of DVT. *Homan's sign* is the reproduction of calf discomfort with passive dorsiflexion of the foot with DVT. *Bancroft's sign* is tenderness on

TABLE 19.4

DIFFERENTIAL DIAGNOSIS OF ULCERATION

Features	Arterial Ulcer	Venous Ulcer	Neuropathic	Vasculitis	Pyoderma Gangrenosum
1. Location	Distal foot (plantar surface) over bony prominences (head of first and fifth metatarsal joints); trauma may localize ulcers more proximally	"Gaiter area" of the medial aspect of the leg	Over bony prominences in the foot (metatarsophalangeal joints)	Medial aspect of lower leg	Lower extremities and trunk
2. Appearance	Round or punched out with a sharply demarcated borders and pale base	Irregular margins that are either flat or with a steep elevation; base is shallow and often covered with exudate	Destructive ulcers with deep ulcer bases; may often be combined with vascular insufficiency (as in diabetes)	Necrotic base; irregular margin	Lesions begin as pustules with development of necrosis and multiple ulcerations; well-defined, raised, purple, serpiginous, and undermined border; lesions may coalesce to form reticulated or cribiform pattern with intervening intact skin
3. Pain	Painful	Minimal to mild pain	Painless	Painful	Painful
4. Associated features	Prolonged capillary refill time (>4–5 s) and change in limb color with limb elevation	Hyperpigmentation, dermatitis and indurated skin and scarring in the middle and lower portions of the leg (lipodermatosclerosis)	Foot numbness, burning, and paresthesias may be seen; often asymptomatic; abnormal, thickened callus in pressure areas with marked abnormalities in sensory perception	Sclerodactyly (PSS) and joint deformities (rheumatoid arthritis)	50% occur with ulcerative colitis, Crohn's disease, chronic active hepatitis, rheumatoid arthritis, lupus, or malignancies
5. Additional testing	Low ankle-brachial index or toe-brachial index	History of CVI and deep venous thrombosis	Failure to perceive the pressure of a 10-g monofilament is a proven indicator of peripheral sensory neuropathy	Serologic testing for collagen-vascular disease	Serologic testing and blood cultures

anteroposterior but not lateral compression of the calf. *Lowenberg's sign* is prompt pain in the calf caused by inflation of a sphygmomanometer cuff around it to a pressure of 80 mm Hg. Indeed, DVT should only be diagnosed using contemporary imaging modalities including duplex ultrasound, computed tomogram venography (CTV), magnetic resonance venography (MRV), or conventional phlebography.

Examination for Venous Reflux

While this can be performed in the office using a handheld Doppler and tourniquet, it is time consuming and thus has fallen out of favor. It has become routine practice to refer these patients to the vascular laboratory for a complete duplex ultrasound assessment of reflux.

Differential Diagnosis

The symptoms of venous disease may be unilateral or bilateral. Unilateral swelling and/or pain of the lower extremity may indicate deep venous thrombosis; however, a number of other conditions should be included in the differential diagnosis:

- Leg trauma (hematoma, muscle injury)
- Cellulitis
- Ruptured Baker's cyst
- Arthritis of the knee or the ankle joint
- Swelling following recent hip surgery, knee surgery or trauma
- Pelvic venous obstruction or external compression of iliac vein
- Superficial venous thrombosis
- Venous insufficiency (varicose veins). Critical limb ischemia due to peripheral arterial disease (swelling only occurs if the patient's leg has been dependent to alleviate rest pain)
- Chronic regional pain syndrome
- Lymphedema

Bilateral swelling is usually related to a systemic process (liver disease, renal disease, cardiovascular disease or medications), central venous obstruction, or bilateral venous disease. The edema of CVI must be distinguished from the edema of congestive heart failure, nephrotic syndrome, and cirrhosis by careful history and physical examination. Chronic lymphedema is also in the differential diagnosis for causes of lower extremity edema, either unilateral or bilateral. It causes thickening of the skin and firmness of the subcutaneous tissue as well but is infrequently associated with ulceration at the medial and lateral malleolar levels. Commonly, this type of edema can occur in the forefoot and extend into the area of the toes (square toe sign), a pattern distinct from the edema of CVI. The ulceration that occurs in the setting of venous disease should be distinguished from other causes of ulcers (Table 19.4). An uncommon but significant cause of nonhealing ulceration is squamous cell carcinoma (SCC). SCC can occur *de novo*, or within the setting of chronic inflammation such as chronic venous stasis ulcers (Marjolin's ulcer), and must be considered in the differential diagnosis, if healing is unusually slow.

DIAGNOSTIC EVALUATION AND APPROACH

Chronic Venous Insufficiency and Varicose Vein Evaluation

The following questions should be answered when evaluating a patient with suspected CVI and/or trunk vein varicosity of the lower extremity: (i) Is there reflux? (ii) Is there obstruction? (iii) Are both present? (iv) What is the severity of reflux and obstruction? (v) Is there a calf or musculoskeletal problem? (vi) Are the abnormalities that are detected enough to explain the patient's presentation or are there additional factors? (vii) What is the prognosis of the patient?

Approach to CVI and Varicosities: Using the CEAP Clinical Class

The "CEAP" classification system was initially developed to communicate results of a comprehensive venous evaluation in a succinct manner (Table 19.5). The main purpose of the "CEAP" system was to help clinicians and researchers communicate with respect to the C (clinical), E (etiology),

TABLE 19.5

CEAP CLASSIFICATION

Clinical (C)	Etiology (E)	Anatomy (A)	Pathophysiology (P)
No signs of venous disease (C_0)	Congenital (E_c)	Superficial (A_s)	Reflux (P_R)
Telangiectasia or spider veins (C1)	Primary undetermined cause (E_p)	Deep (A_D)	Obstruction (P_O)
Varicose veins (C2)	Secondary—known cause (E_s)	Perforator (A_p)	Reflux and obstruction (P_{RO})
Edema due to venous disease (C3)	• Postthrombotic		
Skin changes and lipodermatosclerosis (C4)	• Posttraumatic		
Healed ulcers (C5)			
Active ulcers (C6)			

This classification is designed to define the clinical class (C), etiology (E), anatomic distribution of the veins (A), and its pathologic mechanism (P).
(Modified from The Consensus Group. Classification and grading of chronic venous disease in the lower limbs. A consensus statement. *Vasc Surg* 1996;30:5–11.)

A (anatomic), and P (pathophysiologic) basis for chronic venous disease. This is of utmost importance in clinical research. The clinical classes are summarized by C0 (no visible disease) through C6 (presence of an active venous stasis ulcer) followed by a subscript for symptomatic (s) or asymptomatic (a) patients. The etiology (E) may be primary (Ep) or secondary (Es). The anatomy localizes the areas involved and could be superficial (As), deep (Ad), or perforater (Ap). Finally, the pathophysiologic mechanism, P, is defined as reflux (Pr), obstruction (Po), or both (Pr, o). Although the entire CEAP classification is commonly perceived as being too laborious for clinical practice, an abbreviated form based on the clinical class of CEAP is extremely effective in directing testing in patients presenting with suspected CVI. Thus, placing a patient in a clinical class aids in subsequent diagnostic test selection. For class 3 and beyond, the additional definition of etiology, anatomy, and pathophysiologic involvement helps define management.

Designating Etiology (E), Anatomy (A), and Pathophysiology (P): This is applicable only to class 3 and beyond. *Etiology (E):* Skin changes or swelling may be either due to primary, secondary, or congenital causes. The differentiation begins with a duplex scan with careful attention to perforator incompetence, which may underlie skin changes or swelling and help elucidate reflux and/or obstruction as potential etiologies. Determining the etiology may require additional testing including invasive ascending and descending venography in cases that cannot be defined by simpler tests. *Anatomy (A):* Duplex ultrasound scanning can help delineate the site of involvement as superficial, perforating, and/or deep venous system. *Pathophysiology (P):* Differentiation of reflux from obstruction is important. With primary disease, there is only reflux. In secondary disease, there may be contribution from obstruction. In these cases, elucidation of the predominant mechanism using additional testing such as air plethysmography (APG), which tends to be a good test for global reflux, may be important for assessing treatment options.

Decision Making Based on the Clinical Class of CEAP Classification

The clinical CEAP class can be helpful in apportioning diagnostic testing into three levels. However, in any given patient, testing should be determined by eventual management strategies. If management will revolve around conservative measures, there is little to be gained by doing more sophisticated studies. On the other hand, if surgical options are being considered, additional evaluation by duplex ultrasound, APG (Chapter 22), and venography should be considered.

In *Level 1 testing*, studies include clinical evaluation (history, physical examination) and evaluation of the venous system with handheld Doppler or duplex ultrasound. *Level 2 testing* includes noninvasive investigations such as duplex scanning and APG. *Level 3 testing* includes investigations such as MRV or invasive tests such as phlebography (ascending and descending).

A simple problem such as telangiectasia is always superficial in location and the etiology (E) is primary in cause. A simple designation as C-1 is sufficient to show that the clinical problem is telangiectasia, modified by whether it is symptomatic or asymptomatic (C1a or C1s).

Testing in class 0/1: No visible or palpable signs or venous disease; telangiectasia or reticular veins: In asymptomatic patients, level 1 investigation is often sufficient. In patients presenting with symptoms of CVI such as aching, tiredness, and heaviness, duplex scanning of the lower extremity to detect reflux in the saphenofemoral, saphenopopliteal junctions (SPJs), superficial veins, and the deep veins (femoral and popliteal veins) may be considered. Additionally, obstruction in the deep venous system may be considered and ruled out. If these tests are negative, then no further testing is necessary.

Testing in class 2: Varicose veins presenting without edema or skin changes: Level 1 investigation may be sufficient in some patients, although most individuals require level 2 studies. In the patient with varicosities confined to the long saphenous system with reflux at the SFJ (and absence of reflux at the saphenopopliteal fossa), level 1 tests alone may be sufficient. In most cases, careful duplex Doppler ultrasound examination is required to evaluate the popliteal fossa (small saphenous, gastrocnemial, or popliteal veins). Duplex ultrasound scanning is also required to determine whether reflux or obstruction in the deep veins is responsible for incompetent perforators. Patients with recurrent varicose veins and those with prior DVT require duplex ultrasound scanning. An additional indication for duplex ultrasound scanning is the presence of unusual varicosities arising from atypical sites such as the pelvis.

Testing in Class 3: Edema with or without varicose veins and without skin changes: The presence of edema (especially unilateral) helps direct attention to the veins of the lower extremity as a potential etiology. Level 3 testing may be considered if duplex scan shows deep venous reflux or obstruction and for the determination of etiology (E), anatomy (A), and establishing pathophysiology (P) that then guides management.

Testing in Class 4/5/6: Skin changes suggestive of venous disease, including healed or open ulcerations with or without edema and varicose veins: With the appearance of skin changes due to venous disease, suggesting advanced venous dysfunction, a thorough history and physical examination and duplex evaluation are mandatory. Most individuals with these changes usually have deep and/or perforating venous reflux with or without concomitant obstruction. Isolated superficial venous reflux in this category of patients is uncommon. Duplex scanning is recommended for all patients with skin changes. Additional evaluation by APG and venography should be selectively performed on patients who are potential candidates for surgery (see Fig. 19.9). Venography is usually required in cases where the contribution of obstruction versus reflux is not readily apparent. Usually, ascending venography is sufficient. In some cases, descending venography may be needed to identify the sites of the valves that are involved in the reflux.

Vascular Laboratory Testing in Chronic Venous Insufficiency/Varicose Veins

Level 1 Testing.

Ultrasound evaluation of reflux. The purpose of this evaluation is to determine the presence of reflux in communication points between superficial and deep venous systems, namely the SFJ and the SPJ. This can be accomplished with a handheld device but far more efficiently by duplex evaluation, as color-flow duplex provides directionality of blood flow and allows for discrimination between obstruction with valvular incompetence and primary reflux. For reflux evaluation, the patient is examined in the standing position, with his or her weight on the contralateral extremity. The probe is placed at an angle of 45 degrees to the horizontal. The femoral vein is identified medial to the artery in the femoral triangle. Confirmation of probe placement is obtained by augmentation of blood flow with compression of the thigh, the calf, or the varicosity itself. After confirmation of optimal signal, the patient is asked to cough or perform the Valsalva maneuver followed by abrupt release. If immediately following these maneuvers there is abrupt cessation of flow (within 0.5 to 1.5 seconds), there is no reflux. When SFJ incompetence is present, this increase in flow during the performance of any of these maneuvers is followed by prolonged backflow signal. Figure 19.4 demonstrates SFJ incompetence using color flow Doppler. This test is then repeated at the SPJ level. For this, the knee is evaluated in a slightly flexed position. The Doppler probe is positioned carefully at a 45-degree angle to the horizontal in the popliteal fossa. The popliteal vein is located lateral to the midline of the knee, adjacent to the popliteal artery. Augmentation of the venous signal by calf compression helps the identification. Light, constant compression of the calf for 2 to 3 seconds followed by sudden release once again confirms the presence or absence of reflux in the popliteal vein or small saphenous vein. Compression of the distal calf is the best way to demonstrate reflux at this level, and the Valsalva needs not be performed.

Photoplethysmography. Photoplethysmography (PPG) is a noninvasive technique that can aid in characterizing CVI. Local changes in blood flow to the skin are detected by a probe placed on the leg with an infrared diode, and reception of the backscatter by an adjacent photoreceptor (Fig. 19.5). This technique allows the continuous recording of instantaneous changes in cutaneous capillary blood and relies on the fact that red blood cells within the dermis absorb maximum light when the pressure is high and the capillaries are full. It identifies reflux by determining the time for the capillaries to refill after they are emptied. PPG performed as a screening test has a sensitivity ranging from 50 to 85% depending on the criteria used (sensitivity of 50% if venous refill time (VRT) of 15 seconds used, higher if 23 seconds used) and a specificity of 80%. Thus, some have abandoned its usage. A number of practices still use the PPG as a screening tool. If the test is positive for reflux, typically further characterization is necessary to determine the presence and degree of obstruction and/or reflux. If negative, it may be predictive of the absence of venous reflux. To perform the test, the patient sits and maintains the legs in a vertical position in order to empty the veins. The patient is then asked to stand and the venous filling time is assessed. A normal refilling time suggests a normal venous system. If the VRT is abnormally short (less than 23 seconds), then the test is repeated with a cuff at the level of the ankle to occlude the perforators. If the VRT remains short, then the insufficiency involves the deep venous system, as the cuff is occluding the superficial venous system and the perforators. If the VRT normalizes, then the cuff is placed higher on the calf to occlude the superficial

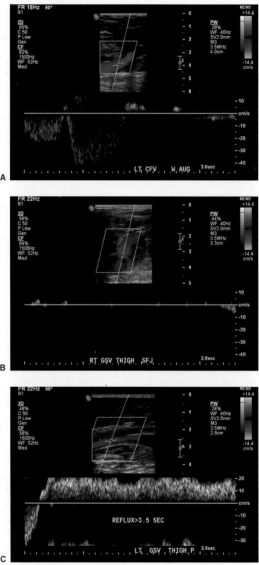

FIGURE 19-4. Demonstration of competency of the SFJ by duplex ultrasound. During quiet respiration (**A, B**), blood flows cephalad in the greater saphenous and the common femoral veins as indicated by the arrows. With performance of the Valsalva, there is complete cessation of flow (**B**) with a competent SFJ. In contrast, in (**C**), there is blood flow in the opposite direction with the Valsalva suggesting reflux of the SFJ. (From Zwiebel WJ. *Introduction to vascular ultrasonography*, 4th ed. Philadelphia: W. B. Saunders, 2000:356–357.) (See color insert.)

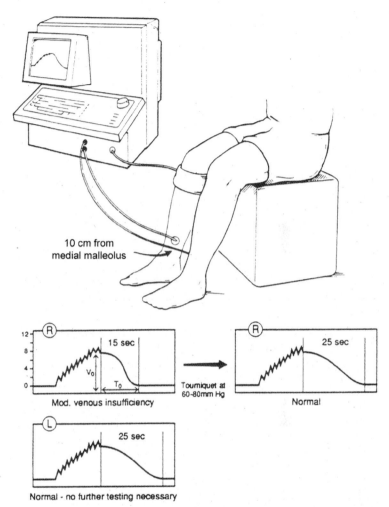

FIGURE 19-5. Photoplethsmographic measurements. The examination is performed with the patient sitting with the sensor placed as demonstrated in the figure. The calf veins are emptied by repeated dorsiflexion and plantarflexion of the ankle joint ten times. With cessation of ankle flexion, the time to veins to fill is the VRT. In this example, the left leg is normal, while the right leg has venous insufficiency. The test is repeated with an above-knee tourniquet at approximately 80 to 100 mm Hg; repeat tracing obtained now shows correction of VRT. (Adapted from Goldman MP, Weiss RA, Bergan JJ, et al. Diagnosis and treatment of varicose veins: a review. *J Am Acad Dermatol* 1994;31(3):393–413.)

veins only and differentiate the insufficiency between the perforators and the superficial veins. This test is considered qualitative and is not precise in quantifying the severity of deep venous insufficiency.

Air plethysmography. A more discriminating diagnostic study is the APG, which has the ability to measure venous reflux, calf muscle pump function, and, to a lesser degree, the presence or absence of outflow obstruction (Fig. 19.6). This test has both high sensitivity and high specificity (100% sensitivity and 90% specificity for reflux if VFI is used—see below). The concept of APG is that the leg is surrounded by a polyurethane sleeve containing expandable chambers that can be filled with air. The air chambers are connected to a very

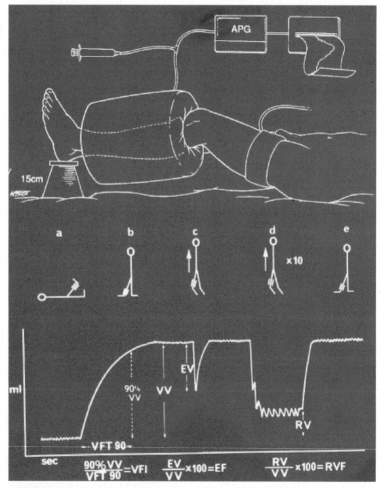

FIGURE 19-6. Diagrammatic representation of the APG apparatus and the methods of deriving the measurements. Also refer to Chapter 22.

sensitive pressure transducer. This allows volume measurements to be made with accuracy based upon pressure transduction calibrations. The benefit of APG in clinical practice is that it gives the physician an understanding of the different components contributing to CVI (reflux versus obstruction) and provides an idea of global venous function. It can be a useful test in objective evaluation of nonoperative therapies, or preoperative and postoperative hemodynamic assessments. For example, APG assessment of compression stocking function has shown that such garments are more effective in controlling reflux than in improving calf muscle function for patients with less severe CVI (CEAP class 4), while patients with more severe CVI (CEAP class 5) benefited more from improved calf muscle pump function than reflux control. APG can also be an important part of patient selection and predicting who will benefit most from surgical therapy. In general, patients with no outflow obstruction and intact calf muscle pump function should have a high likelihood of success with surgical treatment of venous reflux.

Technique. The first of several measurements made with APG is the functional VV. The patient is first placed in a supine position with the leg elevated at 45 degrees and the knee slightly flexed. The patient is then asked to stand up, and the VV measured. In normal limbs, the average VV is 80 to 150 mL, whereas in patients with severe CVI the volume might be close to 400 mL. The venous filling index (VFI) is defined as the ratio between 90% VV and the time taken for 90% filling (VFT90) to occur (VFI = 90%VV/VFT90). In normal limbs, veins should fill slowly from the arterial side with a VFI less than 2 mL/s. In limbs with severe reflux, this number may increase up to 30 mL/s. Increasing VFI is highly associated with the prevalence of skin changes and ulceration. Calf muscle pump function is also assessed. The patient is asked to do tiptoe movements and the recorded decrease in pressure represents the ejected volume (EV). Thus, the ejection fraction (EF) can be measured with the formula EF = [(EV/VV) × 100]. A normal EF is greater than 60%. Severe deep venous disease can result in an EF below 10%. The EF, like the VFI, is an important predictor of which patients will develop skin ulceration. The evaluation of venous outflow with APG is performed with the patient supine. A thigh tourniquet is placed proximally and inflated to 80 mm Hg. With the tourniquet suddenly deflated, the outflow fraction at 1 second (OF_1) is measured. This is expressed as a percentage of the total VV, and an OF_1 below 28% indicates severe obstruction while 30 to 40% indicates moderate obstruction. In patients without significant obstruction, the OF_1 is greater than 40%.

Evaluation of Suspected Deep Vein Thrombosis and Superficial Thrombophlebitis

Testing for DVT or SVT needs to be readily available and accurate. The following questions should be answered when evaluating a patient with suspected DVT or superficial thrombophlebitis: (i) Is there a thrombus? (ii) Is the thrombus acute or chronic? (iii) What is the anatomic extent of clot? (iv) Is there concomitant reflux? (v) Are the abnormalities that are detected enough to explain the patient's presentation or are there additional factors? (vi) What is the prognosis of the patient?

Vascular Laboratory Testing for the Diagnosis of Venous Thrombosis

Duplex ultrasound testing has become a common technique for venous imaging in patients with suspected DVT. Several criteria are used to evaluate for DVT including compressibility of the vein, respirophasic flow characteristics, color flow patency, appearance of an echogenic band (Fig. 19.7), and change in diameter during Valsalva (Table 19.6). Prospective studies demonstrated that the lack of compressibility of a vein

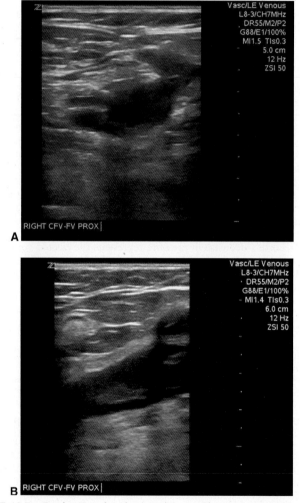

FIGURE 19.7.   Duplex Doppler ultrasound image of a noncompressible vein (**A**) consistent with acute DVT. The same vein (**B**) in longitudinal imaging demonstrating a free-floating echogenic band also consistent with DVT.

TABLE 19.6
DUPLEX CRITERIA FOR ACUTE DVT

Diagnostic Criteria
Thrombus
Noncompressibility
Absent or decreased spontaneous flow
Absent or decreased respiratory variation
Absent or incomplete color opacification of lumen
Additional Criteria
<50% increase in diameter with Valsalva maneuver
Increased venous diameter

with the ultrasound probe is highly sensitive and specific for proximal DVT (sensitivity and specificity greater than 95%). The presence of an echogenic band is very sensitive but not specific (specificity of 50%). The variation of venous size with Valsalva has a low sensitivity and specificity for the presence of DVT. Color flow imaging, in addition to duplex Doppler ultrasound, provides for a less demanding study and is highly accurate for the diagnosis of above-the-knee DVT. The chronicity of the thrombus can frequently be determined from the echogenicity of the clot; an older clot is more echodense (Table 19.7). Duplex ultrasound is slightly less sensitive and specific for diagnosing calf-vein DVT. However, in skilled hands, the sensitivity and specificity approaches that for proximal DVT. Duplex ultrasound has a low sensitivity in diagnosis of DVT in asymptomatic postoperative patients and is therefore not recommended for this purpose.

Impedance plethysmography (IP) has fallen out of favor and is rarely used in most centers. In symptomatic patients, it is both sensitive and specific for diagnosis of proximal DVT rivaling venous duplex ultrasound (sensitivity of 93% and specificity of 97%; positive and negative predictive values of 82 and 97%, respectively). However, IP is insensitive to calf-vein thrombosis. Similar to duplex Doppler ultrasound, IP also has a relatively low sensitivity and specificity in asymptomatic postoperative patients (sensitivity of 12% for thigh thrombi in asymptomatic total hip replacement patients). The accuracy of IP is decreased in conditions where arterial inflow

TABLE 19.7
DUPLEX DIFFERENTIATION OF ACUTE VERSUS CHRONIC DVT

Diagnostic Criteria	Acute Thrombus	Chronic Thrombus
Echo characteristics	Echolucent, homogenous	Echogenic, heterogenous
Lumen	Smooth	Irregular
Compressibility	Spongy	Firm
Diameter of vein	Dilated	Decreased or normal
Collaterals	Absent	Present
Flow channel	Confluent	Multiple

and/or venous outflow are impaired, such as in patients with congestive heart failure, severe arterial occlusive disease, and venous compression.

Ascending venography has long been considered the "gold standard" for diagnosis of DVT. However, venography is not recommended as an initial screening because of several limitations including discomfort to the patient and difficulty in executing the study adequately. Heijboer et al. in their study comparing IP and ultrasound to venography noted that venography could not be performed in 20% (25 of 127) of patients because of contraindications or inability to undergo the contrast study. Venography is currently used when other means of testing are not clinically feasible or to supplement equivocal noninvasive studies. It is performed by injecting contrast into a dorsal foot vein and directing the contrast into the deep venous system by using an ankle tourniquet. This technique can provide useful anatomic information about the location and extent of venous obstruction. However, the profunda femoris veins and internal iliac veins are not typically well visualized with this technique.

Descending venography is an invasive technique used to assess venous reflux and valvular anatomy. This test is performed on a fluoroscopic table tilted 60 degrees, while contrast is injected through a catheter with the tip placed at the distal external iliac vein. Gravity and a Valsalva maneuver propel contrast distally in limbs with incompetent valves. This allows grading of phlebographic reflux, as well as delineating competent valve cusps, which are clearly outlined with this technique. Reflux is graded by the Kistner classification (0, no reflux; 1, reflux confined to upper thigh; 2, reflux extends to lower thigh; 3, reflux extends to the popliteal fossa with extension into the calf). Descending venography requires an experienced imaging team to perform and is costly. Duplex scanning obviates the need for this test in many circumstances.

Magnetic resonance venography: Advances in magnetic resonance technology and MR contrast agents have made MRV the preferred alternative to conventional contrast venography. Not only can the presence of intravenous thrombi be detected with MRV, but this technique can also provide information on perivascular anatomy and assessment of blood flow. MRV has been found to be useful in diagnosing May-Thurner syndrome, a clinical entity of left iliac vein compression by the right iliac artery, which results in isolated left lower extremity swelling and may be a precipitating factor for iliofemoral DVT. MRV is the best technique for evaluation of gonadal vein thrombosis. MRV may be performed with or without gadolinium-based contrast agents (see Chapter 4). Gadolinium may also be used to differentiate acute versus chronic DVT. Acute DVT typically shows perithrombus enhancement (Fig. 19.8, bottom panel). Simple protocols that incorporate 2D time-of-flight (TOF) acquisitions are highly accurate for the diagnosis of DVT involving the femoral, popliteal, or iliac veins. The sensitivity and specificity for above-knee clots with TOF-MRV are 97 and 95%, respectively, while for detecting calf-vein thrombi, the sensitivity and specificity are 85 and 96%, respectively. Figure 19.8 demonstrates a thrombus in the left common femoral vein by TOF imaging. In *contrast-enhanced magnetic resonance* (CE-MR) *venography*, the veins are directly imaged by injection of diluted contrast. A bolus-chase (floating table approach) akin to lower

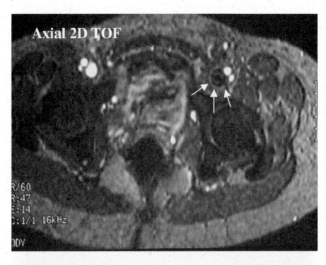

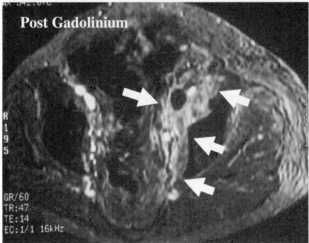

FIGURE 19-8.   MRV depicting a thrombus in the left femoral vein by TOF in the top panel. The bottom panel depicts contrast enhancement of the perithrombotic tissue with gadolinium enhancement.

extremity arterial exams with contrast may be used for veins as well with two to three separate stations (calf, thighs, and pelvis).

Spiral Computed Tomography Venography

Spiral CTV of the leg has shown promise for the diagnosis of DVT and other soft-tissue diseases in patients with leg swelling. It may be combined with computed tomography pulmonary angiography (CTPA) during the evaluation of PE. In a pooled meta-analysis, the sensitivity and specificity of CTV compared to duplex ultrasound were 95.9 and 95.2%, respectively. CTV especially when combined with CTPA may offer benefits in intensive care unit patients in whom bedside imaging may be compromised or patients in whom injury or surgical procedures may limit the use of duplex ultrasound. One consideration for widespread use of CTV is the radiation dose added to the CTPA. Since the diagnostic accuracy among duplex ultrasound, MRV and CTV is comparable, the choice among these testing modalities should be based on clinical grounds.

CONCLUSIONS

The initial approach to the patient with acute or chronic venous disease involves a detailed history, physical examination, and office-based noninvasive assessment with a handheld Doppler and/or referral to the vascular laboratory in order to determine if the symptoms are due to an acute or chronic process. A noninvasive approach is usually used to confirm the clinical suspicion of DVT. The initial diagnostic imaging evaluation of patients with suspected DVT in most centers should be duplex ultrasound with color flow imaging. X-ray contrast venography, MRV, or CTV should not be considered as an initial diagnostic technique but obtained when equivocal results are seen with aforementioned noninvasive techniques or further information is needed, that is, is May-Thurner syndrome the cause of thrombus? For suspected venous reflux, PPG may be a reasonable screen followed by venous duplex ultrasound if venous reflux is positive or in equivocal cases and will allow for localization of the problem. Further testing is warranted with duplex ultrasound, APG, MRV, or contrast venography to determine if treatment strategies are feasible. Figure 19.9 provides an approach to assess venous disorders.

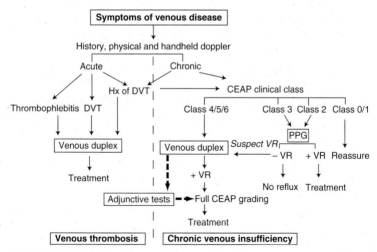

FIGURE 19-9. Diagnostic approach to a patient with venous symptoms. Adjunctive testing may include the following studies: contrast venography, APG, and MR venography. (VR, Venous reflux; PPG, photoplethysmograph)

PRACTICAL POINTS

■ Toe swelling (square toe sign) typically indicates lymphedema instead of venous edema.

■ Suspect May-Thurner syndrome (compression of left iliac vein by right common iliac artery) when left iliofemoral DVT is present.

■ Clinical clues to DVT such as Homan's sign are not specific for diagnosis of DVT and thus should not be used to confirm or discount the presence of DVT.

■ The presence of pigmentation and eczematous changes in the medial aspect of the lower leg ("stasis dermatitis") is pathognomonic for CVI.

■ Lack of compressibility of a vein with the ultrasound probe is highly sensitive and specific for DVT (sensitivity and specificity greater than 95%).

■ APG is extremely sensitive (greater than 95%) for reflux and provides information on outflow obstruction and calf pump function.

■ CEAP class is very helpful to adjudicate investigations in patients presenting with venous symptoms.

■ Most individuals with CEAP class 4/5/6 changes usually have deep venous reflux with or without concomitant obstruction. Isolated superficial venous reflux in this category of patients is uncommon.

RECOMMENDED READING

Barnes RW, Nix ML, Barnes CL, et al. Perioperative asymptomatic venous thrombosis: role of duplex scanning versus venography. *J Vasc Surg* 1989;9:251–260.

Butty S, Hagspiel KD, Leung DA, et al. Body MR venography. *Radiol Clin North Am* 2002;40(4):899–919.

Davidson BL, Elliott CG, Lensing AW. Low accuracy of color Doppler ultrasound in the detection of proximal leg vein thrombosis in asymptomatic high-risk patients. The RD Heparin Arthroplasty Group. *Ann Intern Med* 1992;117:735–738.

Gloviczki Lohr J, Griffith NM. Acute deep venous thrombosis: clinical and diagnostic evaluation. In: Cronenwett JL, ed. *Rutherford's vascular surgery*, 7th ed. Philadelphia, PA: W. B. Saunders, 2010, Chapter 49.

Goodman LR, Sostman HD, Stein PD, et al. CT venography: a necessary adjunct to CT pulmonary angiography or a waste of time, money, and radiation? *Radiology* 2009;250:327–330.

Heijboer H, Cogo A, Buller HR, et al. Detection of deep vein thrombosis with impedance plethysmography and real-time compression ultrasonography in hospitalized patients. *Arch Intern Med* 1992;152:1901–1903.

Jacobson AF. Diagnosis of deep venous thrombosis. A review of radiologic, radionuclide, and non-imaging methods. *Q J Nucl Med* 2001;45(4):324–333.

Kistner RL, Masuda EM. A practical approach to the diagnosis and classification of chronic venous disease in management of venous disease. In: Rutherford RB, ed. *Vascular surgery*, 5th ed. Philadelphia, PA: W. B. Saunders, 2000.

Lensing AW, Doris CI, McGrath FP, et al. A comparison of compression ultrasound with color doppler ultrasound for the diagnosis of symptomless postoperative deep vein thrombosis. *Arch Intern Med* 1997;157:765–768.

Lensing AW, Prandoni P, Brandjes D, et al. Detection of deep-vein thrombosis by real-time B-mode ultrasonography. *N Engl J Med* 1989;320:342–345.

Mattos MA, Londrey GL, Leutz DW, et al. Color-flow duplex scanning for the surveillance and diagnosis of acute deep venous thrombosis. *J Vasc Surg* 1992;15:366–375.

Meissner MH, Eklof B, Coleridge Smith P, et al. Secondary chronic venous disorders. *J Vasc Surg* 2007;46:68S–83S.

Meissner MH, Gloviczki P, Bergan J, et al. Primary chronic venous disorders. *J Vasc Surg* 2007;46:54S–67S.

Meissner MH, Moneta G, Burnand K, et al. The hemodynamics and diagnosis of venous disease. *J Vasc Surg* 2007;46:4S–24S.

O'Shaughnessy AM, FitzGerald DE. Organization patterns of venous thrombus over time as demonstrated by duplex ultrasound. *J Vasc Invest* 1996;2:75–81.

Prince MR, Grist TM, Debatin JF, eds. *3D contrast MR venography in 3D contrast MR angiography*, 2nd ed. Berlin, Germany: Springer Verlag, 1999.

Raffetto JD, Eberhardt RT. Chronic venous disorders: general considerations. Chapter 53. In: Cronenwett JL, ed. *Rutherford's vascular surgery*, 7th ed. Philadelphia, PA: Saunders, 2010.

Thomas SM, Goodacre SW, Sampson FC, et al. Diagnostic value of CT for deep vein thrombosis: results of a systematic review and meta-analysis. *Clin Radiol* 2008;63:299–304.

Wolpert LM, Rahmani O, Stein B, et al. Magnetic resonance venography in the diagnosis and management of May-Thurner syndrome. *Vasc Endovasc Surg* 2002;36(1):51–57.

Zweibel WJ. Extremity venous examination and venous thrombosis. In: Zweibel WJ ed. *Introduction to vascular ultrasonography*, 4th ed. Philadelphia, PA: W. B. Saunders, 2000.

CHAPTER 20 ■ Approaches to and Management of Varicose Veins

Bhagwan Satiani and Maria Litzendorf

Varicose veins are a common problem with one quarter to one third of all adults in the western world affected by this disorder. Varicose veins can be asymptomatic (with purely aesthetic connotation) or can directly impact quality of life when associated with symptoms of heaviness, fatigue, or throbbing pain. Although usually found on the lower extremities, varicose veins can also be located in the upper extremity, trunk, vulva, spermatic cords (varicoceles), rectum (hemorrhoids), and esophagus (esophageal varices). Although primarily an adult condition, in rare cases, children can be affected, most commonly when associated with underlying vascular malformations such as Klippel-Trenaunay syndrome. Other congenital conditions such as Maffucci's syndrome, cutis marmorata telangiectatica congenita, or diffuse neonatal hemangiomatosis may manifest with telangiectasia during childhood.

Varicose veins are generally identified by their tortuous, twisted, bulging, superficial appearance and can be grouped as truncal, reticular, or telangiectasia. Truncal varices (also known as *stem* or *axial veins*) refer to larger vessels including the great and small saphenous veins and their branches. Reticular veins are the smaller, superficial, blue-green, flat, tortuous vessels, while telangiectasias are the small blue-black or red veins that are less than 1 mm in diameter (Figs. 20.1 to 20.3).

The symptoms of varicose veins have often been ignored or underestimated by physicians in the past. In addition, treatment options were often limited. Fortunately, with the advances in our understanding of the pathophysiology of venous disorders and the addition of newer diagnostic and treatment modalities, we are now better equipped to treat patients with varicose veins.

CLINICAL FEATURES

Incidence and Prevalence

Varicose veins are the most common clinical manifestation of chronic venous disease. However, the differing terminology and diagnostic criteria used in many epidemiological data sets make it difficult to accurately determine the prevalence of varicose veins in the general population. In addition, it is estimated that up to one third of patients never seek treatment for their varicose veins. Given these limitations, the incidence of varicose veins may be grossly underestimated. Despite this, most prevalence figures for pronounced disease range from 10 to 15%, and for all types of disease range from 30 to 50%. In the widely referenced Framingham study, the 2-year incidence of varicose veins was 39.4 new cases per

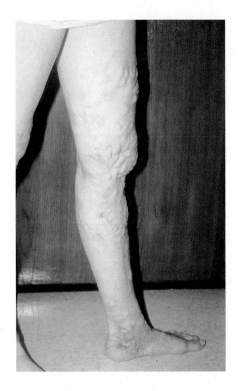

FIGURE 20-1. Varicose veins involving the entire leg of this 32-year-old pregnant woman. There is a strong family history of varicose veins. Varicose veins are graded as class 2 according to the CEAP Clinical Classification System.

1,000 men and 51.9 cases per 1,000 women. While it is generally conceded that women are more likely to seek medical attention for varicose veins, most population studies still agree that varicose veins are two to three times more common in women, occurring in 25 to 46% of women and 7 to 19% of men.

In addition, there are geographical, social, and ethnic factors that impact the prevalence of varicose veins. Industrialized populations tend to have higher prevalence rates than developing countries. In North and Sub-Saharan Africa, rates are one fourth to one fifth of that seen in European women. While these differences have been observed in epidemiologic studies, they are inconsistent in immigrant populations, suggesting that cultural factors including diet and exercise may play a more important role than genetics and geography.

Risk Factors

Table 20.1 lists risk factors that have been implicated in the development of varicose veins. A number of these factors are believed to mediate their effects through increases in lower extremity hydrostatic pressure directly or through an increase in intra-abdominal pressure with resultant compromise

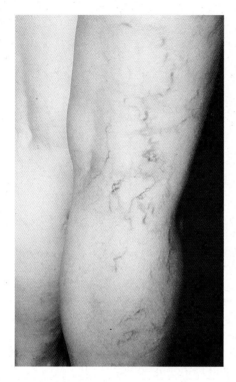

FIGURE 20-2. Reticular veins involving the posterior thigh and calf in this 58-year-old female. They are flat, blue or green in appearance, and are graded class 1 according to the CEAP Clinical Classification System.

in blood return to the iliac veins. The genetics of varicose veins is not understood, although it is believed that there is a genetic component that affects predilection. Commonly believed associations of varicose veins with high systolic blood pressure, congestive heart failure, diabetes, serum lipids, tight undergarments, and hernias have not been supported by population-based studies. However, there is strong evidence that occupations involving prolonged standing including nurses, teachers, assembly-line workers, surgeons, and beauticians are associated with the development of varicosities. A BMI of greater than 30 kg/m^2 carries a fivefold increase in the prevalence of varicose veins in women. Pregnancy is also frequently reported as a risk factor for the development of varicose veins. Although the enlarging uterus is believed to obstruct venous return and contribute to the formation of varicose veins, most women report an increase in varicose veins during their first trimester, when the gravid uterus is not yet large enough to cause mechanical obstruction. The role of estrogen on smooth muscle relaxation has been well described. Thus, women on oral contraceptives or those who are pregnant have increased venous distensibility and decreased venous tone, which may contribute to the development of venous disease. Women with multiple pregnancies also appear to have a higher prevalence of varicose veins.

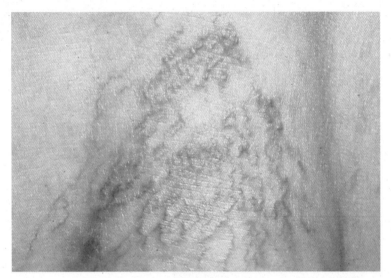

FIGURE 20-3. Example of extensive venous telangiectasia found on the posterior thigh of this 48-year-old woman. Telangiectasias are typically red, or blue-black, in appearance and more commonly referred to as *spider veins* or *hyphen webs*. They usually measure less than 1.0 mm in diameter. They are considered class 1 according to the CEAP Clinical Classification System.

Anatomy and Pathophysiology

The terminology of the major veins in the lower extremities has been revised (Table 20.2) (Fig. 20.4). The venous system of the legs is divided into deep and superficial vessels. Perforator veins link the superficial to the deep veins and enable blood flow during muscle relaxation when pressure in the deep veins falls below that of the superficial vessels. Varicose veins are a common symptom of chronic venous insufficiency (CVI, see

TABLE 20.1
RISK FACTORS FOR VARICOSE VEINS

Heredity

Age

Gender

Occupation (prolonged standing)

Sedentary lifestyle

Obesity

Pregnancy (increase with parity)

Heat (ultraviolet light, sunlight, x-rays)

Hormones (oral contraceptives or hormone replacement therapy)

TABLE 20.2
OLD AND NEW TERMINOLOGY OF LOWER EXTREMITY VEINS

Old	New
Greater saphenous vein	Great saphenous vein
Lesser saphenous vein	Small saphenous vein
Superficial femoral vein	Femoral vein
Hunterian's perforator	Midthigh perforator
Cockett's perforator	Paratibial perforator
	Posterior tibial perforators
May's perforator	Intergemellar perforator

Chapter 22) that develops as a result of a structural or functional defect in the venous system. These defects lead to ambulatory venous hypertension and can be classified as either primary or secondary. Primary disorders affect the venous wall or valves and lead to reflux and venous dilatation without evidence for previous venous thrombosis. They are more common in women and most patients will report a strong family history for varicose veins. Secondary defects are the result of venous thrombosis that leads to obstruction, reflux, or a combination of the two. Venous hypertension is defined as end-exercise venous pressure at the ankle greater than 30 mm Hg (normal is 15 mm Hg) and can be measured (but is rarely done) using a 21-gauge needle. Measurements are made in a dorsal foot vein following 10 tiptoe movements at a rate of one per second as the venous pressures are lowest at the end of exercise. The severity of venous disease correlates excellently with the degree of venous hypertension. At pressures of less than 30 mm Hg, ulceration is rare, while at pressures of greater than 90 mm Hg, there is nearly a 100% incidence of ulceration.

Histologic examination of varicose veins demonstrates disorganization of the muscular layers, with a thickened intima, and fibrosis between the intima and the adventitia. In addition, there is atrophy of the elastic fibers. These histologic changes reiterate the importance of these structural alterations in mediating the functional consequences of reduced contractility and loss of compliance. Subsequent dilatation causes a separation of valve cusps within the vein and results in valvular incompetence or reflux. Secondary defects are a result of valve cusp damage from previous thrombotic episodes. Varicose veins are more likely to develop where the superficial and deep systems communicate, for example, at the saphenofemoral or saphenopopliteal junctions or where perforator veins connect the two systems.

Symptoms and Signs

Table 20.3 lists the presenting symptoms and signs. Varicose veins are associated with varying degrees of pain and swelling. The pain is often described as aching, tingling, or cramping in nature. Common complaints include fatigue, restlessness, burning, stinging, itching, tension, or heaviness in the legs.

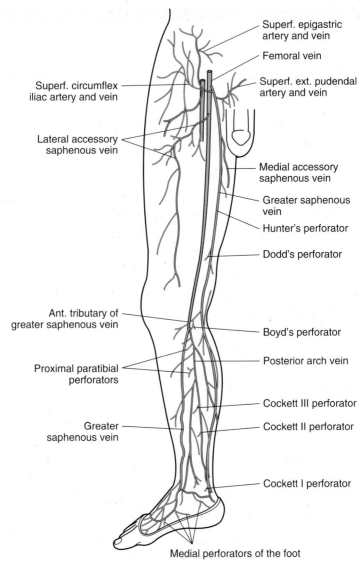

FIGURE 20-4.   Anatomy and terminology of lower extremity veins.

Symptoms are generally less severe in the morning but exacerbated with prolonged standing or sitting throughout the day. Consequently, symptoms tend
to resolve with rest and elevation. The most common symptom reported by
women is aching, while men report cramping pain more often. Varicose veins
may be exacerbated during menses or first noted with pregnancy. Women

TABLE 20.3

SIGNS AND SYMPTOMS OF VARICOSE VEINS

Symptoms
  Cramping pain
  Burning pain
  Heaviness
  Fatigue
  Itching
  Tension
  Throbbing pain
  Restless legs
  Tingling
Signs
  Dermatitis
  Hemorrhage
  Superficial thrombophlebitis
  Ulceration
  Lipodermatosclerosis
  Atrophie blanche

may experience pelvic pain or dyspareunia due to vulvar varices. Symptoms do not always correlate with the size or number of veins and, at times, may seem inconsistent with the physical examination. Patients with small varicosities may complain of a severe burning pain, heaviness, or swelling, while patients with larger varices may be asymptomatic. Patients without symptoms often seek medical attention for cosmetic reasons or simply reassurance about their condition. Approximately 5 to 7% of patients with venous disease seek medical attention because of complications, including superficial venous thrombosis (SVT), bleeding, and ulceration. When bleeding does occur, it is often profuse and may be mistaken for an arterial bleed because of high venous pressure. It is often spontaneous, although it can occur after such minor trauma as shaving the legs.

Physical findings that frequently accompany varicose veins include edema, ulceration, dermatitis, hyperpigmentation, lipodermatosclerosis, atrophie blanche, hemorrhage, and SVT. Hyperpigmentation and ulceration are classically found on the medial side of the ankle (gaiter area) but may also occur in the lateral aspect of the leg above the malleolus (associated with small saphenous vein incompetence). Hyperpigmentation results from hemosiderin deposition within dermal macrophages after the breakdown of red blood cells.

Venous ulcers may be difficult to heal and are frequently recurrent (Fig. 20.5). Lipodermatosclerosis, also known as *stasis cellulitis*, is characterized by edema, erythema, pain, increased warmth, and indurated skin. Atrophie blanche refers to atrophic, circular, white areas of skin that develop in patients with CVI. These ulcerations are extremely painful,

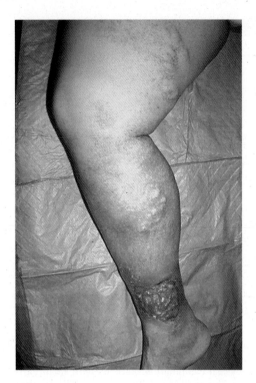

FIGURE 20-5. An example of hyperpigmentation and venous ulceration due to CVI and varicose veins. The extravasation of red blood cells over time into the surrounding tissue leaves the characteristic brown discoloration. Venous ulcers are the most common type of leg ulcers. They generally occur on the medial aspect of the leg, just above the malleolus, and are found in approximately 0.3% of Western adult populations.

small in size, and typically heal with great difficulty (Fig. 20.6). SVT may occasionally develop in varicose veins (Fig. 20.7). Patients usually complain of pain over the varicosity, and physical examination reveals warmth, swelling, and erythema over the varicosity.

Classification of Varicose Veins

A number of classification systems have been used to describe chronic venous insufficiency. The most currently accepted classification system is known as the *CEAP Clinical Classification*. CEAP stands for clinical presentation, etiology, anatomy, and pathophysiology and was established in an effort to better address all aspects of chronic venous disease (see Chapter 22, Table 22.2 for the CEAP classification system). Under this system, varicose veins and chronic venous insufficiency are classified according to their clinical presentation (telangiectasias, reticular veins, pigmentation or ulceration), etiology (congenital, primary, or secondary), anatomy (superficial, perforator, or deep veins), and pathophysiology (reflux or obstruction or both). The CEAP clinical classification is very helpful in adjudicating diagnostic strategies and treatment modalities. In addition, the Villalta and Venous Clinical Severity Score (VCSS) scoring systems have been described in order to objectively describe the clinical response (Table 22.3).

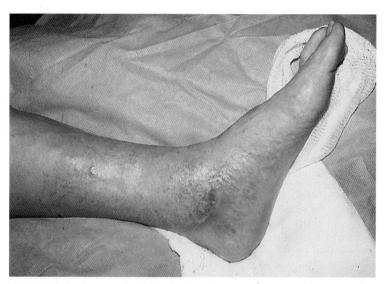

FIGURE 20-6. An example of CVI manifested by varicose veins and the ulceration(s) of atrophie blanche. Note the varicose vein along the medial aspect of the calf and the areas of hypopigmentation and small ulcerations.

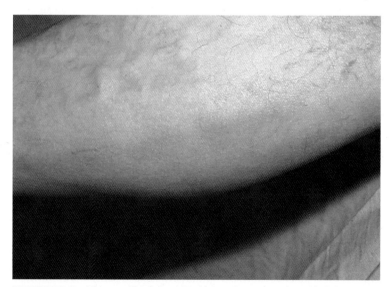

FIGURE 20-7. The superficial thrombophlebitis located on the calf of this patient is characterized by pain, erythema, rubor or heat, and swelling.

DIAGNOSIS

A complete review of the patient's current and past medical history is important with careful attention to the risk factors detailed above. The physical examination should include inspection and palpation of the arterial system, abdomen, and both legs (or arms) with the patient sitting and standing. The location, size, color, and configuration of any varicose, reticular, or telangiectasia vein should be recorded. Any skin changes or ulcerations should also be noted, as well as the presence of edema. Specific techniques for assessing varicose veins during the initial physical examination have included the cough test, percussion or Schwartz' test, Brodie-Trendelenburg test, and Perthes' test. Many of these tests are of value only when noninvasive technology is not available for a precise diagnosis. The most widely used clinical test, the Trendelenburg test, has a 91% sensitivity for identifying superficial and perforator disease but is only 15% specific. The lower extremities are elevated to 45 degrees draining the veins, and a tourniquet is then applied below the saphenofemoral junction. The patient is then asked to stand. If there is rapid filling of distal veins with the tourniquet in place, this suggests perforator incompetence, while rapid filling upon removal of the tourniquet suggests saphenofemoral incompetence.

Laboratory Testing

Duplex ultrasound scanning (DUS) should be part of the initial examination. This has largely replaced venography as the preferred imaging technique for varicose veins in all but a few exceptions. Ascending and descending venography have long been considered the standard methods for the evaluation of valvular reflux and incompetency and for surgical management of varicose veins. Unfortunately, these tests are expensive, painful, and not without complications including deep vein thrombosis and contrast allergic reactions. They remain useful when other noninvasive studies are inadequate or equivocal.

DUS is the test of choice for the evaluation of varicose veins (Chapter 22). Some practitioners may still utilize photoplethysmography (PPG) and air plethysmography (APG), although these are much less sensitive and specific. PPG is used by a number of practices to evaluate leg swelling and to rule out reflux or retrograde flow of blood down the veins. PPG performed as a screening test has a sensitivity ranging from 50 to 85% depending on the criteria used (sensitivity of 50% if venous refill time of 15 seconds used, higher if 23 seconds used) and a specificity of 80%. Owing to the modest sensitivity, the absence of reflux by PPG may still not rule out this diagnosis. APG uses a recording pneumatic cuff placed on the calf and is a physiologic study to measure venous reflux, calf muscle pump function, and venous obstruction. This is detailed further in Chapter 22.

MANAGEMENT

There are a number of treatment options available to patients with varicose veins. Treatment is dependent on the overall health of the individual and the magnitude of symptoms. Treatment options may be considered noninvasive, interventional, or surgical (Table 20.4).

TABLE 20.4

TREATMENT OPTIONS FOR VARICOSE, RETICULAR, AND VENOUS TELANGIECTASIA VEINS

External compression (bandages, support hose, external compression devices)
Sclerotherapy
Laser therapy or light therapy
Endovenous obliteration of the saphenous vein
Transilluminated powered phlebectomy
Ambulatory phlebectomy or stab avulsion phlebectomy
Ligation and stripping

Noninvasive Treatment Options

These include the usage of support or graduated compression hose in addition to regular exercise, elevation, and good skin hygiene. Patients with CEAP class 1 or 2 and many with class 3 may require these options alone.

External Compression Therapy

External compression devices remain the mainstay of treatment for most cases of varicose veins and CVI. The term *graduated* compression implies that the intrinsic pressure generated by the stockings is greater in the lower part of the leg compared to the upper portion. This method is extremely effective in treating the swelling, pain, and ulcers that may develop as complications of varicosities and CVI. Compression may be applied in the form of bandages, elastic stockings, or intermittent pneumatic compression devices. They can be used alone, or in conjunction with other therapies including sclerotherapy and surgery. Contraindications for compression therapy include arterial insufficiency [ankle-brachial index (ABI) less than 0.6 and/or ankle pressures less than 60 mm Hg], active skin disease, or allergy to any of the stocking components. Compression therapy is less expensive than other therapeutic approaches including surgery and sclerotherapy in the short term, although over time these expenses can add up. Unfortunately, many patients are unable or unwilling to use compression hose because they are tight, uncomfortable, and difficult to put on and take off, so compliance is often an issue. Stockings vary in amount of compression, generally ranging from 15 to 50 mm Hg depending on the severity of symptoms and underlying pathology. They can be custom fitted for certain individuals, and correct measurement by a professional such as an orthotist is essential. Compression garments need to be replaced from time to time because they lose their elasticity and can easily be torn or damaged.

More severe disease, including venous ulceration, may mandate more aggressive compression with a rigid compression system. Adequate compression is the foundation for healing with venous ulcerations. The most common methods for applying topical wound treatments and compression include Unna's boots, compression hose with wound covers, and multilayer compression bandages. The Unna's boot, the best-known rigid compression system, alleviates compliance concerns as this compression remains on for up to 1 week and is in general removed and applied by health care professionals. The Unna's boot is a three-layer system. The innermost layer is a medicated paste gauze of calamine, magnesium aluminum silicate, zinc oxide, glycerin, and sorbitol. Next is a gauze layer followed by an outermost elastic compression wrap. In cases of cellulitis, the rigid device may need to be changed more frequently. A multilayer dressing system is typically considered more comfortable than an Unna boot and has the following layers: (i) a natural orthopedic wool, which absorbs exudate and protects bony prominences from excessive pressure; (ii) a crepe bandage adding absorbency and acting to smooth the orthopedic wool layer; (iii) a light compression bandage, which is highly conformable to accommodate a difficult limb shape; and (iv) a cohesive flexible bandage that also applies pressure, maintaining effective levels of compression for up to 1 week. In one study, nearly 80% of patients had ulcer healing by 12 weeks using this therapy.

Medications

There are very few medications available that are beneficial to the patients with varicose veins. Diuretics are commonly prescribed but generally do little to remove the pain or discomfort caused by varices. They may help in the short term with resolution of edema but do not correct the underlying problem. Herbal remedies such as *Horse chestnut extract* (sold as Venastat), *butcher's broom* or *Ruscus aculeatus* have been used for relief of symptoms. *Daflon*, a micronized purified flavonoid fraction, is a venotropic drug that has also been used for the treatment of venous disease. The relative value of these interventions is not supported by randomized controlled clinical trials.

Sclerotherapy

This is an excellent treatment option for patients with venous telangiectasias, reticular veins, and small varicose veins (1 to 3 mm diameter) and is often performed for cosmetic reasons alone. Sclerotherapy is indicated and helpful in eliminating the pain and discomfort caused by superficial varicose veins and, if used appropriately, may be useful in the prevention of complications related to varicose veins including venous hemorrhage and ulceration. Smaller varicosities such as venous telangiectases and reticular veins respond best to sclerotherapy, while treatment of saphenous-related varicose veins, although possible, has demonstrated a higher recurrence rate when compared to surgery in randomized trials. A thorough history and physical examination should precede sclerotherapy. Any suspected underlying reflux should be identified and corrected before sclerotherapy is attempted. There are several different agents used for injection purposes. They include sodium tetradecyl sulfate (Sotradecol); hypertonic saline (11.7 to 23.4%); hypertonic saline (10%) and dextrose (25%) (Sclerodex); and sodium morrhuate 5%, ethanolamine oxalate, and polidocanol (Aethoxysklerol, not FDA approved). Varicose veins are treated similarly to venous telangiectases and reticular veins except that larger volumes and/

TABLE 20.5

COMPLICATIONS OF SCLEROTHERAPY

Pain or cramping
Hyperpigmentation
Telangiectatic matting
Blistering or necrosis
Superficial venous thrombosis
Deep vein thrombosis
Urticaria
Edema

or greater concentrations of the solution may be required. Care must be taken to avoid extravasation of the solution into the surrounding skin. Sclerotherapy has been used in conjunction with DUS to enhance its effectiveness. It is reported to improve therapeutic success rates and reduce complications. Table 20.5 lists complications noted with sclerotherapy. Anaphylaxis has rarely been reported with Sotradecol, ethanolamine, and sodium morrhuate. Pain or cramping is reported to occur with the hypertonic solutions (saline and dextrose). Following sclerotherapy, patients should be placed in a compression garment immediately to decrease the incidence of pigmentation, reduce the incidence of telangiectatic matting, improve the efficacy of the solution, and more rapidly dilute the sclerosing agent, thereby reducing the risk for deep vein thrombosis. Most physicians recommend at least 1 to 3 weeks of compression therapy. Table 20.6 lists some of the contraindication for sclerotherapy.

Sclerotherapy is a viable treatment option when bleeding is the presenting sign and pressure with elevation fails to control it.

TABLE 20.6

ABSOLUTE OR RELATIVE CONTRAINDICATIONS FOR SCLEROTHERAPY

Acute deep vein thrombosis
Bedridden or immobile patient
Acute infections including cellulitis
Allergy to the sclerosant
Uncontrolled diabetes
Blood dyscrasias or thrombophilia
Cancer patients undergoing chemotherapy
Use with caution with arterial disease
Use with caution in women on oral contraceptives or hormone replacement therapy
Pregnant patients
Breastfeeding

Laser Therapy and Intense Pulse Light Therapies

Laser and high-intensity pulsed light therapies have grown in popularity over the past few years. Laser therapy was first introduced in the 1970s, while intense pulse light (IPL) sources were introduced in the 1990s. Unlike sclerotherapy, where vessels are directly injected, laser and light sources are applied indirectly over the superficial vessel. Their effectiveness is dependent on the depth of the vessel, flow, and their size. Early results were often unsatisfactory because of the above conditions and inexperience of the operators. Subsequently, a number of newer lasers and light sources have been developed to enhance clinical efficacy. The recent development of lasers with longer wavelengths and pulse durations has eliminated many of the earlier problems and improved outcomes. Both laser and the light sources are generally more expensive (cost of equipment) than sclerotherapy.

Laser therapy is considered a first-line approach for isolated, superficial, fine-caliber telangiectasia and telangiectatic matting. It is also an option for patients who are afraid of needles, have responded poorly to sclerotherapy, or have had untoward side effects with sclerotherapy (Table 20.7). Larger feeder vessels including reticular veins and incompetent perforators should be typically treated with sclerotherapy prior to laser therapy. Pain is a common side effect, and therefore, topical anesthesia and cooling (e.g., using a water-based gel) are needed when treating many of the larger vessels. Superficial scabbing and hypopigmentation or hyperpigmentation can occur. There are a number of lasers available commercially, and it may be confusing to know which are most effective. Physicians interested in laser therapy should thoroughly familiarize themselves with these devices prior to initiating therapy.

High-intensity pulsed light (PhotoDerm VL, ESC Medical, Inc., Needham, MA) was developed in 1993. This technique differs from laser therapy by emitting a spectrum of light, rather than a single wavelength. Venous telangiectasias respond well to this technology, although hyperpigmentation, blistering, and superficial erosions have been reported.

Surgical and Endovascular Therapy

The most important aspect of managing varicosities is the determination of who will benefit from an intervention and what type of intervention most appropriate. An understanding of the pathophysiology of varicose veins is essential. Determining the anatomical site and degree of valvular reflux

TABLE 20.7

INDICATIONS FOR SURFACE LASER THERAPY

Superficial, fine-caliber venous telangiectasia
Telangiectatic matting
Patient afraid of needles
Poor responders to sclerotherapy
Adverse side effects from sclerotherapy

and ruling out obstruction and deep venous reflux are both critical steps in careful patient selection. All patients ideally should be categorized using the CEAP (clinical presentation, etiology, anatomy, pathophysiology) classification system prior to any operative intervention. Surgery and endovascular approaches remain the preferred treatment for managing symptomatic large or truncal varicose veins that are unresponsive to "conservative" therapy. Indications for surgery include advanced skin changes, ulceration, bleeding, pain, and swelling. In addition, intervention is often performed for cosmetic reasons. The goals of interventional procedures including surgery should be the elimination of the need for support hose, prevention of recurrent ulcers and skin changes, and returning the patient to a near-normal lifestyle.

Great or Small Saphenous Vein Ligation

In cases of GSV or small saphenous vein incompetence, methods of treatment involve removal of the refluxing veins. Ligation of the great saphenous vein at the saphenofemoral junction alone leads to a high recurrence rate. However, when performed in conjunction with removal or ablation of the thigh portion of the saphenous vein ligation at the saphenofemoral junction, it is an acceptable alternative. One of the few randomized studies using duplex scanning comparing ligation alone versus stripping of the great saphenous vein of 133 legs with a minimum follow-up of 5 years showed a 6% recurrence with stripping compared to a 25% recurrence with ligation alone. Ligation of the GSV at the saphenofemoral junction in conjunction with ablation of the thigh portion of the saphenous vein by sclerotherapy is another option, especially followed in Europe.

Ambulatory Phlebectomy (Microphlebectomy/Hook Phlebectomy) of Superficial Varicosities

Ambulatory phlebectomy is a relatively easy, effective, and inexpensive method for removal of superficial varicose vein tributaries that can be performed in the office setting. It may be performed in conjunction with either surgical removal or ablation of the great or small saphenous veins. Ambulatory phlebectomy of tributaries is less effective if untreated reflux is present at the saphenofemoral or saphenopopliteal junctions. With this procedure, the varicosity is hooked and pulled through a small surgical incision and then excised in tiny pieces. It is frequently described as a tedious procedure that is time intensive but allows for satisfactory removal of these veins. Complications are unlikely but do include bleeding and hematomas. Occasionally, transient hyperpigmentation, infection, pain, and telangiectatic matting may also occur.

Endovenous Saphenous Vein Ablation of Superficial Veins

Endovenous ablation or occlusion of the saphenous vein employing radiofrequency or laser energy provides a new and minimally invasive approach for treatment. Using radiofrequency ablation (VNUS Medical Technologies, Inc., Sunnyvale, CA), RF pulses are used to heat the vessel wall resulting in closure and fibrosis. The second-generation RFA catheter ClosureFAST (VNUS Medical Technologies) has been available since 2008.

It uses a higher operating temperature of (120°C) and conducts heat evenly and directly to the vein wall through a 7-cm-long heating coil at the end of the catheter. Endovenous laser treatment uses a laser probe to induce thermal damage (Venacure EVLT, AngioDynamics, Queensbury, NY). The laser wavelength is a major determinant of tissue injury. The first-generation lasers used for venous insufficiency typically employed wavelengths of 810 to 1,064 nm that are absorbed by the hemoglobin of red blood cells. This leads to the formation of steam bubbles that produce convective heat transfer to the vein wall damaging endothelium and subendothelial collagen, causing shrinkage of the vein wall, inflammation, thrombosis, and subsequent fibrosis. If the tip of the laser catheter is in contact with the vein wall, high-energy absorption by small volumes of tissue can lead to tissue vaporization, resulting in vein perforation. Blood leaking from these microperforations often leads to ecchymoses. Higher laser wavelengths (1,320-nm) that are water specific are now available for targeting the water content of the vein wall and may avoid steam bubbles from boiling blood associated with the lower wavelength lasers. Higher wavelengths reduced postoperative bruising and pain compared with the 940-nm hemoglobin-specific wavelength system. More recently, a trial of the 1,470-nm system with an even higher affinity for water absorption showed successful vein ablation with lower energy densities, and perioperative comfort was similar to RFA. A radial-emitting laser fiber design may also have a future role in achieving the ideal system because the light is distributed circumferentially 360 degrees for more symmetrical treatment of the vein wall.

Endovenous vein ablation (VNUS Medical Technologies, Sunnyvale, CA) requires the use of DUS for safely guiding the catheter near the saphenofemoral junction. Access to the great saphenous vein is obtained just below the knee crease by direct vein puncture with a fine-bore needle or a venous cut down. High ligation of the great saphenous vein is not necessary, although some physicians perform ligation prior to ablation. The advantages of this approach include the avoidance of general anesthesia required for most surgical procedures, a shorter convalescence time, and minimal side effects. Patient satisfaction is also reported as very high. Follow-up over a 2-year period has revealed success rates (defined by a lack of recanalization or patients seeking further treatment) of between 84 and 93%. Adverse effects have been reported and include skin burns, paresthesias due to saphenous nerve injury, hematoma, burning or stinging pain, and superficial and deep vein thrombosis. A recent prospective, randomized study from Switzerland comparing endovenous laser ablation and surgery for treatment of primary great saphenous varicose veins after 2 years showed 98% to be symptom free in both groups. However, the laser group had two saphenous veins reopened and five partially opened out of 104 limbs compared to none in the surgery group.

A recent randomized controlled clinical trial evaluated the VNUS closure device (ClosurePLUS) with laser treatment with the Venacure device (810 nm) and tested the treatment of superficial venous insufficiency due to GSV incompetence ($n = 118$ patients). Early postoperative results of pain, bruising, erythema, and hematoma, duplex vein patency and VCSS scores, CEAP clinical class and quality of life was assessed. VCSS score and QOL scores improved in both groups and were no different at 12 months between groups. A higher percentage of patients had patent GSV at the end of 12 months in the RFA group compared with the EVL group (11 RFA patients vs. 2 EVL patients, $p = 0.002$) although. An interesting finding was that anatomic failure at 1 year did not correlate with QOL. This may be partly explained by the reduction in vein diameter, which occurred in nearly all treated patients in this trial, as well as by the benefits they may have received from simultaneous microphlebectomy of branch varicosities (occurred in both groups) and perhaps better compliance with compression.

Transilluminated Power Phlebectomy

This involves the endoscopic resection or ablation of superficial varices using a powered vein resector, an irrigated illuminator, and tumescent anesthesia. It requires fewer incisions when compared to other phlebectomy procedures. If reflux is present, correction is necessary but can be performed at the same time.

CONCLUSION

Varicose veins are a common medical problem and patients may present with symptoms including pain, fatigue, restlessness, and heaviness in the legs. Symptoms are less severe in the morning, are generally exacerbated with prolonged standing or sitting through the day, and are usually relieved with elevation of the legs, or with walking. Physical findings that frequently accompany varicose veins include edema, ulceration, and lipodermatosclerosis. DUS has largely replaced venography as the preferred imaging technique for identifying the underlying physiologic abnormality in patients with varicose veins. There are a number of treatment options available to the patient who presents with varicose veins. The majority of patients can be treated with noninterventional measures including gradient pressure stockings. Intervention with sclerotherapy, endovenous ablation, and surgery is recommended for patients with complications or those not responding to noninvasive measures. Almost all interventions can be safely performed in the outpatient arena.

PRACTICAL POINTS

- The physical examination should include examination of the arterial system, abdomen, and both legs (or arms) in the sitting and standing positions.

- DUS is the method of choice in identifying underlying venous reflux and assists in choosing the type of intervention.

- It is important to rule out deep venous thrombosis in a patient presenting with SVT.

- Most patients with venous disorders can be managed with noninterventional methods.

- Smaller varicosities such as venous telangiectasia and reticular veins respond best to sclerotherapy. Larger varicosities are safely treated surgically or by endovenous ablation.

RECOMMENDED READING

Almeida JI, Kaufman J, Gockeritz O, et al. Radiofrequency endovenous ClosureFAST versus laser ablation for the treatment of great saphenous reflux: a multicenter, single-blinded, randomized study (RECOVERY study). *J Vasc Interv Radiol* 2009;20:752–759.

Bradbury A, Evans C, Allan P, et al. What are the symptoms of varicose veins? Edinburgh vein study cross sectional population survey. *Br Med J* 1999;318:353–356.

Bradbury A, Evans CJ, Allan P, et al. The relationship between lower limb symptoms and superficial and deep venous reflux on duplex ultrasonography: The Edinburgh Vein Study. *J Vasc Surg* 2000;32:921–931.

Christenson JT, Gueddi S, Gemayel G, et al. Prospective randomized trial comparing endovenous laser ablation and surgery for treatment of primary great saphenous varicose veins with a 2 year follow-up. *J Vasc Surg* 2010;52(2010):1234–1241.

Diehm C, Trampisch HJ, Lange S, et al. Comparison of leg compression stocking and oral horse-chestnut seed extract therapy in patients with chronic venous insufficiency. *Lancet* 1996; 347:292–294.

Dwerrhouse S, Davies B, Harradine K, et al. Stripping of the long saphenous vein reduces the rate of reoperation for recurrent varicose veins: five year results of a randomized trial. *J Vasc Surg* 1999;29:589–592.

Fernandez CF, Roizental M, Carvallo J. Combined endovenous laser therapy and microphlebectomy in the treatment of varicose veins: efficacy and complications of a large single-center experience, *J Vasc Surg* 2008;48:947–952.

Gale SS, Lee JN, Walsh ME, et al. A randomized, controlled trial of endovenous thermal ablation using the 810-nm wavelength laser and the ClosurePLUS radiofrequency ablation methods for superficial venous insufficiency of the great saphenous vein. *J Vasc Surg* 2010;52(3): 645–650. [Epub 2010 Jul 17.]

London NJM, Nash R. Varicose veins. *Br Med J* 2000;320:1391–1394.

Lurie F, Creton D, Eklof B, et al. Prospective randomized study of endovenous radiofrequency obliteration (closure procedure) versus ligation and stripping in a selected patient population (EVOLVeS Study). *J Vasc Surg* 2003;38:207–214.

Meissner MH, Moneta G, MD, Burnand K, MD, et al. The hemodynamics and diagnosis of venous disease. *J Vasc Surg* 2007;46:4S–24S.

Meissner MH, Eklof B, Smith PC, et al. Secondary chronic venous disorders. *J Vasc Surg* 2007; 46(Suppl S):68S–83S.

Meissner MH, Gloviczki P, Bergan J, et al. Primary chronic venous disorders. *J Vasc Surg* 2007; 46(Suppl S):54S–67S. [Review.]

Min RJ, Khilnani NM, Golia P. Duplex ultrasound evaluation of lower extremity venous insufficiency. *J Vasc Interv Radiol* 2003;14(10):1233–1241.

Neumann HAM. Compression therapy with medical elastic stockings for venous diseases. *Dermatol Surg* 1998;24:765–770.

O'Donnell TF. The role of perforators in chronic venous insufficiency. *Phlebology* 2010;25(1): 3–10. [Review. Erratum in: *Phlebology* 2010;25(4):21.]

Raju S, Neglén P. Clinical practice. Chronic venous insufficiency and varicose veins. *N Engl J Med* 2009;360(22):2319–2327.

Rautio T, Ohinmaa A, Perala J, et al. Endovenous obliteration versus conventional stripping operation in the treatment of primary varicose veins: a randomized controlled trial with comparison of the costs. *J Vasc Surg* 2002;35:958–965.

CHAPTER 21 ■ Venous Thromboembolism

Cynthia Wu and Mark A. Crowther

Venous thromboembolism (VTE) comprises of both deep vein thrombosis (DVT) and pulmonary embolism (PE). VTE is associated with significant morbidity and mortality. Fully 10% of symptomatic PE is fatal within the first hour of presentation. Because there are extremely effective therapies to both prevent and treat VTE, it is important to be able to recognize the signs and symptoms of DVT and PE, to be aware of the clinical situations in which a high index of suspicion is warranted, to have a simple and accurate diagnostic algorithm, and to understand the various options for treatment.

VTE is age dependent, varying from an annual incidence of 0.03% in subjects under 50 years of age to 0.4% in those over 50 years (incidence of 1 per 10,000 at age 25 to 1 per 1,000 at age 65). Most studies have reported an equal incidence for both sexes. The majority of DVT is diagnosed in the lower extremities, often starting in the calf veins. Proximal DVT has a much stronger association with PE, and it is estimated that 50% of patients with untreated proximal DVT or PE develop recurrent VTE within 3 months. Isolated calf vein thrombi rarely cause clinically significant complications such as PE, and the majority of calf vein thrombi (when detected using screening techniques) resolve spontaneously even in the absence of anticoagulant therapy. About 25% of untreated calf DVT extends proximally, usually within a week of presentation. About half of patients with symptomatic proximal DVT have evidence of PE on imaging studies even without clinically evident respiratory symptoms, and about 70% of patients with symptomatic PE have DVT (2/3 are proximal).

CLINICAL FEATURES OF VENOUS THROMBOEMBOLISM

The clinical findings in DVT and PE are both insensitive and nonspecific. Physical examination must be used in conjunction with a thorough history to rule out alternative diagnoses. The diagnosis requires an evaluation of VTE risk factors and the appropriate use of diagnostic tools. Occasionally, events are entirely asymptomatic and found incidentally on imaging studies done for other reasons. Common clinical presentations for DVT and PE include the following:

Deep Vein Thrombosis

■ leg swelling +/– pitting edema
  ○ particularly if unilateral or involving the whole leg
  ○ objective measurement of circumference best taken 10 cm below the tibial tuberosity and compared to the unaffected leg

- leg pain
  - distribution of the deep veins—within the calf and medial thigh
  - localized tenderness, particularly over a palpable cord or visible group of vessels, may be more in keeping with superficial phlebitis
- redness and warmth
- pallor or cyanosis (rarely)
  - may be associated with massive occlusive iliofemoral DVT
- Homan's sign (calf pain with forced dorsiflexion of the foot) is neither sensitive nor specific for DVT

Other diseases may present with the same symptoms. Some of these include leg trauma, cellulitis, ruptured Baker's cyst, venous insufficiency, external compression of local vessels or lymphatics, and superficial phlebitis. Patients with postphlebitic syndrome from previous DVT may also have chronic leg swelling and pain.

Pulmonary Embolism

- chest pain, particularly pleuritic, sudden in onset and persistent
- sudden onset of shortness of breath
- preceding symptoms of DVT
- tachycardia, cyanosis, signs of right-sided heart failure
- hemoptysis (rare)
  - secondary to pulmonary infarction
- syncope/shock (rare)
  - secondary to obstruction of right-sided cardiac output

Other causes for dyspnea and chest pain should be promptly ruled out (e.g., myocardial infarction, congestive heart failure, pneumonia) as many of these also carry significant morbidity and mortality in the absence of appropriate treatment. Patients with previous PE who develop pulmonary hypertension that does not resolve after the acute event may also suffer from chronic chest pain and shortness of breath.

RISK FACTORS FOR VENOUS THROMBOEMBOLISM

When a patient presents with symptoms suggestive of DVT or PE, it is often useful to determine the background risk for developing VTE as this not only guides further diagnostic testing but also may affect the aggressiveness and the duration of any subsequent treatment. Approximately 25 to 50% of first events are idiopathic in nature with no obvious provoking incident. Despite this, there exists a wide spectrum of known factors that increase the risk of VTE. In 1856, German physician Rudolf Virchow devised a simple framework for categorizing these factors. This is commonly known as Virchow's triad and consists of three pathophysiological mechanisms: stasis, endothelial injury, and hypercoagulability. Thrombotic risk can alternatively be seen as either inherited or acquired. Common risk factors for VTE can be summarized using these approaches (Table 21.1). It is also important to determine whether or not the contributing risk factors are transient or permanent and if any can be attenuated with other

TABLE 21.1

RISK FACTORS FOR VTE

Venous Stasis
　Prolonged immobility
　　Hospitalization, stroke, paralysis
　Fracture with cast/non–weight-bearing status
　External compression of local vasculature and lymphatic channels
Endothelial Injury
　Major trauma
　Major surgery
　Intravenous catheters (central venous access)
Hypercoagulability
　Acquired
　　Cancer and chemotherapy
　　Pregnancy
　　Hormone therapy (oral contraceptive, hormone replacement)
　　Antiphospholipid antibody syndrome
　　Heparin-induced thrombocytopenia
　Inherited
　　Factor V Leiden
　　Prothrombin 20210 gene mutation
　　Protein C deficiency
　　Protein S deficiency
　　Antithrombin deficiency

VTE-unrelated interventions. Controlling or eradicating underlying risk factors can decrease the chances of treatment failure and thrombotic recurrence and can possibly shorten the duration of anticoagulation.

Special Patient Groups

Hospitalized Medical Patients

Most hospitalized medical patients have at least one risk factor for VTE (usually immobility), and most have multiple risks relating to their reason for admission and other comorbid diseases. Without prophylaxis, venographically detected DVT can occur in 10 to 20% of such patients, and when symptomatic, VTE may contribute significantly to in-hospital morbidity, mortality, and length of stay. Preventative measures should be considered in all patients without contraindications to anticoagulation, and a high index of suspicion should be maintained for VTE in these patients.

Hospitalized Surgical Patients

Surgical patients generally have a higher risk of VTE than medical patients, especially trauma patients and those requiring orthopedic procedures such as hip or knee replacements. In such patients, the rate of venographically detected VTE may be as high as 40 to 60% without prophylaxis. After hemostasis is achieved postoperatively, DVT prophylaxis should be initiated in all patients with an important risk of DVT. In some situations, prophylaxis may extend beyond discharge. A high index of suspicion must be maintained if any symptoms of VTE occur.

Cancer Patients

Cancer and its treatment are independent risk factors for VTE and increase the risk fourfold to sixfold. About 15 to 20% of patients with acute VTE concurrently have a diagnosis of cancer, and 10% of patients with idiopathic VTE are diagnosed with cancer within the first year after their thrombotic event. VTE in cancer patients is associated with a more aggressive course, more frequent treatment failures, increased bleeding risk, and shortened life expectancy. Diagnosis may be delayed due to multiple competing alternative explanations for the presenting symptoms. As the risk of VTE is high in these patients, VTE is often considered in the differential diagnosis.

Antiphospholipid Antibody Syndrome

Antiphospholipid antibody syndrome (APLAS) can be a powerful stimulus for both large and small vessel arterial and venous thromboses. DVT is one of the common presenting manifestations of APLAS. The diagnostic criteria for APLAS are provided below and require one clinical criterion and one laboratory criterion. Treatment may also be complicated in patients with concurrent moderate or severe thrombocytopenia.

Clinical Criteria

1. Vascular thrombosis (venous/arterial/small vessel) in any tissue/organ. Superficial venous thrombosis is not included in clinical criteria.
2. Pregnancy morbidity

Laboratory Criteria

1. Lupus anticoagulant present in plasma/serum ≥2 occasions at least 12-weeks apart
2. Anticardiolipin antibodies (IgG and IgM) in plasma/serum ≥ 2 occasions at least 12-weeks apart
3. Anti-β2 glycoprotein 1 antibodies (IgG and IgM) in plasma/serum ≥ 2 occasions at least 12-weeks apart

Hereditary Thrombophilia

The list of inherited conditions that increase the risk of thrombosis continues to grow. More common conditions such as Factor V Leiden are usually associated with an excess of procoagulant proteins and are generally weaker risk factors for the development of VTE. Rarer conditions such as protein C, protein S, and antithrombin III (AT III) deficiencies are usually associated with deficiencies of anticoagulant proteins and are generally stronger risk factors for the development of VTE. While most of these conditions have been shown to increase the risk of a first venous thrombotic event, not all are strongly linked to an increased risk of recurrent events. Thus, caution must be used while interpreting the results of these tests, and widespread screening in all patients with VTE is not recommended.

Testing for thrombophilia may be considered in the following situations:

- First presentation at a young age
- Strong family history of VTE
- Recurrent idiopathic VTE and VTE in unusual sites (portal, splenic, mesenteric, or cerebral vein thromboses)
- Extensive VTE

It is also important to note that anticoagulant use can interfere with accurate interpretation of some thrombophilia testing (e.g., use of warfarin will decrease the normal levels of protein C and protein S even without a hereditary deficiency), and thus timing of testing should also be considered carefully. Other medical conditions such as nephrotic syndrome, liver failure, and pregnancy may also alter the normal levels of procoagulant and anticoagulant proteins even in the absence of hereditary deficiencies. In such patients, thrombophilia testing should either not be done or be done and the results interpreted with extreme caution.

DIAGNOSIS OF VENOUS THROMBOEMBOLISM

The accurate diagnosis of VTE relies on the appropriate use of a combination of tools starting from clinical assessment (focused history and physical examination) to determine the "pretest probability" of DVT or PE and judicious use of laboratory investigations and imaging modalities (Figs. 21.1 and 21.2).

Clinical Assessment

The most commonly used clinical prediction models for VTE are the Well's Criteria for DVT and PE (Tables 21.2 and 21.3). Using a few simple and objective features from the patient's history and physical exam, the clinician can stratify patients as low, moderate, or high probability for VTE. The only room for subjectivity lies in the score for "alternative diagnosis." If no clearly defined alternate diagnosis can be given, patients should be scored accordingly. These clinical prediction models have been incorporated into many diagnostic algorithms to aid in deciding what, if any, further testing should be done (Figs. 21.1 and 21.2).

Laboratory Investigations

The only currently available and widely used laboratory test for the diagnosis of VTE is the D-dimer assay. All D-dimer assays rely on the use of monoclonal antibodies to d-dimer molecules. The d-dimer, two covalently bound D-domains of cross-linked fibrin monomers, is a product of fibrin degradation. They can be found circulating at low levels under physiologic conditions as well as at elevated levels in a number of disease states associated with fibrin formation and fibrinolysis. Thus, the presence of d-dimer

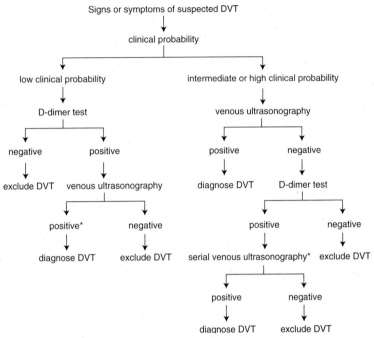

FIGURE 21-1. Diagnostic algorithm for deep vein thrombosis. (From Hirsh J, Lee AYY. How we diagnose and treat deep vein thrombosis. *Blood* 2002;99:3102–3110.)

is not specific for venous thrombosis with the specificity reduced in patients with cancer, pregnant women, and hospitalized and elderly patients. Techniques that detect d-dimer include enzyme-linked immunosorbent assays, latex agglutination and immunoturbidimetric tests, and whole blood agglutination methods. Specific assays that have been validated for use in VTE diagnosis include (i) SimpliRED d-dimer (Agen Biochemical Ltd., Brisbane, Australia), (ii) Vidas d-dimer (bioMérieux, France), (iii) MDA d-dimer (bioMérieux, Durham, NC), and (iv) Tiniquant d-dimer (Roche Diagnostics, The Netherlands). Results of each test cannot be generalized to other methods of d-dimer quantification due to the wide variety of assay techniques. Generally, though, all are characterized by an intermediate to high sensitivity coupled with an intermediate to low specificity. This allows a negative d-dimer, in combination with a low clinical pretest probability, to effectively rule out acute VTE (less than 1% chance that a patient has VTE). Positive d-dimer results, however, do not equate to a diagnosis of VTE, and further testing is required.

Biomarkers in Risk Stratification of Venous Thromboembolism

Use of D-dimer testing to stratify patients for their risk of recurrent events is still being investigated, although preliminary results in this area are

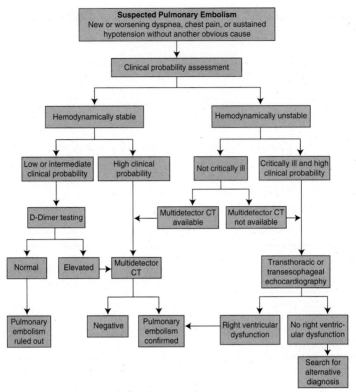

FIGURE 21-2. Diagnostic algorithm for PE. The initial assessment of the clinical probability of PE is based on either clinical judgment or clinical decision rules (e.g., Well's Criteria). Patients are considered to be hemodynamically unstable if they are in shock or have a systolic blood pressure of less than 90 mm Hg or a drop in pressure of more than 40 mm Hg for more than 15 minutes (in the absence of new-onset arrhythmia, hypovolemia, and sepsis). In cases in which multidetector CT is not available or in patients with renal failure or allergy to contrast dye, the use of ventilation–perfusion scanning is an alternative. In patients with a high clinical probability and an elevated d-dimer level but with negative findings on multidetector CT, venous ultrasonography should be considered. Among critically ill patients with right ventricular dysfunction, thrombolysis is an option; multidetector CT should be performed when the patient's condition has been stabilized if doubts remain about clinical management. In patients who are candidates for percutaneous embolectomy, conventional pulmonary angiography can be performed to confirm the diagnosis of PE immediately before the procedure, after the finding of right ventricular dysfunction. (From Agnelli G, Beccatini C. Current concepts. Acute pulmonary embolism. *N Engl J Med* 2010;363:266–274, with permission.)

promising. D-dimer testing may help to make decisions on whether to stop or discontinue anticoagulation therapy. Troponin and BNP measurements may help to stratify patients with PE for their risk, with several studies

TABLE 21.2

CLINICAL PREDICTION RULE FOR PREDICTING DVT

Clinical Feature	Score
Active cancer (treatment ongoing or within previous 6 mo or palliative)	1
Paralysis, paresis, or recent plaster immobilization of the lower extremities	1
Recently bedridden for more than 3 d or major surgery, within 4 wk	1
Localized tenderness along the distribution of the deep vein system	1
Entire leg swollen	1
Calf swelling by >3 cm when compared with the asymptomatic leg (measured 10 cm below tibial tuberosity)	1
Pitting edema (greater in the symptomatic leg)	1
Collateral superficial veins (nonvaricose)	1
Alternative diagnosis as likely or greater than that of DVT	−2
	Total:

In patients with symptoms in both legs, the more symptomatic leg is used. Pretest probability calculated as the total score: high ≥ 3; moderate 1 or 2; low ≤ 0.
(Adapted from Wells PS, Anderson DR, Bormanis J, et al. Value of assessment of pretest probability of deep-vein thrombosis in clinical management. *Lancet* 1997;350:1795–1798.)

showing an association between elevation and short-term risk for dying and recurrent PE. Conversely, the absence of elevation in these parameters is a favorable prognostic factor, with limited studies suggesting an almost 100% negative predictive value for complications if plasma BNP levels are normal. The use of troponin with RV functional abnormalities may also be helpful with the absence of right ventricular dysfunction and a normal troponin level identifying patients who are eligible for early discharge or even outpatient treatment.

TABLE 21.3

CLINICAL PREDICTION RULE FOR PREDICTING PE

Variable	Points
Immobilization or surgery in the previous 4 wk	1.5
Malignancy (treatment ongoing or within previous 6 mo or palliative)	1.0
Previous DVT/PE	1.5
Hemoptysis	1.0
Heart rate > 100 beats/min	1.5
Clinical signs and symptoms of DVT (leg swelling and pain with palpation of deep veins)	3.0
An alternative diagnosis is less likely than PE	3.0
	Total:

Low probability < 2.0; moderate probability 2.0–6.0; high probability ≥ 6.0.
(Adapted from Wells PS, Anderson DR, Rodger M, et al. Derivation of a simple clinical model to categorize patients probability of pulmonary embolism: increasing the models utility with the SimpliRED D-dimer. *Thromb Haemost* 2000;83:416–420.)

Imaging Modalities

Reference Standard Tests

In order to standardize the approach in evaluating diagnostic tools for VTE, it is often useful to think about the probability of developing VTE if the test was negative. For a test to be helpful, the diagnostic modality should have excellent negative predictive value with a ≤1% chance of subsequently developing symptomatic VTE over a 3-month observation period if testing is negative. Sensitivity and specificity of all other imaging modalities are measured against these standards.

Contrast Venography for Deep Vein Thrombosis

The high sensitivity and specificity of combining other diagnostic tools have made use of venography less frequent for proximal DVT. It remains a fairly reliable test to diagnose calf DVT, but this is offset by its invasiveness and exposure of patients to the adverse effects of IV contrast dye and radiation. Venography is reserved for patients with otherwise nondiagnostic testing where the test results may change the management.

Pulmonary Angiography for Pulmonary Embolism

As with venography, pulmonary angiography is also being used less frequently. The disadvantages include the invasiveness and adverse effects related to contrast-dye and radiation exposures. Rarely, complications such as acute renal failure from contrast-dye mortality may occur. This test is therefore reserved in situations where other diagnostic options have been exhausted and where the diagnosis would result in change of treatment options.

Noninvasive Imaging Modalities

Compression Ultrasonography for Deep Vein Thrombosis. Compression ultrasonography (CUS) is the most commonly used imaging modality for the diagnosis of DVT. The test relies on the ability of the operator to locate the vessel of interest and then to be able to appreciate compressibility. This requires the vascular anatomy of the examined area to be generally consistent between individuals and the visualized vessels to be of large enough caliber to evaluate accurately. For proximal DVT, the sensitivity and specificity of this test are 95 and 96%, respectively, and for distal DVT, the sensitivity and specificity are 60 and 70%, respectively. In combination with a low clinical suspicion, when the CUS is negative for proximal DVT, the sensitivity and specificity approach 100%. If the suspicion for DVT remains high after a negative test, or if isolated calf DVT is suspected, various approaches can be taken, including serial CUS in 5 to 7 days (Fig. 21.1). About 1 to 2% of patients will convert to positive CUS findings during this period of time, and the estimated risk of dying from PE while awaiting repeat testing is 0.06%. If venous ultrasonography of the lower limbs is performed first, lung scanning or multidetector computed tomography (CT) can be avoided in about 10% of patients with suspected PE.

Ventilation Perfusion Scanning for Pulmonary Embolism. The ventilation perfusion (VQ) scan is a noninvasive imaging modality that relies on perfusion/ventilation mismatch for diagnosis. In the ventilation phase of the test, a gaseous radionuclide such as xenon or technetium DTPA in an aerosol form is inhaled by the patient through a mouthpiece or mask that covers the nose and mouth. The perfusion phase of the test involves the intravenous injection of radioactive technetium macroaggregated albumin (^{99m}Tc-MAA). A gamma camera acquires the images for both phases of the study. Its use can be considered in cases in which multidetector CT is not available or in patients with renal failure or allergy to contrast dye. A normal VQ scan essentially rules out PE, with a negative predictive value of 97%. A lung scan with findings that suggest high probability has a positive predictive value of 85 to 90%. However, VQ scanning is diagnostic in only 30 to 50% of patients with suspected PE, with the remainder with indeterminate scans requiring further testing.

Spiral/Helical Computed Tomography Scan for Pulmonary Embolism. CT scans are now the test of choice for the evaluation of suspected PE in most centers. This test depends on the opacification of the pulmonary arteries with IV contrast dye to visualize filling defects indicative of intraluminal thrombus. Earlier CT scanners with single detectors were found to be roughly equivalent to VQ scanners in assessing the main or lobar pulmonary arteries, but positive predictive value markedly dropped off when segmental and subsegmental arteries were involved. Multidetector row CT scanners have substantially improved visualization of these smaller yet clinically relevant vessels. In patients with negative findings on multidetector CT who did not receive anticoagulation therapy, the incidence of thromboembolic events is approximately 1.5% at 3 months; the incidence is 1.5% in patients with a high d-dimer level and about 0.5% in patients with a normal d-dimer level. The negative predictive value of CT pulmonary angiography has been marginally improved (from 95 to 97%) by performing concomitant lower-limb CT venography. However, CT venography of the proximal iliofemoral veins increases the overall radiation exposure and should therefore be avoided. In patients with a high clinical probability of PE and negative findings on CT, the value of additional testing is controversial. Venous ultrasonography shows a DVT in less than 1% of such patients. Overall sensitivity of multidetector spiral CT scan is 83% and specificity 96%, giving a positive predictive value of 92% and a negative predictive value of 96%. This is comparable to the reference standard tests. Disadvantages of CT scanning largely revolve around the need for IV contrast dye, significant radiation exposure, and its associated complications. Advantages of the CT scan are its availability, rapid completion, and the possibility of seeing other intrathoracic details (pulmonary parenchyma, pleura, mediastinal structures) that may help determine alternate or concurrent diagnoses.

If all testing for PE is nondiagnostic, one indirect approach is to do bilateral CUS of the legs to look for DVT (70% of patients with symptomatic PE have DVT, two thirds of which are proximal). This strategy has been incorporated into various diagnostic algorithms (Fig. 21.2).

Contrast-Enhanced Magnetic Resonance Angiography for Pulmonary Embolism. In the Prospective Investigation of Pulmonary Embolism Diagnosis III (PIOPED III) trial (ClinicalTrials.gov number, NCT00241826), magnetic resonance angiography (MRA) was shown to have insufficient sensitivity and a high rate of technically inadequate images when used for the diagnosis of PE. However, technically well-performed MRA had a sensitivity of 78% and a specificity of 99%. Contrast-enhanced magnetic resonance angiography (CE-MRA) may be used in patients with a strong suspicion of PE in whom the results of other tests are equivocal or for whom iodinated contrast material and ionizing radiation are relatively contraindicated.

Other Adjunctive Tests. Right ventricular hypokinesis and dilatation are independent predictors of 30-day mortality in VTE patients. This can be assessed by 2D echocardiography or by TEE in patients with inadequate chest windows. The presence of RV dysfunction can serve as confirmatory evidence of PE in those patients who are critically ill and have high clinical probability and can help guide decisions related to thrombolysis or endarterectomy (Fig. 21.2). Right ventricular dysfunction, as assessed by means of multidetector CT, has been suggested also to be of help but warrants EKG gating when doing CT-PE studies.

TREATMENT OF VENOUS THROMBOEMBOLISM
General Considerations

Prompt initiation of the appropriate anticoagulant therapy is the most effective treatment for VTE. When testing cannot be completed promptly, it is prudent in patients with a high pretest probability for VTE to administer a dose of anticoagulation while waiting to confirm the diagnosis, as long as bleeding is not a concern. In the absence of anticoagulation, the rate of recurrent VTE in the first month after diagnosis is approximately 40% and in the 2-month period after the event is approximately 10%. Therapeutic anticoagulation affords a risk reduction of 80%. The annual risk of recurrent VTE while on anticoagulation is estimated to be about only 1%. The goal of treatment in the first 3 months is to prevent thrombus embolization, extension, and early recurrence and to control acute symptoms. Treatment beyond 3 months is targeted at preventing late recurrence. In patients who have PE with hemodynamic compromise, more aggressive measures such as thrombolysis may need to be considered. Conversely, in patients with active bleeding or an absolute contraindication to anticoagulation (Table 21.4), mechanical interventions such as a temporary inferior vena cava (IVC) filter may need to be used. Low-risk situations that may require either no anticoagulant treatment or shorter duration treatment include calf DVT, superficial phlebitis (thrombosis of a superficial vein) and central venous catheter–related DVT (treatment course may be shorter if the catheter can be removed and no other risk factors persist), and some cases of single isolated subsegmental PE (no DVT on bilateral CUS of the legs and no ongoing strong risk factors for VTE). Both initial and

TABLE 21.4

CONTRAINDICATIONS TO ANTICOAGULATION

Absolute	Relative
Active hemorrhage	Recent gastrointestinal hemorrhage or stroke (<14 d)
Neurosurgery or intracranial bleeding within 7 days (including hemorrhagic stroke)	Recent major surgery (<1–2 d)
Severe thrombocytopenia (<20 × 10⁹/L)	Moderate thrombocytopenia (20–50 × 10⁹/L)
	Uncontrolled hypertension
	Inherited or acquired clinically significant coagulopathy/bleeding disorders

long-term treatments must take into account the thrombotic and bleeding risks of individual patients with continual reassessment as these risks may change over time.

Treatment Approach and Special Considerations

Initial Treatment

In patients with objectively confirmed DVT or PE, anticoagulant therapy with subcutaneous (SC) low-molecular-weight heparin (LMWH), unfractionated heparin (UFH), or SC fondaparinux may be used for at least 5 days. The most recent such analysis included 17 studies that compared LMWH with IV heparin, with the analysis showing that LMWH was associated with fewer thrombotic complications, less major bleeding, and fewer deaths. The mortality advantage is, however, confined to those with cancer. Thrombolysis is recommended for patients with PE who have evidence of hemodynamic compromise (see separate section).

Maintenance

Coumadin is initiated on the first treatment day, with discontinuation of heparin preparations when the international normalized ratio (INR) is ≥2.0 for at least 24 hours. In patients with acute nonmassive PE, initial treatment with LMWH is preferable. In patients with massive PE, in other situations where there is concern about SC absorption, in patients with significant impairment in GFR, or in patients for whom thrombolytic therapy is being considered or planned, IV UFH is preferable over SC LMWH or fondaparinux.

Intensity and Duration of Anticoagulation

Duration of anticoagulation is largely based on balancing the risks and benefits of anticoagulation. For those with provoked VTE, the risk of recurrence is estimated to be 5% in the first year after discontinuing anticoagulation and 15% over the first 5 years. After a major transient, risk of recurrence would not justify long-term anticoagulation. Patients with idiopathic DVT have a risk of recurrence of 10% in the first year after discontinuing anticoagulation and 30% over 5 years. This risk outweighs that of major bleeding, and these patients would benefit from ongoing therapy. Patients with chronic strong risk factors are also considered to be at very high risk for recurrence and generally remain on indefinite duration therapy. Other considerations that might factor into the decision-making process include patient compliance, patient preference, previous VTE, strong family history of VTE, other comorbid conditions, and age.

For patients with DVT or PE secondary to a transient (reversible), risk factor treatment with Coumadin for 3 months over treatment for shorter periods is recommended. For patients with unprovoked DVT or PE, indefinite anticoagulant therapy is recommended when the risk of bleeding is low and when this is consistent with the patient's preference and for most patients with a second unprovoked DVT. The dose of vitamin K antagonists (VKA) is adjusted to maintain a target INR of 2.5 (INR range, 2.0 to 3.0) for all treatment durations. The results of two randomized trials indicate that after initial conventional-intensity therapy for 3 months, although low-intensity warfarin therapy is more effective than placebo, it is less effective than conventional-intensity therapy and does not appear to reduce the incidence of bleeding. However, for patients who may desire the convenience of less frequent INR monitoring, this may be an option. For patients with cancer and DVT/PE, at least 3 months of treatment with LMWH is recommended followed by treatment with LMWH or Coumadin as long as the cancer is active. In patients with PE/DVT secondary to a temporary risk factor, therapy with VKA should be given for 3 months.

Catheter-Directed Thrombolysis and Pharmacomechanical Thrombolysis

In selected patients with extensive proximal DVT (iliofemoral) with duration less than14 days, low bleeding risk, good functional status, and life expectancy greater than 1 year, catheter-directed thrombolysis (CDT) may be considered to reduce acute symptoms and reduce postthrombotic syndrome (PTS). Pharmacomechanical strategies such as thrombus aspiration/disruption in addition to CDT may be considered if appropriate expertise exists.

Thrombolysis

Use of thrombolysis for VTE remains controversial. The ACCP consensus document recommends thrombolysis in PE with hemodynamic compromise where the bleeding risk is low. Hypotension and shock are associated with a very high mortality, and there is evidence to support better outcomes in this subgroup of patients if they receive thrombolytic therapy. There may also be a role for thrombolytic therapy in hemodynamically stable patients who demonstrate evidence of severe right heart strain including elevated troponin levels (suggestive of right-sided myocardial infarction), right ventricular dysfunction on echocardiography, or right ventricular enlargement on CT. Some select patients with "massive" proximal DVT can be considered for catheter-directed thrombolysis and possibly systemic thrombolysis (in centers where CDT is unavailable). Characteristics of such patients include extensive DVT with symptoms less than 14 days, good baseline functional status, and suitable life expectancy. The bleeding risk is higher with thrombolytic therapy, and a clinical assessment of bleeding risk and contraindications to thrombolysis needs to be undertaken prior to administering the drug. Concurrent and ongoing anticoagulation also needs to be administered.

Inferior Vena Cava Filters

There is no role for the routine use of IVC filters in patients with uncomplicated DVT. A filter should be considered in patients with absolute contraindications to anticoagulation and an acute, objectively confirmed, DVT. It is important to remember that insertion of a filter does not relieve the underlying prothrombotic condition and does not treat the preexisting thrombus. It should be thought of as a temporary mechanism to decrease the risk of PE when administration of anticoagulation must be delayed or deferred. Anticoagulant therapy administered to a patient with an IVC filter decreases the short- and long-term risks of PE, but the long-term risk of DVT is increased. Thus, the overall thrombotic events are comparable, and there is no overall survival benefit despite the decreased risk of PE. If a filter is placed, continual reassessment of bleeding risk is warranted, and prompt resumption of anticoagulation should occur when those risk factors have resolved. Temporary filters reduce the risk of long-term complications associated with IVC filters if they are truly temporary; however, in large series, less than 25% of "temporary filters" are actually removed.

Prevention of Postthrombotic Syndrome

For the prevention of PTS after proximal DVT, the use of an elastic compression stocking is important.

Selected patients with lower-extremity DVT may be considered for thrombus removal, generally using catheter-based thrombolytic techniques.

Superficial Vein Thrombosis

Superficial vein thrombosis (SVT) related to intravenous infusion may not require anticoagulation and can be managed with topical heparin gel or diclofenac gel applied locally until resolution of symptoms. For patients with spontaneous SVT, the ACCP guidelines now recommend prophylactic or intermediate doses of LMWH or intermediate doses of heparin for a duration of 4 weeks. As an alternative, Coumadin (INR 2.0 to 3.0) can be overlapped with 5 days of UFH and LMWH and continued for 4 weeks.

Antiphospholipid Antibody Syndrome

There is currently no evidence based on randomized control trials that higher intensity anticoagulation is associated with a lower frequency of recurrent thromboembolism. Thus, regular intensity anticoagulation is recommended indefinitely in these patients.

Prevention of Venous Thromboembolism

High-risk situations for the development of VTE have been well established, and these include hospitalized medical and surgical patients. Primary thromboprophylaxis is known to reduce the rate of DVT, PE, and fatal PE. Rates of bleeding and other complications during the use of prophylactic dose anticoagulation are low. Despite this, thromboprophylaxis is uniformly underused worldwide. Pharmacologic prophylaxis is the preferred approach in almost all settings with low-dose UFH and LMWH being most commonly used. If there is active bleeding, mechanical prophylaxis such as graded compression stockings and intermittent pneumatic compression devices can be implemented. A combination of both pharmacologic and mechanical methods of prophylaxis may be warranted in very high-risk patients.

Pharmacology of Anticoagulants in Venous Thromboembolism

Unfractionated Heparin

UFH is a highly sulfated glycosaminoglycan with a heterogeneous molecular weight ranging between 3,000 and 30,000. Its anticoagulant effect is mediated by AT, and interaction with AT occurs via its pentasaccharide sequence. Together, the UFH/AT complex inactivates the serine protease–containing clotting factors including IIa (thrombin), Xa, IXa, XIa, and XIIa. The majority of UFH is cleared through intracellular depolymerization after heparin bound to macrophages and endothelial cells is internalized. UFH can be administered either intravenously or subcutaneously. For the treatment of acute VTE, IV UFH should be given as an initial bolus of 80 U/kg followed by an 18 U/kg/h infusion. This is designed to target a heparin level of 0.2 to 0.4 units by protamine titration or 0.3 to 0.7 units measured by an anti-Xa assay. This usually correlates to a prolongation of the aPTT by two to three times normal, and IV UFH nomogram adjustments are based on aPTT levels measured at regular intervals. SC UFH can also be given with equal efficacy and safety using a dosing scheme of either an initial 5,000 U IV bolus followed by 250 U/kg SC b.i.d. or an initial dose of 333 U/kg SC followed by 250 U/kg SC b.i.d. The prophylactic dose of UFH is 5,000 U SC b.i.d. or t.i.d.

Low-Molecular-Weight Heparin

LMWH formulations are similar to UFH formulations except that these formulations contain smaller fragments produced by controlled enzymatic or chemical depolymerization. The average molecular weight of LMWH is 5,000. The anticoagulant effect is also mediated by AT, but because inactivation of IIa (thrombin) requires a longer chain, LMWH has a much greater anti-Xa effect compared with its anti-IIa effect. The anticoagulant response of LMWH is more predictable than that of UFH due to its higher bioavailability, longer half-life, and dose-independent clearance. This allows LMWH to be administered at lower doses and subcutaneously without the need for monitoring. LMWH is primarily cleared through the kidneys, so these agents have limited use in patients with moderate to severe renal impairment. For the treatment of acute VTE, once daily or twice daily injections are administered depending on the type of LMWH with an aim to target an anti-Xa level of approximately 0.6 to 1.0 U/mL. There is no need to monitor anti-Xa levels in most circumstances with LMWH. Table 21.5 provides dosing considerations for commonly used LMWH. Prophylactic dose regimens of LMWH are once again drug specific.

Warfarin/Vitamin K Antagonists

VKAs interfere with the interconversion of vitamin K and its 2,3 epoxide form. This inhibits the γ-carboxylation of the Gla-residues on vitamin K–dependent clotting factors (II, VII, IX, X), a step required for their procoagulant effect. The anticoagulant effect of VKAs is thus delayed and dependent on the half-life of any already γ-carboxylated factors in the circulation. Vitamin K–dependent anticoagulant proteins such as protein C have a shorter half-life, and a slightly procoagulant state occurs in the first 24 to 48 hours of VKA use. The effect of VKA is monitored through its ability to prolong the prothrombin time (PT). To allow comparison between laboratories, the PT is usually converted to the INR to target a level between 2.0 and 3.0. If immediate anticoagulant effect is required, such as in the treatment of VTE, overlapping treatment with UFH or LMWH must be used until the INR is in the therapeutic range. Usual starting dose is 5 mg orally daily, but this can be adjusted on a patient-to-patient basis. In select patients who are young (less than 40 years) and who have stable VTE, a higher dose of 10 mg may be used. Subsequent dosing is titrated to the INR level, and continuous regular monitoring is required for the duration of VKA treatment as the anticoagulant effect can fluctuate. There are three

TABLE 21.5

LMWH INITIAL TREATMENT REGIMENS FOR VTE

	Enoxaparin	Dalteparin	Nadroparin	Tinzaparin
Dose	1 mg/kg q12h SQ or 1.5 mg/kg/d SQ. Single dose should not exceed 180 mg	200 anti-Xa IU/kg q.d. SQ	86 anti-Xa IU/kg SQ b.i.d. or 171 anti-Xa IU/kg	175 anti-Xa IU kg SQ q.d.
Adjustment in renal failure	Dosing adjustment required for GFR < 30	Dosing adjustment required for GFR < 30	Dosing adjustment required for GFR < 30	Use contraindicated in the elderly and/or GFR < 30

commonly used VKAs: warfarin, phenprocoumon, and acenocoumarol. Only warfarin is routinely available in the United States.

Other Anticoagulants

Fondaparinux (a synthetic anti-Xa agent made up of only the pentasaccharide sequence found in UFH that catalyzes AT-dependent inactivation of activated clotting factors) can also be used for DVT prophylaxis and for the treatment of VTE, including in the setting of heparin-induced thrombocytopenia (HIT). In patients with acute symptomatic DVT and in patients with acute symptomatic PE, the recommended dose of fondaparinux is 5 mg (weight < 50 kg), 7.5 mg (weight 50 to 100 kg), or 10 mg (weight > 100 kg) by SC injection once daily. No dose adjustment is required with hepatic impairment, but its use is contraindicated with creatinine clearance less than 30 mL/min.

Less commonly used parenteral anticoagulants include danaparoid (an anti-Xa agent made up of a mixture of glycosaminoglycans, not available in the United States), hirudin/lepirudin (an irreversible direct thrombin inhibitor), bivalirudin (a reversible direct thrombin inhibitor), and argatroban (a reversible direct thrombin inhibitor). Often, the use of these agents is as alternate anticoagulants in patients diagnosed with or suspected of having HIT.

Emerging Oral Anticoagulants

Several new oral anticoagulants have recently been developed. The most extensively studied and available agents are the direct thrombin inhibitor dabigatran and the Xa inhibitor rivaroxaban (Table 21.6). Advantages of these new oral agents include ease of administration, no need for monitoring, rapid onset of action, and minimal food and drug interactions. The main disadvantages are the inability to reverse these agents in case of emergency and the lack of a monitoring test making compliance assessment difficult or impossible.

COMPLICATIONS OF ANTICOAGULATION

Bleeding

The main adverse side effect of all anticoagulants is that of bleeding. The annual incidence of major or fatal bleeding on full-dose anticoagulation is approximately 3%, but many factors including comorbidities, concurrent use of antiplatelet agents, increasing age, and anticoagulant control can impact on the bleeding risk. The overall case fatality from major bleeding while on anticoagulants is about 15%, and the risk of bleeding is substantially higher in the first month of anticoagulation compared with later on in treatment. In the absence of active bleeding, the immediate benefits of anticoagulation in the setting of newly diagnosed acute VTE usually far outweigh the immediate risks of bleeding. As time passes and the initial thrombotic event heals and dissipates, the risk of bleeding on

TABLE 21.6

NEWER ANTICOAGULANTS

	Dabigatran	Rivaroxaban	Apixaban
Mechanism of action	Direct IIa inhibitor	Direct Xa inhibitor	Direct Xa inhibitor
Activation	Prodrug (dabigatran etexilate)	None	None
Ki	4.5 nM	0.4 nM	0.08 nM
T1/2	12–14 h	5–9 h	8–15 h
Metabolism	Non-CYP pathways Conjugation	Oxidation (via CYP3A4 and CYP2J2) and hydrolysis	Oxidation (via CYP3A4) and conjugation
Renal excretion of active drug	>80%	<40%	<30%
Dose	150 mg once daily and then 220 mg	10 mg q.d.	2.5 mg b.i.d.
Manufacturer	Boehringer-Ingelheim	Bayer with Ortho McNeil	Pfizer with BMS
Approval status	Approved in EU. Approval in 2010 in the United States	Approved in EU. Approval in the United States in 2011	Approval pending

ongoing anticoagulant therapy may eventually outweigh the thrombotic risk. Periodic reevaluation of the risk/benefit profile of anticoagulation in individual patients is necessary.

Management of Major Bleeding While on Anticoagulation

Several general measures apply to all patients. These include cessation of the anticoagulant. Any other medication that may alter hemostasis (antiplatelet therapy, nonsteroidal anti-inflammatories) should also be discontinued until bleeding is controlled. Patients may require hospitalization and prompt evaluation of the need for resuscitative measures including IV fluids. Some anticoagulants have specific antidotes. These are summarized below (also see Table 21.7).

Warfarin/Vitamin K Antagonists

1. Vitamin K PO or IV. Vitamin K should never be given SQ due to an unpredictable and possibly delayed response. IV dosing (2.5 to 5 mg) should be slow over 30 minutes to avoid side effects with oral dosing being considered wherever possible. The full effect of vitamin K occurs

TABLE 21.7

COMPARISON OF ANTICOAGULANTS[a]

Drug	Target	Half-Life	Clearance/ Metabolism	Route	Reversal
UFH	Xa/IIa	30 min	Binding to endothelial cells and macrophages	IV/SQ	Protamine sulfate
LMWH	Xa(IIa)	3–4 h	Renal	SQ	Protamine sulfate (Partial)
Warfarin	II, VII, IX, X	36–42 h	Hepatic	PO	Vitamin K PCC FFP

[a]at therapeutic dose.
PCC, prothrombin complex concentrates; FFP, fresh frozen plasma.

over 12 to 24 hours, so if rapid reversal is required, another agent should be given concurrently.
2. Fresh frozen plasma (FFP) or prothrombin complex concentrates (PCC). FFP—15 mL/kg of body weight with 5 to 8 mL/kg for nonurgent reversal of high INR. Disadvantages include preparation delay, volume overload, and small risk of transmissible infections. PCC contain approximately 25 times the amount of factors (typically II, IX, X, and/or factor VII) compared to an equivalent volume of plasma. 1 U/kg IV of PCC will raise the plasma concentration of vitamin K–dependent factors by 1%.

Unfractionated Heparin and Low-Molecular-Weight Heparin

1. Protamine sulfate reverses the effect of heparin by binding to the molecules and forming stable salt complexes. It is only partially effective against LMWH. The dose required to reverse 100 U of heparin is approximately 1 mg. It is administered IV and should not exceed 50 mg per 10 minutes as more rapid infusions can induce histamine release causing hypotension and bronchospasm.

Reversal of Newer Anticoagulants

In general, the newer anticoagulants such as factor X inhibitors (e.g., fondaparinux) have no direct antidotes. The agents below are experimental with some anecdotal and in vitro data suggesting efficacy.

1. Recombinant factor VIIa (rFVIIa) may play a role in the treatment of life-threatening bleeding in anticoagulated patients. Factor VIIa is a powerful stimulus of the clotting cascade, and both a lack of evidence for efficacy and the potential for thrombotic complications should temper

enthusiasm for its use. In healthy volunteers given fondaparinux, rFVIIa normalized coagulation times and thrombin generation with effects.

2. Desmopressin acetate (DDAVP) stimulates the release of factor VIII and von Willebrand's factor from endothelial cells. It is commonly used to treat and prevent bleeding in bleeding disorders such as von Willebrand's disease and platelet function disorders. There are in vitro data suggesting efficacy with direct thrombin inhibitors.

3. Antifibrinolytic therapy such as tranexamic acid and ε-aminocaproic acid has also been used to attenuate bleeding in other bleeding disorders but has not been studied in anticoagulant-related bleeding.

4. Hemodialysis, hemofiltration, and plasmapheresis have been entertained as possible ways of removing small molecule anticoagulants such as the new oral agents, but efficacy and feasibility of such techniques, particularly in the emergency setting, are unknown.

Heparin-Induced Thrombocytopenia

HIT is a rare but serious complication of heparin-based treatment. It is characterized by an immune-mediated thrombocytopenia in patients exposed to heparin characterized by a prothrombotic state despite falling platelet counts due to platelet-activating IgG antibodies against heparin-platelet factor 4 (PF4). The target antigen is a complex of heparin and PF4 resulting either from charge neutralization of cationic PF4 or from conformational changes in PF4. HIT is highly thrombotic with approximately 50% of affected patients developing thrombosis involving veins, arteries, or the microcirculation. Typical onset of HIT is 5 to 10 days after heparin exposure; HIT can occur in less than 5 days in patients with preexistent antibodies (to heparin given within 5 to 100 days) rechallenged with heparin. HIT diagnosis requires (a) one or more clinical events and (b) the presence of HIT-Abs (Table 21.8). Thus, a patient suspected to have HIT but in whom antibodies cannot be detected does not have this diagnosis. Rarely, patients develop a syndrome that mimics HIT on both clinical and serologic grounds but without a preceding exposure to heparin. Thrombocytopenia is the most common manifestation with greater than 50% decrease in platelet count seen in approximately 90% of patients (in 5 to 10% of patients, the platelet decrease is only 30 to 50%) typically after day 7 with the thrombotic event shortly thereafter. However, the decrease in platelets may evolve contemporaneously with decrease in platelet counts; risk factors of HIT include female sex, postoperative state, and initiation of heparin prophylaxis postsurgery rather than presurgery. Treatment: Management involves two dos, two don'ts, and two diagnostic tests (Table 21.9). Simply stopping heparin may be insufficient to prevent the development of thrombosis due to (a) loss of heparin anticoagulant effect, (b) progressive increase in HIT-Ab levels that activate platelets even in the absence of heparin, (c) procoagulant platelet microparticles, and (d) thrombin generation.

Three nonheparin anticoagulants, danaparoid, lepirudin, and argatroban, are approved for the treatment of HIT. Bivalirudin is approved for use in patients with, or at risk of, heparin-induced thrombocytopenia/

TABLE 21.8

DIAGNOSTIC CRITERIA FOR HIT

CLINICAL
- Thrombocytopenia
- Thrombosis (e.g., venous: DVT, PE, venous limb gangrene, adrenal hemorrhage, arterial thrombosis, visceral, cerebral venous thrombosis, stroke, MI, microvascular thrombosis)
- Necrotizing skin lesions at heparin injection sites
- Acute anaphylactoid reactions that follow within 30 min of IV or SQ heparin

PATHOLOGIC
Heparin-dependent, platelet-activating IgG
- Positive platelet activation assay (e.g., serotonin-release assay)[a]
- Positive anti-PF4/polyanion-IgG EIA[b]

[a]Platelet activation assays detect HIT-Abs based on their ability to activate platelets at therapeutic (0.1–0.3 U/mL) but not supratherapeutic (10–100 IU/mL) concentrations of UFH.
[b]Not all patients with positive EIA have HIT (Only 25–50% of patients with positive EIA also have positive platelet activation assays). In general, the more abnormal the EIA results, the more likely the patient has HIT.

heparin-induced thrombocytopenia thrombosis syndrome (HIT/HITTS) undergoing PCI. Fondaparinux is marketed for non-HIT indications but has a strong rationale for HIT therapy and may even be preferred in view of its long half-life, ability to perform anti-Xa monitoring, and lack of interference with thrombin-mediated beneficial effects including activation of protein C (Table 21.10).

TABLE 21.9

TIPS FOR THE MANAGEMENT OF HIT

Two Do's
- Do stop all heparin, including heparin "flushes" and LMWH.
- Do give an alternative nonheparin anticoagulant (therapeutic dose) on cessation of heparin.

Two Don'ts
- Don't give warfarin (give vitamin K if warfarin has already been given). Warfarin does not block HIT hypercoagulability; it increases thrombosis risk via protein C depletion.
- Don't give platelet transfusions. Platelets might increase the risk for thrombosis.

Two Diagnostics
- Test for HIT-Abs: Negative tests rule out HIT; strong positive tests are usually seen in "true" HIT.
- Image for lower-limb DVT: DVT is the most common complication of HIT.

(From Warkentin T. Agents for the treatment of heparin-induced thrombocytopenia. *Hematol Oncol Clin N Am* 2010;24:755–775, with permission.)

TABLE 21.10

ANTICOAGULANTS FOR TREATMENT OF THROMBOSIS IN HIT

	Lepirudin (Refludan)	Argatroban	Bivalirudin	Fondaparinux
Mechanism	Recombinant derivative of hirudin	Small molecule arginine derivative	C-terminal of hirudin linked by spacer to peptidereactive with thrombin active site	Synthetic pentasac-charide
	Factor IIa inhibitor	Factor IIa inhibitor	Factor IIa inhibitor	Factor Xa inhibitor
Dose	0.05–0.10 mg/kg/h	0.5–2 μg/kg/min	0.10–0.20 mg/kg/h	5–10 mg SQ
Clearance	Renal	Hepatobiliary	Enzymatic (renal is minor)	Renal
Monitoring	aPTT	aPTT	aPTT	aPTT

CONCLUSIONS

1. VTE has a significant impact on morbidity and mortality.
2. Risk factors are well-known, and prevention of VTE should be a high-priority issue for all patients at high risk.
3. A combination of clinical assessment, laboratory studies, and diagnostic imaging is required for the accurate diagnosis of VTE.
4. Anticoagulation is the cornerstone of treatment and prevention of VTE, with LMWH and fondaparinux being equivalent and more convenient than IV heparin.
5. The diagnosis of HIT requires the demonstration of PF4 antibodies that activate platelets and typically occurs 5 to 10 days following exposure to heparin.

PRACTICAL POINTS

■ Homan's sign (calf pain with forced dorsiflexion of the foot) is neither sensitive nor specific for DVT.

■ 10% of patients with idiopathic VTE are diagnosed with cancer within the first year after their thrombotic event.

■ Never use an abnormal d-dimer to diagnose VTE. Confirmatory testing is required as the d-dimer is a nonspecific assay.

■ The negative predictive value of CT pulmonary angiography is only marginally improved (from 95 to 97%) by performing concurrent lower-limb CT venography and increases overall radiation exposure. Consequently, adjunctive CT venography of the proximal iliofemoral veins is not recommended.

■ If testing cannot be promptly completed, patients with a high pretest probability for VTE should be administered a dose of anticoagulation while waiting to confirm the diagnosis, assuming bleeding is not a concern.

■ For patients with cancer and DVT/PE, at least 3 months of treatment with LMWH is recommended followed by treatment with LMWH or warfarin as long as the cancer is active.

■ When treating patients with antiphospholipid antibody syndrome, no evidence-based medicine exists that higher intensity anticoagulation is associated with a lower frequency of recurrent thromboembolism. Thus, regular intensity anticoagulation is recommended indefinitely in these patients.

RECOMMENDED READING

Agnelli G, Beccatini C. Current concepts. Acute pulmonary embolism. *N Engl J Med* 2010;363:266–274.

Crowther MA, Warkentin TE. Bleeding risk and the management of bleeding complications in patients undergoing anticoagulant therapy: focus on new anticoagulant agents. *Blood* 2008;111(10):4871–4879.

Eikelboom JW, Weitz JI. Update on antithrombotic therapy. Newanticoagulants. *Circulation* 2010;121(13):1523–1532.

Executive Summary: American College of Chest Physicians Evidence-Based Clinical Practice Guidelines (8th ed.). *Chest* 2008;133:71S–109S.

Geerts WH, Bergqvist D, Pineo GF, et al. Prevention of venous thromboembolism. *Chest* 2008;133(6):381S–453S.

Hirsh J, Lee AYY. How we diagnose and treat deep vein thrombosis. *Blood* 2002;99: 3102–3110.

Kearon C. Natural history of venous thromboembolism. *Circulation* 2003;107:I-22–I-30.

Kearon C. Diagnosis of pulmonary embolism. *CMAJ* 2003;168:183–194.

Kearon C. Long-term management of patients after venous thromboembolism. *Circulation* 2004;110(Suppl I):I-10–I-18.

Kearon C, Crowther MA, Hirsh J. Management of patients with hereditary hypercoagulable dirorders. *Annu Rev Med* 2000;51:169–185.

Kearon C, Kahn S, Agnelli G, et al. Antithrombotic therapy for venous thromboembolic disease. *Chest* 2008;133(6):454S–545S.

Kelton JG, Warkentin TE. Heparin-induced thrombocytopenia: a historical perspective. *Blood* 2008;112(7):2607–2616.

Lee AYY. Management of thrombosis in cancer: primary and secondary prophylaxis. *Br J Haematol* 2004;128:291–302.

Lee AYY, Rickles FR, Julian J, et al. Randomized comparison of low molecular weight heparin and coumarin derivatives on the survival of patients with cancer and venous thromboembolism. *JCO* 2005;23(10):2123–2129.

Lim W, Crowther MA, Eikelboom JW. Management of antiphospholipid antibody syndrome. A systematic review. *JAMA* 2006;295(9):1050–1057.

Linkins LA, Choi PT, Douketis JD. Clinical impact of bleeding in patients taking oral anticoagulant therapy for venous thromboembolism. A meta-analysis. *Ann Int Med* 2003;139(11): 893–900.

PRÉPIC study group. Eight-year follow-up of patients with permanent vena cava filters in the prevention of pulmonary embolism. The PREPIC (Prevention du Risque d'Embolie Pulmonaire par Interruption Cave) randomized study. *Circulation* 2004;112:416–422.

Righini M, Perrier A, de Moerloose P, et al. D-dimer for venous thromboembolism diagnosis: 20 years later. *J Thromb Haemost* 2008;6:1059–1071.

Schulman S, Bijsterveld NR. Anticoagulants and their reversal. *Transfus Med Rev* 2007;21(1): 37–48.

Stein PD, Chenevert TL, Fowler SE, et al. Gadolinium-enhanced magnetic resonance angiography for pulmonary embolism: a multicenter prospective study (PIOPED III).PIOPED III. *Ann Intern Med* 2010;152(7):434–443, W142–W143.

Stein PD, Fowler SE, Goodman LR, et al. Multidetector computed tomography for acute pulmonary embolism. PIOPED II. *N Engl J Med* 2006;354(22):2317–2327.

van Dongen CJ, van den Belt AG, Prins MH, et al. Fixed dose subcutaneous low molecular weight heparins versus adjusted dose unfractionated heparin for venous thromboembolism [update of Cochrane Database Systematic Review 2000]. *Cochrane Database Syst Rev* 2004;4:CD001100.

Warkentin T. Agents for the treatment of heparin-induced thrombocytopenia. *Hematol Oncol Clin N Am* 2010;24:755–775.

Weitz JI. New oral anticoagulants in development. *Thromb Haemost* 2010;103:62–70.

CHAPTER 22 ■ Approach to and Management of Chronic Venous Insufficiency

Justin B. Hurie and Thomas W. Wakefield

Chronic venous insufficiency (CVI) is a pathologic condition of lower-extremity venous hypertension often due to dysfunction of the vein walls or valves. The most common etiologies of vein dysfunction are primary valvular incompetence and secondary dysfunction due to a prior deep vein thrombosis (DVT), with DVT occurring in more than 350,000 patients annually. The incidence of CVI after appropriate anticoagulation may be as high as 23% after 2 years and 28% after 5 years. Less common causes include cavernous hemangiomas, congenital arteriovenous fistulas, and pelvic tumors. Varicose veins are the most common manifestation of CVI, affecting an estimated 20 million people. Other symptoms include edema, hyperpigmentation, lipodermatosclerosis, and ulceration. The overall incidence of venous stasis syndrome is 76 per 100,000 person-years and rises with increasing age. Although advanced CVI symptoms such as venous ulcers are much less common, having an incidence of 18 per 100,000 person-years, the economic impact is nonetheless significant with an estimated $200 million to $1 billion per year being spent on their treatment in the United States. The prevention, diagnosis, and treatment of this disease process, therefore, become highly relevant.

CLINICAL FEATURES

History and Physical Examination

Symptoms of CVI are variable and include leg tiredness, cramping, itching, burning, and swelling. Physical findings may include prominent dilated superficial veins, edema, skin changes, and ulceration.

Presenting Features

The typical presentation of a patient with CVI is one of edematous lower extremities (unilateral or bilateral) with hyperpigmentation, eczema, and/or lipodermatosclerosis (scarring of the skin and fat). Accompanying varicose veins or skin ulceration may also be present. Edema is the initial finding and most commonly occurs at and above the ankle, without involvement of the forefoot or toes. It usually responds to leg elevation and is typically worse in the evening. When ulcers occur, they are most often large, irregular, and associated with a shallow moist granulation base (Fig. 22.1). They are often very painful and occur on the medial or lateral surface of the leg in the supramalleolar position. Because of the significant variability in the manifestations and severity of CVI, several classification schemes have been designed to help categorize patients. Two such schemes will be briefly reviewed later in this chapter.

439

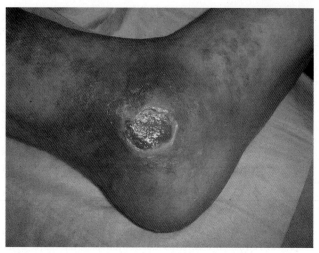

FIGURE 22-1. Chronic venous stasis ulcer with location in the medial paramalleolar position.

Differential Diagnosis

The symptoms of CVI (pain, edema, skin changes, and ulcerations) must be distinguished from other etiologies of these symptoms. Likewise, venous ulcers can be mistaken for other lesions such as squamous cell carcinoma (Marjolin's ulcers).

Pathophysiology

The pathophysiology of CVI can be broken down into changes occurring at the level of the large venous vessels, the microvasculature, and the tissue. CVI occurs as a result of valvular dysfunction within the large veins of the leg. The resulting standing column of blood leads to venous hypertension. Venous hypertension is defined as end-exercise venous pressure at the ankle greater than 30 mm Hg (normal is 15 mm Hg). This, in turn, leads to capillary dysfunction and tissue injury. Common causes of valvular dysfunction include primary valvular incompetence and secondary valvular incompetence after DVT. In patients with no history or evidence of DVT, primary valve abnormalities such as valvular agenesis or aplasia are most likely, although vein wall abnormalities can also lead to valvular insufficiency. Contemporary data in DVT patients suggest that the incidence of severe CVI after 8 years follow-up is approximately 30% and may be even higher if associated with ipsilateral recurrent DVT. It has also been shown that valvular dysfunction occurs more commonly if there is delayed DVT resolution and if the more proximal veins are involved in the initial venous thrombosis. Skin ulceration is also more common in patients with recurrent DVT. Risk factors for DVT formation can be inherited, acquired, or multifactorial (Table 22.1). Once valvular dysfunction occurs, the ensuing chronic venous hypertension has profound effects at the microvascular level. Capillaries become dilated and

TABLE 22.1

RISK FACTORS FOR DVT

Congenital	Acquired	Situational	Mixed
Factor VII excess	HIV infection	Surgery	Hyperhomocysteinemia
Protein C deficiency	Age	Trauma	Increased factor VIII levels
Protein S deficiency	Immobilization	Pregnancy	Increased factor IX levels
Factor V Leiden	Malignancy	Oral contraceptives	Increased factor XI levels
Antithrombin deficiency	Heparin-induced thrombocytopenia	Hormone replacement therapy	
Prothrombin G20210A	Behçet's disease		
	Nephrotic syndrome		
	Antiphospholipid antibodies		
	Myeloproliferative disorders		
	Polycythemia vera		
	Paroxysmal nocturnal hemoglobinuria		
	Inflammatory bowel disease		

(From Gloviczki P, ed. *Handbook of venous disorders*. London, UK: Arnold, 2009:95, with permission.)

tortuous, allowing extravasation of fluid, red blood cells, and macromolecules. There is an increase in white blood cell adhesion to the endothelium as well as leukocyte activation. Increased microvascular blood flow is seen initially, but there can be late findings of capillary thrombosis leading to tissue hypoxia. Within the tissues, the extravasated red blood cells break down to produce a dark pigment called hemosiderin. The perivascular space becomes surrounded by intracellular matrix proteins. Chronic accompanying inflammation leads to scarring and fibrosis of the subcutaneous tissues. Macrophages, mast cells, and T lymphocytes are the cell types most commonly involved in tissue destruction. As skin perfusion decreases, the resulting ischemia can lead to skin breakdown and ulceration.

Classification

As illustrated in the previous section, there are many manifestations of venous hypertension. Due to the variety of presentations, it is important to standardize the classification of degree of CVI. The most commonly used classification is the CEAP system illustrated in Table 22.2. In addition, the Villalta

TABLE 22.2

CEAP CLASSIFICATION

Clinical Classification		
	C0	No visible or palpable signs of venous disease
	C1	Telangiectasias or reticular veins
	C2	Varicose veins
	C3	Edema
	C4a	Pigmentation and/or eczema
	C4b	Lipodermatosclerosis and/or atrophie blanche
	C5	Healed venous ulceration
	C6	Active venous ulceration
	S	Symptoms including pain, tightness, skin irritation, heaviness, or muscle cramps
	A	Asymptomatic
Etiologic Classification		
	E_c	Congenital
	E_p	Primary
	E_s	Secondary (postthrombotic)
	E_n	No venous etiology identified
Anatomic Classification		
	A_s	Superficial veins
	1	Telangiectasias/reticular veins
	2	Great saphenous vein (above knee)
	3	Great saphenous vein (below knee)
	4	Small saphenous vein
	5	Nonsaphenous veins
	A_d	Deep veins
	6	Inferior vena cava
	7	Common iliac vein
	8	Internal iliac vein
	9	External iliac vein
	10	Pelvic veins (gonadal, broad ligament, other)
	11	Common femoral vein
	12	Deep femoral vein
	13	Femoral vein
	14	Popliteal vein
	15	Crural vein (anterior tibial, posterior tibial, peroneal)
	16	Muscular vein (gastrocnemial, soleal, other)
	A_p	Perforating veins
	17	Thigh perforator veins
	18	Calf perforator veins
Pathophysiological Classification		
	P_r	Reflux
	P_o	Obstruction
	$P_{r,o}$	Reflux and obstruction
	P_n	No venous pathophysiology identified

(From Gloviczki P, ed. *Handbook of venous disorders*. London, UK: Arnold, 2009:38–39, with permission.)

scoring system and Venous Clinical Severity Score (VCSS) system have been described in order to objectively describe the clinical response. The Villalta scale gives 0 (none) to 3 (severe) points for five patient-given symptoms and six physician-observed signs. A score greater than 5 is consistent with the postthrombotic syndrome and has been shown to correlate with quality of life. The VCSS also awards 0 (none) to 3 (severe) for ten different complaints (see Table 22.3). These systems are recommended by various organizations including the American Venous Forum in order to standardize reporting and allow more objective observation of clinical benefit and improved research.

DIAGNOSIS

Diagnostic Modalities

Several diagnostic studies may be employed in the evaluation of CVI, and they can be divided into invasive and noninvasive tests. A careful history and physical examination including arterial evaluation form the cornerstone of diagnostic evaluation. Within the last 10 years, duplex ultrasound has become the primary noninvasive diagnostic modality due to high sensitivity and specificity rates greater than 95%. Duplex ultrasound is safe during pregnancy and may also elucidate other causes of the patients' symptoms. Additional noninvasive tests may be performed selectively and include air plethysmography (APG). Magnetic resonance venography or invasive testing such as phlebography is usually reserved for the evaluation of proximal venous structures in patients in whom surgical treatment is being considered. Historically, the Brodie-Trendelenburg test has been performed as an in-office evaluation for patients with prominent varicose veins. This tourniquet-based test, which helps discriminate saphenofemoral junction (SFJ) incompetence from deep-to-superficial communication via incompetent perforators, has been supplanted by the use of ultrasound-based testing and is not usually performed in modern practice. The duplex evaluation helps localize specific perforators that may be contributing to the varicosities along with other points of reflux and may discriminate obstruction from valvular incompetence and reflux.

Duplex Ultrasound

Duplex ultrasound scanning is the modality of choice for the diagnosis of both acute and chronic DVT as well as to evaluate the presence of reflux. Compression maneuvers and examination of flow patterns with augmentation can allow systematic evaluation of the saphenofemoral and saphenopopliteal junctions and deep, superficial, and perforating veins. Venous reflux is identified by having the patient do Valsalva maneuver while in the 15-degree reverse Trendelenburg position or by using rapidly deflating pneumatic cuffs below the level being evaluated to elicit reflux. Some recommend that this technique be performed in the upright position. Incompetent perforator veins are identified and their size is measured by holding the transducer directly over the vein while squeezing and releasing the leg. Bidirectionality of flow with compression and release indicates an incompetent perforating vein. Limitations of duplex ultrasound scanning

TABLE 22.3

VENOUS CLINICAL SEVERITY SCORE

Attribute	Absent = 0	Mild = 1	Moderate = 2	Severe = 3
Pain	None	Occasional, not restricting activity or requiring analgesics	Daily, moderate activity limitation, occasional analgesics	Daily, severe limiting activities or requiring regular use of analgesics
Varicose veins[a]	None	Few, scattered; branch veins	Multiple; GS veins confined to calf or thigh	Extensive; thigh and calf or GS and SS distribution
Venous edema[b]	None	Evening ankle edema only	Afternoon edema, above ankle	Morning edema above ankle and requiring activity change, elevation
Skin pigmentation[c]	None or focal, low intensity (tan)	Diffuse, but limited in area and old (brown)	Diffuse over most of gaiter distribution (lower 1/3) or recent pigmentation (purple)	Wider distribution (above lower 1/3) and recent pigmentation
Inflammation	None	Mild cellulitis, limited to marginal area around ulcer	Moderate cellulitis, involves most of gaiter area (lower 1/3)	Severe cellulitis (lower 1/3 and above) or significant venous eczema
Induration	None	Focal, circummalleolar (<5 cm)	Medial or lateral, less than lower third of leg	Entire lower third of leg or more
No. of active ulcers	0	1	2	>2
Active ulceration, duration	None	<3 mo	>3 mo, <1 y	Not healed > 1 y
Active ulcer, size[d]	None	<2-cm diameter	2-6-cm diameter	>6-cm diameter
Compressive therapy	Not used or not compliant	Intermittent use of stockings	Wears elastic stocking most days	Full compliance: stockings + elevation

[a]"Varicose" veins must be >4-mm diameter to qualify so that differentiation is ensured between C1 and C2 venous pathology.

[b]Presumes venous origin by characteristics [e.g., Brawny (not pitting or spongy) edema], with significant effect of standing/limb elevation and/or other clinical evidence of venous etiology (i.e., varicose veins, history of DVT). Edema must be a regular finding (e.g., daily occurrence).

[c]Focal pigmentation over varicose veins does not qualify.

[d]Largest dimension/diameter of largest ulcer.

GS, great saphenous; SS, small saphenous.

(Reproduced from Rutherford RB, Padberg FT, Comerota AJ, et al. Venous severity scoring: an adjunct to venous outcome assessment. *J Vasc Surg* 2000;31:1307–1312, with permission.)

include the need for an experienced vascular technologist to perform the exam, interoperator variability, and the inability to accurately visualize the venous system above the inguinal ligament. Duplex ultrasound provides direct evaluation of the veins in the lower extremity and indirect evaluation of the pelvic vasculature. The evaluation of the iliac veins through ultrasound relies on indirect evidence of obstruction such as loss of characteristic cessation of venous flow with Valsalva maneuver and loss of respiratory variation, indicating a more proximal obstruction.

Air Plethysmography

An additional diagnostic study is APG, which is a physiologic study to measure venous reflux, calf muscle pump function, and venous obstruction. APG testing makes precise volume measurements with air-filled polyurethane sleeves that surround the legs. The first of several measurements that can be made with APG is the functional venous volume (VV). In normal limbs, the average VV is 80 to 150 mL, while in patients with severe CVI, the volume might be close to 400 mL. In order to measure VV, the patient is asked to stand from a supine position, and the VV is measured within the context of the venous filling index (VFI). The VFI is defined as the ratio between 90% VV and the time taken for 90% filling (VFT90) to occur (VFI = 90%VV/VFT90). In the normal situation, veins should fill slowly from the arterial side with a VFI less than 2 mL/s. In limbs with severe reflux, this number may increase up to 30 mL/s. VFI has been shown to correlate with the prevalence of skin changes and ulceration. Calf muscle pump function is also assessed by APG. The patient is asked to do tiptoe movements, and the recorded decrease in pressure represents the ejected volume (EV). Thus, the ejection fraction (EF) can be measured with the formula EF = [(EV/VV) × 100]. A normal EF is above 60%. Severe deep venous disease can result in an EF below 10%. The EF, like the VFI, is an important predictor of which patients will develop skin ulceration. Finally, APG can also be used to measure obstruction using a thigh tourniquet. The benefit of APG in clinical practice is that it gives the physician an understanding of the different components contributing to the overall severity of patients' CVI. APG can also be an important part of patient selection and predicting who will benefit most from surgical therapy. However, the most reliable part of APG is the assessment of reflux.

Phlebography

Ascending phlebography, once considered the "gold standard" in the assessment of chronic venous obstruction, is infrequently used given the advances in noninvasive testing. Phlebography is performed by injecting contrast into a dorsal foot vein and directing the contrast into the deep venous system by using an ankle tourniquet. This technique can provide useful anatomic information about the location and extent of venous obstruction. However, the profunda femoris veins and internal iliac veins are not typically well visualized with this technique.

An invasive technique used to assess venous reflux and valvular anatomy is descending phlebography. This test is performed on a fluoroscopic table tilted 60 degrees, while contrast is injected through a catheter with the tip placed at the distal external iliac vein. Gravity and a Valsalva maneuver propel the contrast distally in limbs with incompetent valves. This allows grading of phlebographic reflux as well as delineating competent valve cusps, which are clearly outlined with this technique. Reflux grades include 0, no reflux; 1, reflux into the femoral vein to the level of the proximal thigh; 2, reflux into the femoral vein but not through the popliteal vein; 3, reflux to a level just below the knee; and 4, reflux through to the level of the calf or ankle. However, descending phlebography requires an experienced imaging team to perform and is costly. Duplex scanning obviates the need for this test in many circumstances, although phlebograms are often performed in conjunction with therapeutic maneuvers such as venoplasty and stenting as well as thrombolysis.

MANAGEMENT

Nonoperative Management of Chronic Venous Insufficiency

The goals of nonoperative management of CVI are symptom control, prevention of ulceration, and promotion of ulcer healing. Patient education is extremely important and should emphasize the sequela of uncontrolled lower-extremity edema, including skin ulceration and infection. Patients should be encouraged to elevate their legs, exercise (to improve calf muscle function), and maintain good hygiene. There are currently no effective pharmacologic agents for the prevention of venous ulceration that are approved by the U.S. Food and Drug Administration. The mainstay of preventative treatment, therefore, is compression therapy, which may reduce the incidence of postphlebitic pain and swelling by 50%. Prior to implementing compression therapy, patients should be evaluated for concomitant peripheral arterial disease. Palpable pulses in the patient without symptoms of intermittent claudication typically require no further investigation. If pulses are not palpable, or the patient gives a strong history of intermittent claudication, then lower-extremity arterial Doppler studies with waveforms and ankle-brachial indexes (ABIs) should be performed to evaluate for arterial disease. There have been some preliminary reports that treatment of concomitant arterial disease will allow quicker healing of the venous stasis ulcers. The recommended compression stockings for patients with CVI are 30 to 40 mm Hg pressure at the ankle with graded compression up the leg. A randomized clinical trial comparing compression stockings to no-compression stockings in patients following acute DVT revealed that approximately 60% of patients with first-episode DVT develop post-thrombotic syndrome within 2 years. Sized-to-fit compression stockings reduced this rate by approximately one half. Compression stockings can be difficult to apply, and compliance is often a problem. If patients need assistance putting on their stockings, devices are available to aid in their application. Alternatively, nonelastic compression such as the CircAid orthosis can be used as an effective alternative with easier application. In addition to compression, we emphasize good exercise to improve calf muscle pump function and intermittent leg elevation above the level of the heart.

Management of the Venous Ulcer

Adequate compression is the foundation for healing with venous ulcerations. The most common methods for applying topical wound treatments and compression include Unna boots, compression hose with wound covers, and multilayer compression bandages. Unna boots are made with a paste containing zinc oxide, gelatin, sorbitol, magnesium sulfate, and glycerin, and this mixture dries to a semirigid consistency when wrapped. However, many patients find Unna boots uncomfortable. If compression hose and wound coverings are utilized, patients typically require intermittent leg elevation until the edema is lessened enough to allow appropriately fitting graded compression hose. The combination of wound covering and compression allows for frequent ulcer healing, up to 90% by approximately 5 months.

A multilayer dressing system is typically considered more comfortable than an Unna boot and has the following layers: (i) a natural orthopedic wool, which absorbs exudate and protects bony prominences from excessive pressure; (ii) a crepe bandage adding absorbency and acting to smoothen the orthopedic wool layer; (iii) a light compression bandage, which is highly conformable to accommodate a difficult limb shape; and (iv) a cohesive flexible bandage that also applies pressure, maintaining effective levels of compression for up to 1 week. In one study, nearly 80% of patients had ulcer healing by 12 weeks using this therapy.

It should be emphasized that meticulous local wound care and careful attention to the skin surrounding the ulcer are paramount in allowing ulcer healing. Multiple topical wound-care agents are available. Many are costly, and efficacy beyond standard compression with wound covering has been difficult to demonstrate. In most situations, combinations of local wound dressings (especially occlusive dressings) with support are most useful. For large venous ulcers expected to have slow rates of healing, cultured human skin equivalent or split-thickness skin grafting can be considered. In general, the care for venous ulcers should be in the setting of a skilled wound-care provider with regular patient contact to aid in compliance and ongoing patient education. Also, the best prevention for recurrent ulceration once healing has occurred is ongoing control of lower-extremity edema with graded compression stockings.

Surgical Management

General Principles

The most difficult aspects of the surgical management of CVI are determining who will benefit from an operation and what surgical intervention is most appropriate. An understanding of the mechanism of CVI in each individual patient is essential. Duplex is recommended for all patients with C2 or higher disease, because it determines the presence and location of outflow obstruction and documents the degree and anatomical site of valvular reflux. Without a complete understanding of the pathology, an operation intended to help the patient can quickly worsen his or her venous disease. Patients should be categorized with their CEAP (clinical presentation,

Venous insufficiency protocol

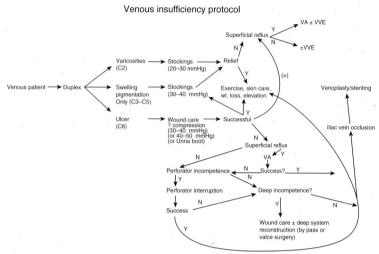

FIGURE 22-2. Diagnostic and therapeutic approach to a patient with venous symptoms based on CEAP classification. (VVE, varicose vein excision; Success, ulcer healed; VA, vein ablation; C2–C6, CEAP clinical classification.)

*e*tiology, *a*natomy, *p*athophysiology) classification system (Table 22.2) prior to operative intervention (see Fig. 22.2). Additionally, the VCSS system allows for the assessment of changes in the patients' venous condition with therapy (Table 22.3). Briefly, patients with varicosities are treated with compression stockings (20 to 30 mm Hg) and conservative measures such as exercise, skin care, elevation, and weight loss. Patients without symptomatic relief are recommended to undergo varicose vein excision (VVE). Those patients found to have superficial reflux should undergo great saphenous ablation (VA) at the same time as VVE. Patients found to have C3-C5 disease are also treated with conservative measures and compression stockings (30 to 40 mm Hg). Patients without improvement should be treated with VVE and VA if they are found to have superficial reflux. Symptomatic patients without reflux may benefit from additional testing such as CT, APG, or MR to evaluate other potential etiologies. Finally, patients with C6 disease should undergo initial treatment with compression (30 to 40 mm Hg, 40 to 50 mm Hg, or Unna boots). Even if conservative measures are successful, these patients may benefit from a decreased risk of ulcer recurrence with the treatment of superficial reflux through VVE and VA. In patients with a recalcitrant ulcer, additional treatment with VA, perforator interruption, or deep system reconstruction may be recommended depending on the suspected origin of venous hypertension.

Laser Therapy

Percutaneous laser treatments may be used in telangiectasias up to 0.7 mm diameter. Given the uptake by melanin, laser treatments should not be undertaken in patients with a sun tan because of the fear of long-lasting hyperpigmentation.

Sclerotherapy

Sclerotherapy damages the vessel wall causing inflammation and is an excellent technique for the treatment of superficial venules (venous spiders/telangiectasias) and small varicosities (1 to 3 mm diameter). There are several FDA-approved sclerosing agents available, including hypertonic saline. Sodium morrhuate is commonly used, although its use predates the approval process by the FDA. In the United States, 0.5 to 3% sodium tetradecyl sulfate is most commonly used for treating varicose veins. Small volumes (0.25 to 0.5 mL) of a sclerosing agent are injected into the problem venous segment under good lighting and two to three times magnification. Foam sclerotherapy is being increasingly used, although cerebrovascular events are one potential side effect (although rarely these events have been reported). Graduated external compression is then applied to produce apposition of the inflamed vein walls and avoid thrombus formation. Potential complications include pigmentation, pain, skin necrosis, DVT (rare), and anaphylactic reactions (extremely rare).

Treatment of Great Saphenous Vein

Duplex ultrasound plays a pivotal role in the preoperative workup prior to treatment for great saphenous vein (GSV) reflux. The duplex scan can determine the competence of the GSV as well as evaluate the deep system for adequate outflow capabilities. In cases of GSV incompetence, methods of treatment involve removal of the refluxing veins. Historically, removal of the GSV was accomplished through high ligation of the GSV at the SFJ and removal of the vein to the knee. This has traditionally resulted in a rate of recurrence less than 25% at 2 years but increases to 41% after 5 years. Saphenous vein stripping from ankle to groin has largely been abandoned now that duplex scanning permits localization of the site of origin of the varicosities and determination of points of reflux. Also, most perforating veins in the leg enter the posterior arch vein rather than the GSV, rendering stripping of the anterior continuation of the greater saphenous vein below the knee unnecessary. Newer endovascular means of treatment of the GSV have evolved over the last ten years, including radiofrequency ablation (RFA) and laser ablation. RFA involves the percutaneous insertion of a 7-cm heating probe into the GSV. The probe is then sequentially removed while heated in stages to ablate the vein by heating it to 120 degrees Celsius for 20-second periods. Laser ablation causes thermal injury to the vein wall. Both methods involve the infusion of tumescent anesthesia with a small amount of epinephrine to isolate the vein segment from the surrounding tissue in order to decrease the injury to surrounding structures and to shrink the vein onto the catheter. Complications are rare but include infection, DVT, nerve damage, and hematoma formation. Randomized controlled trials have demonstrated that treatment of GSV results in a significantly decreased rate of ulcer recurrence but does not increase the rate of healing of current venous ulcers.

Superficial Vein Resection

Vascular surgeons have variable degrees of enthusiasm for superficial vein resection, but most would agree that short-term and midterm results are good. The objectives of these operations are to treat locally advanced varicose veins. Although removal of the saphenous vein is no longer performed by surgical excision in most cases, the branch varicosities still need to be surgically resected. Stab avulsion is performed using small 2- to 3-mm incisions over the individual varicosities followed by removal of the varicose vein clusters. Complications from vein stripping include recurrence of varicose veins (early and late), ecchymosis, lymphocele, wound infection, and transient numbness both in the saphenous nerve distribution and in the general distribution of skin nerves. There are newer, minimally invasive methods to remove superficial varicose veins. One method involves the use of powered phlebectomy, Trivex, which uses transillumination of the varicose veins. Tumescent anesthesia is infiltrated through a separate port to allow improved pain control, to allow constriction of veins, and to flush blood from the subcutaneous space. The Trivex machine then cuts and evacuates the vein clusters. Separate 1.5-mm punch holes are used to evacuate the buildup of fluid and retained blood. Preliminary reports indicate a low risk of infection and a high rate of patient satisfaction greater than 99%. This can be performed as an isolated procedure or in concert with treatment of the greater saphenous system. These are currently done as outpatient procedures.

Perforator Ligation

The role of incompetent perforating veins in the development of venous stasis ulcers is an area of continued debate. The identification of bidirectional flow and location of the perforating veins are performed preoperatively using duplex ultrasound. Linton developed a technique for ligating perforating veins using a medial calf incision in the 1930s. This operation has since been employed with several modifications, variable success (Table 22.4), and significant morbidity. More recently, a less invasive approach to perforator ligation has become popularized. This subfascial endoscopic perforator surgery (SEPS) has been shown to be effective in combination with saphenous vein surgery (Table 22.5). A surgical endoscope is introduced beneath the fascia, as is a working port, and under gas insufflation, the perforating veins are individually identified and either ligated or ligated and divided. This technique is well suited for the treatment of class 4 to 6 CVI. However, recurrence or new ulcer development is still a significant problem, especially in postthrombotic limbs. Given the improvements in endovascular intervention, many perforator interruptions can be approached intraluminally using laser or RFA, but this is a technique in evolution.

Valvuloplasty

This operation may be performed at any incompetent major venous valve site. Valvuloplasty operations should only be used to treat venous reflux in the absence of outflow obstruction. Various techniques for repairing

TABLE 22.4

CLINICAL RESULTS OF OPEN PERFORATOR INTERRUPTION FOR THE TREATMENT OF ADVANCED CHRONIC VENOUS DISEASE

Author, Year	No. of Limbs Treated	No. of Limbs with Ulcer	Wound Complications No. (%)	Ulcer Healing No. (%)	Ulcer Recurrence[a] No. (%)	Mean Follow-Up (Years)
Silver, 1971	31	19	4 (14)	—	— (10)	1–15
Thurston, 1973	102	0	12 (12)	[b]	11 (13)	3.3
Bowen, 1975	71	8	31 (44)	—	24 (34)	4.5
Burnand, 1976	41	0	—	[b]	24 (55)	—
Negus, 1983	108	108	24 (22)	91 (84)	16 (15)	3.7
Wilkinson, 1986	108	0	26 (24)	[b]	3 (7)	6
Cikrit, 1988	32	30	6 (19)	30 (100)	5 (19)	4
Bradbury, 1993	53	0	—	[b]	14 (26)	5
Pierik, 1997	19	19	10 (53)	17 (90)	0 (0)	1.8
Sato, 1999	29	19	13 (45)	19 (100)	13 (68)	2.9
Total	594 (100)	203 (34)	126/497 (25)	157/176 (89)	110/471 (23)	—

[a]Recurrence calculated where data available and percentage account for patients lost to follow-up.

[b]Only Class 5 (healed ulcer) patients admitted in study.

(From Gloviczki P, ed. *Handbook of venous disorders*. London, UK: Arnold, 2009:529 ,with permission.)

TABLE 22.5

CLINICAL RESULTS OF SEPS FOR THE TREATMENT OF ADVANCED CHRONIC VENOUS DISEASE

Author, Year	No. of Limbs Treated	No. of Limbs with Ulcer[a]	Concomitant Saphenous Ablation No. (%)	Wound Complications No. (%)	Ulcer Healing No. (%)	Ulcer Recurrence[b] No. (%)	Mean Follow-Up (Months)
Jugenheimer, 1992	103	17	97 (94)	3 (3)	16 (94)	0 (0)	27
Pierek, 1995	40	16	4 (10)	3 (8)	16 (100)	1 (2.5)	46
Bergan, 1996	31	15	31 (100)	3 (10)	15 (100)	(0)	—
Wolters, 1996	27	27	0 (0)	2 (7)	26 (96)	2 (8)	12–24
Padberg, 1996	11	0	11 (100)	—	c	0 (0)	16
Pierek, 1997	20	20	14 (70)	0 (0)	17 (85)	0 (0)	21
Gloviczki, 1999	146	101	86 (59)	9 (6)	85 (84)	26 (21)	24
Illig, 1999	30	19	—	—	17 (89)	4 (15)	9
Sato, 1999	27	20	17 (63)	2 (7)	18 (90)	5 (28)	8
Nelzen, 2001	149	36	132 (89)	11 (7)	32 (89)	3 (5)	32
Kalra, 2002	103	42	74 (72)	7 (6)	38 (90)	15 (21)	40
Iarati, 2002	51	29	33 (65)	3 (6)	22 (76)	6 (13)	38
Baron, 2004	98	53	36 (42)	—	53 (100)	0 (0)	—
Total no. of limbs (%)	836 (100)	395 (47)	535/789 (68)	50/680 (7)	355/395 (90)	62/580 (11)	—

[a]Only Class 6 (active ulcer) patients are included.
[b]Recurrence calculated for Class 5 and Class 6 limbs only, where data available and percentage account for patients lost to follow-up.
[c]Only Class 5 (healed ulcer) patients were admitted in this study.
(From Gloviczki P, ed. *Handbook of venous disorders*. London, UK: Arnold, 2009:530, with permission.)

TABLE 22.6

FOLLOW-UP DATA FOR INTERNAL VALVULOPLASTY PROCEDURES

Author, Year	No. of Limbs	Follow-Up (Months)	Clinical Success (%)[a]	Valve Competence (%)[b]
Eriksson and Almgren, 1988	17	6–84	62	—
Masuda and Kistner, 1994	32	48–252	73	77
Raju, 1997	68	12–144	62	—
Sottiurai, 1997	143	9–168	—	75
Lurie, 1997	52	36–108	73	—
Perrin, 1997	75	24–96	75	73

[a]Percentage of patients with good to excellent results defined by sustained ulcer healing and absent or minimal symptoms.
[b]Percentage of patients with minimal to no reflux assessed by ultrasound or venography.
(Reproduced from Gloviczki P, Yao JS, eds. *Handbook of venous disorders*. London, UK: Arnold, 2001:334, with permission.)

the incompetent valve have been employed. Some involve a venotomy (internal valvuloplasty) (Fig. 22.3A), while other techniques rely on external sutures alone (external valvuloplasty) (Fig. 22.3B). A number of methods for venotomy and valve exposure during internal valvuloplasty have been described. A semiclosed repair has also been described where external sutures are placed under angioscopic guidance (Fig. 22.3C). All of these operations attempt to bring the two valve attachment lines into proximity, either by suturing the valve attachments alone or by including the valve cusp edges in the repair. Follow-up of these patients is greater than 15 years in some series, and clinical success is achieved in 60 to 75% of patients (Table 22.6). Postoperative complications occur in approximately 10% of patients and are primarily related to bleeding and thrombosis. Only a few centers in the world have performed a number of these procedures.

Venous Segment Transfer

Transposition of a venous segment to one containing a competent proximal valve is another option for the surgical treatment of venous reflux. This procedure relies on competent valves in either the great saphenous or the profunda femoris proximal venous segments. The most straightforward technique involves division of the femoral vein with proximal ligation and an end-to-end anastomosis of the distal transected segment to the proximal GSV segment that contains the competent valve(s). Alternatively, if the GSV is diseased, the femoral vein can be anastomosed in an end-to-side pattern to the competent profunda femoris vein or end-to-end pattern to its first branch. The competency of the newly constructed venous segment is assessed intraoperatively by stripping the vein or with duplex scanning.

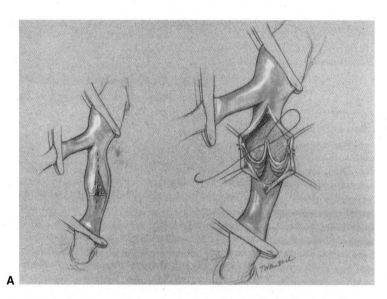

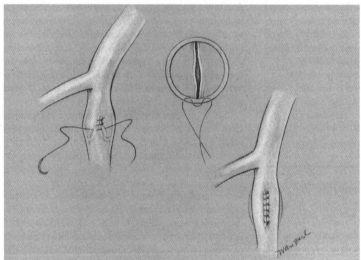

FIGURE 22-3.   A: Longitudinal incision for internal valvuloplasty. B: External valvuloplasty.   (*Continued*)

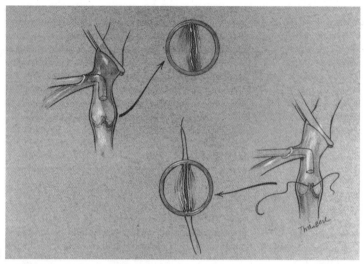

C

FIGURE 22-3. (*Continued*) C: External valvuloplasty under angioscopic guidance. (Reproduced from Gloviczki P, Yao JS, eds. *Handbook of venous disorders*. London, UK: Arnold, 2001:331, with permission.)

This operation is associated with an ulcer recurrence rate of 35% and an ulcer-free interval shorter than that achieved with primary valvuloplasty. Also, surgical site thrombosis occurs in approximately 10% of patients.

Vein Valve Transplantation

Another effective method in restoring valve competency is vein valve transplantation (VVT). This operation is usually performed in clinical classification 5 to 6 patients by taking a segment of axillary vein after its competency has been proven by duplex scanning or phlebography. The popliteal vein is exposed through a standard above-knee approach, or, alternatively, a groin approach is used to expose the femoral vein below the profunda femoris vein junction. A short segment of vein is excised in either location, and the axillary vein segment is interposed with interrupted suture technique (Fig. 22.4). Patency and competency of the transplanted segment are then assessed, and if incompetence is noted, a valvuloplasty is then performed. A summary of the results of 15 large, published series reveals that nearly 80% of patients have ulcer healing, but ulcer recurrence occurs in nearly 30% (Table 22.7). Objective hemodynamic improvement is less frequent than ulcer healing, occurring in approximately 30% of patients. Although objective testing results are inferior to those found after valvuloplasty, the clinical outcomes are comparable. The reason for this discrepancy is not clear. More recent studies using the large axillary vein valve rather than the smaller brachial vein valve (as used in the past) have been very promising. The problem with this technique is the development of recurrent valvular

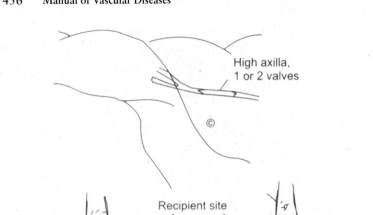

FIGURE 22-4.   Axillary vein segment harvest for venous valve transposition to above-knee popliteal vein. (Reproduced from O'Donnell TF, Mackey WC, Shepard AD, et al. Clinical, hemodynamic and anatomic follow-up of direct venous reconstruction. *Arch Surg* 1987;122:474–482, with permission.)

incompetence in the majority of cases over a short 2-year follow-up. As a consequence, some groups recommend routine wrapping of the vein segment with material (such as ePTFE) to prevent vein dilatation and resulting valvular incompetence.

Venous Bypass

The treatment of postthrombotic venous obstruction with venous bypass is an important option in a small subgroup of patients who have failed conservative measures. The crossover femorofemoral venous bypass

TABLE 22.7

RESULTS OF 15 VEIN VALVE TRANSPLANTATION SERIES (420 LIMBS, 1982–2000)

	Preoperative Characteristics						
	CEAP Classification	Ulcers C5/C6	Age (Years)	Gender Ratio M:F	Phlebography Asc/Desc	Hemodynamic Studies	Superficial Venous Surgery
Number of series reporting	10/15	15/15	8/15	8/15	9/15	7/15	8/15
Mean OR proportion	—	62%	47	1.27	—	—	85%

	Postoperative Outcome Measures					
	Ulcer Healing	Ulcer Recurrence	Follow-Up Length (Mean)	Phlebography Asc vs. Desc	Hemodynamics	Complications
Number of series reporting	11/15 (157 limbs)	6/15 (53 limbs)	8/15	13/15 vs. 11/15	12/15	6/15
Mean OR proportion	79%	28%	3 series, 5 years	5.6% occluded vs. 25% reflux	27% improved over preop	1 death, 5% hematoma

(Reproduced from Gloviczki P, Yao JS, eds. *Handbook of venous disorders.* London, UK: Arnold, 2001:342, with permission.)

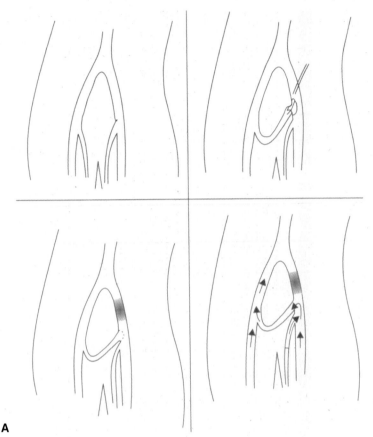

A

FIGURE 22-5.   A: Autogenous vein femorofemoral crossover bypass for iliofemoral outflow obstruction.   (*Continued*)

(Fig. 22.5A) is utilized to bypass an obstructed iliac vein segment, while the saphenopopliteal venous bypass relieves femoral venous occlusion (Fig. 22.5B). Both of these operations require a single venovenous anastomosis. However, they both require a patent greater saphenous vein without varicosities as well as unobstructed iliofemoral and caval runoff. For the femorofemoral bypass, the contralateral saphenous vein is used, whereas for the saphenopopliteal bypass, the ipsilateral saphenous vein is used. In these specific cases, the clinical improvement can be as high as 70 to 80% with both operations. Long-term patency is better for femorofemoral bypass (70%) than saphenopopliteal bypass (50%). The morbidity of these operations ranges from 5 to 10% with minimal risk of mortality.

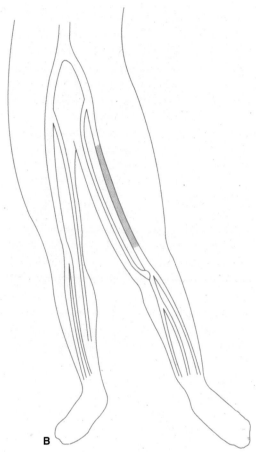

B

FIGURE 22-5. (*Continued*) **B:** Autogenous vein saphenopopliteal venous bypass for femoropopliteal outflow obstruction. (Reproduced from Gloviczki P, Yao JS, eds. *Handbook of venous disorders*. London, UK: Arnold, 2001:367–369, with permission.)

Bypasses of iliac venous obstruction are rapidly being supplanted by iliac vein venoplasty and stenting.

Endovascular Treatment of Chronic Venous Occlusion

Percutaneous treatment of chronic venous occlusion is most commonly performed in the setting of May-Thurner syndrome, in which a left-sided iliofemoral DVT or venous obstruction is caused by the repetitive pulsatile

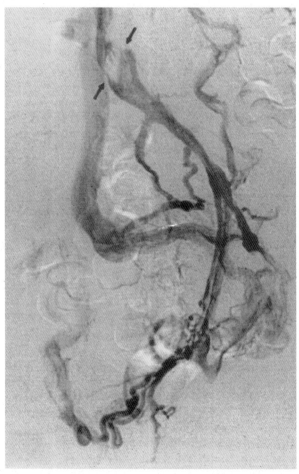

A

FIGURE 22-6.   A: Oblique view of a descending phlebogram demonstrating overlying right common iliac artery with compression and obstruction of the left common iliac vein (*arrows*).   (*Continued*)

trauma of the crossing right common iliac artery. This is most common in young women, especially after pregnancy. Venous access may be obtained from the jugular vein or popliteal vein. A guidewire is advanced across the obstructed segment, and a balloon venoplasty is performed to the appropriate diameter with concomitant stent placement (Fig. 22.6A–D). Midterm follow-up of treated patients reveals freedom from symptoms of venous obstruction and ongoing patency in the majority of cases, with a low incidence of neointimal hyperplasia. The primary and assisted primary patency rates for iliac vein stenting are 75% and 92% at 3 years and 69% and 89% at 6 years.

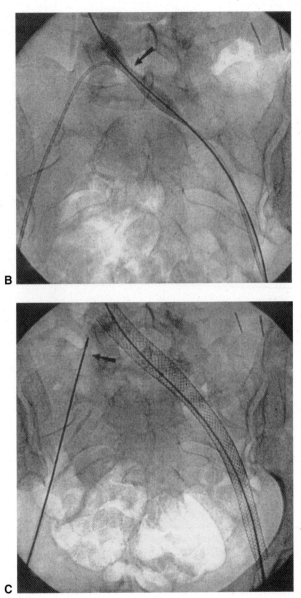

FIGURE 22-6. (*Continued*) **B:** Balloon angioplasty of left common iliac vein stenosis (*arrow*) with 10 × 4-mm balloon catheter. **C:** Postdeployment radiograph of 14/40 mm, 10/68 mm, and 10/38 mm Wallstents in the left common and external iliac veins with reduction of gradient from 4 to 0 mm Hg. Note IVUS catheter in right common iliac vein (*arrow*), which was used to monitor placement of the caval end of the common iliac vein stent.   (*Continued*)

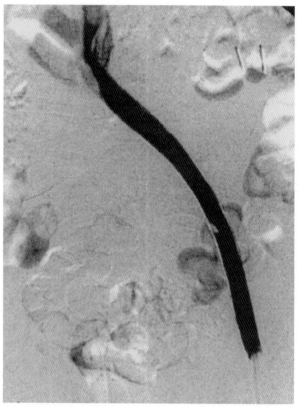

D

FIGURE 22-6. (*Continued*) **D:** Postdeployment venogram demonstrating widely patent left common and external iliac veins with no residual stenosis. (Reproduced from Hurst DR, Forauer AR, Bloom JR, et al. Diagnosis and endovascular treatment of iliocaval compression syndrome. *J Vasc Surg* 2001;34:106–113, with permission.)

CONCLUSIONS

CVI is a common disorder and is a consequence of chronic venous reflux and venous obstruction leading to venous hypertension. Varicose veins are the most common manifestation of CVI. Untreated lower-extremity edema in CVI is a prelude to more serious sequelae such as ulceration. Goals of management of CVI are education, symptom control, prevention of ulceration, and promotion of ulcer healing. Prevention of skin ulceration is preferably achieved by nonoperative measures using graded compression stockings. Patients with CVI should be categorized using the CEAP classification and the VCSS system prior to any intervention. It is critical to determine who will benefit from an operation and what surgical intervention is most appropriate prior to surgical consideration. Surgical treatment of CVI should be reserved for those patients failing nonoperative treatment. Figure 22.2 provides an approach to the diagnosis and management of CVI.

PRACTICAL POINTS

■ CVI commonly occurs in the setting of prior DVT but may occur as a primary idiopathic phenomenon.

■ Varicose veins are the most common manifestation of CVI.

■ Chronic venous ulcers typically occur on the medial surface and less frequently on the lateral surface of the leg in the supramalleolar position.

■ Venous hypertension is defined as end-exercise venous pressure at the ankle above 30 mm Hg (normal is 15 mm Hg).

■ An uncommon but significant cause of nonhealing ulceration that may mimic venous ulcer is squamous cell carcinoma (Marjolin's ulcer).

■ APG has high sensitivity and specificity for the diagnosis of any reflux.

■ CEAP clinical classification is helpful in adjudicating diagnostic tests.

■ CEAP classification is recommended prior to any invasive treatment approach, and results of therapy can be followed up by either VCSS or Villalta score.

RECOMMENDED READING

Barwell JR, Davies CE, Deacon J, et al. Comparison of surgery and compression with compression alone in chronic venous ulceration (ESCHAR study): randomized controlled trial. *Lancet* 2004;363:1854–1859.

Bergan JJ, Yao JS, Flinn WR, et al. Surgical treatment of venous obstruction and insufficiency. *J Vasc Surg* 1986;3:174–181.

Brandjes DP, Büller HR, Heijboer H, et al. Randomized trial of effect of compression stockings in patients with symptomatic proximal-vein thrombosis. *Lancet* 1997;349:759–762.

Caggiati A, Bergan JJ, Gloviczki P, et al. and the International Interdisciplinary Consensus Committee on Venous Anatomical Terminology. Nomenclature of the veins of the lower limbs: an international interdisciplinary consensus statement. *J Vasc Surg* 2002;36:416–422.

Coleridge Smith PD, Thomas P, Scurr JH, et al. Causes of venous ulceration: a new hypothesis. *Br Med J* 1988;296:1726–1727.

Crowther MA, Kelton JG. Congenital thrombophilic states associated with venous thrombosis: a qualitative overview and proposed classification system. *Ann Intern Med* 2003;138: 128–134.

Franz RW, Knapp ED. Transilluminated powered phlebectomy surgery for varicose veins: a review of 339 consecutive patients. *Ann Vasc Surg* 2009;23:303–309.

Gloviczki P, Bergan JJ, Rhodes JM, et al. Mid-term results of endoscopic perforator vein interruption for chronic venous insufficiency: lessons learned from the North American Subfascial Endoscopic Perforator Surgery registry. *J Vasc Surg* 1999;29:489–502.

Heit JA, Rooke TW, Silverstein MD, et al. Trends in the incidence of venous stasis syndrome and venous ulcer: a 25-year population-based study. *J Vasc Surg* 2001;33:1022–1027.

Hurst DR, Forauer AR, Bloom JR, et al. Diagnosis and endovascular treatment of iliocaval compression syndrome. *J Vasc Surg* 2001;34:106–113.

Iafrati MD, Pare GJ, O'Donnell TF, et al. Is the nihilistic approach to surgical reduction of superficial and perforator vein incompetence for venous ulcer justified? *J Vasc Surg* 2002;36:1167–1174.

Jull A, Waters J, Arrol B. Pentoxifylline for treatment of venous leg ulcers: a systematic review. *Lancet* 2002;359:1550–1554.

Killewich LA, Martin R, Cramer M, et al. Pathophysiology of venous claudication. *J Vasc Surg* 1984;1:507–511.

Markel A, Manzo RA, Bergelin RO, et al. Valvular reflux after deep venous thrombosis: incidence and time of occurrence. *J Vasc Surg* 1992;15:377–382.

Meissner M. Proceedings of the International Summit of the 5th Pacific Vascular Symposium. *J Vasc Surg* 2007;46:S1–S94.

Neglen P, Raju S. Intravascular ultrasound scan evaluation of the obstructed vein. *J Vasc Surg* 2002;35:694–700.

Nicolaides AN. Investigation of chronic venous insufficiency: a consensus statement. *Circulation* 2000;102:e126–e163.

Villalta S, Prandoni P, Cogo A, et al. The utility of non-invasive tests for detection of previous proximal-vein thrombosis. *Thrombos Haemost* 1995;73:592–596.

Wilkinson LS, Bunker C, Edwards JC, et al. Leukocytes: their role in the etiopathogenesis of skin damage in venous disease. *J Vasc Surg* 1993;17:669–675.

Wright DD. The ESCHAR trial: should it change practice? *Perspect Vasc Surg Endovasc Ther* 2009;21(2):69–72. [Epub 2009 Jul 14.]

Zajkowski PJ, Proctor MC, Wakefield TW, et al. Compression stockings and venous function. *Arch Surg* 2002;137:1064–1068.

CHAPTER 23 ■ Upper-Extremity Deep Vein and Superior Vena Cava Thrombosis

Emile R. Mohler III, Debabrata Mukherjee, and Sanjay Rajagopalan

Upper-extremity deep vein thrombosis (UEDVT) is an increasingly common clinical problem with potential for considerable morbidity. UEDVT usually refers to thrombosis of the axillary and/or subclavian veins, can rarely involve the brachial vein, and may be primary or secondary (Table 23.1). The presence of UEDVT is brought to medical attention due to upper-extremity pain and swelling. Extension of the clot to the brachiocephalic veins may result in a syndrome identical to the superior vena cava (SVC) syndrome. In this chapter, the approach to subclavian- axillary and brachiocephalic vein thromboses will be addressed in the first section, while the approach and management of SVC syndrome will be addressed separately in order to deal with etiologic and management features that are specific to these entities. However, it must be recognized that secondary thrombosis of the subclavian and central veins of the neck, such as due to indwelling catheters and lines, is dealt with in a very similar fashion.

CLASSIFICATION OF UPPER-EXTREMITY DEEP VEIN THROMBOSIS

UEDVT typically occurs in the axillary, subclavian, and brachiocephalic veins and is increasingly common owing to the usage of catheters and devices routed through the upper-extremity veins. UEDVT may be classified as primary or secondary (Table 23.1).

Primary Upper-Extremity Thrombosis

Primary UEDVT is characterized as idiopathic or effort thrombosis (Paget-Schroetter syndrome). Patients presenting with idiopathic UEDVT have no immediate underlying disease but may have occult or undetected cancer. The etiology is believed to be repetitive microtrauma to the vein with subsequent thrombosis. The acute thrombosis invariably occurs in an area of chronic compression and stricture of the axillosubclavian vein due to compression between the hypertrophied scalene or subclavius tendon and the first rib. The syndrome typically develops in the dominant arm after strenuous activity such as weight lifting, rowing, or baseball pitching in otherwise healthy young individuals. The repeated trauma to the vein is thought to activate the coagulation cascade, especially if a mechanical compression of the vessel is also present. Occasionally, patients with thoracic outlet obstruction [thoracic outlet syndrome (TOS), compression of the neurovascular bundle involving the brachial plexus, subclavian artery, and subclavian vein] may present with venous thrombosis.

TABLE 23.1
CAUSES OF UPPER-EXTREMITY DVT

Primary (idiopathic)
　　Effort thrombosis of the axillary and subclavian veins (Paget-Schroetter syndrome)
　　Occult cancer
　　Thrombophilia
Secondary
　　Central venous catheters
　　Pacemakers/defibrillators
　　Local head/neck malignancy

Secondary Thrombosis

Secondary UEDVT occurs due to intravenous catheters or pacemakers or external compression from a malignancy. Patients may present with limb swelling and discomfort but may be completely asymptomatic and only found to have deep venous thrombosis upon incidental imaging. High fever in the setting of UEDVT suggests septic thrombophlebitis, and an infectious disease evaluation is indicated to identify the infectious cause.

Central Venous Thrombosis Associated with Long-Term Central Venous Instrumentation

Central venous thrombosis is a frequent event in the presence of indwelling central venous catheters, with partial thrombosis occurring in 30 to 45% of cases and complete thrombosis in 5 to 10%. Long-term transvenous access for hemodialysis, chemotherapy, total parenteral nutrition, and transfusions likely accounts for the majority of causes of central venous occlusive disease. Central venous thrombosis rates are equal with long-term and short-term central venous catheters, with the most important determinants of clot formation being the caliber of the catheter, the use of subclavian access route, and the presence of underlying central venous stenosis. Patients undergoing hemodialysis are at a particularly increased risk for the development of central venous thrombosis, much of which is caused by multiple central venous catheterizations and possibly by a downstream effect of the ipsilateral arteriovenous fistula.

CLINICAL FEATURES

Symptoms and Signs of Upper-Extremity Deep Vein Thrombosis

Table 23.2 lists the presenting signs and symptoms of UEDVT. Axillary or subclavian vein thrombosis may sometimes be completely asymptomatic. More often, patients complain of vague shoulder or neck discomfort and arm edema. If thrombosis causes complete obstruction of the SVC, the patient may complain of arm and facial edema, head fullness, blurred vision, or shortness of breath. Patients with TOS may have pain that radiates into

TABLE 23.2

PRESENTING SIGNS AND SYMPTOMS OF UEDVT

	Symptoms	Signs
Axillary or subclavian vein thrombosis	Vague shoulder or neck discomfort Arm or hand edema	Supraclavicular fullness Palpable cord Arm or hand edema Extremity cyanosis Dilated cutaneous veins Jugular venous distension Unable to access central venous catheter
Thoracic outlet syndrome	Pain radiating to arm/forearm Hand weakness	Brachial plexus tenderness Arm or hand atrophy Positive Adson's[a] or Wright's[b] maneuver
SVC syndrome	Fullness and ache in head and neck increased by dependent postures and with exertion (increases venous return) Swelling of the face, neck, and eyelids	Engorged neck and upper-extremity veins

[a]Adson's maneuver: The examiner extends the patient's arm on the affected side, while the patient extends the neck and rotates the head toward the same side. The test is positive if there is weakening of the radial pulse with deep inspiration and suggests compression of the subclavian artery.

[b]Wright's maneuver: The patient's shoulder is abducted and the humerus is externally rotated. The test is positive if symptoms are reproduced and there is weakening of the radial pulse.

(Adapted from Joffe HV, Goldhaber SZ. Upper-extremity deep vein thrombosis. *Circulation* 2002;106(14):1874–1880.)

the fourth and fifth digits via the medial arm and forearm, attributable to injury of the brachial plexus. Symptoms may be position dependent and worsen with hyperabduction of the shoulder or lifting. If TOS is suspected, the examiner should palpate the supraclavicular fossa for brachial plexus tenderness, inspect the hand and arm for atrophy, and perform provocative tests, such as Adson's and Wright's maneuvers (Table 23.2; also see Chapter 1). Patients with UEDVT may have mild cyanosis of the involved extremity, a palpable tender cord, arm and hand edema, supraclavicular fullness, jugular venous distension, and possibly dilated cutaneous collateral veins over the chest or upper arm. If a central venous catheter is present, one or multiple ports may be occluded. One should remember that the signs and symptoms of UEDVT are nonspecific and may often occur in patients with lymphedema, neoplastic compression of the blood vessels, muscle injury, or superficial vein thrombosis. Therefore, it is important to confirm or exclude the diagnosis with objective testing, as appropriate diagnosis is crucial to management of these patients.

DIAGNOSIS

Diagnostic Imaging

The initial diagnostic evaluation technique of choice for diagnosing UEDVT is duplex ultrasound as this technique is noninvasive with a high sensitivity and specificity. A limitation of this technique is potential acoustic shadowing from the clavicle, which may impair visualization of a short segment of the subclavian vein and result in a false-negative study. Further, extension of a clot to the SVC may be inadequately visualized. CT may enable visualization of a proximal clot. An increasingly utilized alternative to x-ray contrast venography is magnetic resonance venography (MRV), which affords an accurate method to noninvasively detect thrombosis in the central thoracic veins, such as the SVC and brachiocephalic veins. The relative advantages and disadvantages of various imaging modalities are listed in Table 23.3. Usually, x-ray contrast venography is considered the gold standard for evaluation of upper-extremity venous thrombosis, but it has limitations. These limitations include the use of iodinated contrast agent with all the associated problems, potential difficulty in cannulating the vein in an edematous arm, and exposure to radiation, especially if this occurs in pregnant women. Venography is typically done as a prelude to an intervention, such as catheter-directed thrombolysis (CDT) or venoplasty.

TABLE 23.3

IMAGING MODALITIES USED TO DIAGNOSE UEDVT WITH RELATIVE ADVANTAGES AND DISADVANTAGES

	Advantages	Disadvantages
Ultrasound	Inexpensive Noninvasive Reproducible	May fail to detect central thrombus that is directly below the clavicle
CT scan	May detect central thrombus May detect the presence of extrinsic vessel compression	Contrast dye Not fully validated
Magnetic resonance venography	Accurately detects central thrombus Provides detailed evaluation of collaterals and blood flow	Limited availability Claustrophobia Not suitable for some patients with implanted metal

(Adapted from Joffe HV, Goldhaber SZ. Upper-extremity deep vein thrombosis. *Circulation* 2002;106(14):1874–1880.)

MANAGEMENT OF PATIENT

Treatment options depend on whether the UEDVT etiology is primary or secondary. Various treatment options are listed in Table 23.4. The goals of treatment include prevention of further progression of thrombosis, improvement in venous blood flow, and prevention of recurrent thrombosis.

Anticoagulation

Anticoagulation treatment remains the cornerstone of therapy in all patients with UEDVT. Either unfractionated or low-molecular-weight heparin is given initially and followed by warfarin or other anti–vitamin K agents for a minimum of 3 months with a goal of international normalized ratio (INR) of 2.0 to 3.0. Patients with thrombophilia may require more prolonged anticoagulation. If the UEDVT is associated with a venous catheter, the catheter should be removed and anticoagulation administered. Patients with postthrombotic syndrome caused by venous hypertension secondary to outflow obstruction and valvular injury benefit from graduated compression sleeves to reduce symptoms. Although one third of patients with UEDVT have pulmonary embolus, it is rare that a pulmonary embolus secondary to UEDVT is fatal. Of note, catheter removal may cause fibrin sheaths to peel off from the catheter, break loose, and embolize to the lung. Therefore, patients should be observed for any manifestations of pulmonary embolus after catheter removal.

TABLE 23.4

TREATMENT OPTIONS TO CONSIDER FOR UEDVT AND SVC SYNDROME

General measures
    Limb elevation
    Graduated compression arm sleeve
    Physical therapy
    Diuretics (for SVC syndrome)
    Anticoagulation
        Unfractionated heparin as "bridge" to warfarin
        Low-molecular-weight heparin as "bridge" to warfarin
        Low-molecular-weight heparin as monotherapy
Endovascular approaches
    Catheter-directed thrombolysis
    Suction thrombectomy
    Angioplasty ± stenting
Surgical therapy
    Surgical thrombectomy
    Thoracic outlet decompression (in cases of TOS or Paget-Schroetter syndrome with evidence of compression)
    SVC filter

Thrombophilia Testing

The prevalence of coagulation disorders in patients with UEDVT is uncertain. A study of 150 consecutive patients with UEDVT enrolled in the MAISTHRO (MAin-ISar-THROmbosis) registry showed that at least one thrombophilia was present in 34% of those with UEDVT relative to 55% in those with LEDVT (Linnemann B, Meister F, Schwonberg J, Schindewolf M, Zgouras D, Lindhoff- Last E. Hereditary and acquired thrombophilia in patients with upper extremity deep-vein thrombosis: results from the MAISTHRO registry. Thromb Haemost 2008;100:440-6). Routine testing has never been shown to be cost-effective for UEDVT. Testing for a hypercoagulable state may be most worthwhile in patients with idiopathic UEDVT, a family history of DVT, a history of recurrent miscarriage, or a prior personal history of DVT.

Thrombolytics

In the absence of contraindications, all patients presenting with acute or sub-acute vascular symptoms with venographically documented axillary-subclavi-an-brachiocephalic vein thrombosis should undergo early CDT with or without adjunctive percutaneous mechanical thrombectomy. Early lysis may potentially minimize intimal scarring and fibrosis. Patients presenting with symptom duration less than 7 days have the best response, while those with longer durations have lower response rates to thrombolysis. The most popular choices are recombinant tissue plasminogen activator (rTPA) and urokinase. Catheter-directed rTPA is commonly administered as a continuous infusion of 1 to 2 mg/h of rTPA for at least 8 hours with serial venography to assess the response of treatment. Alternatively, a pulse-wave catheter, centered in the obstructing thrombosis, delivering rTPA over 15 minutes, may be utilized. In addition, per-cutaneous mechanical thrombectomy with devices such as the AngioJet may be used in conjunction with thrombolytic therapy. Heparin is usually given in conjunction with the thrombolytic agent in order to reduce the risk of thrombosis around the catheter. The advantage of the mechanical thrombectomy is that lower doses and duration of thrombolytic therapy may be used. Research is ongoing as to whether the combination of ultrasound and thrombolytics may allow for enhanced fibrinolysis and more efficient dissolution of the thrombus.

Endovascular Treatment

Endovascular approaches have replaced surgical bypass as the primary management modality in symptomatic primary and secondary UEDVT. Figure 23.1 is a simple algorithm for the management of patients with UEDVT. Endovascular approaches with primary UEDVT should be followed by determination of compression and TOS by performance of positional venography, typically during repeat venography at the end of lysis. The presence of compression may represent an indication for surgical correction of TOS (see section on surgical therapy). Virtually all types of secondary central venous obstructions can be effectively treated by endovascular means. Recurrences after endovascular treatment of subclavian and brachiocephalic veins occur commonly (perhaps related to the high mobility of the shoulder joint and the high general prevalence of positional compression at the thoracic outlet)

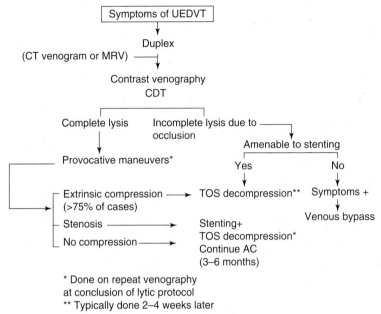

FIGURE 23-1. A simple algorithm for the management of patients with UEDVT. (MRV, magnetic resonance venography; CDT, catheter-directed thrombolysis; TOS, thoracic outlet syndrome)

but are usually readily amenable to additional endovascular interventions, with good secondary patency rates. Patients undergoing hemodialysis with subclavian vein stenosis have a high rate of restenosis after stent placement, and repeated balloon dilation or surgical bypass options may be more durable options. In patients with recurrent restenosis after stent implantation, brachytherapy or drug-eluting stents may provide a viable option.

Surgery

Surgery is usually reserved for eradicating vein compression in patients with primary UEDVT to reduce the risk of recurrent thrombosis and postthrombotic syndrome. Patients should be assessed for venous compression after successful thrombolysis using either repeat ultrasound or venography when the patient is in the neutral and shoulder-abducted position. Those with confirmed extrinsic vein compression may benefit from resection of the first rib or clavicle and/or lysis of dense adhesions around the subclavian vein if this is occurring due to repeated trauma to the vessel. Patients who do not have an adequate response to surgery may undergo venoplasty and/or stenting to maintain patency of the vein. Surgical thrombectomy is reserved for refractory cases, as it carries the risk of general anesthesia, pneumothorax, and brachial plexus damage. Joffe and Goldhaber recommend a trial of conservative therapy rather than early surgical decompression for patients with TOS. The conservative measures include structured physical therapy program to loosen muscles compressing the subclavian vein, weight loss if indicated, and nonsteroidal anti-inflammatory medication.

Timing of Surgical Decompression

Some practitioners advocate an interval period of anticoagulation after initial thrombolytic therapy, followed by delayed surgical decompression, while others favor early surgical decompression shortly after successful thrombolysis, even during the same admission. In most cases, the timing of surgery may be individually determined based on flow quality in the subclavian-axillary vein and severity of residual symptoms after lytic therapy. For instance, when high-grade residual stenosis and sluggish flow persist after successful thrombolytic therapy, the risk of rethrombosis with adequate anticoagulation therapy is high and early decompressive surgery would be beneficial, whereas a more delayed approach may be justified in patients in whom minimal underlying abnormality persists after successful thrombolysis.

Prophylaxis

Some clinicians prescribe a "minidose" (1 mg) of warfarin daily to their cancer patients with central venous catheters to potentially reduce the risk of developing subsequent UEDVT. This low dose usually does not prolong the prothrombin time or cause clinical bleeding. Patients with poor nutrition, those receiving broad-spectrum antibiotics, or those with advanced liver disease or liver metastases may not be suitable candidates for warfarin prophylaxis, because in these situations, even the tiny dose of 1 mg may be sufficient to elevate the prothrombin time excessively and result in clinical bleeding. Low-molecular-weight heparin is an alternative to warfarin for UEDVT prophylaxis in cancer patients with central venous catheters. One study showed that once-daily subcutaneous administration of 2,500 IU of dalteparin starting 2 hours before catheter insertion greatly reduces the frequency of UEDVT. There were no bleeding complications, even when patients received chemotherapy that caused bone marrow suppression. Low-molecular-weight heparin is a safer choice than warfarin for prophylaxis of patients with liver dysfunction or malnutrition but should be avoided in patients with renal dysfunction.

SPECIAL ISSUES

Postthrombotic Syndrome

This is caused by venous hypertension secondary to outflow obstruction and valvular injury. It varies from mild edema with little discomfort to incapacitating limb swelling with pain and ulceration. Graduated compression stockings markedly reduce the rate of postthrombotic syndrome in patients with lower-extremity DVT. Therefore, graduated compression sleeves for all symptomatic patients with acute UEDVT are recommended. Those with refractory swelling may need to use these sleeves indefinitely.

The frequency of postthrombotic syndrome in UEDVT patients treated only with conventional anticoagulation is uncertain, because studies are small and report conflicting results. As few as one half to as many as three fourths of these patients may develop this long-term complication. Thrombolytic therapy during initial presentation may prevent these symptoms in the majority of patients. Patients with primary UEDVT are usually young and healthy, are more active, live longer, and do not have chronic medical conditions. Therefore, they should receive more aggressive treatment, such as thrombolysis and correction of outlet obstruction, to reduce the risk of chronic venous insufficiency. Patients with secondary UEDVT are less bothered by symptoms and are often not candidates for surgery or thrombolysis, so conservative treatment with anticoagulation alone is generally recommended. These patients have very high short-term mortality rates compared with patients who have lower-extremity DVT. Most die from underlying medical problems such as infection, cancer, or multisystem organ failure rather than from complications of the UEDVT, and conservative therapy appears reasonable.

Superior Vena Cava Thrombosis

Etiology

Table 23.5 lists the underlying etiologies associated with an SVC thrombus. Malignant disease is associated with more than 85% of cases.

Clinical Features

Patients with SVC syndrome typically present with fullness in the head and neck that is characteristically worsened in the recumbent posture. Physical activity or exertion also typically worsens the symptom, and this may also be accompanied by headaches that can be intense and throbbing. The other symptoms related to venous hypertension include confusion, dizziness, and orthopnea. Swelling of the face and eyelids is characteristic and, if extensive, may be accompanied by swelling of the upper extremity. Physical exam findings include venous engorgement in the neck and visible collaterals over the chest. Malignant SVC syndrome (especially that associated with lung cancer) may be associated with hemoptysis, hoarseness (recurrent laryngeal nerve palsy), weight loss, and swelling of lymph nodes.

TABLE 23.5

ETIOLOGIES OF SVC THROMBOSIS

Malignancies
    Adenocarcinoma of the lung
    Thyroid carcinoma
    Mediastinal etiologies (lymphoma, teratoma, thymoma, etc.)
Nonmalignant (benign)
    Mediastinitis and mediastinal fibrosis
    Indwelling lines (such as central venous catheters)
Pacemakers/defibrillators

Diagnostic Imaging

The diagnosis of SVC syndrome is typically made by contrast CT of the chest. Diagnostic evaluation should include a thorough evaluation to rule out malignancy. The findings include nonopacification of the SVC along with obvious collaterals (azygos system, lateral thoracic and thoracoepigastric and internal mammary pathways). An adjunctive finding may be opacification of the medial segment of the left lobe of the liver (due to collaterals). Duplex scanning is inadequate to visualize the SVC but may be important for operative/intervention planning. Adjunctive findings on duplex may suggest an SVC thrombosis (lack of respiratory variation of the subclavian and the internal jugular veins). MRV is an attractive option and may be used instead of CT scanning. Venography is usually required prior to intervention.

Management of Superior Vena Cava Syndrome

General Management Measures

These measures include general instructions to sleep using pillows, avoidance of heavy activity and tight-fitting garments, and institution of a diuretic if edema is severe. SVC syndrome presenting acutely should be managed with thrombolysis if there are no contraindications.

Approach to Superior Vena Cava Thrombosis

Figure 23.2 summarizes the approach to a patient presenting with characteristic symptoms and signs of SVC syndrome. Institution of radiation therapy (XRT) with or without chemotherapy for malignancies responsive to these modalities is often sufficient to reduce tumor bulk and provide relief. These same patients often may present several months later with chronic SVC symptoms. Venography is necessary prior to any planned intervention and if performed bilaterally through access obtained via the basilic veins (femoral vein access if this is not feasible). Bilateral venography is performed to document the extent of clot and extension to the brachiocephalic veins. CDT should be performed in acute clot and for chronic clot where guidewire passage is not feasible. The methods are identical to those described for axillary-subclavian vein thrombosis. Thrombolytic therapy is contraindicated in those with metastatic disease (especially to the brain and spinal cord).

Endovascular Approaches to Superior Vena Cava Syndrome

Endovascular approaches should be generally considered in all patients. Patients with advanced malignancy may derive considerable benefit with such treatment. An earlier limitation of SVC angioplasty was restenosis caused by elastic recoil of the vein and venous compression from the mass or fibrosis that remains after the angioplasty. Several studies have now reported excellent short- and intermediate-term outcomes after angioplasty followed by venous stenting. Both self-expanding (Wall Stent, Schneider, SMART, J&J Inteventional Systems and Gianturco Z-stent, Cook) and

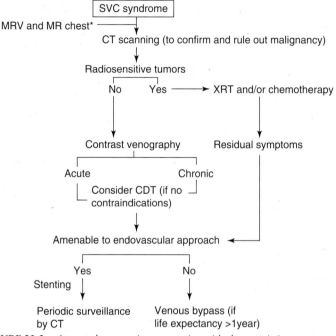

FIGURE 23-2. Approach to a patient presenting with characteristic symptoms and signs of SVC syndrome.

non–self-expanding stents (Genesis, J&J Inteventional Systems) have been used. A choice of a particular stent is dependent on patient factors (self-expanding stents in the subclavian-axillary veins), anatomic considerations, and physician preference. Primary patency rates for SVC stents range from 50 to 75% at 1 year, while secondary patency rates are between 25 and 85%. Adjunctive CDT is required in 25% of patients with a high rate of technical success (more than 95% of procedures) with no major complications and prompt resolution of symptoms in nearly all treated patients. A number of other series also support the value of stent placement with provisional thrombolytic therapy as a primary treatment modality in malignant SVC syndrome. Endovascular treatment with stent placement is effective both in SVC syndrome with benign causes and in cases secondary to malignancy where it results in rapid resolution of symptoms. Super-imposed thrombosis occurs commonly with SVC syndrome with intrinsic central venous causes such as central venous catheters, stenotic lesions, and transvenous pacemakers. Cross-sectional imaging modalities have an important place in preinterventional planning to evaluate for the presence of central venous thrombus and to rule out extrinsic compression. In the case of superimposed thrombosis, pharmacothrombolytic therapy and/or percutaneous mechanical thrombectomy are initially performed and are usually followed by balloon angioplasty and stent placement of the underlying occlusive pathology. Endovascular treatment is also highly relevant to SVC syndrome with benign causes, given the efficacy and safety of this approach, the lack of effective medical therapeutic alternatives, and the high morbidity rate of surgical alternatives.

Surgical Approaches

Surgical treatment of SVC syndrome should be attempted in individuals with a life expectancy of more than 1 year and is usually a consideration in individuals with extensive thrombosis. A left internal jugular vein–right atrial spiral vein graft or a PTFE graft from the left innominate vein to the right atrium may be performed.

CONCLUSIONS

UEDVT is a common problem because of increased use of central venous catheters for chemotherapy, bone marrow transplantation, dialysis, and parenteral nutrition. The underlying concern is that of pulmonary embolism, but fatal pulmonary embolism is quite rare in UEDVT. If UEDVT is suspected based on history and physical examination, it should be confirmed or excluded with imaging studies. Duplex ultrasonography is the best initial evaluation, because it is noninvasive and has a high sensitivity and specificity. Anticoagulation, with agents such as warfarin, remains a key therapy for patients with UEDVT. Endovascular therapy has replaced surgery as the primary modality of therapy in patients with UEDVT. Surgical thrombectomy is usually only considered when other options fail. Low-dose warfarin may be effective prophylaxis in patients with central venous catheters.

PRACTICAL POINTS

- UEDVT has been reported in up to 25% of patients with central venous catheters.

- The prevalence of coagulation disorders in patients with UEDVT is uncertain, and routine testing has never been shown to be cost-effective.

- Testing for a hypercoagulable state may be most worthwhile in patients with idiopathic UEDVT, a family history of DVT, a history of recurrent miscarriage, or a prior personal history of DVT.

- Patients presenting with acute or subacute vascular symptoms with venographically documented axillary-subclavian-brachiocephalic vein thrombosis should undergo early CDT with or without adjunctive percutaneous mechanical thrombectomy.

- Endovascular options including angioplasty and stenting are the primary modalities of therapy in patients with UEDVT and SVC syndrome.

- Endovascular techniques are also helpful adjuncts to prolong the patency of grafts implanted for SVC occlusion.

RECOMMENDED READING

AbuRahma AF, Sadler DL, Robinson PA. Axillary subclavian vein thrombosis. Changing patterns of etiology, diagnostic, and therapeutic modalities. *Am Surg* 1991;57(2):101–107.

Becker DM, Philbrick JT, Walker FB. Axillary and subclavian venous thrombosis. Prognosis and treatment. *Arch Intern Med* 1991;151(10):1934–1943.

Brandjes DP, Buller HR, Heijboer H, et al. Randomized trial of effect of compression stockings in patients with symptomatic proximal-vein thrombosis. *Lancet* 1997;349(9054):759–762.

Chan AW, Bhatt DL, Wilkoff BL, et al. Percutaneous treatment for pacemaker-associated superior vena cava syndrome. *Pacing Clin Electrophysiol* 2002;25(11):1628–1633.

Chang R, Horne MK III, Mayo DJ, et al. Pulse-spray treatment of subclavian and jugular venous thrombi with recombinant tissue plasminogen activator. *J Vasc Intervent Radiol* 1996;7(6):845–851.

Francis CW, Suchkova VN. Ultrasound and thrombolysis. *Vasc Med* 2001;6(3):181–187.

Fraschini G, Jadeja J, Lawson M, et al. Local infusion of urokinase for the lysis of thrombosis associated with permanent central venous catheters in cancer patients. *J Clin Oncol* 1987;5(4):672–678.

Girolami A, Prandoni P, Zanon E, et al. Venous thromboses of upper limbs are more frequently associated with occult cancer as compared with those of lower limbs. *Blood Coagul Fibrinolysis* 1999;10(8):455–457.

Haire WD, Lynch TG, Lund GB, et al. Limitations of magnetic resonance imaging and ultrasound-directed (duplex) scanning in the diagnosis of subclavian vein thrombosis. *J Vasc Surg* 1991;13(3):391–397.

Hartnell GG, Hughes LA, Finn JP, et al. Magnetic resonance angiography of the central chest veins. A new gold standard? *Chest* 1995;107(4):1053–1057.

Hicken GJ, Ameli FM. Management of subclavian-axillary vein thrombosis: a review. *Can J Surg* 1998;41(1):13–25.

Horattas MC, Wright DJ, Fenton AH, et al. Changing concepts of deep venous thrombosis of the upper extremity—report of a series and review of the literature. *Surgery* 1988;104(3):561–567.

Joffe HV, Goldhaber SZ. Upper-extremity deep vein thrombosis. *Circulation* 2002;106(14):1874–1880.

Kasirajan K, Gray B, Ouriel K. Percutaneous AngioJet thrombectomy in the management of extensive deep venous thrombosis. *J Vasc Intervent Radiol* 2001;12(2):179–185.

Lindblad B, Tengborn L, Bergqvist D. Deep vein thrombosis of the axillary-subclavian veins: epidemiologic data, effects of different types of treatment and late sequelae. *Eur J Vasc Surg* 1988;2(3):161–165.

Machleder HI. Evaluation of a new treatment strategy for Paget-Schroetter syndrome: spontaneous thrombosis of the axillary-subclavian vein. *J Vasc Surg* 1993;17(2):305–315.

Mukherjee D, Wilkoff BL, Yadav JS. Angioplasty and stenting of a patient with superior vena cava syndrome. In: White C, ed. *Fifty cases in peripheral intervention.* London, UK: Martin Dunitz, 2002:61–65.

Parziale JR, Akelman E, Weiss AP, et al. Thoracic outlet syndrome. *Am J Orthop* 2000;29(5):353–360.

Prandoni P, Bernardi E. Upper extremity deep vein thrombosis. *Curr Opin Pulm Med* 1999;5(4):222–226.

Prandoni P, Polistena P, Bernardi E, et al. Upper-extremity deep vein thrombosis. Risk factors, diagnosis, and complications. *Arch Intern Med* 1997;157(1):57–62.

Urschel HC Jr, Razzuk MA. Paget-Schroetter syndrome: what is the best management? *Ann Thorac Surg* 2000;69(6):1663–1668.

Zell L, Kindermann W, Marschall F, et al. Paget-Schroetter syndrome in sports activities—case study and literature review. *Angiology* 2001;52(5):337–342.

CHAPTER 24 ■ Vasculogenic Erectile Dysfunction

Gregory Lowe and Robert Bahnson

Erectile dysfunction (ED) is defined as the persistent inability to achieve and maintain penile erection sufficient for sexual intercourse. The incidence of ED increases with age. Approximately 1 to 10% of men aged 40 to 59 years have ED compared to 20 to 30% of men greater than 60 years of age. This prevalence has been confirmed in multiple international studies. ED is now well recognized as an early marker for systemic vascular and coronary disease and indeed shares many of the same risk factors (Table 24.1). As research emerges correlating ED with the future risk of coronary artery disease and systemic vascular disease, these patients represent a group for preventative care. With the introduction of oral treatment for ED, public awareness and the number of men seeking treatment have risen. The initiation of medical therapy for ED is increasingly being administered in the primary care physician's office, with those patients failing oral therapy obtaining specialist referral.

CLINICAL FEATURES

Physiology and Pathophysiology of an Erection

Vascular Supply and Innervation of the Penis

An understanding of the anatomy and physiology of normal penile erection is crucial to appropriate identification of likely etiologies and planning treatment strategies. Attainment of an erection results from multiple influences converging on the penile smooth muscle. An erection requires adequate blood flow to the paired corpora cavernosae surrounding the penile urethra and the corpus spongiosum at the glans penis (Fig. 24.1).

The central nervous system plays an important role in erectile function. The hypothalamus (medial preoptic area) is the integration point for the central control of erection. This area receives rich sensory impulses from a multitude of brain areas. Auditory stimuli, visual stimuli, and fantasy-initiated impulses project to this area and then travel down the spinal cord to peripheral nerves that innervate the penile vasculature initiating an erection. The penis is innervated by the sympathetic (T11-L2), parasympathetic (S2–S4), and somatic (S2–S4) nervous systems. Sympathetic input is antierectile, whereas parasympathetic and somatic inputs are proerectile. Both sympathetic and parasympathetic fibers reach the inferior hypogastric plexus in the pelvis, where the autonomic input to the penis is integrated and penile innervation via the cavernous nerves originates. The lesser cavernous nerves travel along the penis to supply the penile urethra and erectile tissue of the corpus spongiosum, while the greater cavernous nerves innervate the helicine arteries in the erectile

TABLE 24.1

RISK FACTORS ASSOCIATED WITH ED

Hypertension
Hyperlipidemia
Coronary artery or peripheral arterial disease
Diabetes
Metabolic syndrome
Hypogonadism
Endocrine disorders
Smoking
Depression
Alcohol and drug abuse
Peyronie's disease
Trauma or surgery to the pelvis or spine
Vascular surgery

tissue. The somatic component, the pudendal nerve, through the dorsal nerve branches is responsible for penile sensation and the contraction and relaxation of the extracorporeal striated muscles (bulbocavernous and ischiocavernous).

Erection Phase

In response to sexual stimulation, parasympathetic neural activity predominates, resulting in increased blood flow into the cavernous sinuses and achievement of erection due to smooth muscle relaxation. The main neurotransmitter mediating smooth muscle relaxation is nitric oxide, which is released from the endothelium of the corpus cavernosa during nonadrenergic, noncholinergic neurotransmission. Nitric oxide, in turn, activates soluble guanylyl cyclase, which increases intracellular concentrations of cyclic guanosine monophosphate (cGMP). cGMP, in turn, results in the activation of cGMP-dependent protein kinase, which, in turn, phosphorylates specific proteins and ion channels. The consequence is a decrease in intracellular calcium concentration and relaxation of the smooth muscle. The rapid filling of the penile sinusoids results in expansion of the sinuses with resultant compression of the subtunical venular plexuses, resulting in near total occlusion of venous outflow. This results in trapping of blood within the corpus cavernosum raising the penis from a dependent position to an erect position. Resultant intracavernosal pressures may exceed 90 mm Hg during the full phase of penile erection. During the course of sexual intercourse or masturbation, the bulbocavernous reflex results in forcible compression of the base of the blood-filled corpora cavernosa, resulting in the penis becoming harder with intracavernous pressures exceeding several 100 mm Hg. During this maintenance phase of penile erection, both blood entering and blood leaving the penis temporarily seize.

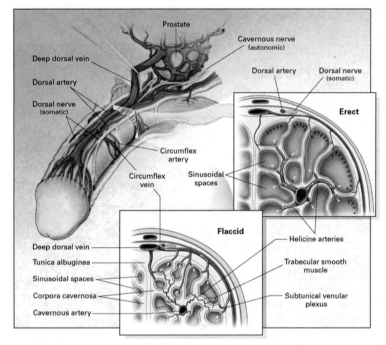

FIGURE 24-1. Anatomy and mechanism of penile erection. The mechanisms of erection and flaccidity are shown in the upper and lower inserts, respectively. During erection, relaxation of the trabecular smooth muscle and dilatation of the arterioles result in an increase in blood flow, which expands the sinusoidal spaces to lengthen and enlarge the penis. The expansion of the sinusoids compresses the subtunical venular plexus against the tunica albuginea and simultaneously compresses the emissary veins, reducing the outflow of blood to a minimum. (From Lue TF. Erectile dysfunction. *N Engl J Med* 2000;342:1802–1813, with permission.)

Detumescence Phase

This results from the sudden suppression of neurotransmitter release, breakdown of second messenger products, or discharge of sympathetic stimuli during ejaculation. Constriction of the trabecular smooth muscles reopens the venous channels resulting in expulsion of the trapped blood and return of a flaccid state. ED may result in abnormalities in one or several of these steps involved in the initiation or maintenance of an erection.

Future Cardiovascular Risk in Patients with Erectile Dysfunction and Cardiovascular Risk of Sexual Activity

The Second Princeton Consensus Panel is a practice guideline for the management of ED in patients with significant cardiac risk, which stratifies patients according to the presence or severity of conventional cardiovascular risk factors [low risk (<10%), intermediate (10 to 20%), and high risk

(>20%)]. A careful assessment of subclinical and/or asymptomatic cardiovascular disease should be considered, especially in patients with ED and an estimated cardiovascular risk greater than 10%.

Several studies have looked at the risk of cardiovascular events with sexual activity. After correcting for chance, only 0.9% of cases presenting with acute MI are currently felt to relate to antecedent sexual activity. This risk is exceedingly low in patients able to exert at least six metabolic equivalents of oxygen consumption (METS). Man-on-top intercourse leads to the highest heart rate with a mean peak heart rate of 127 beats/min. Overall vigorous sexual activity is estimated to equate to about 5 to 6 METS, with a mean 3.3 METS at orgasm for men-on-top intercourse. Masturbation and woman-on-top position are associated with lower metabolic demand.

Differential Diagnosis

The differential diagnosis of ED includes a variety of etiologies (Table 24.2). Aside from organic psychiatric causes of ED, a number of well-recognized stressors can trigger performance anxiety including anger, alienation, and depression. Mental illness and drugs used to treat them can commonly cause ED. Commonly prevalent risk factors that are implicated in atherosclerosis such as smoking, high cholesterol, and diabetes mellitus can all cause ED. Systemic disorders such as diabetes, chronic renal failure, and even aging can commonly contribute to ED via a combination of factors including neuronal and vascular dysfunctions.

Organic Causes of Erectile Dysfunction

Neurologic. Damage to the CNS from cerebrovascular accidents and degenerative processes such as Alzheimer's or Parkinson's disease may all result in ED. Similarly, damage to the peripheral nervous system as may ensue from spinal cord injury, diabetic neuropathy, and vascular or prostate surgery are common causes of ED.

Endocrine. Testosterone deficiency causes both decreased libido and an inability to maintain an erection secondary to low levels of nitric oxide synthase. In addition, hyperprolactinemia, hyperthyroidism, and hypothyroidism can all cause ED. In these settings, normalizing hormonal levels often results in return of normal male sexual function.

Vasculogenic. Anatomic defects in the arterial and venous systems may cause ED. Arterial stenosis and vasodilator dysfunction secondary to atherosclerosis can prevent adequate blood flow to the penis for an erection and are the most common causes of ED. Arterial stenosis involving the aortoiliac blood vessels resulting in claudication in one or both legs, diminution in femoral pulses, and ED is referred to as *Leriche's syndrome*. Venous dysfunction causing failure of veins to close during an erection may prevent the maintenance of an erection. Causes of abnormal venous drainage include Peyronie's disease, aging, and diabetes mellitus.

TABLE 24.2

RISK FACTORS ASSOCIATED WITH ED DIFFERENTIAL DIAGNOSIS OF ED

	Common Disorders	Pathophysiology
Psychogenic		
	Depression	Decreased libido
	Anxiety disorder	Treatment side effects
	Schizophrenia	
	Relationship conflict	
	Stress	
Organic		
Neurologic	Cerebrovascular accident	Failure to initiate or transmit
	Alzheimer's or Parkinson's disease	nerve impulses
	Spinal cord injury	
	Diabetic neuropathy	
	Radical pelvic surgery	
Hormonal	Hypogonadism	Decreased libido
	Thyroid disease	Endothelial dysfunction
	Hyperprolactinemia	
Vascular	Atherosclerosis	Endothelial dysfunction
	Peyronie's disease	Decreased arterial blood flow
	Trauma	Impaired veno-occlusion
Drug induced	Antidepressants	Central suppression
	Antihypertensives	Decreased libido
	Diuretics	
	Alcohol and cigarette abuse	
Multifactorial		
Systemic disease	Diabetes mellitus	Vascular dysfunction
	Chronic renal failure	Neural dysfunction
	Coronary artery disease	
Mixed psychogenic and organic	Mixture of above	Multifactorial

(Adapted from Lue TF. Erectile dysfunction. *N Engl J Med* 2000;342:1802–1813.)

Medications. Table 24.3 lists common medications that should be considered during the evaluation of ED.

Erectile Dysfunction and Vascular Risk Factors

ED and lower-extremity arterial disease share many of the same risk factors. These include diabetes mellitus, metabolic syndrome, smoking, hypertension, dyslipidemia, obesity, and age, all of which are well-known

TABLE 24.3

DRUGS IMPLICATED IN ED

Category	Class

Antihypertensives/heart failure/antiarrhythmics	*β Blockers*
	    Selective and nonselective (atenolol, metoprolol, propranolol, labetalol, carvedilol)
	Diuretics
	    Thiazide agents
	    Loop diuretics (less than thiazides)
	Vasodilators
	    Hydralazine
	    Verapamil, nifedipine
	    Diazoxide
	    Minoxidil
	Antiarrhythmics
	    Disopyramide
	Aldosterone Receptor Antagonists
	    Spironolactone, eplerenone

Antidepressants	*Selective Serotonin Reuptake Inhibitors*
	    Citalopram, escitalopram, fluoxetine, fluvoxamine, paroxetine, sertraline
	Tricyclic Antidepressants
	    Amitriptyline, imipramine, nortriptyline
	Monoamine Oxidase Inhibitors
	    Phenelzine, isocarboxazid, tranylcypromine
	Selective Serotonin and Norepinephrine Reuptake Inhibitors
	    Venlafaxine, desvenlafaxine, duloxetine
	    Lithium

Antipsychotics	Phenothiazines (chlorpromazine, thioridazine, fluphenazine)
Antiepileptics	Diphenylhydantoin, carbamazepine, valproic acid
Lipid lowering	Gemfibrozil
Ulcer healing	H_2 antagonists
Antigout	Allopurinol Indomethacin
Antiparkinson agents	l-Dopa, biperiden Benztropine, trihexyphenidyl, procyclidine Bromocriptine, levodopa (Sinemet)
Miscellaneous	Antihistamines (phenothiazines), cyclobenzaprine
Hormonal agents	Estrogens, androgens, cyproterone acetate; luteinizing hormone–releasing hormone analogues

risk factors for vascular disease. Patients with ED have abnormalities in a number of atherosclerosis risk surrogates including higher high-sensitivity C-reactive protein level, lower brachial artery flow-mediated dilation, and coronary calcium score. These associations typically persist even after adjustment for Framingham risk score, diabetes, or body mass index. ED has been associated with coronary artery disease, cerebrovascular disease, and lower-extremity arterial disease. Many studies have been published in the last decade related to the association of coronary artery disease and ED. ED predicts cardiovascular risk even after adjustment for other conventional risk factors. The Olmsted County Study of Urinary Symptoms and Health Status among Men cohort was utilized to assess the future risk of coronary disease in patients with and without ED (Inman et al., 2009). The prevalence of ED amplified as age increased, with approximately 5% of the population developing new ED every 2 years. Overall, 11% of patients developed coronary events over the 10-year period. After multivariate analysis, ED was associated with an 80% higher risk of subsequent coronary events. This finding was particularly prominent in younger men diagnosed with ED. In men aged 40 to 49 years, there was a 50-fold increase in the 10-year incidence of coronary artery disease. As patients aged, this increased risk was attenuated. Currently, patients diagnosed with ED should be stratified based on risk factors to determine the need for noninvasive coronary or vascular workup.

DIAGNOSTIC EVALUATION

Figure 24.2 summarizes a clinical approach to the evaluation of ED.

History

Evaluation of a patient with ED often begins with simply inquiring about the presence of ED. Patients vary in their willingness to bring ED to the clinician's attention and, therefore, may need direct questioning for initial diagnosis. The inquiry should include a clarification of what the patient interprets ED to mean and whether there is difficulty attaining, maintaining, or in both aspects of an erection. Patients may also report ejaculatory problems or diminished libido as ED. It is important to clarify these aspects to prevent unnecessary testing. An important step in evaluation includes common questioning regarding the onset and duration, maximal rigidity, penetration (vaginal) ability, morning or nocturnal erections, sexual arousal/libido, erections with masturbation, penile curvature, relationship problems, anxiety, or stress. If possible, a psychologic component should be separated from organic etiologies. Thorough medical, surgical, and social histories are necessary, including trauma, exercise habits, smoking, and medication usage. Often, performance anxiety becomes problematic for patients who have suffered difficulty with erectile function on prior intercourse attempts. The Sexual Health Inventory for Men (SHIM) and International Index of Erectile Function (IIEF-15) are validated patient questionnaires excellent for evaluating ED symptoms. The SHIM consists

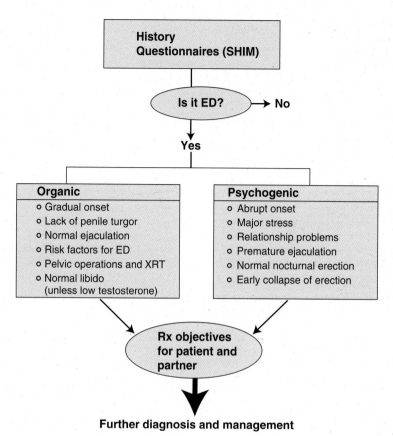

FIGURE 24-2. Initial approach to ED and differentiating psychogenic form organic ED.

of five questions, each rated on a five-point scale (Fig. 24.3). There are four questions dealing with the quality of erection and a final question focused on erectile satisfaction. The score reflects severity of ED, with scores lower than 21 indicating the presence of ED. The IIEF-15 questionnaire is more commonly associated with specific ED evaluation or research and consists of 15 questions, each rated on a five-point scale.

Physical Examination

The physical exam should focus on external genitalia, testes size, secondary sexual characteristics, palpable penile plaques, and peripheral pulses. Peripheral neuropathy, central obesity, and other signs of systemic disease should be observed. Less commonly, galactorrhea or gynecomastia may be encountered, or visual field defects may all indicate a pituitary etiology.

Over the past 6 months:					
1. How do you rate your confidence that you could get and keep an erection	Very low	Low	Moderate	High	Very high
	[1]	[2]	[3]	[4]	[5]
2. When you had erections with sexual stimulation, how often were your erections hard enough for penetration?	Almost never/never	A few times (much less than half the time)	Sometimes (about half the time)	Most times (much more than half the time)	Almost always/always
	[1]	[2]	[3]	[4]	[5]
3. During sexual intercourse, how often were you able to maintain your erection after you had penetrated (entered) your partner?	Almost never/never	A few times (much less than half the time)	Sometimes (about half the time)	Most times (much more than half the time)	Almost always/always
	[1]	[2]	[3]	[4]	[5]
4. During sexual intercourse, how difficult was it to maintain your erection to completion of intercourse?	Extremely difficult	Very difficult	Difficult	Slightly difficult	Not difficult
	[1]	[2]	[3]	[4]	[5]
5. When you attempted sexual intercourse, how often was it satisfactory for you?	Almost never/never	A few times (much less than half the time)	Sometimes (about half the time)	Most times (much more than half the time)	Almost always/always
	[1]	[2]	[3]	[4]	[5]

FIGURE 24-3. The Sexual Health Inventory for Men or SHIM index. (Adapted from Rosen RC, Cappelleri JC, Smith MD, et al. Development and evaluation of an abridged 5-item version of the International Index of Erectile Function (IIEF-5) as a diagnostic tool for erectile dysfunction. *Int J Impot Res* 1999;11:319–326.)

Laboratory Testing

This is used to screen for systemic illness. Recommended testing includes measurement of serum glucose, complete blood count, cholesterol, triglycerides, testosterone (total and free levels), and prostate-specific antigen. Some authors recommend screening serum thyroid, hepatic, prolactin, cortisol, or luteinizing hormone levels based on physical exam findings. Free testosterone levels should be obtained in preference to total testosterone levels and preferably in the morning hours to prevent misinterpretation.

Specialized Testing

Patients may often be referred for specialized testing based on the findings of the above studies. A more thorough review of specialized tests is presented in the "Recommended Reading" section of this chapter; however, a brief introduction will follow. Multiple measures of nocturnal penile tumescence and rigidity testing exist and are useful to evaluate for psychogenic components of ED. Most men experience at least three to six nocturnal erections a night, with fewer erections occurring as men age. Nocturnal erections do not correlate well with sexual performance and therefore are often not sufficient as a solitary diagnostic test. In-office injection of a vasodilator compound into the corporal bodies provides a more thorough evaluation and may be combined with duplex ultrasound for the evaluation of both arterial and venous flows. A simple vasodilator injection with sexual stimulation may provide sufficient information to rule out a venous occlusion disorder but does not indicate sufficient arterial inflow. When penile injection is combined with duplex ultrasonography, a more detailed assessment of penile arterial input is obtained. Peak penile systolic velocity should be greater than 35 cm/s, but this varies with age. Levels below this value indicate an arterial component to ED. The dosage of intracavernosal injection is not standardized, and patient sympathetic discharge from anxiety may limit the true estimate of arterial vascular status. An added benefit of intracavernosal injection is that patients are able to experience a potential treatment option. A penile-brachial index can be obtained and calculated to assess for adequacy of arterial flow, with values below 0.7 indicating arteriogenic ED. Pudendal and inferior epigastric arteriography is still the gold standard for demonstrating arterial stenosis/ occlusion and planning possible revascularization. Such a workup is typically only indicated in young men with suspected vascular disease usually resulting from pelvic trauma.

TREATMENT

Figure 24.4 summarizes the current treatment approach to ED.

Initial Approach

Management of the patient with ED should begin with the treatment of potentially reversible causes and reevaluation. Counseling may be beneficial for psychogenic components and, although time-consuming, may significantly improve subsequent treatments if not reversing the ED completely. A central spinal cord or brain disorder should be referred for neurologic evaluation. Following the treatment of reversible causes, it is not uncommon to find patients still experience some degree of ED. Prior to medical therapy, the clinician should not overlook common lifestyle modification that can improve the overall health of the patient. This provides an excellent opportunity to promote weight loss, smoking cessation, and increasing physical activity. Increased physical activity and weight loss have been shown to independently improve erectile function. Medication changes may not be feasible; however, when possible, it is best to consult the prescribing physician for such changes. Patients should be encouraged to use alcohol in moderation or stop excessive use as this has been shown to cause ED. Hypogonadism may promote ED, and androgen replacement should be reserved only for symptomatic patients. Low testosterone alone often does not cause ED but is associated with fatigue and loss of libido. Testosterone appears to play a facilitative role in normal erections. Prior to initiating testosterone

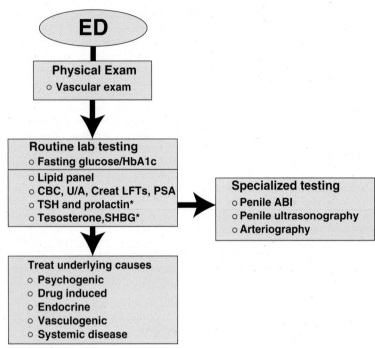

FIGURE 24-4.   Recommended diagnostic approach in ED. *Asterisk* indicates testing that may be considered if there is sufficient clinical evidence. (SHBG, sex hormone–binding globulin)

replacement, existing cardiovascular risk, a digital rectal exam, serum prostate-specific antigen, hematocrit, liver panel, and lipid profile should be obtained. Recent studies have demonstrated that supplementation with testosterone is associated with a small but significant risk for cardiovascular events, and this should be taken into consideration. Patients on testosterone should be monitored at least yearly with emphasis to evaluate for hepatic disease or polycythemia.

Oral Phosphodiesterase Inhibitors

After treating reversible causes and correction of modifiable risk factors including treatment of lipids and potentially diabetes, first-line therapy involves treatment with phosphodiesterase type 5 inhibitors (PDE5-i). These medications selectively target the phosphodiesterase degradation of cGMP. By limiting the loss of cGMP, the nitric oxide response is maintained, enhancing vasodilation and subsequent erection. These medications will not lead to direct erection without the sexual stimulation and nitric

TABLE 24.4

PHARMACOLOGY OF PHOSPHODIESTERASE TYPE 5 INHIBITORS

PDE5 Inhibitor	Dosages	Half-Life	Common Adverse Events	Notes
Sildenafil	25, 50, 100 mg Usual starting 50 mg	$T_{1/2} = 4$ h Peak plasma levels in 1 h	Headache, abnormal color vision, flushing	Efficacious, safe, longest clinical experience
Vardenafil	2.5, 5, 10, 20 mg Usual starting 5 mg	$T_{1/2} = 4$–5 h Peak plasma levels in 0.7 h	Headache, flushing, rhinitis	Similar efficacy and safety to sildenafil, highest potency
Tadalafil	5, 10, 20 mg Usual starting 10 mg	$T_{1/2} = 17.5$ h Peak plasma levels in 2 h	Headache, dyspepsia, myalgia	Longest half-life may improve spontaneity, less visual side effects, increased incidence of back pain and myalgias

oxide influence. Medications in this class include sildenafil, vardenafil, and tadalafil (Table 24.4). These medications act in a similar fashion and are all contraindicated currently in patients taking nitrates or nitric oxide donors. Sildenafil (Viagra, Pfizer) is the most extensively studied PDE5-i. The time to onset of action is between 15 and 60 minutes with a half-life of 3 to 5 hours. Vardenafil (Levitra, Bayer and GlaxoSmithKline, Inc.) has a time to onset similar to sildenafil. The half-life is 4 to 5 hours. Tadalafil (Cialis, Lilly) has a longer time to peak concentration at 2 hours and a longer half-life of 17.5 hours. Onset of action is reported to occur as early as 30 minutes but likely requires closer to 60 to 120 minutes for most patients. Sildenafil and vardenafil are affected by fatty meal as it reduces absorption. This does not appear to be an issue with tadalafil. Side effects associated with PDE5-i include flushing, headache, dyspepsia, myalgias, nasal congestion, or potentiation of blood pressure lowering with nitrates and α-antagonist therapy. Sildenafil may cause abnormal vision with a blue hue secondary to slight inhibition of nonpenile phosphodiesterases. A very rare nonarteritic anterior ischemic optic neuropathy has been reported to occur, causing sudden vision loss as well.

PDE5-i has a well-established record of effectiveness and can be used as on-demand therapy or nightly low-dose therapy. Cost may be an issue for some patients with this treatment plan, as pills are expensive if paid out of pocket. Patients who fail initial trials with PDE5-i should be encouraged to attempt up to eight doses, with clinical response rates increasing through the eighth trial. Ensuring patients are using the medication appropriately with adequate time prior to sexual arousal is also important.

Intraurethral Delivery and Intracavernous Injections

Intraurethral prostaglandins [alprostadil or prostaglandin E1 (PGE1) Medicated Urethral System for Erection (MUSE); Astra] help with vasodilation of the penile vasculature locally. In response to intraurethral delivery of PGE1, 60 to 70% of patients experience an erection sufficient to engage in sexual intercourse. The effect usually occurs in 5 to 20 minutes. The main adverse reaction associated with intraurethral PGE1 application includes penile pain in up to 36% of patients, which limits patient compliance. Other adverse reactions include urethral bleeding, hypotension, headache, or dizziness. It is recommended that the first dose be administered in the physician office to assess for hypotension. Intraurethral alprostadil should not be used in patients at risk for priapism or with a distal urethral stricture.

Intracavernous injection of alprostadil (PGE1, Caverject, Pharmacia-Upjohn) is frequently effective in men who fail to respond to a PDE5-i. In comparison with intraurethral PGE1, a randomized, multicenter study demonstrated that intracavernous injection is more efficacious, better tolerated, and preferred over transurethral application. Trimixture (Trimix) consists of a mixture of papaverine, phentolamine, and PGE1. Phentolamine does not induce an erection but does assist to inhibit detumescence. Papaverine acts as a nonspecific inhibitor of phosphodiesterases and has been associated with priapism. As previously mentioned, PGE1 is often associated with penile pain. Therefore, the combination therapy is popular owing to its high efficacy and limited side effects via utilization of lower dosages of each medication. Most clinicians treating ED reserve this mixture for patients who fail therapy with PDE5-i, intraurethral alprostadil, and the papaverine/phentolamine combination (Bimix) or who experience severe penile pain with PGE1 injections. Potential adverse reactions with intracavernous injections include penile hematoma, penile edema, and fibrotic changes within the tunica albuginea in the form of plaques and nodules. Priapism is an adverse reaction patients should be warned about, consisting of an erection lasting greater than 4 hours. Often, these prolonged erections are painful and may be associated with fibrosis of the corpora cavernosum, leading to further ED.

Miscellaneous Treatments

Vacuum erection devices work through creation of a negative pressure in a cylindrical pump placed over the penis. The negative pressure draws blood into the penis, allowing placement of an occlusive ring at the penile base to maintain an erection. This therapy has shown very high efficacy; however, many patients find the process cumbersome. Potential side effects include penile hematoma, penile pivoting at the ring due to lack of corporal rigidity proximal to this point, sensation of a cold penis, and lack of ejaculation. This therapy is contraindicated in patients on anticoagulation or with a bleeding disorder.

Surgical Therapies

For the majority of patients, the primary surgical option consists of implantation of a penile prosthesis. These prosthetic devices can be either malleable

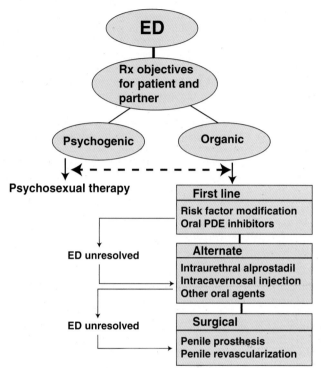

FIGURE 24-5. Treatment approaches in ED.

(noninflatable) or inflatable. Patient and partner satisfaction rates typically are greater than 60 to 80%. At 2 years, a surgical revision rate of 2.5% exists, with removal rates of 4.4%. This procedure is not limited by arterial inflow or preventing venous outflow. Complications include infection, hematoma, mechanical failure, or erosion.

Penile vascular surgery deserves special mention. Many surgical techniques exist, and much of the literature is impressive at first evaluation. Frequently, these studies are limited by a small patient population and short follow-up. Vascular surgery does have the potential benefit of being curative in cases of vasculogenic ED. Prior to consideration for penile revascularization, specialized testing with duplex penile ultrasonography and pharmacologic arteriography are necessary. Most revascularization surgeries utilize the inferior epigastric artery to supplement inflow to the cavernosal or dorsal penile arteries. Long-term follow-up of these patients frequently reports success rates between 25 and 80% in those studies that have examined success rate. The particular patient populations and surgical indications are not uniform between studies. Complications of these procedures include hyperemia of the glans (7 to 13%), hematomas, thrombosis of vascular anastomosis, or infection.

Hyperemia of the glans may lead to tissue desquamation and sloughing. The best outcomes have been obtained in patients younger than 30 years, having less than two vascular/coronary risk factors, and with no history of smoking, diabetes mellitus, hypertension, or dyslipidemia. A recent meta-analysis reviewed the evidence for penile revascularization. There were few randomized controlled or prospective studies included, preoperative workup was not standardized between studies, the definition of surgical success varied, and studies mostly included patients less than 50 years. The most common cause of failure was inappropriate patient selection and misdiagnosis, with other risk factors being smoking, diabetes mellitus, hypertension, dyslipidemia, prior radiation therapy, coronary artery disease, obesity, and distal-extremity arteriogenic disease. Currently, penile revascularization is reserved for a few select men who appear to have only a vasculogenic etiology of ED.

CONCLUSIONS

Figure 24.5 summarizes the source of ED and treatment course.

ED is a common diagnosis among men as they age. Diagnostic tests exist to better define the role of vascular disease in ED for each patient, but frequently, patients are given PDE5-i as first-line treatment prior to evaluation. The clinician should utilize this opportunity to impact lifestyle factors promoting better long-term patient health and potentially even improving erectile function. While this often works well and limits unnecessary testing for ED, more attention should be placed on the role of ED as a marker for future vascular or coronary disease. ED is treated with PDE5-i as first-line therapy, reserving more invasive treatments for those not responding to medical therapy. Rarely, a patient presenting with ED is a candidate for penile revascularization.

PRACTICAL POINTS

- The five-item IIEF (also known as the Sexual Health Inventory for Men, or SHIM) can be filled out in the office prior to examination and is a quick way to screen for ED.

- Nearly all patients should be evaluated with noninvasive cardiac testing when presenting with ED, especially when associated with cardiac risk factors.

- Sexual activity is generally associated with a similar MET equivalent of moderate exercise.

- Hypogonadism is generally an uncommon cause of ED in the vascular clinic. Other symptoms often associated with hypogonadism include low libido, fatigue, and low-force bone fractures. Testosterone replacement may improve response to treatment.

- A true vascular stenosis causing reduced blood flow should be suspected in a patient with claudication and absent femoral pulses (Leriche's syndrome).

- PDE5 inhibitors are an effective treatment for ED and should be considered first-line therapy. Nitrates are contraindicated with the use of PDE5 inhibitors.

■ Trimix consists of a mixture of papaverine, phentolamine, and PGE1. Many clinicians reserve this mixture for patients who have failed therapy with PDE5 inhibitors and intraurethral alprostadil or who experience severe penile pain with PGE1 injections.

■ Mechanical options for the treatment of ED include vacuum-assisted devices and penile prosthesis.

RECOMMENDED READING

Arruda-Olson A, Mahoney D, Nehra A, et al. Cardiovascular effects of sildenafil during exercise in men with known or probable coronary artery disease. *JAMA* 2002 Feb 13;287(6):719–25.

Babaei A, Safarinejad M, Kolahi A. Penile revascularization for erectile dysfunction. *Urol J* 2009 Winter;6(1):1–7. Review.

Bhasin S, Cunningham G, Hayes F, et al. Testosterone therapy in adult men with androgen deficiency syndromes: an endocrine society clinical practice guideline. *J Clin Endocrinol Metab* 2006 Jun;91(6):1995–2010.

Bocchi E, Guimaraes G, Mocelin A, et al. Sildenafil effects on exercise, neurohormonal activation, and erectile dysfunction in congestive heart failure: a double-blind, placebo-controlled, randomized study followed by a prospective treatment for erectile dysfunction. *Circulation* 2002 Aug 27;106(9):1097–103.

Chai S, Barrett-Connor E, Gamst A. Small-vessel lower extremity arterial disease and erectile dysfunction: the Rancho Bernardo study. *Atherosclerosis* 2009 Apr;203(2):620–5

Cheitlin M. Sexual activity and cardiovascular disease. *Am J Cardiol* 2003 Nov 6;92(9A): 3M–8M.

DeBusk R. Erectile dysfunction therapy in special populations and applications: coronary artery disease. *Am J Cardiol* 2005 Dec 26;96(12B):62M–66M.

Esposito K, Giugliano F, Di Palo C, et al. Effect of lifestyle changes on erectile dysfunction in obese men. *JAMA* 2004 Jun 23;291(24):2978–84.

Foresta C, Caretta N, Corona G. Clinical and metabolic evaluation of subjects with erectile dysfunction: a review with a proposal flowchart. *Int J Androl* 2009 Jun;32(3):198–211. Epub 2008 Dec 9.

Gazzaruso C, Pujia A, Solerte S, et al. Erectile dysfunction and angiographic extent of coronary artery disease in type II diabetic patients. *Int J Imp Res* 2006 May-Jun;18(3):311–5.

Herrmann H, Chang G, Klugherz B, et al. Hemodynamic effects of sildenafil in men with severe coronary artery disease. *N Engl J Med* 2000 Jun 1;342(22):1622–6.

Inman B, St. Sauver J, Jacobson D, et al. A population-based, longitudinal study of erectile dysfunction and future coronary artery disease. *Mayo Clin Proc* 2009 Feb;84(2):108–13.

Jackson G, Montorsi P, Cheitlin M. Cardiovascular safety of sildenafil citrate (Viagra®): an updated perspective. *Urology* 2006 Sep;68(3 Suppl):47–60.

Jackson G, Rosen R, Kloner R, et al. The Second Princeton Consensus on sexual dysfunction and cardiac risk: new guidelines for sexual medicine. *J Sex Med* 2006 Jan;3(1):28–36.

Kawanishi Y, Kimura K, Nakanishi R, et al. Retinal vascular findings and penile cavernosal artery blood flow. *BJU Int* 2003 Dec;92(9):977–80.

Lue T. Physiology of penile erection and pathophysiology of erectile dysfunction. In: W. et al, *Campbell-Walsh Urology*, Vol. 1. Philadelphia: Elsevier, 2007:718–749.

Manolis A, Doumas M. Sexual dysfunction: the 'prima ballerina' of hypertension-related quality-of-life complications. *J Hypertens* 2008 Nov;26(11):2074–84.

Montorsi F, Briganti A, Salonia A, et al. Erectile dysfunction prevalence, time of onset, and association with risk factors in 300 consecutive patients with acute chest pain and angiographically documented coronary artery disease. *Eur Urol* 2003 Sep;44(3):360–4; discussion 364–5.

Montorsi P, Ravagnani P, Galli S, et al. The artery size hypothesis: a macrovascular link between erectile dysfunction and coronary artery disease. *Am J Cardiol* 2005 Dec 26;96(12B): 19M–23M.

Montorsi P, Ravagnani P, Galli S, et al. Association between erectile dysfunction and coronary artery disease. Role of coronary clinical presentation and extent of coronary vessels involvment: the COBRA trial. *Eur Heart J* 2006;2632–2639.

Rao D, Donatucci C. Vasculogenic impotence; arterial and venous surgery. *Urol Clin North Am* 2001.

Thadani U, Smith W, Nash S, et al. The effect of vardenafil, a potent and highly selective phosphodiesterase-5 inhibitor for the treatment of erectile dysfunction, on the cardiovascular response to exercise in patients with coronary aretery disease. *J Am Coll cardiol* 2002; 2006–2012.

Thompson IM, Tangen CM, Goodman PJ, et al. Erectile dysfunction and subsequent cardiovascular disease. *JAMA* 2005;2996–3002.

Vicari E, Di Pino L, La Vignera S, et al. Peak systolic velocity in patients with arterial erectile dysfunction and peripheral arterial disease. *Int J Impot Res* 2006;175–179.

CHAPTER 25

■ Approach to and
Management of Inflammatory Vasculitis
Wael Jarjour

The primary vasculitides are idiopathic diseases that present with constitutional features, limb or organ ischemia, and/or tissue inflammation. While multiorgan dysfunction should heighten the suspicion for the presence of systemic vasculitis, single-organ involvement can be the result of an inflammatory vasculitis and multisystem diseases can result from nonvasculitic disorders. Clinicians faced with such clinical scenarios are plagued by multiple problems, including the following: first and foremost the need to identify the presence of a primary vasculitis; the overlap and the variability in expression patterns of the different vasculitic disorders; the controversy over the diagnostic criteria for specific vasculitis syndromes and the limitations of the present classification systems; the difficulty in obtaining tissue for the "gold standard" histopathologic diagnosis; and the lack of explicitly diagnostic serologic tests. Thus, the diagnosis is usually based on compatible clinical features along with consistent biopsies or angiography results that may not be diagnostic until other disorders have been diligently excluded (i.e., infections, malignancies).

CLASSIFICATION OF PRIMARY VASCULITIDES

The classification of the primary vasculitides in the clinical setting serves only as a framework for the diagnostic workup; response to treatment should never be used as a way to rule in/out the presence of a vasculitis. Several different classification schemes have been published. The major components have been the distinction between primary vasculitis and secondary vasculitis, the recognition of dominant blood vessel size (Fig. 25.1), and the presence or absence of antineutrophil cytoplasmic antibodies (ANCA). In 1990, the American College of Rheumatology (ACR) published criteria for the diagnosis of polyarteritis nodosa (PAN), Churg-Strauss syndrome (CSS), Wegener's granulomatosis (WG), hypersensitivity vasculitis (HV), Henoch-Schönlein purpura (HSP), giant cell arteritis (GCA), and Takayasu's arteritis (TA). In 1993, an international consensus conference was convened in Chapel Hill to develop definitions for the nomenclatures of different inflammatory vasculitides based on clinical and laboratory features (Table 25.1). This updated classification scheme clarified the definitions of the major vasculitides. Although quite useful in defining these syndromes, when used in clinical practice, these schemes may be overly restrictive since specificity rather than sensitivity is emphasized. Thus, many patients may not fit neatly into any of the "classically" defined syndromes, particularly early in the course of their illness. In this chapter, clinical features of each disorder will be discussed, followed by the

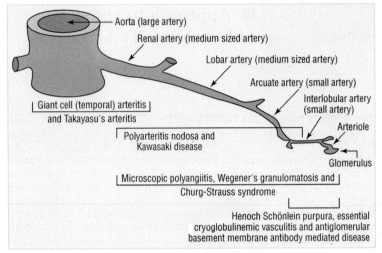

FIGURE 25-1.   Classification of systemic vasculitides. (Adapted from Jennette JC, Falk RJ, Andrassy K, et al. Nomenclature of systemic vasculitis. Proposal of an international consensus conference. *Arthritis Rheum* 1994;37:187–192.)

presentation of a general diagnostic strategy that may be employed when vasculitis is suspected and several heuristic clinical vignettes.

LARGE-VESSEL VASCULITIS

Takayasu's Arteritis

TA is a chronic granulomatous panarteritis affecting large elastic arteries such as the aorta and its main branches, the coronary arteries, and occasionally the pulmonary arteries. Inflammation results in stenosis, occlusion, or aneurysm formation and potentially secondary thrombosis. Early reports emphasized a "triphasic" disease process: a "prepulseless" phase characterized by nonspecific inflammatory symptoms, followed by painful arteries, and ending in "burned-out disease" with vessel occlusion and distal ischemia. Prospective evaluation of patients with TA, however, has revealed significant variability in disease course rather than these distinct stages of disease.

Epidemiology

The prevalence rates and distribution of involved vessels differ between ethnic groups. High prevalence rates are reported in Asian countries, such as Japan, Korea, China, and India. TA is less common among white populations. The estimated peak age of disease onset is in the third decade, and the disease is more common in women.

TABLE 25.1

NAMES AND DEFINITIONS OF VASCULITIDES ADOPTED BY THE CHAPEL HILL CONSENSUS CONFERENCE ON THE NOMENCLATURE OF SYSTEMIC VASCULITIS

Type of Vasculitis	Definition
Large-vessel vasculitis	
Giant cell arteritis	Granulomatous arteritis of the aorta and its major branches, with a predilection for the extracranial branches of the carotid artery. Often involves the temporal artery. Usually occurs in patients older than 50 y and is often associated with polymyalgia rheumatica.
Takayasu's arteritis	Granulomatous inflammation of the aorta and its major branches. Usually occurs in patients younger than 50 y. Constitutional features may not be present.
Medium-sized vessel vasculitis	
Polyarteritis nodosa	Necrotizing inflammation of medium-sized muscular arteries, with few or no immune deposits, without glomerulonephritis or vasculitis in arterioles, capillaries, or venules.
Kawasaki's disease	Arteritis involving large-, medium-, or small-sized arteries and associated with mucocutaneous lymph node syndrome. Coronary arteries are often involved, and large coronary aneurysms can be associated with early or delayed myocardial infarction. Usually occurs in children.
Small-vessel vasculitis	
Wegener's granulomatosis	Granulomatous inflammation, with few or no immune deposits, involving the respiratory tract and necrotizing vasculitis affecting small and medium vessels (capillaries, venules, arterioles, and arteries). Necrotizing glomerulonephritis is common.
Churg-Strauss syndrome	Eosinophilic rich and granulomatous inflammation involving the respiratory tract, necrotizing vasculitis affecting small- to medium-sized vessels, with few or no immune deposits and associated with asthma and eosinophilia.
Microscopic polyangiitis	Necrotizing vasculitis, with few or no immune deposits, affecting small vessels (i.e., capillaries, venules, arterioles). Necrotizing vasculitis affecting small- and medium-sized arteries may be present. Necrotizing glomerulonephritis is very common. Pulmonary capillaritis is common.
Henoch-Schönlein purpura	Vasculitis, with immunoglobulin A–dominant immune deposits, affecting small vessels (i.e., capillaries, venules, arterioles). Typically involves skin, gut, and glomeruli and is associated with arthralgia or arthritis.
Essential cryoglobulinemic vasculitis	Vasculitis, with cryoglobulin immune deposits, affecting small vessels (i.e., capillaries, venules, arterioles) and associated with cryoglobulins in serum. Skin and glomeruli are often involved.
Isolated cutaneous leukocytoclastic angiitis	Cutaneous leukocytoclastic angiitis without systemic vasculitis or glomerulonephritis.

(Adapted from Jennette JC, Falk RJ, Andrassy K, et al. Nomenclature of systemic vasculitis. Proposal of an international consensus conference. *Arthritis Rheum,* 1994;37:187–192.)

Clinical Features

Musculoskeletal and constitutional findings are present in 30 to 40% of patients. Since 20% of all TA patients are completely asymptomatic, the disease may be discovered with the finding of an asymptomatic bruit (widespread bruits are common in TA) or diminished pulses. Other patients may present with claudication of arms or legs, cerebrovascular accidents, myocardial infarction, renovascular hypertension, congestive heart failure secondary to myocardial infarction, or aortic insufficiency. Vascular ischemic symptoms with findings of stenosis or occlusion are the hallmarks of the disease. Table 25.2 lists the ACR criteria for the diagnosis of TA. Delay in diagnosis has been attributed to the nonspecific nature of the initial symptoms and the clinical presentation, which may be quite similar to that of patients suffering from atherosclerotic disease. TA should be suspected in any young patient with bruits, atypical distribution of ischemic symptoms (i.e., upper extremities), and age-inappropriate vascular disease (congestive heart failure, aortic aneurysm, myocardial infarction, or aortic insufficiency). Table 25.3 lists the angiographic classification of TA. This may be helpful in intervention planning if indicated but is of no prognostic significance. Aneurysms are relatively uncommon features of TA in the United States. This is different from the experience in the Far East, where both abdominal and thoracic aortic aneurysms frequently develop as long-term sequelae of TA.

TABLE 25.2

1990 ACR CRITERIA FOR THE CLASSIFICATION OF TAKAYASU'S ARTERITIS

Criterion	Findings
Age at disease onset 40 y	Development of symptoms or findings related to Takayasu's arteritis at the age of 40 y
Blood pressure difference >10 mm Hg	Difference of >10 mm Hg in systolic blood pressure between arms
Claudication of extremities	Development and worsening of fatigue and discomfort in muscles of one or more extremity while in use, especially the upper extremities
Decreased brachial artery pulse	Decreased pulsation of one or both brachial arteries
Bruit over subclavian arteries or aorta	Bruit audible on auscultation over one or both subclavian arteries or abdominal aorta
Arteriogram abnormality	Arteriographic narrowing or occlusion of the entire aorta, its primary branches, or large arteries in the proximal upper or lower extremities, not caused by arteriosclerosis, fibromuscular dysplasia, or similar causes; changes usually focal or segmental

Diagnosis of TA requires that at least three of the six criteria be met.
(Adapted from Arend WP, Michel BA, Bloch DA, et al. The American College of Rheumatology 1990 criteria for the classification of takayasu arteritis. *Arthritis Rheum* 1990;33:1129–1134.)

TABLE 25.3

ANGIOGRAPHIC CLASSIFICATION OF TAKAYASU'S ARTERITIS, TAKAYASU CONFERENCE 1994

Type I: Branches from the aortic arch

Type IIa: Ascending aorta, aortic arch, and its branches

Type IIb: Ascending aorta, aortic arch, and its branches, thoracic descending aorta

Type III: Thoracic descending aorta, abdominal aorta, and/or renal arteries

Type IV: Abdominal aorta and/or renal arteries

Type V: Combined features of types IIb and IV

(According to this classification system, involvement of the coronary or pulmonary arteries should be designated as C (+) or P (+), respectively.)

(Adapted from Moriwaki R, Makoto N, Yajima M, et al. Clinical Manifestations of Takayasu Arteritis in India and Japan–New Classificaion of Angiographic Findings. *Angiology* 1997;48:369–379.)

Diagnosis

Acute-phase reactants such as erythrocyte sedimentation rate (ESR) and C-reactive protein (CRP) may be elevated in more than 50% of patients with TA. All patients with suspected TA should have blood pressures in four extremities (by Doppler if necessary). Subclavian artery stenosis is very common, and blood pressure in the upper extremities may be unreliable. Renal artery stenosis may produce extreme hypertension, and in the presence of bilateral subclavian disease, this may not be recognized until occurrence of stroke, myocardial infarction, or congestive heart failure. Leg pressures should always be evaluated, renal artery disease should be screened for, and a central pressure should be evaluated if there is any question regarding the reliability of pressure readings.

Confirmation of diagnosis and staging requires comprehensive evaluation of the aorta and its main branches by angiography or magnetic resonance angiography (MRA). Three-dimensional (3D) contrast-enhanced MRA can be utilized to evaluate anatomy; T2-weighted sequences and double inversion recovery (DIR) (black-blood) sequences can be used to evaluate vessel wall thickening; delayed postgadolinium sequences can be used to assess vessel wall enhancement as a potential sign of inflammation. Positron emission tomography (PET) can also be useful in the evaluation of patients with large cell vasculitis. x-Ray angiography may provide definitive information in diagnostically challenging cases and allows for measurement of central pressure, surgical planning, and/or intervention. CT angiography is also widely used and can provide useful information including the location and severity of stenosis/aneurysm and can provide accurate measurement of the blood vessel wall thickness at least during the initial evaluation. The need for ionizing radiation, particularly in young patients, and use of nephrotoxic contrast limit the use particularly in young women and those with concomitant renovascular disease and consequent renal dysfunction.

Follow-up of patients is frequently quite difficult because of the lack of reliable measures of disease activity, including acute-phase reactants. MR-derived surrogate information, such as vessel wall thickening, along with 3D MRA may be used in the absence of serum markers. Carotid and renal duplex may be used selectively as adjunctive modalities in the follow-up of patients. The role of intravascular ultrasound in determining disease activity remains to be defined.

Treatment

Glucocorticoids are the mainstay of treatment in TA with resolution of symptoms in 25 to 100% of the patients. Different regimens of steroids have been advocated in the initial treatment of TA. To date, there have been no comparative trials to determine the optimal dose and length of glucocorticoid regimen. In a retrospective analysis of patients who received an initial dose of 30 mg of prednisone with active arteritis, 51% had an improved quality of life, 37% experienced no change, and 12% worsened. In the largest prospective standardized experience with glucocorticoid in TA, patients received 1 mg/kg/d for the first 1 to 3 months. When disease activity decreased, the prednisone was tapered to an alternate-day schedule and further tapered. In this regimen, initial remission was achieved in 52% of the patients. Although such data support the use of an initial high dose of prednisone (1 mg/kg/d), a lower dose may be selected in individuals at high risk for steroid toxicity in cases where there is no immediate threat of tissue ischemia.

Cytotoxic therapy is considered in patients with TA when there are signs of progressive disease despite the use of adequate glucocorticoid therapy, relapse upon tapering of glucocorticoid, and major organ's risk or when there is an especially high rate of complications from glucocorticoid therapy. The greatest published experience with cytotoxic medications in TA has been with methotrexate and, to a lesser degree, with cyclophosphamide. Methotrexate may be an effective means of inducing remission and minimizing glucocorticoid toxicity in resistant TA patients.

Empiric adjunctive use of statins has been advocated by virtue of their potential immunomodulatory and anti-inflammatory effects. Antiplatelet therapy with aspirin or dipyridamole has been used in retrospective studies, but the potential benefits remain unclear.

Several studies have reported that angioplasty with or without stenting can be used successfully to treat patients with segmental arterial stenosis caused by TA, especially after the acute inflammatory phase has resolved. In the future, drug-coated stents may afford benefits. Surgical revascularization may be required in patients with diffuse disease, but surgical planning must take into consideration the relative likelihood of involvement of the proximal (source) vessel with TA in the future. Vascular tissue samples, to document disease activity, should be obtained whenever possible.

Giant Cell Arteritis of the Elderly

GCA (temporal arteritis, cranial arteritis) is an inflammatory vasculopathy that affects medium and large vessels. Activated macrophages and CD4+ T cells are found in all vessel layers, presumably entering through the vasa-vasorum. Giant cells may or may not be found in the vessel wall.

Epidemiology

GCA is a common form of primary vasculitis in the United States and Europe with incidence rates reaching 15 to 25 cases per 100,000 in persons aged 50 years and older. GCA is uncommon in Southern Europeans (6 cases/100,000) and in African Americans and Hispanics (1 or 2 cases/100,000). GCA typically affects patients older than 50 years of age with a mean age of 70 years. The female:male ratio is 2:1.

Clinical Features

GCA may present with various signs and symptoms. Table 25.4 lists some of the clinical features in GCA. Constitutional symptoms are frequent and may be the presenting features. Polymyalgia rheumatica (PMR) is a clinical syndrome closely linked to GCA, characterized by the presence of symmetrical proximal aching and morning stiffness due to low-grade proximal synovitis, bursitis, and tenosynovitis. PMR is present in 40% of patients with GCA and may be the only presenting feature; however, most patients with PMR do not have clinical GCA. Headache, usually of sudden onset, is the most frequent symptom of GCA. It is usually localized to the temporal areas but may be frontal, occipital, or more diffuse. Prominent and enlarged temporal arteries and jaw claudication (due to masseter ischemia) constitute relatively specific signs for GCA. Loss of vision is the most feared complication of GCA. It is usually secondary to ischemia of the optic nerve due to arteritis of the branches of the ophthalmic or posterior ciliary arteries and occasionally due to occlusion of the retinal arterioles. The incidence of permanent loss of vision in recent series is about 20%. Stroke and/or transient ischemic attacks are the most common neurological findings and are present in 30% of the cases. Occlusive lesions of large proximal

TABLE 25.4

SPECIFICITY AND SENSITIVITY OF SIGNS AND SYMPTOMS IN PATIENTS WITH SUSPECTED GCA

Sign or Symptom	Sensitivity (95% CI)[a]	Positive Likelihood Ratio (95% CI)[b]
Jaw claudication	0.34 (0.29–0.41)	4.2 (2.8–6.2)
Diplopia	0.09 (0.07–0.13)	3.4 (1.3–8.6)
Prominent/enlarged temporal artery	0.47 (0.40–0.54)	4.3 (2.1–8.9)
Synovitis		0.4 (0.2–0.7)
Headaches	0.76 (0.72–0.79)	1.2 (1.1–1.4)
Elevated ESR	0.96 (0.93–0.97)	1.1 (1.0–1.2)

[a]Defined as the frequency in patients with biopsy-proven GCA.
[b]Defined as the frequency of the sign or symptom in patients with biopsy-positive GCA compared with the frequency in patients who had a negative result on temporal artery biopsy. (Adapted from Smetana J, Schmerling RH. Does This Patient Have Temporal Arteritis? *JAMA* 2002;287:92–101.)

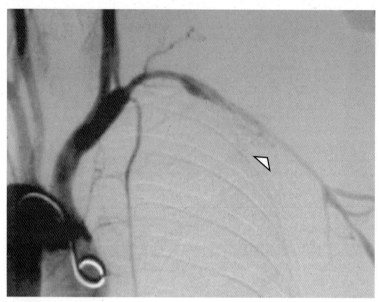

FIGURE 25-2. Angiogram in a patient with GCA showing diffuse stenoses involving the subclavian artery (*arrowhead*).

extremity arteries occur in about 15% of the cases (affecting mainly the subclavian, axillary, and brachial arteries) and result in arm claudication with reduced pulses (Fig. 25.2). Patients with GCA are 17.3 times more likely to develop thoracic aneurysms compared to age- and sex-matched normal population.

Patients who present with PMR without symptoms of GCA may have a positive temporal artery biopsy and/or vascular complications including aortic branch stenoses and thoracic aortic aneurysms.

Diagnosis

GCA is usually considered in patients older than 50 years who present with a new headache, abrupt visual loss, or fever of unknown etiology or in patients with PMR who have vascular manifestations as described earlier. Exclusion of atherosclerotic disease of the carotid, aorta, and aortic branches, which can also present with acute loss of vision, and of aortic aneurysm is an essential step in the workup of these patients. The "at-risk" age group for both entities is similar; however, the presence of elevated acute-phase reactants and other features of the disease, including PMR, favor the diagnosis of GCA over atherosclerotic diseases. A normal ESR or CRP level does not exclude the diagnosis of GCA. However, the diagnosis of GCA should be confirmed by temporal artery biopsy and/or angiographic studies when it involves arteries other than the temporal arteries.

Tissue Examination

The superficial temporal artery is the most commonly biopsied artery, and biopsy is a simple procedure performed under local anesthesia. Glucocorticoid therapy may be initiated before performance of the biopsy; even a week of steroid therapy prior to biopsy is not likely to influence the results. The diagnosis of GCA is confirmed by the presence of inflammatory cells in the vessel wall, often with destruction of the inner elastic membrane. Giant cells are not necessary to make the diagnosis. False-negative biopsies occur due to the patchy involvement of the vessel and can be minimized by sampling larger pieces and the contralateral temporal arteries.

Treatment

GCA is exquisitely sensitive to steroids, and prompt initiation markedly reduces the likelihood of vascular complications. Most patients respond to 40 to 60 mg of prednisone once daily. Response within 3 to 5 days is often quoted as a characteristic feature. If patients do not respond to initial therapy of 40 to 60 mg/d, the dose can be temporarily increased by 10 to 20 mg/d.

In patients with immediate threatening symptoms such as visual loss, intravenous pulses of glucocorticoid have been used initially and then switched to oral therapy, although there are no prospective data directly comparing the visual outcome using these two regimens. By contrast, some patients clearly respond to lower initial doses, but currently there are no reliable clinical or laboratory markers available to identify these patients before starting therapy. Furthermore, there is insufficient evidence to support efficacy of immunosuppressive agents other than glucocorticoids in GCA, although this issue has not been thoroughly studied.

After response to initial steroid therapy, dosage can be reduced every 2 weeks by 10% of the daily dose as long as the patient and the laboratory tests are normal. Below the daily dose of 20 mg/d, the length between decrements can be increased to 2 to 4 weeks depending on the patient's course and an even slower tapering regimen when the dose is below 10 mg/d. A significant number of patients with GCA will not tolerate such tapering without a flare in their disease. Therefore, careful monitoring of clinical and laboratory inflammatory parameters is necessary [ESR, CRP, and interleukin 6 (IL-6) levels, if available]. Decisions on tapering the treatment regimen should take into consideration the inflammatory markers but should rely mainly on the clinical evaluation of the patient, since the former tend to be unreliable later on in the course of the disease. A common relapsing manifestation of GCA is PMR, which may often respond to small incremental doses of steroids. Another potential, yet silent, complication is the development of aortic aneurysms.

Aspirin and statins may be of some benefit as adjunctive therapies as protection against ischemic cardiovascular events. Furthermore, aspirin has been shown to reduce the risk of visual loss. Osteoporosis is a major concern in elderly patients on long-term steroids.

MEDIUM-VESSEL VASCULITIS

Polyarteritis Nodosa

PAN is a necrotizing vasculitis of medium muscular arteries. Destruction of the blood vessel wall by inflammatory cells will lead to fibrinoid necrosis, with consequent aneurysmal bulges of the vessel wall, which may be visible in gross specimens.

Epidemiology

PAN is an uncommon disease that affects persons of any age but most often those between 40 and 60 years. Male:female ratio is 2:1. The association of PAN with viral hepatitis B and C is well described, and these disorders should always be excluded.

Clinical Features

Constitutional features including malaise, weight loss, fever, myalgias, and arthralgias are the most frequent presenting symptoms. Clinical manifestations of the disease are protean but with some predilection for certain organs, particularly the peripheral nerves, gastrointestinal tract, and muscular renal arteries (not glomerulonephritis). Mononeuritis multiplex or polyneuropathy is common. Gastrointestinal manifestations result from ischemic lesions and may present as "intestinal angina" with postprandial abdominal pain. Bleeding and bowel perforation due to infarction of the bowel are devastating complications of PAN. Renin-mediated hypertension is the most clinically recognized sign of renal involvement, but renal infarction and pericapsular hematoma can also occur. Other findings include livedo reticularis, subcutaneous nodules, ulcers, and digital gangrene. Complications due to PAN should be differentiated from a more common cause of abdominal ischemia and renal artery stenosis (RAS): atherosclerosis. The presence of constitutional symptoms, tempo of disease progression, peripheral neuropathy, and otherwise unexplained elevation of acute-phase reactants should alert the treating physician to an underlying vasculitis.

Diagnosis

The diagnosis of PAN is ideally confirmed by documenting the presence of necrotizing vasculitis in an affected organ. Short of biopsy, angiograms can help in the diagnosis by demonstrating the formation of microaneurysms (Fig. 25.3), but microaneurysms are not specific for PAN. Biopsy of clinically normal tissue should be avoided. Patients usually have elevated ESR and CRP, anemia, leukocytosis, and thrombocytosis. Positive ANCA is very rare.

Treatment

Glucocorticoids are an important part of therapy and have increased the survival of patients with PAN. There is a role for additional immunosuppressant therapy in patients with severe disease, and cyclophosphamide is a valuable adjunct treatment.

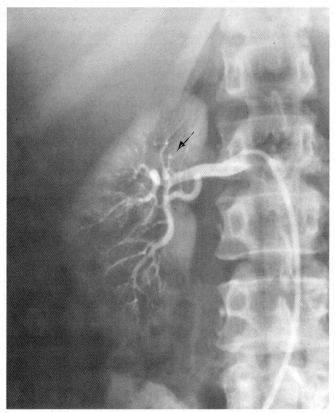

FIGURE 25-3.   Angiogram showing aneurysms (*arrow*) in the muscular arteries of kidneys in a patient with polyarteritis nodosa.

Kawasaki's Disease

Kawasaki's disease (KD), or mucocutaneous lymph node syndrome, is a necrotizing vasculitis involving small- and medium-sized muscular arteries, with a predilection for the coronary arteries in a specific pediatric clinical setting.

Epidemiology

KD usually affects children younger than 12 years. In Japan, the incidence exceeds 100/100,000 in children younger than 5 years but is less than 5/100,000 in this age group in the United States.

Clinical Features

KD is an acute febrile illness that usually affects infants and small children. Patients may present with fever, conjunctivitis, cervical lymphadenopathy,

TABLE 25.5

FEATURES OF KAWASAKI'S DISEASE

Fever for >5 d

Conjunctival congestion

Changes to lips and oral cavity: dry, red, fissured lips; strawberry tongue; reddening of oral and pharyngeal mucosa

Changes of peripheral extremities: red palms and soles; indurative edema; desquamation of fingertips during convalescence

Macular polymorphous rash on trunk

Swollen cervical lymph nodes

At least five features must be present for a diagnosis.

(Adapted from Savage CO, Harper L, Cockwell P, et al. ABC of arterial and vascular disease: vasculitis. *Br Med J* 2000;320:1325–1328.)

erythematous desquamating rash, oral mucositis, and arthritis. Myocarditis and coronary artery aneurysm formation may result in myocardial infarction early or late in the course of the disease, or even years later.

Diagnosis

The diagnostic criteria for KD are listed in Table 25.5. Five of the six criteria, with a fever, must be present for diagnosis. In addition, the illness should not be explained by other known disease processes. "Atypical" cases may be diagnosed with fewer criteria when coronary artery aneurysms are identified.

Treatment

Intravenous gamma globulins (IVGGs) have been shown to reduce the incidence of coronary artery aneurysm formation as well as abate the fever and reduce myocardial inflammation. IVGG is administered as a single infusion (2 g/kg) concurrently with aspirin 80 to 100 mg/kg/d until the fever subsides. After the child becomes afebrile, the dose of aspirin is reduced to 3 to 5 mg/kg/d, which is sufficient for the antiplatelet effect. This dose is usually continued for 6 to 8 weeks if there is no evidence of coronary artery abnormalities and indefinitely if coronary abnormalities have been identified. Referral to a pediatric cardiologist should be initiated for long-term follow-up of patients with coronary artery disease. If the fever persists despite the initial IVGG therapy, another IVGG dose may result in defervescence.

SMALL- TO MEDIUM-VESSEL VASCULITIS

Wegener's Granulomatosis

WG is a systemic vasculitis characterized by involvement of medium-sized and predominately small vessels with prominent necrotizing and/or granulomatous inflammation in selected organs.

Epidemiology

WG affects approximately 1 in 20,000 to 30,000 people.

Clinical Features

WG is a form of systemic vasculitis that primarily involves the upper and lower respiratory tracts and the kidneys, often with extensive necrotic inflammation. Pulmonary hemorrhage can be a fatal complication of the disease. However, many patients present with indolent upper airway symptoms that can be chronic and atypical. Clinical findings isolated to the upper respiratory tract or the lungs occur in approximately one fourth of cases. However, a majority of such patients eventually have renal involvement. Other organ systems that may become involved include musculoskeletal (myalgias, arthralgias, and arthritis), eyes, skin (palpable purpura, ulcers, and panniculitis), nervous system (mononeuritis multiplex, cranial nerve abnormalities, central nervous system mass lesions, ophthalmoplegia, and hearing loss), heart (pericarditis, myocarditis, and conduction system abnormalities), gastrointestinal tract, subglottis, trachea, or lower genitourinary tract. Even if glomerulonephritis does not occur, involvement of other organs may be serious and life threatening. Since renal involvement is common, regular screening by frequent urinalysis is essential to detect involvement of the kidneys by glomerulonephritis, which is almost invariably a silent process.

Diagnosis

The diagnosis of WG is generally confirmed by tissue biopsy at a site of active disease. The characteristic pathological feature of WG is necrotizing granulomatous inflammation. Vessels can be involved in the form of non-granulomatous or granulomatous arteritis or perivasculitis. All pathologic features may not be seen if only a small amount of tissue can be sampled, as in the case of nasopharyngeal tissue. Proliferative crescentic focal glomerulonephritis, with minimal immune deposits, is a common pathologic finding on renal biopsy but is not diagnostic of WG. Lung biopsy most often requires an open or thoracoscopic approach and has the highest yield to establish a definitive diagnosis (90%). Transbronchial biopsy is useful in excluding infection but rarely provides sufficient tissue to make the diagnosis of WG.

ANCAs have been associated with WG. The most clear-cut association of a disease with ANCA is the association of active generalized WG and PR3-ANCA (c-ANCA). There is some evidence, however, that in some ethnic groups, WG can be more associated with MPO-ANCA (p-ANCA). Furthermore, there appear to be important differences between MPO-associated WG and PR3-associated WG clinically.

Treatment

There are marked variations in the disease presentation in WG as well as in the course of illness. As such, treatment should be tailored to the unique clinical circumstances that include disease activity, severity of the organ involvement, and the presence of renal or hepatic dysfunction.

Glucocorticoids alone are insufficient therapy for patients with generalized WG. Induction therapy with prednisone (1 mg/kg/d) and cyclophosph-amide (2 mg/kg/d) has dramatically improved survival from 15–50% to 85%. Weekly methotrexate therapy in addition to glucocorticoids can be used as induction therapy in patients who do not have immediately life-threatening disease and do not have significant renal dysfunction. Once remission has been successfully induced by cyclophosphamide for several months, converting to either methotrexate or azathioprine (after thiopurine s-methyltransferase or TPMT genetic testing) has led to persistent remis-sion in perhaps 60% of cases. In a recent trial, B-cell depletion with ritux-imab (375 mg/m²/wk for 4 weeks) was compared with cyclophosphamide (2 mg/kg/d) for remission induction. Glucocorticoids were tapered off; the primary end point was remission of disease without the use of prednisone at 6 months. Rituximab therapy was not inferior to daily cyclophosph-amide treatment for induction of remission in severe ANCA-associated vasculitis and may be superior in cases of relapsing disease. Additional less well-studied options include mycophenolate mofetil.

Important aspects of the care of patients with WG include educating patients about the importance of nasal and sinus "hygiene" to minimize crusting and secondary sinus infection. The management of subglottic stenosis requires an otolaryngologist skilled in intralesional injection of long-acting glucocorticoids. Adjunctive therapy with trimethoprim-sulfa is advantageous as prophylaxis against PCP and may reduce the frequency of upper airway flares in WG.

Churg-Strauss Syndrome

CSS, or allergic granulomatosis and angiitis, is a multisystem disorder characterized by allergic rhinitis or asthma, prominent peripheral blood eosinophilia, and a small- and medium-sized vessel vasculitis.

Epidemiology

The estimated annual incidence of CSS is 4 per million, and people of any age can be affected.

Clinical Features

The clinical elements of CSS may occur in three phases. A prodromal phase occurs among individuals in the second and third decades of life and is characterized by atopic disease, allergic rhinitis, and asthma. An eosino-philic phase can include peripheral blood eosinophilia and eosinophilic infiltration of multiple organs, especially the lungs and gastrointestinal tract. The vasculitic phase is characterized by vasculitis of the medium and small vessels and is often found with extravascular granulomatosis. Asthma (or atopy) is the cardinal feature of CSS and often precedes the vasculitic phase by approximately 8 to 10 years. Two thirds of patients with CSS will develop skin lesions manifested as palpable purpura, macu-lar or papular erythematous rash, hemorrhagic lesions, or tender nodules. Skin involvement is one of the most common features of the vasculitic phase. Other organs frequently involved include the heart (pericarditis, heart failure, and the coronaries with myocardial infarction) and the nervous system (mononeuritis multiplex and polyneuropathy). Kidneys can be involved, but unlike WG, renal failure is less common among patients with CSS. Other manifestations include abdominal pain, gastrointestinal bleeding, and colitis as well as myalgias, migratory polyarthralgias, and frank arthritis. Lung involvement usually presents with infiltrates; cavitary nodules are much less common than in WG.

Diagnosis

The diagnosis of CSS is suggested by the clinical findings and then confirmed by biopsy of clinically affected tissues. Histologic findings include eosinophilic infiltrates, necrosis, eosinophilic giant cell vasculitis, and necrotizing granuloma. The main laboratory finding in CSS is eosinophilia (above $1,500/mm^3$). ANCAs are present in 47 to 85% of CSS cases and are usually perinuclear, rarely cytoplasmic, and directed against myeloperoxidase (MPO) more so than proteinase 3.

Treatment

CSS responds well to glucocorticoids. Glucocorticoids are usually given at an initial dose of 1 mg/kg/d with further tapering according to disease course. Higher doses of glucocorticoids and/or additional cytotoxic agents are usually reserved for patients who are resistant to treatment or those with major organ involvement. Late relapses after a successful response to treatment are seemingly less common than in microscopic polyangiitis (MPA) or WG. As a result, treatment can be discontinued in most patients. However, premature withdrawal of treatment can result in recurrence.

Microscopic Polyangiitis

MPA is a necrotizing vasculitis affecting small and medium vessels (i.e., muscular arteries, arterioles, and capillaries) with dominant involvement of glomerular and pulmonary capillaries.

Epidemiology

The annual incidence of MPA ranges from 3.5 to 5.2 cases/million. MPA occurs more often in the white population and has a slight predilection to males (male:female—1.8:1).

Clinical Features

Necrotizing glomerulonephritis is very common, and pulmonary capillaritis is not an infrequent complication. Patients may thus present with a pulmonary-renal syndrome that must be distinguished from antiglomerular basement membrane disease. Older case series clubbed MPA together with PAN, which is why some series include alveolar hemorrhage or glomerulonephritis as a feature of PAN. MPA has many similarities to WG, but prominent involvement of the upper respiratory tract is uncommon. Skin involvement such as purpura, livedo reticularis, or subcutaneous nodules occurs in two thirds of the patients. More than 60% have neurologic involvement, particularly mononeuritis multiplex.

Diagnosis

The characteristic histopathologic finding includes focal thrombosis with fibrinoid necrosis of capillaries. Kidney biopsies show 15 to 20% crescent formation with sparse glomerular immune deposits. ANCA is found in 85% of patients. It is usually of perinuclear pattern and is MPO specific.

Treatment

MPA is a serious disease with a significant risk of either death or end-stage renal failure. The initial treatment of active disease is aggressive and follows the same therapeutic approach as in WG. Maximal disease suppression is advocated for the initial active phase followed by a less aggressive, less toxic regimen once disease activity is controlled. There is a significant risk of relapse; thus, long-term maintenance therapy should be considered.

Henoch-Schönlein Purpura

HSP is a systemic vasculitis with a prominent cutaneous component. Unlike the previously discussed vasculitides, which are not associated with immune complex (IC) deposition, HSP affects small-sized vessels, with immunoglobulin A–dominant immune deposits.

Epidemiology

The annual incidence is about 20 per 100,000 children. HSP occurs more often in children than in adults, and many cases follow an upper respiratory tract infection.

Clinical Features

Clinical manifestations include fever, palpable purpura on the lower extremities and buttocks (Fig. 25.4), arthritis, and abdominal pain. Complications include bowel ischemia (intussusception in children) and glomerulonephritis.

Diagnosis

The characteristic tetrad of nonthrombocytopenic purpura, knee arthritis, abdominal pain, and microscopic hematuria in a child is virtually pathognomonic of HSP. Confirmation of the diagnosis of HSP requires evidence of IgA deposition by immunofluorescence microscopy in the skin or kidney tissue. Biopsy of skin lesions reveals inflammation of the small blood vessels, leukocytoclastic vasculitis. This finding is not specific for HSP, but dominant IgA deposition in addition to the previously described data is quite suggestive of the diagnosis.

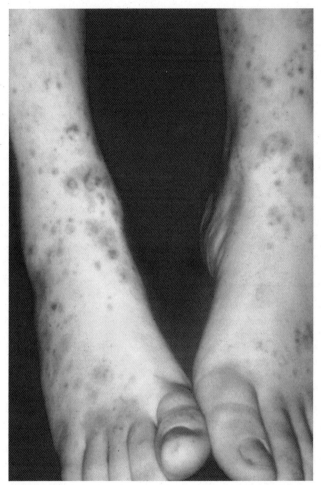

FIGURE 25-4. Palpable purpura in a patient with cutaneous vasculitis.

Treatment

Complete recovery occurs in 94% and 89% of children and adults, respectively. Treatment is either supportive or with short courses of low-moderate dose of prednisone. Recurrences are common, occurring in approximately one third of patients; recurrences are more likely in patients with nephritis. More aggressive treatment should be considered in patients with marked proteinuria and/or impaired renal function during the acute episode.

Cutaneous Leukocytoclastic Angiitis

This can occur as a part of other vasculitic syndromes (WG, MPA, CSS, or HV) or as an isolated cutaneous process without evidence of systemic vasculitis. IC-associated cutaneous vasculitis is frequently associated with bacterial or viral infections, systemic autoimmune diseases [systemic lupus erythematosus (SLE), Sjögren's syndrome], and malignancy (myeloproliferative, solid-cell carcinomas, and lymphoproliferative diseases) and is secondary to drug exposure. Thus, these etiologies need to be excluded prior to attributing cutaneous vasculitis to a primary vasculitic disease. Cryoglobulinemic vasculitis results from the deposition of IC in the small vessels of the skin and other areas. The most common cause of cryoglobulinemic vasculitis is infection with hepatitis C virus. Cryoglobulinemic and other small-vessel vasculitides most frequently manifest as recurrent crops of palpable purpura as well as painful ulcers. Other manifestations include peripheral neuropathy, arthralgias, malaise, fatigue, Raynaud's phenomenon, livedo reticularis, and glomerulonephritis. Leg ulcers secondary to cryoglobulinemic vasculitis should be differentiated from other causes of ulcers, including peripheral artery disease and antiphospholipid syndrome (APS), by measuring cryoglobulin levels in the blood and by careful scrutiny of the patient for manifestations of underlying disease, particularly hepatitis C or B-cell lymphomas.

Diagnosis

The clinical findings and the identification of leukocytoclastic vasculitis on skin biopsy confirm the diagnosis. Immunofluorescence should be performed on the skin biopsy to exclude HSP. Cutaneous leukocytoclastic vasculitis is classified as a primary vasculitis only after other etiologies are excluded.

Treatment

Therapy of primary cutaneous vasculitis depends on the severity of disease. Antihistamines have been suggested as a first line of therapy. Nonsteroidal anti-inflammatory agents have been reported to be beneficial in some patients. Some patients with occlusive vasculopathy, such as livedo reticularis, may benefit from pentoxifylline. Other treatment modalities that may offer benefit include dapsone and colchicine. Glucocorticoids are effective; however, in patients with chronic, non–life-threatening disease, their use is discouraged. Immunosuppressive agents such as azathioprine and methotrexate can be used in low doses to limit the dosage of glucocorticoids in particularly difficult cases.

Hypersensitivity Vasculitis

HV includes several entities such as serum sickness and drug-induced vasculitis. Its hallmark is the deposit of immune complexes in capillaries, venules, and arterioles.

Epidemiology

It is the most common type of vasculitis.

Clinical Features

The most important feature is a temporal relationship of symptoms to the inciting agent. Most patients have purpuric lesions and possibly a spectrum of systemic symptoms. In the case of serum sickness, the patient usually has a fever, joint pain, and rash that develop 2 weeks after exposure.

Diagnosis

Skin biopsy would establish the diagnosis of leukocytoclastic vasculitis; however, the critical element is an inciting agent.

Treatment

The identification and removal of the inciting agent are most important. Glucocorticoids may be used for patients with more severe disease and can be tapered relatively quickly once the disease is under control.

Hypocomplementemic Urticarial Vasculitis

Hypocomplementemic urticarial vasculitis (HUV) is a cutaneous vasculitis that is associated with low C_3 and C_4. If associated with systemic features (pleuritis, pericarditis, angioedema, COPD, uveitis, and glomerulonephritis), it is referred to as hypocomplementemic urticarial vasculitis syndrome (HUVS).

Epidemiology

Five percent of patients who present with chronic urticaria have HUV. HUV could also be associated with a variety of illnesses including SLE, Sjögren's syndrome, HCV, and IgG and IgM gammopathy.

Clinical Presentation

The distinguishing features of the urticaria associated with HUV are that it has purpura-like qualities, it may be painful, each lesion can last longer than 24 hours, and it may be associated with arthralgia and myalgia. HUVS has some systemic features that overlap with SLE (pleuritis, pericarditis, and glomerulonephritis).

Diagnosis

Skin biopsy reveals leukocytoclastic vasculitis, and immunofluorescence will show deposits of immune complexes and complement. The deposits occur also at the dermal-epidermal junction in a pattern identical to what is seen in the lupus band.

Therapy

Glucocorticoids are effective. Plaquenil, dapsone, or other immune-modulating drugs can be used as a glucocorticoid-sparing agent. The choice of a particular drug depends on the severity of systemic involvement.

Miscellaneous Vasculitis

Behçet's Disease

Behçet's disease (BD) is a chronic inflammatory disease that is thought to be due to an underlying vasculitis.

Epidemiology

The prevalence varies significantly among various ethnic groups and is the highest in people from a middle-eastern background. The prevalence in North America is five cases per hundred thousand. It is more common in women than in men in North America but not in the Middle East.

Clinical Features

Clinical features include recurrent oral and genital ulcers, anterior or posterior uveitis, retinal vasculitis, and multiple skin lesions that include acne-like nodules, erythema nodosum, pseudofolliculitis, and papulopustular lesions. Other organ involvement includes CNS, peripheral nerves, gastrointestinal tract, joints, kidney, and epididymis. BD is associated with a significant risk of thrombosis and aneurysm formation. Vascular abnormalities occur in 7 to 29% of patients, mostly men. Histologic findings include media thickening, elastic fiber splitting, and perivascular round cell infiltration. The types of vascular lesions recognized in persons with BD are arterial occlusions, venous occlusions, aneurysms, and varices. Affected sites of the venous system are the superior vena cava, inferior vena cava, deep femoral vein, and subclavian vein. Aneurysmal dilation and stenosis are the most common arterial abnormality with the subclavian and pulmonary arteries being the most common arteries occluded. Depending on the site, arterial occlusions can have different clinical presentations with hypertension ensuing from RAS, loss of pulses, and arm claudication with subclavian artery occlusion and intermittent claudication due to femoral artery involvement. Aneurysm rupture accounts for most vascular deaths in BD with common sites of aneurysms being the thoracic/abdominal aorta and femoral artery. Because the vascular involvement of BD can be significant and life threatening, diagnosing and treating vascular involvement early are vital.

Diagnosis

BD diagnosis is made based on the identification of a constellation of clinical features that is seen in the same patient but which may be separated in time. Pathergy (an exaggerated reaction to minor trauma such as the prick of a needle characterized by the development of a pustule), although not very sensitive, is reasonably specific for BD.

Treatment

Treatment should be tailored to the severity of organ involvement. In mucocutaneous disease, colchicine may be effective. However, in neurological disease, glucocorticoid and cytotoxic drugs may be used. In ocular disease, glucocorticoids, cytotoxic drugs, and anti-TNFα inhibitors may be effective.

Primary Angiitis of the Central Nervous System

Primary angiitis of the central nervous system (PACNS) is a chronic inflammatory disease process that is limited to the CNS. The inflammatory process may be granulomatous and involves the arteries and, less commonly, the veins of the brain and the leptomeninges.

Epidemiology

The annual incident rate is 2.4 cases per million. It is more common in males.

Clinical Features

The symptoms range depending on the anatomic location of the inflammatory process, and almost any area of the CNS could be affected including the spinal cord. The most common symptom is headache.

Diagnosis

Diagnosis is best established based on histologic examination of a brain biopsy; however, a negative biopsy does not rule out the possibility of PACNS because of the segmental nature of the disease. Angiographic evidence of vasculitis in the proper clinical setting could be diagnostic. Magnetic resonance imaging (MRI) is almost always abnormal in PACNS and may assist in the localization of an area to be targeted (if possible) for biopsy. MRA may be normal in PACNS because the vessels involved are below the resolution for the study.

Treatment

Glucocorticoids and cytotoxic drugs are the appropriate therapy for this usually progressive and often fatal disease.

DIAGNOSIS

Approach to Diagnostic Testing

The intrigue in the diagnostic workup for vasculitis comes largely from the fact that there is no single test that can completely rule out the possibility of vasculitis. Furthermore, when ordering blood tests, bear in mind that there are no specific blood tests to diagnose "vasculitis" and that the relative utility of each laboratory test, including invasive biopsies, depends on the pretest likelihood of the specific disease that is being sought. Rates of "false positives" are higher when the pretest probability of the specific disease is low. Initial examination and testing should be used to document the pattern and the degree of organ involvement, to exclude mimics of vasculitis, to identify disorders causing a secondary vasculitis, and to support the diagnosis of a specific primary vasculitis (Table 25.6).

TABLE 25.6

SELECTED LABORATORY TESTS IN THE EVALUATION OF PATIENTS WITH POSSIBLE PRIMARY VASCULITIS

Test	Comments
Platelet count	Thrombocytosis may parallel the acute-phase response. Thrombocytopenia is not expected in primary vasculitides. Consider SLE, marrow infiltration, hairy cell leukemia, TTP, DIC, hypersplenism, APLS, HIV scleroderma renal crisis, and heparin-induced thrombocytopenia.
WBC count	Leukopenia not expected in autoimmune vasculopathies. Consider SLE, leukemia, hypersplenism, sepsis, myelodysplasia, and HIV. Eosinophilia common in Churg-Strauss syndrome; may occur in WG, rheumatoid arthritis, and scleroderma renal crisis.
ESR, CRP	Nonspecific measurement of acute-phase response. Usually high in autoimmune vasculopathies. Can be elevated in infection and malignancies. May not be elevated in TA and GCA and frequently low in HSP.
Transaminases	Elevated ALT or AST in liver disease, myositis, rhabdomyolysis, hemolysis, myocardial infarction.
Ant-GBM	Evaluation of alveolar hemorrhage, with or without GN. Evaluation of normocomplementemic GN.
ANA	Order when there is clinical suspicion of SLE, not a general screening test.
ANCA	Order when there is a clinical suspicion of WG, MPA, drug-induced vasculitis, or unexplained normocomplementemic GN without extensive tissue immune deposits. Both immunofluorescence and antigen-specific ELISA are important to evaluate patients with a high test probability for vasculitis.
Drug screen	Unexplained CNS symptoms, myocardial ischemia, vascular spasm, panic attacks with systemic features, tachycardia. Urine screen should be done.
Blood cultures	Febrile, multisystem or wasting illness, pulmonary infiltrates, focal ischemia/infarction. Have low threshold to obtain cultures.
APLA	Unexplained venous or arterial thrombosis, thrombocytopenia.
PPD (±anergy) or quantitative T-cell responses to the *Mycobacterium tuberculosis*–specific antigens	Anyone who may require steroid therapy, has unexplained sterile pyuria or hematuria, granulomatous inflammation, chronic meningitis, or possible exposure to TB. Alternatively, (especially if BCG vaccinated) use the QuantiFERON-TB Gold test or T-SPOT.TB.

TABLE 25.6

SELECTED LABORATORY TESTS IN THE EVALUATION OF PATIENTS WITH POSSIBLE PRIMARY VASCULITIS (*Continued*)

Test	Comments
Examination of *fresh* urinary sediment	Perform in everyone with unexplained febrile or multisystem illness.
Hepatitis serologies	Abnormal transaminases or elevated hepatic alkaline phosphatase, or portal hypertension, PAN or MPA syndrome. Unexplained cryoglobulinemia, polyarthritis, cutaneous vasculitis.

GN, glomerulonephritis; ANA, antinuclear antibody; ANCA, antineutrophil cytoplasmic antibody; APLA, antiphospholipid antibody; TTP, thrombotic thrombocytopenic purpura; DIC, disseminated intravascular coagulopathy; WG, Wegener's granulomatosis; MPA, microscopic polyangiitis; PAN, polyarteritis nodosa; SLE, systemic lupus erythematosus; TB, tuberculosis; HSP, Henoch-Schönlein purpura.
(Adapted from Mandell BF. General approach to the diagnosis of vasculitis. In: Hoffman GS, Weyand CM, eds. *Inflammatory diseases of blood vessels.* New York: Marcel Dekker, 2002:239–253.)

Acute-phase Responses in Vasculitis

Elevation of CRP and ESR is by no means specific to vasculitis; infections and other concurrent illnesses are also accompanied by rises of CRP or ESR. In addition, up to 20% of GCA patients may present with ESR values that are not considered elevated. Some clinicians consider the CRP and IL-6 levels to be more reliable than the ESR as markers of inflammation; this has not been rigorously demonstrated in the literature. It is important to recognize that elevation of CRP (hsCRP) in vasculitis is far greater than the elevations described in atherosclerotic cardiovascular disease. Furthermore, ESR and CRP are notoriously poor markers of disease activity when following up patients with large cell arteritis. Other markers for disease activity are becoming available (e.g., macrophage migration inhibitory factor in WG), but none are universally accepted or validated.

Drug Screening

Screening for drugs, including prescribed, over-the-counter, and illicit drug use, is essential in patients with unexplained multisystem disease.

Complete Blood Count

Complete blood count (CBC) provides important clues in the evaluation of patients. Thrombocytosis may parallel the acute-phase response, but thrombocytopenia is not expected in primary vasculitis. The presence of thrombocytopenia should alert the clinician to other diagnoses including SLE, marrow infiltration, thrombotic thrombocytopenic purpura (TTP), disseminated intravascular coagulopathy (DIC), APS, human immunodeficiency virus (HIV), and scleroderma renal crisis. The white blood count is usually normal or elevated in primary vasculitis. Leukopenia is not expected; if it is present, one should consider SLE, leukemia, HIV, myelo-dysplasia, and sepsis. Eosinophilia is common in CSS and in WG (although usually to a lesser degree), but it can also occur in lymphomas, cholesterol embolization syndrome, and some carcinomas.

Antineutrophil Cytoplasmic Antibodies

This is positive in WG, MPA, and CSS. ANCAs are antibodies directed against specific neutrophil granular proteins. ANCA can be of two different immunofluorescent patterns, either perinuclear (p-ANCA) or cytoplasmic (c-ANCA). The characteristic c-ANCA pattern in WG is usually caused by antibodies against proteinase 3 (PR3), while the pattern of p-ANCA (most frequently in MPA) is usually secondary to antibodies against MPO. The most clear-cut association of a disease with ANCA is the association of active generalized WG and PR3-ANCA. Between 80 and 90% of all ANCAs found in WG are c-ANCA. The association of p-ANCA with MPA is reported to be in the range of 40 to 80%. Both PR3 and MPO have been described as target antigens in patients with CSS. High titers of p-ANCA (anti-MPO) have also been well described in patients with drug-associated vasculitis (e.g., propylthiouracil, hydralazine, and minocycline). To optimize the diagnostic performance of ANCA, a combined ANCA testing system [indirect immunofluorescence ANCA and antigen-specific ANCA (anti-MPO and anti-PR3)] is recommended. Other ANCA antigen specificities include elastase, which has been associated with drug-induced vasculitis.

The clinical utility of ANCA in the diagnosis for particular disease depends on the pretest likelihood of the disease in the patient, published sensitivity, and specificity data. For example, in the setting of isolated sinus-itis, a positive c-ANCA has a posttest probability of predicting WG in only approximately 10% of cases. In this setting, the diagnosis should be guided by histopathologic findings and the entire clinical picture. On the other hand, in a patient with sinusitis, pulmonary infiltrates and/or nodules, and glom-erulonephritis, a positive c-ANCA titer has a posttest probability of 98% for WG. In the latter scenario, if infection has been ruled out, one may take these data to be strong enough circumstantial evidence for the diagnosis of WG to treat the patient without further diagnostic procedures. The limita-tion of such an approach is the uncertainty of the diagnosis if there is a poor response to appropriate treatment or if unexpected complications occur.

The second important query is whether ANCA measurement can pre-dict disease activity and play a role in treatment decision making. This issue remains somewhat controversial, but the current data do not support the use of ANCA levels as a predictor of disease course or activity. Thus, ANCA can be a useful diagnostic adjunct in the evaluation of patients with WG or MPA but does not supplant histopathologic data in atypical cases. ANCA should *not* be used as a screening test for "vasculitis."

There is a growing list of autoantigens that have been identified as tar-gets of autoantibodies in small-vessel vasculitis. The list of autoantibodies described includes anti-B2-glycoprotein I, antiendothelial antibodies (AECA), antienolase antibodies, and antilamin antibodies. Furthermore,

AECA has been associated with large- and medium-size vasculitis such as JCA, TA, PAN, and KW. Interestingly, TA AECA levels have been associated with disease activity.

Urinalysis

This is a crucial test in patients with multisystem disease. The importance of examination of fresh urinary sediment by a physician for the screening of glomerular disease cannot be overstated. It should be performed, more than once, in everyone with an unexplained febrile or multisystem disease to look for glomerulonephritis, which is usually clinically silent.

Radiographic Evaluation

This should be tailored according to the history and physical examination. A chest radiograph is an essential initial evaluation in a patient with pulmonary symptoms. Computed tomography (CT) may play a crucial role if malignancies are expected. In the initial workup for possible WG, a CT scan of the chest should be strongly considered, since it is more sensitive to detect adenopathy, cavitary lesions, and infiltrates in this disease. CT angiography may also be considered in the workup of large-vessel vasculitis.

Angiography

Angiography is a valuable tool in patients with suspected large- or medium-sized vessel pathology. It is performed in situations where MRA is not possible or feasible or in the setting of a planned intervention. Angiography has limitations when used as a test to "rule out" vasculitis, since in the absence of luminal stenosis or aneurysms, the diagnosis may still not conclusively be ruled out (particularly in GCA or in smaller-vessel diseases). The advantage of angiography is in the detection of clinically silent aneurysms such as in the diagnosis of PAN, where microaneurysms are detected in approximately 60% of cases (but also seen with atrial myxoma, bacterial endocarditis, peritoneal carcinomatosis, severe arterial hypertension, and following methamphetamine use). The classic angiographic appearance in large-vessel vasculitides (mainly GCA and TA) is that of stenotic lesions with smooth, elongated tapering of the vessel. Distinction from atherosclerosis is not always possible. Accurate measurements of true central aortic pressures may be obtained, and this information may be invaluable.

Magnetic Resonance Imaging

MRI is a noninvasive diagnostic test most useful in patients with large-vessel vasculitis (such as GCA and TA) and may occasionally be of value in medium-vessel vasculitis if involvement of renal, mesenteric, and extremity arteries is suspected. MRI, using special sequences (3D contrast, T2 weighted, DIR, and postgadolinium), can potentially aid in the diagnosis and follow-up of patients with vasculitis and can assess arterial wall thickening and associated (apparent) edema, a presumed surrogate marker of inflammation. However, further validation of this modality with histopathologic findings is needed.

Positron Emission Tomography

Emerging evidence supports the diagnostic value of using 18F [2'-deoxy-2'-fluoro-D-glucose] (FDG)–PET. The sensitivity of this procedure ranges between 77 and 92% to diagnose large-vessel vasculitis, especially GCA. Specificity ranges between 89 and 100%. The most promising advantage of this technique is that it can demonstrate the onset of vasculitis earlier than other radiological studies. It is also advantageous in monitoring the effectiveness of therapy. However, further validation of this modality with histopathologic findings is needed. Finally, it is useful in identifying areas that are affected so that a biopsy can be targeted to those areas.

Pathologic Diagnosis

The gold standard in the diagnostic evaluation of patients with primary vasculitis remains the histopathologic findings. Several issues must be taken into account when considering tissue sampling. First, the vasculitic process may not affect a vessel or the organ in a uniform way. It is well documented that vessel involvement may occur in a patchy manner. These "skin lesions" pose a diagnostic challenge in sampling of tissue, and a large specimen is desired to avoid sampling error. Excisional tissue biopsies are preferred over needle, endoscopic, and bronchoscopic ones. Second, when multiple organs are involved, the choice of the biopsy site should be dictated not only by the sensitivity of obtaining a positive result but also by the morbidity and mortality of the biopsied site. Sample size and the accessibility of appropriate tissue are the limiting factors in determining the utility of a biopsy. Biopsy of asymptomatic tissue should generally be avoided, especially when pursuing the diagnosis of small- and medium-sized vessel disease.

Differential Diagnosis—General Comments

Primary vasculitides manifest by ischemic symptoms of the involved organs, localized inflammation, and nonlocalized constitutional symptoms. The main challenge is in the earlier stages of disease when the organ involvement is limited, constitutional symptoms predominate, and the list of possible nonvasculitic disorders is vast (Table 25.7). The initial step when approaching a patient with suspected primary vasculitis is to diligently pursue a careful history and physical examination. At this stage of evaluation, the major step is to exclude infections, malignancies, and other mimics and to confirm the diagnosis of a specific primary vasculitis. A careful examination of all apparent organ involvement is critical, especially in identifying silent manifestations, such as the presence of glomerulonephritis, adenopathy, and nasal ulcers. After a careful history and physical examination, directed blood studies may be helpful in the diagnostic process. When interpreting the results of blood testing, take into account that many nonvasculitic disorders cause signs, symptoms, and laboratory findings similar to those that occur in patients with systemic vasculitis. For example, endovascular infections, including infectious endocarditis, present with constitutional symptoms, can cause glomerulonephritis and peripheral ischemic lesions, and can be associated with immunologic

TABLE 25.7

SOME MIMICS OF PRIMARY VASCULITIC SYNDROMES

Infection
  Endocarditis
  Mycotic aneurysms
  Viral hepatitis
  Whipple's disease
Drug toxicity/poisoning
  Cocaine, sympathomimetics
  Allopurinol
  Diphenylhydantoin
  Arsenic
Coagulopathies
  Antiphospholipid antibody syndrome
  Disseminated intravascular coagulation
  Thrombotic thrombocytopenic purpura
Malignancy
  Lymphoma
  Carcinomatosis
  Hairy cell leukemia
  Myelodysplasia
Cardiac myxomas
Generalized atherosclerosis
Cholesterol embolization syndrome
Buerger's disease
Fibromuscular dysplasia
Ehlers-Danlos, vascular type
Thoracic outlet syndrome
Reversible cerebral vasoconstriction syndrome

abnormalities including hypocomplementemia, rheumatoid factor, and, rarely, even ANCA. Malignancies, most commonly leukemias and myelodysplasia, are important causes of secondary vasculitis, including cutaneous small-vessel vasculitis. The presence of thrombocytopenia or leukopenia should increase concern of hematopoietic malignancies.

A number of thrombotic disorders, including TTP and APS, cause ischemic events similar to primary vasculitides. The findings of thrombocytopenia and microangiopathic hemolytic anemia suggest a nonvasculitic process.

Cholesterol embolization syndrome, which manifests as peripheral embolization with ischemia, fever, livedo reticularis, eosinophiluria, eosinophilia, and slowly rising creatinine, can mimic vasculitis. Risk factors for the syndrome include angiographic procedures, lytic therapy, and recent anticoagulation, in the setting of atherosclerotic disease of the aorta.

Definitive diagnosis is made by finding telltale cholesterol clefts occluding small arteries and arterioles on deep muscle biopsy.

Other entities that need to be considered are diseases associated with vasospasms that can mimic vasculitis (e.g., benign angiopathy of the CNS). Finally, other systemic autoimmune disorders including SLE can mimic symptoms of vasculitides. The presence of leukopenia or thrombocytopenia in the setting of a systemic disease warrants the consideration of SLE. The negative predictive value of antinuclear antibodies (ANA) is high, and a negative test usually excludes SLE.

GENERAL MANAGEMENT PRINCIPLES

Treatment of primary vasculitic syndromes should be individualized according to specific forms of vasculitis, the severity of the disease, and the type of organ involvement. Glucocorticoids remain the mainstay of initial therapy of vasculitides with systemic features and/or organs at risk; high-dose glucocorticoids (i.e., prednisone 1 mg/kg/d), occasionally in divided doses, are standard initial therapy for most of the systemic vasculitis syndromes. Glucocorticoid therapy is often administered as intravenous "pulse" steroids (e.g., methylprednisolone in a dosage of 1 g/d for 3 days) in patients who have severe or life-threatening organ involvement; however, this approach has not been well validated. Immunosuppressive therapy, particularly cyclophosphamide, azathioprine mycophenolate, or methotrexate, in combination with glucocorticoids, is widely used for systemic vasculitides. However, combination therapy in a patient with systemic vasculitis should be tailored to the specific type and severity of vasculitis. For example, the addition of oral cyclophosphamide to standard glucocorticoid therapy provides a definite survival advantage in patients with WG. Plasmapheresis can be lifesaving in patients with cryoglobulinemic crisis. The addition of cytotoxic medications may not be essential in the initial management of other vasculitides (e.g., GCA, PAN). When caring for patients with a primary vasculitic syndrome, extensive monitoring and screening for treatment-related morbidity are crucial. Meticulous attention to bone health, glaucoma, and proper antibiotic prophylaxis is essential. Monitoring and screening for cardiovascular disease are also of great importance.

SPECIAL ISSUES
Takayasu's Arteritis

Medical Management

The most important medical aspects of managing patients with TA relate to the management of hypertension and the prevention of thrombosis. Hypertension can be difficult to detect in the presence of subclavian stenosis and hard to manage. Renal function should be carefully monitored, and the use of angiotensin-converting enzyme inhibitors or angiotensin receptor blockers should take into account the existence of possible RAS. Patients with unilateral RAS should be medically managed. Kidney size and/or glomerular filtration rate may be monitored by duplex ultrasound, and if there is a diminution in renal size, consideration may be given to intervention. However, MRI may overestimate the severity of stenosis. Empiric use of statins and aspirin is also encouraged in view of the anti-inflammatory effects of these drugs, but definitive evidence of benefit is lacking.

Percutaneous Therapy

Percutaneous transluminal angioplasty and stenting (PTRAS) is a potentially useful modality for treating TA patients with hemodynamically significant RAS who are not adequately controlled by medical therapy. Bilaterally significant RAS or single kidney with a high-grade stenosis in a patient with TA is an indication to intervene provided inflammatory markers are under control. However, this approach is empirical and not supported by prospective trials. Unlike other arteries involved with TA, the renal artery may have a short segmental lesion and it is a technically easier artery in which to intervene. Percutaneous transluminal angioplasty (PTA) of the subclavian or axillary arteries is increasingly being reported, particularly with the use of stents. The quoted indications for this procedure are usually arm claudication, restoration of the ability to monitor blood pressures, and, rarely, subclavian steal. PTA is less invasive than bypass procedures; however, long-term follow-up studies are needed to determine its utility and the rate of restenosis.

Surgical Management

Indications for surgery include reversible cerebrovascular ischemia or critical stenoses of three or more cerebral vessels (critical stenoses should be corrected to prevent stroke, with grafts originating from the ascending aorta), moderate aortic regurgitation, and coronary ischemia with confirmed coronary artery involvement. In general, surgery should be performed at a time of quiescent disease, but this can be extremely difficult to ascertain. Complications of surgery include restenosis, anastomotic failure, aneurysms, thrombosis, hemorrhage, and infection. Repair of abdominal and thoracic aortic aneurysms is indicated if they are greater than 5 cm. The new endovascular approaches may provide an interesting alternative for patients with abdominal aortic aneurysms from TA. Tissue *should be obtained whenever possible* at time of surgery to assess disease activity.

CASE VIGNETTES IN VASCULITIS

The following case scenarios may be useful in further emphasizing the principles of evaluating patients with potential primary vasculitis.

Case No. 1

A 45-year-old man who had always enjoyed good health developed fever, cough, and lung crackles on physical exam. He was initially diagnosed with pneumonia and treated with antibiotics. Two weeks later, the symptoms were persistent, and a chest radiograph was ordered and revealed bilateral alveolar infiltrates. He was admitted to the hospital for intravenous antibiotics, but with no response.

Discussion

The most likely initial diagnosis as an infectious process was totally reasonable and the diagnosis of primary vasculitis (such as WG and MPA) was far less likely. However, the finding of active urine sediment upon admission to the hospital suggested the presence of glomerulonephritis and the refractoriness to multiple antibiotic regimens modifies the hierarchy of the differential diagnosis list, increasing the likelihood of a primary vasculitis. The patient underwent an open lung biopsy, which revealed granulomatous inflammation with necrosis, and the diagnosis of WG was made after all cultures and special stains were negative.

Case No. 2

A 38-year-old previously healthy man was referred for possible diagnosis of WG. Two months prior to his presentation, he noted intermittent low-grade fevers, generalized fatigue, and polyarthralgias in hands, knees, and feet. He also experienced intermittent nose bleeds and dyspnea on exertion. Evaluation revealed anemia, marked elevation of his acute-phase reactants (CRP and ESR), and red blood cell casts in the urine. Because of the history of "sinusitis," elevation of acute-phase reactants, and polyarthralgia, the patient was initially suspected to have WG. On physical examination, he was found to have a loud aortic murmur, not documented previously. Although WG has been associated with aortic insufficiency, blood cultures were ordered that grew streptococci in 24 hours. An echocardiography revealed vegetations on a bicuspid aortic valve.

Discussion

Nothing piques the internist's diagnostic interests more than a potential case of systemic vasculitis. In this case, WG was considered immediately, given the history of "sinusitis," polyarthralgia, glomerulonephritis, and the elevation of acute-phase reactants. This example illustrates how a careful physical examination and conservative use of diagnostic tests along with the suspicion of the treating physician ended in the right diagnosis of the patient. Nose bleeds and "sinus pain" are common symptoms in the population. In this case, a CT of the sinuses showed normal sinus anatomy with no evidence of "chronic sinusitis." Infective endocarditis is a systemic disease that shares many features with primary vasculitides. Patients should be routinely and diligently evaluated for possible infectious etiologies.

Case No. 3

A 45-year-old woman, who is a heavy smoker, presented for evaluation of possible TA diseases. The patient was previously healthy and had come to the attention of her physician because of left-hand claudication with excessive use. She denied any fever, arthralgia, or constitutional symptoms. An angiogram was performed for the possibility of TA given her age, gender, and symptoms.

Angiography of her major vessels revealed stenotic lesions near the origins of the left vertebral artery and left subclavian artery with small atheromatous plaques at the origins of the innominate and left carotid arteries.

Discussion

This case history illustrates several points. (i) Atherosclerotic disease can present at a younger age, particularly in the setting of risk factors. This patient is a heavy smoker, which predisposes her to premature atherosclerosis. (ii) Careful interpretation of the angiogram is a crucial step in the diagnosis of vascular disease. Atheromatous lesions are characterized by stenotic lesions with an abrupt change in caliber of the artery immediately beyond the stenotic focus. Interpretation of the angiogram is sometimes quite difficult and requires the opinion of an experienced cardiovascular imager. Misreading may result in erroneous diagnosis and wrong treatment. Repeat angiograms, looking for evolution of the lesions, or MRI can, at times, be helpful; however, the clinician must be prepared and willing to reassess the diagnosis over time.

CONCLUSIONS

When confronted with a patient with a possible diagnosis of primary vasculitis, it is imperative to strive for a firm, preferably tissue-confirmed, diagnosis prior to embarking on any treatment regimen. Constant vigilance must be exercised over time to confirm the accuracy of diagnosis by excluding other conditions that may mimic vasculitis (including infection and malignancies). Serologic tests and markers of inflammation often cannot supplant other diagnostic efforts. The diagnostic evaluation depends on the index of suspicion for specific diseases and should be appropriately targeted.

PRACTICAL POINTS

- The three forms of vasculitis most likely to lead to loss of a pulse are TA, GCA, and Buerger's disease.

- Jaw claudication and scalp tenderness in patients older than 50 years are relatively specific for GCA.

- When systemic vasculitis is suspected, the first step in the evaluation is to exclude other processes such as infection, thrombosis, or malignancy. This is particularly true in the presence of cutaneous purpura.

- The ESR and CRP are not accurate gauges of disease activity in TA and GCA. Up to 50% of cases may have no elevation in TA, and GCA in the elderly may present without elevation in ESR.

- Caring for patients with vasculitis should include specific disease treatment and careful monitoring of adverse treatment effects. Adjuvant therapy for osteoporosis, hypertension, infection prophylaxis, hyperglycemia, and atherosclerotic vascular diseases should be instituted.

RECOMMENDED READING

Becker H, Maaser C, Mickholz E, et al. Relationship between serum levels of macrophage migration inhibitory factor and the activity of antineutrophil cytoplasmic antibody-associated vasculitides. *Clin Rheumatol* 2006;25:368–372.

Blanco R, Martinez-Taboada VM, Rodriguez-Valverde V, et al. Cutaneous vasculitis in children and adults. Associated disease and etiologic factors in 303 patients. *Medicine* 1998;77:403–418.

Bley T, Markl M, Schelp M, et al. Mural inflammatory hyperenhancement in MRI of giant cell (temporal) arteritis resolves under corticosteroid treatment. *Rheumatology (Oxford, England)* 2008;47:65–67.

Calabrese L. Cutaneous vasculitis, hypersensitivity vasculitis, erythema nodosum, and pyoderma gangrenosum. *Curr Opin Rheumatol* 1991;3:23–27.

Calamia K, Wilson F, Icen M, et al. Epidemiology and clinical characteristics of Behçet's disease in the US: a population-based study. *Arthritis Rheumat* 2009;61:600–604.

Christodoulou C, Sangle S, D'Cruz D. Vasculopathy and arterial stenotic lesions in the antiphospholipid syndrome. *Rheumatology (Oxford, England)* 2007;46:907–910.

Cotch MF, Hoffman GS, Yerg DE, et al. The epidemiology of Wegener's granulomatosis. *Arthritis Rheumat* 1996;39:87–92.

Davis MD, Brewer JD. Urticarial vasculitis and hypocomplementemic urticarial vasculitis syndrome. *Immunol Allergy Clin North Am* 2004;24:183.

De Groot K, Rasmussen N, Bacon P, et al. Randomized trial of cyclophosphamide versus methotrexate for induction of remission in early systemic antineutrophil cytoplasmic antibody-associated vasculitis. *Arthritis Rheum* 2005;52:2461–2469.

Evans JM, O'Fallon WM, Hunder GG. Increased incidence of aortic aneurysm and dissection in giant cell (temporal) arteritis: a population based study. *Ann Int Med* 1995;122:502–507.

Finkielman J, Merkel P, Schroeder D, et al. Antiproteinase 3 antineutrophil cytoplasmic antibodies and disease activity in Wegener granulomatosis. *Ann Int Med* 2007;147:611–619.

Guillevin L. Advances in the treatments of systemic vasculitides. *Clin Rev Allergy Immunol* 2008;35:72–78.

Guillevin L, Lhote F, Cohen P. Churg-Strauss syndrome: clinical aspects. In: Hoffman GS, Weyand CM, eds. *Inflammatory disease of blood vessels*. New York: Marcel Dekker, Inc,. 2002:399–412.

Guilpain P, Mouthon L. Antiendothelial cells autoantibodies in vasculitis-associated systemic diseases. *Clin Rev Allergy Immunol* 2008;35:59–65.

Hall S, Barr W, Lie JT, et al. Takayasu' arteritis: a study of 32 North American patients. *Medicine (Baltimore)* 1985;64:89–99.

Hind CRK, Savage CO, Winearls CG, et al. Objective monitoring of disease activity in polyarteritis by measurement of serum C-reactive protein concentration. *BMJ* 1984;288:1027–1030.

Hoffman GS. Classification of the systemic vasculitides: antineutrophil cytoplasmic antibodies, consensus and controversy. *Clin Exp Rheumatol* 1998;16:111–115.

Hoffman GS, Ahmed AE. Surrogate markers of disease activity in patients with Takayasu arteritis. A preliminary report from the International Network for the study of the Systemic Vasculitides (INSSYS). *Int J Cardiol* 1998;66:S191–S194.

Hunder GG. Giant cell arteritis and polymyalgia rheumatica. *Med Clin North Am* 1997;81:195–219.

Hunder GG, Arend WP, Bloch DA, et al. The American College of Rheumatology 1990 criteria for the classification of vasculitis. Patients and methods. *Arthritis Rheumat* 1990;33:1068–1072.

Jennette JC, Falk RJ, Andrassy K, et al. Nomenclature of systemic vasculitis. Proposal of an international consensus conference. *Arthritis Rheumat* 1994;37:187–192.

Kerr GS, Hallahan CW, Giordano J, et al. Takayasu arteritis. *Ann Int Med* 1994;120:919–929.

Kumar S, Radhakrishnan S, Phadke RV, et al. Takayasu's arteritis: evaluation with three-dimensional time-of-flight MR angiography. *Eur Radiol* 1997;7:44–50.

Lee MS, Smith SD, Galor A, et al. Antiplatelet and anticoagulant therapy in patients with giant cell arteritis. *Arthritis Rheumat* 2006;54:3306–3309.

Lee TJ, Chun JK, Yeon SI, et al. Increased serum levels of macrophage migration inhibitory factor in patients with Kawasaki disease. *Scand J Rheumatol* 2007;36:222–225.

Lupi Herrera E, Sanchez-Torres G, Marchushamer J, et al. Takayasu arteritis. Clinical study of 107 cases. *Am Heart J* 1977;93:94–103.

Mandell BF. General Approach to the diagnosis of vasculitis. In: Hoffman GS, Weyand CM, eds. *Inflammatory diseases of blood vessels*. New York: Marcel Dekker, Inc.; 2002:239–253.

Martinez Del Pero M, Chaudhry A, Jones R, et al. B-cell depletion with rituximab for refractory head and neck Wegener's granulomatosis: a cohort study. *Clin Otolaryngol* 2009;34:328–335.

Meller J, Grabbe E, Becker W, et al. Value of F-18 FDG hybrid camera PET and MRI in early takayasu aortitis. *Eur Radiol* 2003;13:400–405.

Mendes D, Correia M, Barbedo M, et al. Behçet's disease—a contemporary review. *J Autoimmun* 2009;32:178–188.

Miyata T, Sato O, Koyama H, et al. Long-term survival after surgical treatment of patients with Takayasu's arteritis. *Circulation* 2003;108:1474–1480.

Molloy E, Langford C, Clark T, et al. Anti-tumour necrosis factor therapy in patients with refractory Takayasu arteritis: long-term follow-up. *Ann Rheum Dis* 2008;67:1567–1569.

Murakami R, Korogi Y, Matsuno Y, et al. Percutaneous transluminal angioplasty for carotid artery stenosis in Takayasu arteritis: persistent benefit over 10 years. *Cardiovasc Intervent Radiol* 1997;20:219–221.

Nastri M, Baptista L, Baroni R, et al. Gadolinium-enhanced three-dimensional MR angiography of Takayasu arteritis. *Radiographics* 2004;24:773–786.

Park JH, Han MC, Kim SH, et al. Takayasu arteritis: angiographic findings and results of angioplasty. *Am J Roentgenol* 1989;153:1069–1074.

Patel Y, St. John A, McHugh N. Antiphospholipid syndrome with proliferative vasculopathy and bowel infarction. *Rheumatology (Oxford, England)* 2000;39:108–110.

Rao JK, Allen NB, Pincus T. Limitations of the 1990 American College of Rheumatology classification criteria in the diagnosis of systemic vasculitis. *Ann Int Med* 1998;129:345–352.

Rieu V, Cohen P, Andre MH, et al. Characteristics and outcome of 49 patients with symptomatic cryoglobulinaemia. *Rheumatology* 2002;4:290–300.

Salvarani C, Brown R, Calamia K, et al. Primary central nervous system vasculitis: analysis of 101 patients. *Ann Neurol* 2007;62:442–451.

Savage CO, Harper L, Cockwell P, et al. ABC of arterial and vascular disease: vasculitis. *BMJ* 2000;320:1325–1328.

Sfikakis PP, Markomichelakis N, Alpsoy E, et al. Anti-TNF therapy in the management of Behçet's disease--review and basis for recommendations. *Rheumatology (Oxford, England)* 2007;46:736–741.

Shackelford PG, Strauss AW. Kawasaki syndrome. *N Engl J Med* 1991;324:1664–1666.

Smetana GW, Shmerling RH. Does this patient have temporal arteritis? *JAMA* 2002;287:92–101.

Stone JH, Merkel PA, et al. Rituximab versus cyclophosphamide for ANCA-associated vasculitis. *N Engl J Med* 2010;363(3):221–232.

Tso E, Flamm SD, White RD, et al. Takayasu arteritis: utility and limitations of magnetic resonance imaging in diagnosis and treatment. *Arthritis Rheumat* 2002;46:1634–1642.

Venzor J, Lee W, Huston D. Urticarial vasculitis. *Clin Rev Allergy Immunol* 2002;23:201–216.

Watts RA, Scott D, GI. Classification and epidemiology of vasculitides. *Ballières Clin Rheumatol* 1997;11:191–217.

Weyand CM, Goronzy JJ. Giant-cell arteritis and polymyalgia rheumatica. *Ann Intern Med* 2003;139:505–515.

Weyand CM, Goronzy JJ. Medium- and large-vessel vasculitis. *N Engl J Med* 2003;349:160–169.

Wiik A. Clinical and pathophysiological significance of anti-neutrophil cytoplasmic autoantibodies in vasculitis syndromes. *Mod Rheumatol/Jpn Rheum Assoc* 2009;19:590–599.

Zerizer I, Tan K, Khan S, et al. Role of FDG-PET and PET/CT in the diagnosis and management of vasculitis. *Eur J Radiol* 2010;73:504–509.

CHAPTER 26 ■ Lymphedema

Stanley Rockson and Steven M. Dean

Lymphedema is the broad descriptive term that is employed to describe the clinical presentation of lymphatic vascular insufficiency. In lymphatic disease, there is excessive, regionalized (typically) interstitial accumulation of protein-rich fluid. Such conditions develop when there is an imbalance between the lymphatic load (the amount of lymph generated at the tissue level) and the lymphatic transport capacity; either or both of these variables may contribute to the development of clinically relevant lymphatic edema. Lymphedema can occur as a consequence of heritable disorders of lymphatic vascular development (primary) or as an acquired condition (secondary); the latter typically results as a consequence of traumatic disruption of the structural or functional integrity of the lymphatic circulation. Although lymphedema most typically occurs as a consequence of abnormal regional lymphatic drainage of one or more of the extremities, visceral involvement, particularly in the respiratory and gastrointestinal tracts, is occasionally encountered. Clinically, lymphedema of the extremities will produce chronic volume excess in the affected limbs; with time, irreversible structural changes supervene in the skin and soft tissues of the affected regions. In addition, lymphedema produces a well-documented, detrimental effect on the patient's perceived well-being and quality of life. The associated psychological derangements may, in turn, reduce compliance with recommended therapeutic interventions.

CLINICAL FEATURES

Clinical Classification

The clinical evaluation of lymphedema entails the differentiation of so-called primary and secondary causes (Table 26.1).

Primary lymphedema may be present at birth or develop at predictable points in the patient's natural history. Thus, the primary lymphedemas are typically classified according to the age of onset of edema. *Congenital lymphedema* is detectable at birth or within the first 2 years of life. *Lymphedema praecox* begins at, or shortly after, the onset of puberty but may be delayed for up to two decades. *Lymphedema tarda* most commonly appears after age 35 but is relatively uncommon, accounting for less than 10% of cases. Many of the primary lymphedemas are inherited in an autosomal dominant pattern, although there is, despite the Mendelian form of inheritance, a modest-to-significant female predominance in the clinical presentation. The most common form of congenital lymphedema carries the eponym of *Milroy's disease*, which is typically bilateral in distribution. The molecular basis of this disease has been established in numerous family

TABLE 26.1

CLASSIFICATION SCHEMA FOR LYMPHEDEMA

Primary	Secondary
Congenital	Benign
Familial (e.g., Milroy's disease)	Obesity
	Idiopathic
	Chronic venous insufficiency
Syndrome-associated (usually recessive)	Posttraumatic
Sporadic	Postinfectious
Lymphedema praecox	Postsurgical (e.g., axillary lymph node dissection)
Familial	
Sporadic	Filariasis
Lymphedema tarda	Malignant
	Tumor encroachment
	Primary lymphatic malignancies

cohorts: the disease appears to be the reflection of disordered lymphatic vasculogenesis, since it is determined by the presence of missense mutations in the domain encoding the tyrosine kinase signaling function of the vascular endothelial growth factor receptor 3 (VEGFR3) and the lymphatic endothelial receptor that mediates the effects of VEGF-C and VEGF-D. Other genetically determined syndromes include lymphedema-distichiasis, which has been ascribed to mutations in the nuclear transcription factor FOXC2, and cholestasis-lymphedema syndrome. Lymphedema praecox is the most common form of primary lymphedema, accounting for up to 94% of the cases in large reported series. Here, there is an estimated 10:1 ratio of females to males. The edema is most often unilateral and limited to the foot and calf.

Secondary lymphedemas are much more common than the primary disorders and develop when the lymphatic vascular channels or nodal structures are damaged or obstructed by other processes, most commonly due to surgery, infection, trauma, or radiotherapy. Figure 26.1 demonstrates a case of secondary lymphedema due to axillary lymph node dissection (following breast cancer). In the United States, lymphedema following axillary lymph node dissection is the most common cause of secondary lymphedema (~15% in breast cancer patients). Similar edematous complications in the lower extremities occur following interventions for pelvic and genital cancers, particularly when inguinal and pelvic lymph nodes are dissected or irradiated. Lymphedema is a common sequel after lymph node dissection for malignant melanoma as well. Worldwide, the most common cause of secondary lymphedema is filariasis, where severe forms of lymphatic destruction can lead to the advanced presentations of lymphedema, called elephantiasis. Morbid obesity is an increasingly prevalent, yet underappreciated, secondary cause of lower-extremity lymphedema (Fig. 26.2).

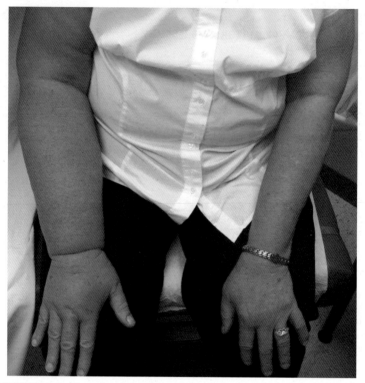

FIGURE 26-1.   Secondary lymphedema of the right upper extremity from a prior axillary lymph node dissection for breast carcinoma.

Physiology and Pathophysiology

The lymphatic vasculature begins, in the skin, in the form of blind-end sinuses, called the *initial* lymphatics. Attached to the surrounding connective tissue by anchoring filaments, and characterized by the absence of tight intercellular junctions, the initial lymphatics are ideally designed to encourage the rapid ingress of extracellular fluid, macromolecules, and cells through the porous basement membrane. The initial lymphatics ultimately coalesce into lymphatic conduit vessels that are invested with unidirectional valvular structures, resembling those of the venous circulation, and a prominent smooth muscle layer that possesses remarkable autocontractile properties. Lymph flow ultimately depends on lymphatic vascular contraction that can, in turn, be influenced by neural and humoral factors. Lymph flow and contractility increase in the presence of increased tissue turgor, upright posture (hydrostatic forces), mechanical stimulation, and exercise. The conduit vessels carry lymph into the lymph nodes, where lymphovenous fluid exchange is able to occur. In the extremities, the superficial (epifascial)

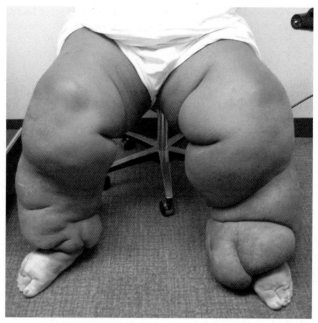

FIGURE 26-2. Morbid obesity is an increasingly prevalent, yet underappreciated, secondary cause of lower-extremity lymphedema.

system collects lymph from the skin and subcutaneous tissues; the deep system carries the lymph that originates in the subfascial structures (muscle, bone, and blood vessels). In the lower extremity, the superficial and deep systems merge within the pelvis, whereas those of the upper extremity coalesce in the axilla. Functional or structural disruption of any component of this intricate drainage system can lead to the accumulation of protein-rich fluid in the interstitium. A variety of anatomic and functional derangements can lead to lymph stasis. Mutations identified in genes that regulate lymphatic development can result in inherited lymphedema. Recent studies in families with inherited forms of lymphedema have identified the following six genes that cause lymphedema: FLT 4 (encoding VEGFR3), FOXC2, SOX18, HGF/MET, HGF, GJC2, and CCBE1. Anatomically, these gene mutations may manifest as lymphatic hypoplasia, functional insufficiency, or anatomic absence of lymphatic valves, leading to lymphangiectasia, or a hypothesized intrinsic derangement in the contractile function of the vasculature. Secondary lymphedema, which is much more common than the primary form, can appear as a by-product of any trauma, inflammation, radiation, or surgical disruption of the lymphatic vascular or nodal structures. Cellulitis may actually be more of a predictor of underlying, initially subclinical, lymphedema as opposed to a cause of the subsequent clinically manifest lymphedema. The significant role of obesity in provoking secondary lymphedema cannot be overemphasized. It must be recognized that patients with "occult" or asymptomatic primary lymphedema are at risk for developing clinical lymphedema when exposed to a "secondary" insult. Primary involvement of the lymphatics with neoplasia is a common setting for the development of secondary lymphedema.

The commonly accepted concepts of lymphedema pathophysiology are derived from observations in experimental animal model systems. When mechanical interruption of lymph vessels is created in the canine limb, lymphedema arises after an elapsed latency phase of months to years. Prior to the appearance of overt edema or any measurable accumulation of interstitial fluid, there is demonstrable anatomic pathology if the conduit lymphatic vessels are angiographically imaged. Scanning electron microscopy demonstrates irreversible loss of competence of the interendothelial junctions. Eventually, the lymph collectors become fibrotic and permeability is lost. In contrast to what is seen in hydrostatic edema, however, chronic lymphedema is not characterized by lymphatic hypertension.

Chronic lymph stasis fosters the extracellular accumulation of protein and cellular metabolites, including hyaluronan and other glycosaminoglycans. The increased tissue colloid osmotic pressure leads to water accumulation and elevation of interstitial hydraulic pressure. Changes in the tissue architecture are common. Lymph stagnation is often accompanied by an increase in the presence of fibroblasts, adipocytes, and keratinocytes in the affected regions. Enhanced populations of mononuclear cells (chiefly macrophages) signal the presence of a chronic inflammatory response. There is an exaggerated deposition of collagen, ultimately accompanied by adipose and connective tissue overgrowth in the edematous skin and subcutaneous tissues. The histopathology of chronic lymphedema may include thickening of the lymphatic basement membranes, fragmentation and degeneration of elastin, prominent ingress of fibroblasts and inflammatory cells, and increased amounts of ground substance and pathological collagen fibers. Clinically, these histologic features contribute to the development of progressive cutaneous and subcutaneous fibrosis. Table 26.2 summarizes the pathophysiology of lymphedema.

TABLE 26.2

PATHOPHYSIOLOGY OF LYMPHEDEMA

Anatomic Derangement	Pathology
Impaired lymphatic contractility	Lymph stasis, with accumulation of protein,
Lymphatic vascular underdevelopment	fluid, and glycosaminoglycans
Primary valvular incompetence	Lymphatic hypertension
Lymphatic vascular disruption or	Secondary contractile impairments
obliteration	Secondary valvular insufficiency

Presentation and Common Clinical Signs and Symptoms

Natural History of Lymphedema

The natural history of lymphedema can be quite variable. A large percentage of the patients with objectively documented lymphatic dysfunction remain asymptomatic. A long phase of latency characterizes both primary and secondary forms of lymphedema. The latent phase terminates when compensatory mechanisms become inadequate to withstand the requirement for lymphatic flow.

The precipitating factors for the transformation to overt lymphedema are not known. Initially, mild increases in limb volume may be intermittent and may, in fact, elude the patient's notice. Nevertheless, in most patients, the maximal increase in girth of the involved limb is determined within the first year after onset, unless there are supervening complications such as recurrent cellulitis. The propensity to recurrent soft tissue infection is one of the most troublesome aspects of long-standing lymphedema. Bacterial growth is encouraged both by the boggy, protein-enriched nature of the interstitium and by the impaired regional immune responses that reflect the abnormal immune traffic of lymphedema. Recurrent attacks of cellulitis further damage the cutaneous lymphatics, worsen the skin quality, and aggravate the edema.

Signs and Symptoms of Lymphedema

The clinical stages of lymphedema are outlined in Table 26.3. In early lymphedema, the edema is often pitting and fully reversible with limb elevation overnight. As lymphedema progresses, the edema no longer reverses with elevation and fails to pit with digital pressure. When progressive lymphedema is complicated by underlying obesity and recurrent soft tissue infection, disfiguring cutaneous changes such as hyperkeratosis, papillomatosis, "cobblestoning," and verrucous-appearing nodules can eventuate in elephantiasis nostras verrucosa (ENV) (Fig. 26.3). Once lymphedema becomes firmly established, the diagnosis is fairly apparent from the clinical presentation. However, the clinical presentation of early lymphedema may pose diagnostic challenges. Intermittent swelling, often described by the patient as a puffy ankle or limb, may not be accompanied by other manifestations to strongly suggest lymphatic malfunction. Of course, a

TABLE 26.3

STAGES OF LYMPHEDEMA

Stage I	Swelling reverses with elevation at night
Stage II	Swelling no longer reverses with elevation; no papillomatous lesions
Stage III	Marked swelling with associated papillomatous and verrucous lesions plus hyperkeratosis; also known as "elephantiasis"

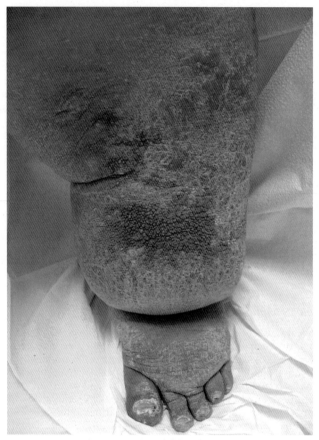

FIGURE 26-3.   Stage III lower-extremity lymphedema: ENV marked by a "mossy" appearance with hyperkeratosis, plaques, and nodules.

family history of lymphedema, or known predisposing factors, including prior infection or cancer history, will strongly suggest an appropriate investigation of potential lymphatic pathophysiology. In all patients, the diagnosis of lymphedema will be strongly supported by the findings on physical examination.

Several physical features distinguish lymphedema from other causes of chronic edema of the extremities. The pathognomonic physical finding of lymphedema is a positive *Stemmer's sign*, which is characterized by the inability to tent the skin on the dorsum of the digits (Fig. 26.4). While Stemmer described this finding in the lower extremity (and the diagnostic sensitivity and specificity of the finding have not been validated), it can certainly be extended to examination of the hand in upper-extremity edema as well. The finding of a Stemmer's sign is based upon the presence of inelastic

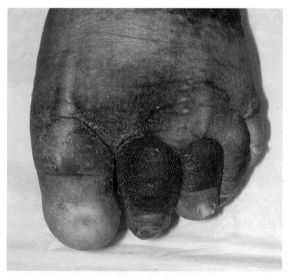

FIGURE 26-4. Hyperkeratotic, papillomatous skin along the dorsum of the second toe prohibits the ability to pinch or "tent" the affected area, thus fulfilling the definition of a *positive Stemmer's sign*. (See color insert.)

skin with increased collagen content, a cutaneous change of edema that fundamentally occurs only when lymph stagnation is present. However, in early lymphedema that is not complicated by dermal fibrosis (Stage I), a Stemmer's sign can be negative. An additional, similar finding, which reflects subcutaneous fibrosis, is so-called *peau d'orange*, a thickening of the skin, with prominent pores, that resembles an orange peel. In the legs, lymphedema often produces preferential swelling of the dorsum of the foot or a "buffalo hump." In addition, there is a characteristic blunt, "squared-off" appearance to the digits (square toe sign or "sausage toes").

Differential Diagnosis

The differential diagnosis of lymphedema encompasses the pathological states that can produce chronic swelling of one or more of the extremities.

Chronic Venous Insufficiency and Postphlebitic Syndrome

Chronic venous insufficiency is the condition that would most likely be confused with lymphedema in the lower extremities. In chronic venous insufficiency, the distinguishing clinical features would include aching discomfort in the lower extremities during sitting or standing and chronic pruritus, particularly overlying the incompetent communicating veins. Physical findings might include cutaneous deposits of hemosiderin, dusky discoloration and venous engorgement with dependence, cutaneous varicosities, and, if advanced, ulceration of the skin with atrophie blanche scarring. These cutaneous findings are most prominent within the distal medial portion of the calf and surrounding the medial malleolus. In contrast to lymphedema, patients with chronic venous insufficiency typically have little, if any, involvement of the feet, and the digits are spared. In the upper extremity, if edema is ascribable to a venous cause, it is more likely to reflect acute or chronic thrombotic occlusion of a proximal venous structure. In both upper and lower extremities, unless there is a secondary lymphedematous component, there should be no cutaneous fibrosis or thickening. However, lymphedema can occur commonly in cases of advanced chronic venous insufficiency (Fig. 26.5).

Lipedema

Lipedema is a disorder that affects women nearly exclusively; when it is seen in men, it occurs only in the setting of a feminizing disorder. In lipedema, the volume excess is caused by the abnormal accumulation of fatty substances in the subcutaneous regions, typically between the pelvis and

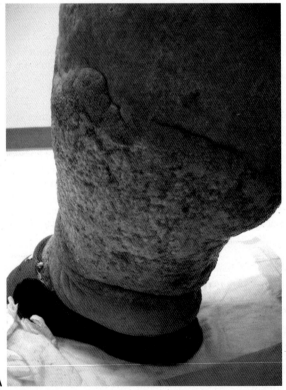

A

FIGURE 26-5. Chronic venous insufficiency is an increasingly recognized secondary cause of lymphedema. Note the constellation of marked venous stasis hyperpigmentation and profound lymphedematous dorsal foot swelling.   (*Continued*)

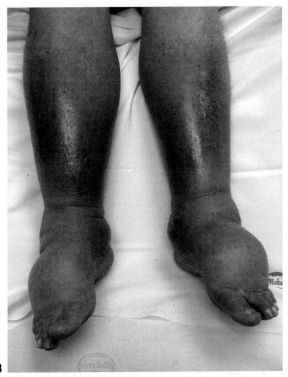

B

FIGURE 26-5. (*Continued*) Multiple malodorous, weeping, refractory lymphostatic ulcerations can rarely complicate ENV. (See color insert.)

the ankle. As opposed to lymphedema, there is sparing of the feet and toes as depicted in Figure 26.6. The pathogenesis of lipedema is not well understood but is known to involve an expanded population of subcutaneous adipocytes, and it is associated with structural alterations in the small vascular structures within the skin. In fact, it is conjectured that regional abnormalities of the circulation may cause the initial accumulation of fat in the affected regions. The characteristic distribution of leg enlargement, with sparing of the feet, should suggest the correct diagnosis. Stemmer's sign is absent, unless there is secondary lymphedema or "lipolymphedema" (Fig. 26.7). Most often, lipedema arises within 1 to 2 years after the onset of puberty. In addition to the near lifelong history of heavy thighs and hips, affected patients often complain of painful swelling and unusual cutaneous hypersensitivity. There is also, commonly, a propensity to bruising, perhaps a result of increased fragility of capillaries within the adipose tissue.

Malignant Lymphedema

In the differential diagnosis of lymphedema, it is appropriate to distinguish benign lymphedema (even if acquired as a consequence of cancer therapy)

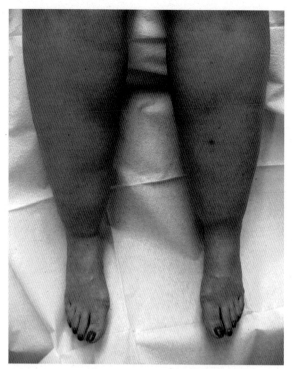

FIGURE 26-6.   Classic lipedema of the lower extremities. Observe the symmetric calf involvement and "ankle cutoff sign" with sparing of the feet and toes. These clinical features delineate lipedema from lymphedema. (See color insert.)

from the lymphatic stagnation that accompanies direct encroachment upon the lymphatic conduits by active neoplastic disease. Thus, in the differential diagnosis of new or worsening lymphedema, the presence or recurrence of cancer, leading to intrinsic or extrinsic obstruction of lymph flow, must be considered. Malignant lymphedema often develops rapidly and displays a pattern of relentless progression. Furthermore, whereas pain is generally absent in benign lymphedema, it is a common presenting feature of the malignant variety. In contrast to the former, malignant lymphedema begins centrally and lacks the early soft consistency seen in the initial presentation of benign lymphedema.

Myxedema

Myxedema is an unusual form of edema that arises in the setting of thyroid disease. It is characterized by the presence of abnormal deposits of mucinous substances in the skin. Hyaluronic acid–rich protein deposition in the dermis produces edema that eventually disrupts the structural integrity and reduces the elasticity of the skin. In thyrotoxicosis, myxedema is a focal process, typically

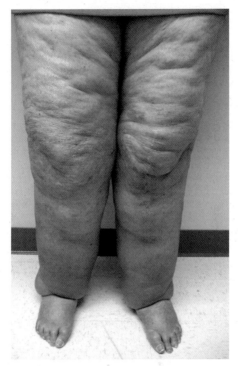

FIGURE 26-7. Lipolymphedema. Rarely, long-standing lipedema can eventuate in secondary lymphedema. Although this female patient experienced a 40-year history of familial symmetric thigh and calf swelling without foot involvement, for the last several years, dorsal pedal edema evolved. (See color insert.)

limited to the pretibial and pedal regions, whereas in hypothyroidism, the myxedema is more generalized. Myxedema can often be recognized by associated physical findings: roughening of the skin of the palms, soles, elbows, and knees; brittle, uneven nails; dull, thinning hair; yellow-orange discoloration of the skin; and reduced sweat production. However, it may, in fact, be difficult to distinguish from lymphedema as the mucin infiltrates the lymphatic system. A rare form known as elephantiasic pretibial myxedema exists.

Factitious Edema

A complete differential diagnosis of lymphedema must include acknowledgment that, rarely, patients may choose to factitiously induce the presence of edema through the habitual application of a tourniquet. This form of edema, if sufficiently chronic, may ultimately acquire some of the cutaneous attributes of lymphedema. Upon close inspection, circumferential depression is often observed along the proximal portion of the limb. The swelling abruptly terminates above this line of demarcation.

DIAGNOSIS

The diagnosis of lymphedema relies heavily upon an appropriate history, coupled with the classic features of this condition as documented by physical examination. However, in cases where edema is multifactorial, or where the diagnosis remains in question, there are ancillary studies that can be undertaken to establish the diagnosis with greater certainty. Available tests include isotope lymphoscintigraphy, indirect and direct lymphography, magnetic resonance imaging (MRI), computed axial tomography (CAT scan), and ultrasonography. Direct lymphography is generally limited to the evaluation of candidates for lymphatic surgery. Figure 26.8 provides a diagnostic approach to lymphedema. The most useful and commonly employed imaging modality is radionuclide lymphoscintigraphy. This minimally invasive procedure simply requires intradermal or subcutaneous injection of an appropriate radiolabeled tracer. ^{99m}Tc-antimony sulfide colloid, ^{99m}Tc-sulfur colloid, ^{99m}Tc-albumin colloid, and ^{99m}Tc-labeled human serum albumin have become the primary agents for clinical use.

Subcutaneous tracer injection is recommended by many investigators, but intradermal injection is preferred by others. Images are recorded with a dual-detector instrument, using high-resolution parallel-hole collimators, in the whole-body scanning mode. Lymphoscintigraphy is usually performed after injection into the web space of the upper or lower extremities, followed by imaging for 30 to 60 minutes. Imaging offers objective evidence to distinguish lymphatic pathology from nonlymphatic causes

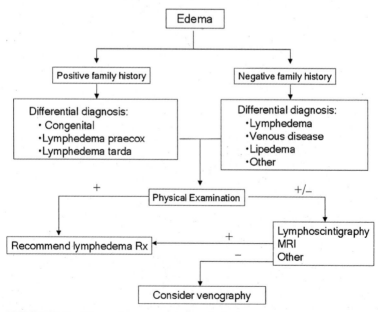

FIGURE 26-8.   Diagnostic approach to lymphedema.

of extremity edema. In addition to providing evidence for a lymphatic mechanism of established edema, lymphoscintigraphy has been utilized to identify patients at high risk for the future development of lymphedema. Criteria for lymphatic dysfunction include delayed, asymmetric, or absent visualization of regional lymph nodes and the presence of dermal backflow, generally felt to represent the extravasation of lymph from the vasculature into the interstitium that accompanies the incompetence of the lymphatics in these conditions. Figure 26.9 provides a good example of an abnormal

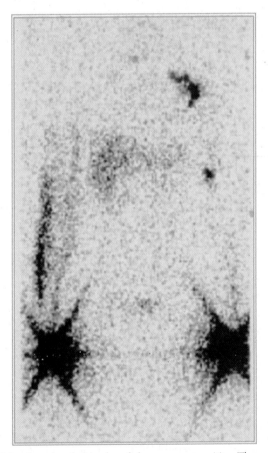

FIGURE 26-9. Lymphoscintigraphy of the upper extremities. The radiotracer is injected into the subcutaneous space on the dorsa of both hands and sequential static images are obtained. On the left, the patient has normal visualization of axillary lymph nodes. On the right, there is a failure to visualize axillary nodes, coupled with "dermal backflow," that is, accumulation of radiotracer in the subcutaneous tissues as a result of reflux from incompetent lymphatic vasculature. This finding is felt to be pathognomonic of lymphedema.

lymphoscintigram that fulfills multiple criteria. Additional findings include asymmetric visualization of lymphatic channels, collateral lymphatic channels, interrupted vascular structures, and visibility of the lymph nodes of the deep lymphatic system, such as the popliteal lymph nodes after web space injection in the lower extremities.

Additional, clinically relevant imaging modalities include MRI and CAT. These techniques permit objective documentation of structural changes of lymphedema. A characteristic absence of edema within the muscular compartment helps to distinguish lymphedema radiographically from other forms of edema. Also, a honeycomb distribution of edema within the epifascial plane, along with thickening of the skin, is characteristic of lymphedema but absent in other forms of edema. These findings serve to complement the functional assessment provided by lymphoscintigraphy.

Additional techniques for the evaluation of lymphedema have not been clinically validated and are usually applied in a research context. These include tissue tonometry and bioelectric impedance analysis. Both of these techniques are designed to detect small changes in tissue turgor and therefore might be utilized to detect subclinical states of lymphatic impairment.

Direct contrast lymphography has largely been abandoned for the objective evaluation of edema patients, not only because the cannulation of the lymphatic vessels is tedious but also because the iodinated contrast agent is toxic to the lining of the lymphatic vasculature and may thus contribute to exacerbation of the presenting edematous state. This modality is reserved for the evaluation of the minority of patients who are considered candidates for potential surgical interventions.

MANAGEMENT OF PATIENTS
Conservative Approaches

Physiotherapy

Lymphedema is a chronic condition that requires lifelong management. Effective therapeutic interventions may retard disease progression and reduce the incidence of soft tissue infections. The accepted mainstay of treatment is physiotherapy. For lymphedema, a complex, multifaceted approach, called complex decongestive physiotherapy (CDPT), is employed. CDPT integrates meticulous skin care, massage, exercise, and the use of compressive elastic garments. Decongestive lymphatic therapy can acutely reduce limb volume as well as provide long-term benefits owing to the acceleration of lymph transport in the edematous limb and the dispersal of accumulated protein. The massage component of CDPT is called manual lymphatic drainage (MLD). It is an empirically designed form of gentle stimulation of the cutaneous afferents that has been demonstrated to enhance lymphatic contractility and to augment and redirect lymph flow through the nonobstructed cutaneous lymphatics. MLD should not be confused with other forms of therapeutic massage that have no effect on lymphatic contractility. The mild tissue compression during MLD produces better filling of the initial lymphatics and enhances transport capacity, through the cutaneous lymphatic dilatation and development of accessory lymph collectors.

During therapies designed to accomplish the initial volume reduction in a previously untreated patient, MLD is coupled with the application of nonelastic, multilayered compressive bandages that should be applied after each massage session and worn during exercise to prevent reaccumulation of fluid and to promote lymph flow during exertion. When maximal volume reduction has been accomplished (typically following 5 to 15 such sessions), the patient can be fitted with an appropriate compression garment (Fig. 26.10), conventionally designed to deliver 40 to 80 mm Hg. Garments must be fitted properly and replaced when they lose their elasticity (every 3 to 6 months). In all phases of treatment, the interventions should be coupled with meticulous skin care and gentle muscular exercise, the latter designed to further augment the activity of the lymphatic pump.

Ancillary modalities can also effectively be employed to increase the efficacy of compression therapy. A variety of compressive garments, including some specifically designed for nocturnal use, have been recommended. Application of intermittent pneumatic compression with single-chamber or multichamber pumps can remove excess fluid from the extremity and

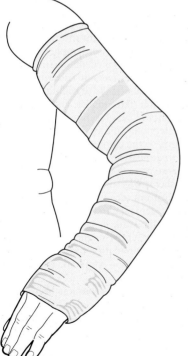

FIGURE 26-10. Compression garment to reduce secondary lymphedema following radical mastectomy.

therefore may be considered as an adjunctive approach to CDPT. Older pneumatic compression techniques, however, cannot clear edema fluid from the adjacent trunk or pelvis, which is critical in the setting of proximal lymph node obstruction. Consequently, as fluid shifts occur during pneumatic compression, the root of the limb must be decompressed with manual techniques. However, several novel advanced programmable pneumatic pumps are now available that can provide preparatory truncal or pelvic clearance, thereby obviating the need for adjunctive MLD. The use of any form of compressive therapy requires a sufficient arterial blood supply to the limb. In cases of limb ischemia, compressive therapy, which can compromise arterial blood flow and promote severe ischemia and necrosis, is contraindicated.

Other forms of physical treatment are under investigation. Low-level laser therapy may be effective in postmastectomy lymphedema, at least on the basis of small, published patient trials. Similar benefits have been ascribed to local hyperthermia and to the intra-arterial injection of autologous lymphocytes. Maintaining ideal body weight is critical. Weight reduction surgery should be considered in the morbidly obese patient with Stage III lymphedema who is unable to lose weight via conservative methods.

Pharmacotherapy

In lymphedema, the only class of drugs with unquestioned, proven efficacy is antibiotics, when they are indicated to treat intercurrent soft tissue infection. The clinical presentation of soft tissue infection in lymphedema can be variable, from very subtle exacerbations of lymphedema characterized by skin changes without fever to rapidly progressive soft tissue infection with high fever and systemic toxicity. Recurrent attacks of cellulitis further damage the cutaneous lymphatics, worsen the skin quality, and aggravate the edema. Broad-spectrum antibiotics should be prescribed promptly at the first sign or suspicion of soft tissue infection. Culture documentation of the pathogen is almost never forthcoming, so the choice of antibiotic is, by design, empiric. Prolonged courses of treatment are frequently necessary; at times, long-term suppression of bacterial growth on the skin necessitates the continuation of systemic antibiotic therapy for months to years.

Aside from this highly focused application, drug therapy has little, if any, role in the current treatment of lymphedema. Diuretics have commonly been employed in such patients, but to little avail; in fact, on theoretical grounds, it is altogether likely that diuretic therapy might exacerbate the deleterious effects of the soft tissue protein accumulation that accompanies lymphedema. It is only in cases of mixed venous and lymphatic edema that diuretic treatment is likely to be useful.

The coumarins represent an additional drug class that has been advocated in lymphedema. However, despite the enthusiasm generated by initial reports of efficacy, these drugs have been determined to possess an unacceptable tendency to adversely affect hepatic function, so that their use has generally not been advocated. The drug class remains unavailable in the United States.

Surgical Approaches

In general, while physical therapies are designed to prevent complications and to retard the progression of lymphedema, the role of surgery is, for the most part, palliative. In addition, a surgical approach may cause further damage to cutaneous lymphatics and may lead to edema exacerbation, skin necrosis, ulceration, and fistula formation. Nevertheless, an invasive strategy may become necessary in patients with unacceptable degrees of subcutaneous adipose hypertrophy and fibrosis. Excisional procedures entail removal of redundant skin and most or all of the lymphedematous epifascial tissue, often with wide excision and split skin grafting. These procedures do not improve lymphatic drainage. Microsurgical approaches utilize the creation of new lymphaticolymphatic, lymphaticovenous, or lymph node–venous anastomoses to improve lymphatic drainage. Although there is enthusiasm for these procedures in some surgical quarters, the long-term results of such interventions have not been uniformly encouraging. Other surgical techniques include treatment with transfer of an omental pedicle or interposition of a vascular pedicle flap to serve as a lymphatic wick.

Recently, reports have appeared documenting the therapeutic benefits to be obtained by liposuction in advanced, stable lymphedema. Surgical liposuction in cases of chronic postmastectomy lymphedema has been reported to produce excellent results, with sustained reduction of excess volume. Liposuction with long-term decongestive compression therapy reduces edema volume more successfully than does compression therapy alone. However, the volume reduction will not be successful unless compression therapy is maintained after the surgical intervention.

Emerging Therapies

Lymphedema currently lacks a cure. Although physiotherapy has proven efficacy, this is accomplished at the expense of tremendous time expenditure and, often, deterioration in the patient's quality of life. The exponential growth in comprehension of the molecular forces that govern lymphatic vascular development has contributed to the expectation that molecular strategies for lymphedema treatment may soon be forthcoming. The receptor-ligand interactions between the VEGFR3 receptor and the VEGF-C and VEGF-D ligands are critical to lymphatic microvascular development; this fact is underscored by the recently demonstrated role of VEGFR3 missense mutations in the pathogenesis of Milroy's disease, the most common form of heritable primary lymphedema. Furthermore, it has quite recently been reported that growth factor therapy with VEGF-C can ameliorate and, to a degree, reverse the lymphatic malfunction in animal models of both primary and acquired forms of lymphedema. These observations create the hope that extension of these molecular strategies to the human disease states may be forthcoming. Intensive future investigation will be required to verify the therapeutic potential of such approaches as well as to establish dose-response relationships and durability of the therapeutic response. As with other forms of angiogenic therapy, the relative virtues of growth factor therapy versus gene therapy must be established.

CONCLUSIONS

Lymphedema produces chronic, painless swelling of one or more limbs when the lymphatic circulation is underdeveloped, has functional abnormalities, or is traumatized. Lymphatic damage may precede overt lymphedema by weeks, months, or years. The hallmark of lymphedema is the progressive induration and inelasticity of the skin and subcutaneous tissues that ensue with disease chronicity.

The pathognomonic physical signs of lymphedema include "Stemmer's sign" and *peau d'orange* changes in the skin.

When the diagnosis cannot be established with certainty, the presence of lymphedema can be confirmed with radioisotope lymphoscintigraphy; contrast lymphography should be avoided, if at all possible. The mainstay of therapy is CDPT, comprising skin care, MLD, bandaging, compressive garments, and exercise. Surgery should be avoided unless an unacceptable degree of soft tissue hypertrophy hinders the patient's limb function.

PRACTICAL POINTS

■ In a patient with leg swelling, pitting edema over the dorsum of the foot and "squared-off" appearance to the digits are almost always signs of lymphatic involvement.

■ Cellulitis is often difficult to recognize in the setting of lymphedema; when in doubt, treat with antibiotics.

■ A standard course of treatment for cellulitis is almost never sufficient for a lymphedema patient; plan on a minimum of 2 to 4 weeks of treatment, using oral doses at the high end of the recommended spectrum.

■ When lymphedema abruptly worsens or ceases to respond to the usual measures, the two most likely explanations are occult soft tissue infection or recurrent cancer.

RECOMMENDED READING

Brorson H, Svensson H. Liposuction combined with controlled compression therapy reduces arm lymphedema more effectively than controlled compression therapy alone. *Plast Reconstr Surg* 1998;102:1058–1068.

Foeldi E, Foeldi M, Weissleder H. Conservative treatment of lymphedema of the limbs. *Angiology* 1985;36:171–180.

Mallon E, Powell S, Mortimer P, et al. Evidence for altered cell-mediated immunity in postmastectomy lymphoedema. *Br J Dermatol* 1997;137:928–933.

Rockson SG. Precipitating factors in lymphedema: myths and realities. *Cancer* 1998;83(Suppl 12):2814–2816.

Rockson SG. Lymphedema. *Am J Med* 2001;110:288–295.

Rockson SG. Primary lymphedema. In: Ernst CB, Stanley JB, eds. *Current therapy in vascular surgery*, 4th ed. St. Louis: Mosby, 2001:915–918.

Rockson SG, ed. The lymphatic continuum: a multidisciplinary conference on mechanisms and therapeutics. *Ann NY Acad Sci* 2002;979:1–235.

Schirger A, Harrison EG, Janes JM. Idiopathic lymphedema. Review of 131 cases. *JAMA* 1962;182:124–132.

Szuba A, Achalu R, Rockson SG. Decongestive lymphatic therapy for breast cancer-associated lymphedema: a randomized, prospective study of a role for adjunctive intermittent pneumatic compression. *Cancer* 2002;95:2260–2267.

Szuba A, Shin WS, Strauss HW, et al. The third circulation: radionuclide lymphoscintigraphy in the evaluation of lymphedema. *J Nucl Med* 2003;44:43–57.

Tammela T, Alitalo K. Lymphangiogenesis: molecular mechanisms and future promise. *Cell* 2010;140(4):460–476.

CHAPTER 27 ■ Hemodialysis Vascular Access

Anil K. Agarwal

INTRODUCTION

An ideal vascular access (VA) would provide adequate blood flow for performance of hemodialysis (HD) treatments on a consistent basis. It would be easy to create, cannulate, and maintain and should be devoid of the complications of bleeding, thrombosis, stenosis, and infection. HD was pioneered during the last century using a VA that has evolved from arterial cutdown and Scribner shunt to the Cimino fistula. Use of newer forms of VA such as arteriovenous grafts (AVGs), subcutaneous ports, and various HD catheters has become common. Despite these advances, the quest for an ideal VA is far from over.

Chronic kidney disease (CKD) of various stages afflicts over 13% of the population of the United States. In 2007, over 360,000 patients required maintenance dialysis with stage V CKD, also known as end-stage renal disease (ESRD) with over 108,000 new patients requiring dialysis, the vast majority as a result of diabetes mellitus and hypertension. Other major causes of kidney failure include various glomerulonephrites, polycystic kidney disease, and obstructive uropathy. People with failed transplant contribute a significant number to the pool of ESRD. The mortality in this population remains very high, from almost 40% during the first 3 months (particularly in older patients) to over 20% per year later. VA not only is the most important determinant of the success of HD process, it also impacts the survival on HD significantly. Specifically, there is a significant body of data showing that arteriovenous fistula (AVF) is associated with the best outcomes with catheter access being associated with a high degree of morbidity and mortality. Considering these factors, the Kidney Disease Outcomes Quality Initiative (K/DOQI) recommends placement of AVF as a priority in patients who may need permanent dialysis. In the United States, Fistula First Initiative, using its "Change Concepts," has been successful in increasing the prevalence of AVF among the prevalent ESRD patients from approximately 30% in 2003 to over 50% in 2009, although the goal of 66% prevalent AVF by 2010 is yet to be achieved.

As the number of patients requiring HD has increased, the number of procedures for VA has increased as well. Access-related procedures are the most common vascular surgery procedure done in the United States. Many of these are done for initiation of dialysis; however, since the lifespan of an access site is limited, many are done to revise existing sites. VA-related complications, especially sepsis and thrombosis, are responsible for 15 to 20% of hospitalizations in the ESRD patients undergoing HD. Access-related procedures cost over $1.8 billion annually in economic costs.

This chapter provides an overview of several important issues related to VA, including making a choice of VA, planning, creation, and maintenance of VA.

Indications for Dialysis and Vascular Access Creation

Dialysis for acute renal failure or CKD is needed to treat the uremic syndrome, medically refractory volume overload, hyperkalemia, and acidosis. Drug overdose and intoxications can sometimes need dialysis.

CHOICE OF VASCULAR ACCESS

The choice of VA for HD depends on several clinical factors. These include the timing (when dialysis will be started), duration (how long it will be continued), and the suitability of the patient's vasculature. The ideal site should have easy access to the circulation, durability, and limited complications and should provide effective dialysis. The access that comes closest to reaching this goal is the autogenous AVF. Despite these obvious advantages, until recently, the most common type of access used in practice has been the polytetrafluoroethylene (PTFE) graft. Although this prosthetic graft suffers from high rates of thrombosis and failure, it was used more commonly than AVF owing to such factors as delayed referral for AVF placement, unsuitable veins, and greater technical expertise required for AVF placement. Additionally, there is a significant risk of failure of maturation of AVF. However, once mature, AVF requires minimal intervention and is associated with the lowest incidence of infection and expense. Catheters and ports constitute the other major type of access but are complicated by a high incidence of infection and thrombosis.

Timing of access placement is immensely important as the maturation time for an AVF is 4 to 6 weeks. The waiting time for cannulation of AVF after placement also varies widely. Given the high rates of delayed or failed maturation, an AVF should be created 6 to 12 months before anticipated dialysis. This requires early referral to nephrologists and surgeons. Once an AVF is planned, it is important to protect the veins of the nondominant arm. The nondominant arm is preferred so that the dominant arm is free during dialysis. Ultimately, however, the quality of the vessels takes priority. AVGs are usually ready for use within 2 to 4 weeks (which accounts partly for their wider usage), are less likely to fail early, but require higher numbers of intervention and have less longevity than AVF. Catheters can be used instantly but are complicated by thrombosis, infection, and central venous stenosis.

ANATOMIC CONSIDERATIONS

Figure 27.1 shows various anatomic sites and most plausible configurations for AVFs and synthetic grafts. AVFs can be in side-to-side (vein to artery), end-to-side, or end-to-end pattern. The basilic and cephalic veins are the most important veins used for VA, because they are subcutaneous and more accessible than deep veins. It is also possible to use perforating

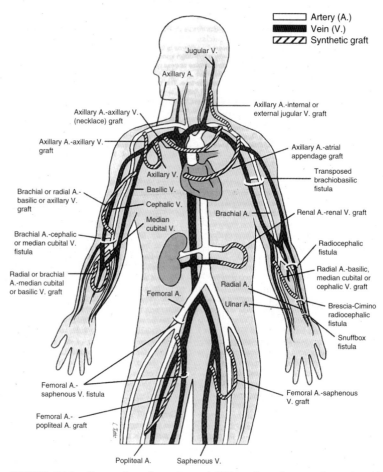

FIGURE 27-1. Sites and configurations of AVFs and synthetic grafts. (Adapted from Paulson WD, Ram SJ, Zibari GB: Vascular access: Anatomy, examination, management. *Semin Nephrol* 22:183–194, 2002.)

veins or transpose veins in the upper extremity. Clinical variables that may predict failure of an AVF include advanced age, female gender, diabetes, and obesity, often due to small vessel size. However, presence of these factors does not necessarily preclude AVF placement and maturation.

VASCULAR ACCESS PLANNING

Physical Examination

A careful preoperative physical examination is extremely important in planning access placement. The inflow artery and the outflow vein must be examined. The inflow artery should be able to provide adequate flow without rendering the extremity ischemic. Physical exam should involve palpation of the brachial, radial, and ulnar pulses. Blood pressures in the arms should be within 20 mm Hg of each other. The Allen test should also be performed in all patients. The examination of the venous system involves inflation of a blood pressure cuff to 5 mm Hg above diastolic pressure for less than 5 minutes. The cephalic vein should be relatively straight from the wrist to the antecubital space. Accessory veins should be identified so that they can be ligated during surgery as these can delay maturation of the fistula by siphoning blood from the outflow vein.

Vessel Mapping

Emphasis should be placed on preoperative vessel mapping, especially in high-risk cases. Duplex studies are commonly used to provide the surgeon a roadmap for creation of a successful AVF. Both the inflow arteries and the veins should be examined. Factors that are considered favorable include minimum venous and arterial lumen diameters of at least 2.5 mm and 2.0 mm, respectively; absence of stenoses; continuity of the vein with the deep venous system; and absence of calcification of the inflow artery. Preoperative venography may be appropriate in those with a history of previous central venous cannulation to demonstrate patency of central veins, which is difficult to detect with duplex study. Use of a small amount of low osmolar radiocontrast agents has been shown to be safe without the occurrence of acute renal failure even in the presence of advanced renal insufficiency. Use of vessel mapping has been shown to be associated with a higher rate of AVF placement, although this does not translate into a higher maturity rate of AVF.

CREATION OF ARTERIOVENOUS FISTULA

The first AVF should be placed as distally in the forearm as possible to maximize the ability to secure future AVFs. This consideration has to be tempered by the realization that the distal vessels are smaller than proximal vessels and less likely to be of adequate caliber. The radio cephalic fistula is the preferred first fistula. It has been modified from its original configuration, which was a side-to-side anastomosis, as this configuration led to excessive venous congestion in the hand from venous hypertension. To avoid this, the vein is ligated distally and an end-to-side anastomosis is created. The second choice is a proximal forearm fistula. A brachiobasilic fistula is technically more time-consuming and has a higher rate of thrombosis than the standard brachiocephalic fistula. Its advantage is that it has a lower early failure rate. Another possible option would be a prosthetic graft as this will allow time for the proximal veins to dilate, so that when the prosthetic graft fails, the proximal veins will be available and suitable for an AVF. The risk of such a strategy is that the proximal veins may become stenotic and unsuitable for AVFs.

Secondary AVFs (SAVFs) are defined as the fistulae created after the failure of previous VA in the same or another extremity. SAVFs provide an important, though underutilized, strategy to improve prevalent AVF rates and must be considered in those with a failing existing VA.

FAILURE OF MATURATION OF ARTERIOVENOUS FISTULA

Soon after the creation of AVF, there is a marked increase in blood flow via the newly created vascular circuit. This is attributed to venous remodeling with dilatation and "arterialization" as well as to arterial dilatation under the influence of changes in shear stress and cytokine expression profile. There are a number of reasons for the AVF's failure to mature. These commonly include presence of accessory veins or stenosis of venous outflow. Presence of stenosis of the juxta-anastomotic segment (the so-called "swing segment") of the outflow vein is not an uncommon finding. Additionally, there may be failure of arterial dilatation. The exact mechanism for non-maturation of AVF in many of the seemingly "adequate" vessels remains unclear at this time.

After the AVF is created, it is important to monitor both the extremity and the fistula. The presence of accessory veins is sought by occluding the fistula with a finger. The presence of a stenosis is suggested by a very strong pulse upstream followed by a decrease in intensity or disappearance of the pulse beyond the stenosis. Also, a normal fistula has a continuous thrill with a soft compressible pulse. The direction of blood flow is determined by occluding the fistula and feeling for a pulse on either side of the occlusion. The inflow side is the one with the pulse.

In general, if an AVF does not show signs of maturation within a month, investigation must be undertaken to identify a cause. Ultrasound or venography should be used to identify accessory veins, stenosis of outflow vein, stenosis at the anastomosis, and CVS. It is important to recognize that many AVFs with failure to mature can be salvaged using percutaneous intervention, including angioplasty of stenosis or coiling of accessory veins.

PROSTHETIC ARTERIOVENOUS GRAFT PLACEMENT CONSIDERATIONS

A PTFE graft should be considered if circumstances are unfavorable for the creation of an AVF. Again, distal vessels should be used first. After upper-extremity vessels have been used, vessels in the chest wall or thigh can be considered. Chest wall grafts can erode through the skin, because of the paucity of subcutaneous tissue overlying the sternum. Thigh grafts can be problematic in patients with peripheral vascular disease and can additionally have high flows, so the patient's cardiac function must also be considered.

MONITORING AND MAINTENANCE OF ARTERIOVENOUS ACCESS

Stenosis occurs more commonly in synthetic AVG than in AVFs. It most commonly occurs in the outflow vein or venous anastomosis and is attributed to the development of neointimal hyperplasia. This may be detected on exam by palpating a localized systolic thrill rather than a continuous thrill. If the stenosis reduces flow enough, blood may recirculate from the venous to the arterial needle. If obstruction is severe, the venous pressure may be high enough to stop the pump. Presence of severe stenosis can cause stagnation of access flow and eventually thrombosis of the access. Clinical signs of dysfunctional AV access include difficulty in cannulation, prolonged bleeding, inadequate dialysis, recirculation of blood during dialysis, and decline in access flow. Presence of strong pulsations and systolic accentuation of the bruit (rather than a continuous bruit) also indicate the presence of obstruction. A weak bruit and thrill over the access may indicate poor inflow. Thrombosis of access is a late sign of dysfunctional access.

The access monitoring can be done in various ways, including periodic physical examination, monitoring of static and dynamic venous pressures before and during dialysis, and flow monitoring using various techniques including duplex, CTA, MRA, or conductivity methods.

Duplex Evaluation of Arteriovenous Graft and Arteriovenous Fistula

Duplex ultrasound is the most commonly used tool to identify HD access dysfunction. Although angiography is the recognized gold standard, ultrasound has the advantage of being noninvasive and providing anatomic and physiologic information. The use of ultrasound is supported by the K/DOQI guidelines. A complete ultrasound study includes a B-mode assessment of the access, inflow, and venous runoff vessels and measurement of blood flow velocities. When interrogating grafts, velocities and flow measurements must be obtained at the arterial anastomosis, throughout the length of the access, at the venous anastomosis, and the venous runoff. If low volume flow is detected in the absence of a stenosis, then arterial inflow must also be imaged. The volume flow is the product of the blood flow velocity and the cross-sectional area.

The accuracy, sensitivity, and specificity of ultrasound compared to angiography for the detection of stenosis have been established. For grafts, the accuracy, sensitivity, and specificity are reported to be 86, 92, and 84%, respectively. For AVFs, the accuracy, sensitivity, and specificity are 81, 79, and 81%, respectively. Venous outflow stenosis is even more readily detectable with 96% accuracy, 95% sensitivity, and 97% specificity.

Surveillance of access with ultrasound has significant implications on treatment and prevention of access thrombosis, although the value has been questioned in recent studies. Grafts with access flow less than 600 mL/min have a high incidence of thrombosis over 6 months. Elective revision of grafts with flows less than 600 mL/min, decline in flow by greater than 25%, and with greater than 50% stenosis has been shown to reduce the 6-month incidence of thrombosis.

Finally, it is important to recognize that the complete access circuit comprises of not only the artery, vein, and anastomosis but also the pump (heart) and the central veins. In difficult or recurrent cases, it may be useful to study these components of the circuit.

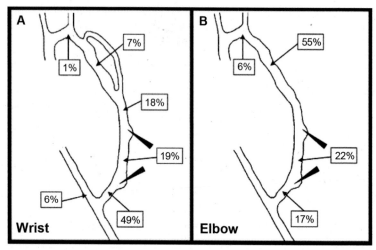

FIGURE 27-2.   Common sites of stenosis of AVF. **A:** Wrist AVF. **B:** Upper arm AVF. (Adapted from Turmel-Rodrigues L, Pengloan J, Baudin S, et al. Treatment of stenosis and thrombosis in haemodialysis fistulas and grafts by interventional radiology. *Nephrol Dial Transplant* 2000;15:2032–2036.)

PERCUTANEOUS ENDOVASCULAR MANAGEMENT OF VASCULAR ACCESS

Stenoses are common in both AVF and AVG and can involve various sites in the VA circuit (Figure 27.2, Turmel-Rodrigues; and Figure 27.3, Roy-Chaudhury). With increasing experience and better technology, endovascular therapy has gained increasing popularity and has become widely accepted as the preferred approach to maintenance and salvage of dysfunctional VA.

Vascular Access Stenosis

Percutaneous transluminal angioplasty is an outpatient procedure that can be performed in both venous and arterial outflow tracts and on anastomotic and proximal lesions. Angioplasty is indicated for venous stenoses (greater than 50%) to improve VA function and prolong access survival. Angioplasty is done under direct fluoroscopy using digital subtraction angiography. Heparinization is not usually required because the flow is occluded for a brief period of time. Clotting of the access occurs very rarely. Venography is required prior to the intervention to localize the stenosis. Access is achieved by inserting a needle antegrade into the fistula or graft and inserting a sheath. Once access is achieved and a fistulogram defines the lesion, angioplasty can be performed. Angioplasty requires introduction of a guidewire that is advanced beyond the stenosis, and a balloon catheter is placed over the guidewire. The balloon should be slightly larger than the affected vein. Usually, 6 to 8 × 4 balloons are used in grafts and peripheral veins. A 12-mm balloon may be used in the central vein. Serial inflations at

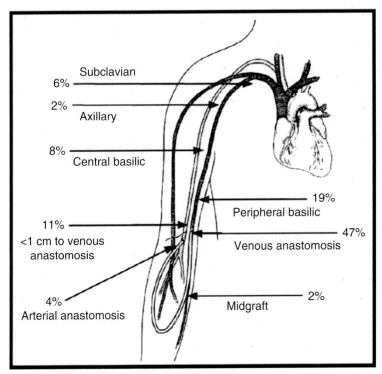

FIGURE 27-3.   Common sites of stenosis in AVG. (Adapted from Roy-Chaudhury P, Kelly B, Melhem M, et al. Vascular access in hemodialysis: issues, management, and emerging concepts. *Cardiol Clin* 2005;23:249–273.)

10 to 20 atmosphere or higher may be required for resistant lesions. Each inflation is usually for 1 to 2 minutes. Resistant lesions are typically treated with multiple dilations. The angioplasty procedure may be complicated by pain or dissection of the vessel wall, leading to extravasation of the contrast, which can usually be treated with prolonged inflation of the balloon.

The initial success rates of percutaneous intervention for either native fistula or PTFE graft range from 80 to 95%. The initial success rates for angioplasty of forearm native fistulas are higher and range from 91 to 99%. The patency rates for percutaneous intervention of native AV fistula range from 67 to 84% at 90 days and 39 to 68% at 1 year. Patency rates with percutaneous techniques for PTFE grafts are lower and range from 37 to 52% at 90 days and 8 to 40% at 1 year. Anastomotic lesions have significantly worse outcomes with 1-year patency as low as 8%.

The role of stents in the management of venous stenosis is less clear than in coronary lesions. Their use is generally accepted for venous rupture after balloon angioplasty, especially when prolonged balloon inflation fails. Use of stents is recommended to treat elastic recoil of central veins after angioplasty. In general, role of routine stenting in peripheral AV stenosis is controversial due to poor long-term patency. Only self-expanding stents are typically used in treating dialysis access stenosis. The diameter of the stent should be 1 to 2 mm larger than the diameter of the largest balloon used for angioplasty to avoid central migration. It should be as short as possible to cover the lesion. The stent should not protrude from the cephalic vein into the subclavian vein or from the subclavian vein into the superior vena cava. The primary patency rate after implantation of a stent into a vein is 20% at 1 year. After aggressive reintervention, the secondary patency rate is 70 to 80% at 1 year. Stents may be maintained by thrombolysis, repeat angioplasty, placement of a new stent, or atherectomy. The main reason for the poor patency after stent placement is the development of intrastent neointimal hyperplasia. Role of drug-eluting stents is unclear at this time. Recently, FDA has approved the use of FLAIR stent (Bard) for venous anastomotic lesions in selected cases.

Vascular Access Thrombosis

Thrombosis is the most common complication of permanent VA. It accounts for 80 to 85% of access loss. Venous outflow stenosis accounts for the majority of thromboses. Other causes include arterial stenoses, fistula compression, hypovolemia, and hypercoagulable states. Thrombosis can be treated with surgical thrombectomy, thrombolysis with thrombolytic agents, or mechanical modalities.

Endovascular therapy can utilize pharmacomechanical or purely mechanical techniques. The pulse-spray technique involves placing two multiside-holed catheters in a criss-cross fashion into the thrombosed graft. A mixture of urokinase and heparin is then infused through a tuberculin syringe every 30 seconds through each catheter. This technique combines thrombolysis with hydromechanical therapy to achieve a 90% success rate. Thrombolytic agents can be infused through catheters continuously over several minutes or hours with or without crushing of any residual thrombus with a balloon catheter. Purely mechanical methods include clot extraction or disruption methods and balloon-based methods. There are several mechanical declotting devices available today, with the Angiojet (Possis Medical, Minneapolis, MN) catheter being the most commonly used. Other devices that have been used include the Amplatz Thrombectomy Device (Microvena, White Bear Lake, MN), the Trerotola-Percutaneous Thrombectomy Device (Arrow International, Reading, PA), and the Hydrolyser (Cordis Europa, Roden, The Netherlands) device. The main concern with purely mechanical techniques is the risk of large pulmonary emboli. To decrease this risk, several devices such as the Hydrolyser pulverize the thrombus into tiny particles.

The initial technical success rates for pharmacomechanical and mechanical methods for both AV fistula and PTFE graft are 89 to 95%; however, the long-term patency rates are low. Native fistulas have better results with reported primary patency rates at 1, 3, 6, and 12 months of 74, 63, 52, and 27%, respectively. Primary patency rates after declotting PTFE grafts are only 8 to 10% per year. Secondary patency rates are approximately 75% with native AVFs and approximately 50% with PTFE grafts. Mortality rates related to the procedure itself are low and typically less than 1%, while complication rates are approximately 9% and include vessel rupture, injection, pseudoaneurysm, and bleeding 1%.

VASCULAR ACCESS–ASSOCIATED HAND ISCHEMIA

Dialysis access–associated hand ischemia is not uncommon occurring in 1 to 20% of VA. This can lead to pain or loss of function, and rarely the loss of limb. There are several mechanisms that can lead to ischemia, including popularly known arterial steal syndrome causing retrograde flow in the distal artery toward the access, arterial stenosis, or distal arteriopathy involving small vessels. It may be corrected by the ligation of the shunt, by reduction of the shunt volume flow rate (banding), or by using distal revascularization interval ligation procedure (i.e., the ligation of the main supplying artery in the direct distal vicinity of the fistula with a widely bridging bypass anastomosed at a sufficient distance from the shunt origin). In refractory cases threatening loss of function or limb, it may be necessary to ligate the access completely.

HEMODIALYSIS CATHETERS AND PORTS

The HD catheter is a VA device that allows blood withdrawal and infusion at high flow rates. The catheters may be used as a bridge to permanent access, as temporary access for patients with acute renal failure, and as permanent access in patients who have exhausted all other options. In 2007, over 80% of the patients initiating HD used catheters, and over 25% of the prevalent patients were using catheters as their permanent access in the United States.

Catheters can be short term (nontunneled, noncuffed) or long term (tunneled, cuffed). The benefits of catheter-based access are that there are no needle sticks and cannulation is easy. The disadvantage is the high frequency of infection and thrombosis. The right internal jugular vein is the preferred site for insertion of the tunneled, cuffed catheter. This is so because it offers a direct route to the right atrium, which is the optimal position for the tip of the catheter and is associated with a lower rate of complications both during insertion and after insertion when compared to the subclavian vein. There is a lower incidence CVS with IJ cannulation when compared to the subclavian vein, although IJ vein cannulation is also associated with a noninsubstantive incidence of CVS (Fig. 27.4). The tip of the catheter should be ideally located in the middle of the right atrium, and the catheter should be able to deliver at least 300 mL/min of flow. The 1997 DOQI recommends real-time ultrasound guidance for catheter insertion. Prospective studies have shown 100% success in internal jugular vein cannulation with the use of ultrasound compared to 88.1% with the use of landmarks.

Catheter Insertion Technique

The cuffed, tunneled catheter should be placed in a maximum barrier environment, similar to an operating room. The ultrasound probe should be used to identify the vein prior to surgical scrub. The surgical scrub should include the insertion site as well as the surrounding area. The area overlying the vein should be insonated using the ultrasound probe in a sterile

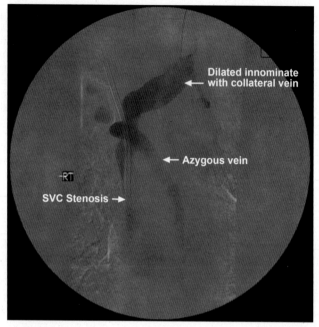

FIGURE 27-4. Severe stenosis of superior vena cava and large dilated azygous vein due to an indwelling right IJ dialysis catheter.

sheath. Once the vein is identified, the insertion site is infiltrated with local anesthesia. Conscious sedation is then administered through a peripheral IV. A 21-gauge micropuncture needle is advanced into the vein under real-time ultrasound guidance. The syringe is removed after entry into the vein, and a 0.018-in guidewire is advanced. The needle is removed, a small stab wound is created, and a 5F coaxial dilator is inserted over the wire. The inner 3F dilator is removed with the wire, and the 5F dilator is attached to a stopcock.

Next, the exit site in the infraclavicular area is identified using the catheter or guidewire on the patient's chest to determine the distance to the right atrium. The exit site is infiltrated with local anesthesia. A number-11 blade is inserted into the exit site parallel to the skin. The tunnel tract is infiltrated with local anesthesia. The tunnel is then created using the tunneling device, and a catheter is tunneled. The 5F dilator in the vein is exchanged over the guidewire (advanced to the inferior vena cava under fluoroscopic guidance) for larger dilators. Ultimately, a dilator with peel-away catheter introducer sheath is inserted over the wire, and the dilator and wire are removed. The catheter is advanced through the peel-away sheath. The sheath is then pulled out and peeled apart. After ensuring that the tip of the catheter is in the right atrium, that there are no kinks in the catheter, and that there is easy withdrawal of blood from the catheter, the venotomy site is closed with sutures. The catheter is anchored to the exit site. Topical antibiotics may be used along with pressure dressing. Finally, the lumen of the catheter is filled with heparin.

A number of catheter designs are approved for use for HD. There are dual catheter designs as well as retrograde catheter designs in which the catheter is first introduced into the right atrium via the sheath and then tunneled retrogradely. Sheathless designs of catheters are also available. Various chemically coated catheters are also available with limited evidence showing reduced incidence of infection or thrombosis.

Catheter Outcomes

Catheters for dialysis are associated with high risk of infection, thrombosis, fibrin sheath formation, and occurrence of CVS. The outcomes after cuffed, tunneled catheter placement have not been rigorously studied; however, there are some short-term studies. One study quoted a 100% technical success rate, infection rate of 0.08 per 100 catheter days, malfunction requiring removal of 0.22 per 100 catheter days, and thrombosis requiring removal of 0.16 per 100 catheter days. Catheter-related bacteremia is common with tunneled, cuffed dialysis catheters (1.6 to 5.5/1,000 catheter days), although less common than with nontunneled, noncuffed catheters (3.8 to 6.6/1,000 catheter days). The average blood flow rates are similar for most cuffed, tunneled catheters.

An alternative to the cuffed, tunneled catheter is the subcutaneous vascular port. This device is implanted within a subcutaneous pocket and is accessed through the skin. One such design was used in the United States during the last decade but was withdrawn from the market due to a high incidence of complications.

FUTURE OF VASCULAR ACCESS

Our understanding of physiology, pathology, and mechanics of VA has evolved significantly in the last decade. There is significant emphasis on the studies of neointimal hyperplasia, which is considered the most important cause of poor maturation of AVF and failure of AVG. New therapies to treat neointimal hyperplasia include locally delivered cellular therapies, perivascular wraps containing antiproliferative agents, gene therapy, percutaneous balloon cryoplasty, and use of ionizing radiation to induce apoptosis. Far infrared therapy has also been experimented with encouraging results. Development of new conduits including venous allografts, femoral arterial allografts, and decellularized bovine xenografts utilizing mesenteric veins or ureters is in progress. Preformed connectors to construct AV anastomosis are also being developed.

Catheters for dialysis, although fraught with complications, remain a necessity in selected patients and in selected clinical scenarios. Use of antibiotic lock therapy for prevention and treatment of catheter-related bacteremia is becoming increasingly popular. Newer coating agents to retard the development of thrombosis, biofilms, or infections are also in research.

CONCLUSIONS

- CKD is prevalent, and the number of patients with ESRD is increasing. Mortality and morbidity in this population remain very high, partly attributed to VA-related complications.

- Referral to nephrologist for evaluation of CKD should be prompt. Referral to surgeon for creation of an AVF must be early—6 months to 1 year before dialysis initiation is expected.

- Preoperative evaluation must include good physical examination and vessel mapping.

- Surgical expertise is essential, and all available surgical techniques should be considered to achieve a mature AVF.

- All currently available HD access types have their unique advantages and disadvantages. Due to its impact on clinical outcomes, AVF is the preferred access in most circumstances and requires least intervention once established.

- The AV graft requires less time to mature, but its lifespan is limited by thrombosis and infection.

- Most dysfunctional VA can be salvaged using endovascular techniques.

- Catheters are implanted with relative ease and are ready to be used immediately after placement. In most cases, they are used on a temporary basis due to their complications and adverse impact on outcomes.

PRACTICAL POINTS

- Optimal access for dialysis is the autogenous AVF.

- If an AVF does not show signs of maturation in 4 to 6 weeks, further investigation and intervention should be planned promptly.

- History and physical examination provide crucial information in deciding location and type of dialysis access.

- Early detection and percutaneous treatment of stenosis of dialysis access can significantly prolong the lifespan of the AV access.

- The tip of percutaneously placed dialysis catheters must be positioned in the mid right atrium.

RECOMMENDED READING

Allon M. Current management of vascular access. *Clin J Am Soc Nephrol* 2007;2:786–800.

Ethier J, Mendelssohn DC, Elder SJ, et al. Vascular access use and outcomes: an international perspective from the dialysis outcomes and practice patterns study. *Nephrol Dial Transplant* 2008;23:3219–3226.

Gibson KD, Gillen DL, Caps MT, et al. VA survival and incidence of revisions: a comparison of prosthetic grafts, simple autogenous fistulas, and venous transposition fistulas from the United States Renal Data System Dialysis Morbidity and Mortality Study. *J Vasc Surg* 2001;34(4):694–700.

National Kidney Foundation. K/DOQI clinical practice guidelines in vascular access: 2006 update. *Am J Kidney Dis* 2006;48:S176–S306.

NephSap. Nephrology Self Assessment Program: Interventional Nephrology. In: Agarwal AK, Asif A, eds. July 2009, The American Society of Nephrology.

Roy-Chaudhury P, Kelly B, Melhem M, et al. Vascular access in hemodialysis: issues, management, and emerging concepts. *Cardiol Clin* 2005;23:249–273. http://www.fistulafirst.org/. Accessed April 25, 2010.

Silva MB, Hobson RW, Pappas PJ, et al. A strategy for increasing use of autogenous hemodialysis access procedures: Impact of preoperative noninvasive evaluation. *J Vasc Surg* 1998;27: 302–307.

Tonelli JM, Wiebe N, Jindal K, et al. Ultrasound monitoring to detect access stenosis in hemodialysis patients: a systematic review. *Am J Kidney Dis* 2008;51:630–640.

CHAPTER 28 ■ Perioperative Management of Patients with Peripheral Vascular Disease

Vineet Chopra and James B. Froehlich

The perioperative period poses unique challenges for the management of patients with peripheral vascular disease (PVD; includes arterial disorders of the peripheral vessels including aortic disease). Cardiovascular complications remain a concern for any patient facing surgery, but those with PVD have a heightened risk of perioperative cardiovascular events and death.

The past 25 years have witnessed a significant research effort both to identify patients who are at an increased risk of perioperative cardiac events and evaluate interventions. These investigations have led to the creation of risk-assessment tools and the establishment of perioperative guidelines. Investigators have also paid greater attention to evaluating interventions that may mitigate perioperative cardiac risk. Such interventions include perioperative and long-term medical therapy and coronary revascularization. This chapter will review evidence-supported perioperative cardiac risk-reduction strategies, current preoperative assessment guidelines, and the studies that have examined the effectiveness of these entities.

PREOPERATIVE CARDIAC RISK ASSESSMENT

Cardiologists and internists are frequently asked to "clear" patients for surgery. This term is a misnomer. The role of the perioperative consultant is to summarize accurately the cardiac risk of surgery while identifying strategies to maximize the odds of a positive surgical outcome. Such assessment is a prerequisite for both the patient and the surgeon when faced with decision making regarding surgery, as this information can facilitate the timing and appropriateness of interventions.

Several studies have established that perioperative cardiac risk is best assessed by clinical evaluation and this is true for patients with PVD. A good history and physical examination can provide a very good estimate of operative risk. This estimate can then be modified and/or improved by selective testing.

The testing of patients prior to noncardiac surgery, whether by treadmill stress testing, treadmill testing with nuclear imaging, or dobutamine stress echocardiography or with MRI stress testing, is most appropriate for patients for whom: (a) stress-testing can effect a change in management and/or alter overall outcome, or (b) cardiac risk for surgery is unclear. In contrast, patients deemed to be at low or high clinical risk of perioperative cardiac events do not benefit from further testing. Such tests are quite effective when applied selectively based on clinical assessment. The use of Bayes theorem (using pre-test probability to assess the predictive value of

TABLE 28.1

AMERICAN SOCIETY OF ANESTHESIOLOGY CLASSIFICATION OF PERIOPERATIVE RISK

1. Normal healthy patient
2. Mild systemic disease
3. Severe systemic disease that limits activity
4. Incapacitating systemic disease that is a constant threat to life
5. Moribund patient not expected to survive >24 h, with or without operation

(Adapted from The 1962 House of Delegates of the American Society of Anesthesiologists, Inc. New Classification of Physical Status. *Anesthesiology* 1963;24:111.)

a test), is thus very much applicable to pre-operative assessment as it is in other medical interventions.

Prior to the 1970s, the only clinical risk classification system widely available for preoperative assessment was that created by the American Society of Anesthesiology; this is still used today (Table 28.1). According to this classification, patients with imminently life-threatening disease are placed into category 4 or 5, whereas those with activity-limiting disease are classified as 3. The overwhelming majority of patients fall into category 2, that is, those with mild systemic disease that is well controlled. The biggest drawback of this instrument is that it poorly defines the perioperative risk faced by a patient, (especially those in categories 1 and 2), and provides little guidance with respect to further management. Furthermore, its lack of specificity meant that wide latitude was given in determining what constitutes a systemic disease, a severe disease, or an incapacitating disease. The ASA classification system thus did little to improve the understanding of perioperative risk. Faced with this dearth of guidance, Goldman et al. identified specific clinical factors that were associated with increased perioperative risk. Based on 1,000 consecutive patients referred for evaluation prior to noncardiac surgery, Goldman et al. identified clinical variables most associated with life-threatening or fatal cardiac complications of surgery. A score was assigned to each of these factors based on the strength of association, allowing for the creation of a risk index. This study was the first comprehensive attempt to identify clinical factors associated with perioperative risk. The authors demonstrated that (within their derivation cohort) calculated risk scores correlated with perioperative complications and death. High-risk clinical features included *severe valvular heart disease, active heart failure, recent myocardial infarction, older age, arrhythmia, and/or a serious medical comorbidity.* Detsky et al. performed a similar analysis on 455 patients prospectively assessed preoperatively. These investigators also demonstrated that a risk-index score could predict the likelihood of a perioperative cardiac event. Interestingly, they included descriptive and remote factors such as *severity of angina, a history of pulmonary edema, or a history of prior myocardial infarction* in their risk model.

More recently, Lee et al. derived and then validated a risk-assessment index for perioperative cardiac complications of noncardiac surgery among 4,315 patients undergoing elective noncardiac surgery at the Brigham and

TABLE 28.2

THE REVISED CARDIAC RISK INDEX

1. High-risk type of surgery (intra-abdominal, intra-thoracic or supra-inguinal vascular)
2. History of Ischemic heart disease
3. History of congestive heart failure
4. History of cerebrovascular disease (prior TIA and/or stroke)
5. Diabetes Mellitus requiring insulin therapy
6. Preoperative serum creatinine > 2.0 mg/dL

(Adapted from Lee TH, Marcantonio ER, Manqione CM, et al. Derivation and prospective validation of a simple index for prediction of cardiac risk of major noncardiac surgery. *Circulation* 1999;100(10):1043–1049.)

Womens' Hospital. Clinical correlates of cardiac complications were modeled using stepwise logistic-regression analysis. The authors identified six clinical markers of risk and then tested these variables in a separate validation cohort of patients (Table 28.2). By assigning one point to each of these six cardiac risk factors, a risk index was derived and found to be highly predictive of perioperative cardiac complications.

L'Italien et al. developed a risk-prediction model specifically for patients undergoing vascular surgery (Table 28.3). The investigators focused on 1,081 consecutive patients with PVD undergoing major vascular surgery, a cohort at increased risk of perioperative cardiac complications. Multivariate analysis identified five clinical variables; *advanced age, angina, history of myocardial infarction, diabetes mellitus, and history of heart failure*, associated with increased perioperative risk. This clinical model stratified patients correctly into low, moderate, and high-risk patients with observed cardiovascular events rate of 3, 8, and 18%, respectively. More importantly, these investigators found that the predictive power of preoperative risk assessment was improved with the combined use of both clinical risk- assessment and selective dipyridamole-thallium testing. They noted no additional benefit from thallium testing in clinically low or high-risk groups.

TABLE 28.3

EAGLE MARKERS OF PERIOPERATIVE CARDIAC RISK

1. Age > 70
2. Diabetes mellitus (on medication)
3. History of angina
4. History of MI, or Q waves on ECG
5. CHF, by history or exam/VEA requiring treatment

(Adapted from Eagle KA, Coley CM, Newell JB, et al. Combining clinical and thallium data optimizes preoperative assessment of cardiac risk before major vascular surgery. *Ann Intern Med* 1989;110(11):859–866.)

TABLE 28.4

CLINICAL ENTITIES ASSOCIATED WITH INCREASED RISK OF PERIOPERATIVE CARDIAC EVENTS

Unstable coronary syndromes [unstable angina, acute myocardial ischemia or infarction, recent myocardial infarction (≥7 d but ≤1 mo).]

Decompensated heart failure (NYHA Class IV, new-onset or deteriorating heart-failure)

Significant arrhythmias (high grade AV-block, symptomatic ventricular arrhythmias, etc.)

Severe valvular heart disease (severe aortic stenosis, symptomatic mitral stenosis, etc.)

(Adapted from Fleisher LA, Beckman JA, Brown KA, et al. 2009 ACCF/AHA Focused Update on Perioperative Beta Blockade Incorporated Into the ACC/AHA 2007 Guidelines on Perioperative Cardiovascular Evaluation and Care for Noncardiac Surgery: A Report of the American College of Cardiology Foundation/American Heart Association Task Force on Practice Guidelines. *Circulation* 2009;120:e169–e276.)

Based on these and other studies, the American Heart Association/American College of Cardiology Foundation (AHA/ACCF) preoperative guidelines have identified clinical markers of risk for perioperative cardiac events. It is informative to note that these risk factors do not include many well-known markers of risk for atherosclerotic disease. For instance, no study has identified elevated cholesterol, high blood pressure, or tobacco use as being associated with increased risk of perioperative events. Although these factors are contributors to the development of atherosclerosis (thus increasing the long-term risk for cardiac events), they do not identify patients at immediate risk for cardiac events (i.e., those at risk for perioperative events). Thus, the clinical factors associated with increased risk of perioperative events appear to be markers associated with increased biological activity of coronary lesions rather than those associated with the initiation and propagation of these entities (Table 28.4).

PREOPERATIVE TESTING

An impressive number of clinical studies in a wide range of patient populations have evaluated the effectiveness of thallium stress testing to predict the risk of perioperative cardiac events. In spite of the varied patient cohorts examined and the time elapsed from the first study to the last, there is a remarkable uniformity of findings in terms of the predictive power of this test in identifying those at risk of perioperative cardiac events. In patients with a history of PVD requiring vascular surgery, numerous studies have shown that the negative predictive value of thallium stress testing remains close to 100%. That is to say, those with a normal thallium stress test have an almost 100% likelihood of being free from perioperative cardiac events. Conversely, the positive predictive value was remarkably and consistently poor at about 12%. Thus, patients with an abnormal thallium stress test only had a 12% chance of having a perioperative cardiac event. This makes thallium testing of questionable utility as a screening test, as many patients facing vascular surgery are likely to have an abnormal thallium test sans perioperative cardiac event.

A review of published papers evaluating dobutamine echocardiogram testing reveals strikingly similar results. Throughout the decade of the 1990s, numerous studies evaluating the ability of dobutamine echocardiography to predict perioperative cardiac events found a near-perfect 99% negative predictive value, but a disappointing 15% positive predictive value. Thus, both modalities seem quite powerful in their ability to identify patients who will be free of perioperative cardiac events, but imprecise in identifying patients at increased risk.

This begs the obvious question: how to apply testing selectively, or which patients should undergo testing? The fundamental concept behind this question is well illustrated by the study by L'Italien et al. These investigators reviewed both the clinical evaluation and thallium test results in 1,081 patients, all of whom underwent thallium testing and vascular surgery. Clinical evaluation accurately stratified patients into those at low, moderate, and high risk of perioperative cardiac events. All those at clinically low-risk did well regardless of thallium test results. Similarly, regardless of thallium testing results, those clinically estimated at high risk experienced high rates of cardiac events. Only those at moderate risk (i.e., having only one or two of the five clinical markers of risk identified by these authors) benefited from thallium testing by further risk stratification. Those in this group with normal thallium test result had a 3% rate of cardiac-events, but those with abnormal test results had a significantly higher 15% complication rate.

Recent data has challenged the paradigm of further testing even in patients at intermediate cardiac risk. Boersma et al. showed that regardless of whether or not intermediate-risk patients underwent preoperative stress testing prior to vascular surgery, immediate or long-term cardiac outcomes were not affected. Again, clinical risk scoring predicted perioperative complications with accuracy. Similarly, in the DECREASE study, Poldermans et al. randomized patients at intermediate and high risk of adverse outcome to receive no revascularization versus revascularization prior to noncardiac surgery. Importantly, all patients received beta-blockers (bisoprolol) titrated to heart rate and blood pressure in the perioperative setting. At 30 days, there was no observed difference in death or MI between groups (1.8 vs. 2.3%, OR 0.781 95% CI 0.28–2.1; $p = 0.62$). Thus, even via a strategy targeting intermediate-risk patients, preoperative testing is not necessarily helpful. If revascularization based on test results makes no difference given the available literature, routine perioperative testing or treatment can no longer be recommended and should be restricted to those conditions where testing clearly improves immediate and delayed outcomes (Table 28.4).

PERIOPERATIVE CARDIAC RISK REDUCTION

The reduction of perioperative cardiac events has been the subject of much research over the past decade. Modalities evaluated to reduce perioperative cardiac risk have included surgical risk reduction via coronary artery bypass grafting (CABG), percutaneous coronary intervention (coronary angioplasty and stenting), and medical treatment.

Medical Treatment

Perioperative Beta-Blockers

Several studies have examined the value of beta-blockers in reducing perioperative cardiac complications. In their original study, Mangano et al. evaluated the effect of beta-blockers on perioperative and long-term cardiac events in patients undergoing noncardiac surgery. Although they observed no difference in perioperative cardiac events, long-term follow-up over 2 years demonstrated a reduced rate of cardiac events among patients receiving perioperative beta-blockers. Though relevant, the study had several limitations including its small size, a heterogeneous group of patients undergoing a variety of surgical procedures, and no control over medications received postoperatively. It was also unclear how short-term perioperative beta-blocker treatment influenced long-term outcomes. Nonetheless, this trial first suggested that beta-blockers during surgery may be associated with a reduction in cardiac events. A subsequent study by Poldermans et al. randomized a more homogeneous group of high-risk patients (those with abnormal dobutamine stress echocardiography facing major vascular surgery) to perioperative treatment with bisoprolol versus placebo. Importantly, perioperative bisoprolol was started at a median of 37 days prior to surgery at a starting dose of 2.5 mg daily. This dose was individually adjusted to achieve a resting heart rate of 50 to 70 beats/min. The investigators found that despite their high-risk cohort, beta-blocker therapy dramatically lowered perioperative rates of death or MI. These data first suggested that perioperative beta-blockers were associated with a reduction in cardiac events in high-risk patients undergoing high-risk surgery.

In a subsequent nonrandomized study, Boersma et al. studied outcomes in 1,351 consecutive patients undergoing major vascular surgery. They compared the cardiac event rate among those receiving perioperative beta-blockers versus those not receiving beta-blocker therapy and found fewer cardiac events among those receiving beta-blockers, irrespective of clinical risk. The benefit was even more pronounced in those with abnormal dobutamine stress echocardiography. These data suggested a protective effect of perioperative beta-blocker therapy at all levels of clinical risk, with greater benefit afforded to those at high-risk of perioperative cardiac events. A subsequent analysis by Poldermans et al. showed that the benefit of beta-blockers was directly related to perioperative heart rate reduction, with an event rate of 1.3% in those whose heart rate was controlled to ≤65 beats/min versus 5.2% in those with heart-rates ≥65 beats/min.

Given these data, should perioperative beta-blockers be applied ubiquitously to patients undergoing operative intervention? In a large meta-analysis, Lindenauer et al. analyzed the effect of perioperative beta-blockers according to Lee's revised cardiac risk index (RCRI) score in 782,969 Medicare beneficiaries, and found that patients with low RCRI scores experience no benefit and possible harm from perioperative beta blockade. They also observed an association between beta-blocker use and lowered mortality in subjects at high risk of cardiac events. These findings called for a strategic approach incorporating clinical risk and selective application of perioperative beta-blocker treatment.

Results from the Perioperative Outcomes Ischemia Study Evaluation (POISE) study have questioned the routine use of perioperative beta-blockers. In POISE, 8,351 patients were randomized to receive either 200 mg long-acting metoprolol daily or placebo. The trial protocol specified that long acting metoprolol be given as a 100 mg oral dose 2 to 4 hours prior to surgery, followed by a second dose of 100 mg 6 hours postoperatively, provided that heart rate was ≥45 beats/min and systolic blood pressure was ≥100 mm Hg. The regimen was then continued at 200 mg daily. POISE showed cardiac benefit form beta blockade. However, the prevention of perioperative cardiac events occurred at the expense of increased mortality, sepsis, and ischemic stroke owing to intraoperative bradycardia and hypotension. A recent meta-analysis by Bangalore et al. incorporating the POISE trial findings confirmed that although perioperative beta-blockers decreased non-fatal MI and myocardial ischemia (NNT = 63), they increased the risk of intraoperative hypotension, bradycardia, and stroke (NNH = 22). The weight of the evidence (largely influenced by POISE), no longer supported the administration of perioperative beta-blockers to reduce cardiac risk given this unacceptable risk.

Largely due to POISE, the 2009 ACCF/AHA Focused Update on Perioperative Beta-Blockers narrowed the Class I indications of perioperative beta blockade to only include those already receiving this therapy (Table 28.5). However, POISE provided several valuable lessons. First, in every case, beta-blockers should only be offered with close attention to hemodynamic parameters. Second, they should be initiated between 7 and 30 days

TABLE 28.5

2009 ACCF/AHA UPDATED RECOMMENDATIONS FOR PERIOPERATIVE BETA-BLOCKER THERAPY

Class I
1. Beta-blockers should be continued in patients undergoing surgery who are receiving beta-blockers for treatment of conditions with ACCF/AHA guideline Class I indications for these drugs.

Class IIa
1. Beta-blockers titrated to heart-rate and blood pressure are probably recommended for patients undergoing vascular surgery who are at high cardiac risk owing to coronary artery disease or the finding of preoperative cardiac ischemia.
2. Beta-blockers titrated to heart-rate and blood pressure are reasonable for patients in whom preoperative assessment prior to vascular surgery identifies high-cardiac risk.
3. Beta-blockers titrated to heart-rate and blood pressure are reasonable for patients in whom preoperative testing identifies coronary artery disease or high cardiac risk, defined by the presence of more than one risk factor, in patients undergoing intermediate risk surgery.

(Adapted from Fleisher LA, Beckman JA, Brown KA, et al. 2009 ACCF/AHA Focused Update on Perioperative Beta Blockade Incorporated Into the ACC/AHA 2007 Guidelines on Perioperative Cardiovascular Evaluation and Care for Noncardiac Surgery: A Report of the American College of Cardiology Foundation/American Heart Association Task Force on Practice Guidelines. *Circulation* 2009;120:e169–e276.)

prior to surgery with dose titration to target a resting heart rate between 60 and 70/min, maintaining systolic blood pressures greater than 100 mm Hg. Third, among those receiving beta-blockers, treatment must be continued throughout the perioperative period, substituting intravenous agents if oral intake is not possible. Finally, post-operative tachycardia should not reflexively call for higher doses of beta-blockers, but investigation and treatment of the underlying cause (e.g., pain, hypovolemia, infection, etc). The optimal duration of beta-blocker therapy is unclear; however, the occurrence of delayed cardiac events and late benefits is incentive enough to continue these agents for months postoperatively. These parameters were incorporated into the ACCF/AHA Focused Update on Perioperative Beta Blockade.

Perioperative Statins

Several observational studies have implied a protective benefit of statin therapy in patients undergoing noncardiac surgery. Lindenauer et al. first reported that perioperative statin users experienced a lower crude mortality (2.13 vs. 3.02%, $p \leq 0.001$), after adjusting for covariates and propensity scores (OR 0.62; 95% CI 0.58–0.67) than non-users. In a retrospective study, Ward et al. also found that statin use was associated with lower all-cause mortality, myocardial infarction, and stroke (6.9 vs. 21.1%, $p = 0.008$) in patients undergoing vascular surgery.

In 2004, Durrazo et al. were the first to prospectively show in a randomized trial that 20 mg of perioperative atorvastatin reduced cardiac events in 100 patients undergoing major vascular surgery (26 vs. 8%; $p = 0.31$). Notably, this effect was seen at immediate follow-up and persisted at 180 days. In the recent double-blinded, placebo-controlled DECREASE-III study, Schouten et al. found that 80 mg fluvastatin significantly reduced death from cardiovascular causes (4.8 vs. 10.1%, HR 0.47; 95% CI 0.24–0.93; $p \leq 0.01$) and postoperative myocardial ischemia (10.8 vs. 19.0%, HR 0.55; 95% CI 0.34–0.88; $p \leq 0.01$) in 497 vascular surgery patients when started 37 days prior to surgery. Importantly, the study also found significant attenuation of inflammatory markers among those treated with fluvastatin (C-Reactive Protein and interleukin-6), implying that statins may have exerted their beneficial perioperative effect through inflammatory pathways. In their study, fluvastatin was well tolerated without significant adverse effects such as rhabdomyolysis, liver injury, etc.

There exist no formal recommendations for perioperative statin use at this juncture. However, several studies have reported that the perioperative discontinuation of statins among patients maintained on this therapy may produce a "rebound" inflammatory state, leading to an increased risk of coronary events. Therefore, continuing perioperative statins in those on this therapy appears reasonable and appropriate. As no intravenous formulations of statins exist, statins with a long half-life (such as rosuvastatin, atorvastatin or fluvastatin) are preferred in the perioperative setting.

Percutaneous Coronary Interventions

Observational studies suggested that preoperative percutaneous coronary interventions (PCIs) were associated with lower rates of perioperative cardiac complications. Although PCI has frequently been performed for the purpose of lowering perioperative cardiac risk, data derived from randomized trials have failed to reveal the benefit from this technique.

Numerous investigators attempted to evaluate the effectiveness of preoperative PCI using observational data. Posner et al. first compared 686 consecutive patients with prior PCI undergoing noncardiac surgery with matched control patients who had coronary disease but had not undergone PCI. They also compared these post-PCI patients with control subjects who did not have coronary artery disease. Perioperative heart failure and angina were more frequent among those who had not undergone PCI but no difference in perioperative death and MI rates was found. The findings suggested that PCI might afford some benefit in the perioperative setting.

In their review of a Medicare database, Fleisher et al. reported death and MI rates among patients undergoing aortic and peripheral vascular bypass surgery. Among patients undergoing aortic surgery, preoperative stress testing followed by PCI was associated with lower perioperative mortality. However, among patients undergoing peripheral bypass surgery, preoperative PCI was associated with higher perioperative mortality than those who did not undergo this intervention. Subsequently, Vicenzi et al. prospectively studied the efficacy of percutaneous stenting (either bare metal or drug-eluting stents) prior to surgical intervention. Importantly, anti-platelet therapy was continued till 3 days prior to surgical intervention. The investigators found that PCI prior to surgery lead to high rates of perioperative myocardial infarction, death and unstable angina likely due to an increase in the risk of stent thrombosis associated with preoperative PCI followed by noncardiac surgery. This may be due to withholding of anti-platelet therapy, and/or increased thrombogenicity surrounding surgery in the setting of a freshly placed, non-endothelialized stent. Finally and most importantly, McFalls et al. randomized patients facing major vascular surgery (n = 510) to either coronary revascularization or no revascularization prior to surgery. PCI was performed in 59% and CABG in 41%. After a mean follow-up of 2.7 years, there was no difference in mortality between the two groups. Furthermore, post-operative MI rates did not differ between the groups at 30 days after vascular surgery.

The 2009 ACCF/AHA guidelines therefore suggest that PCI indications in the preoperative setting should be the same as those in the non-operative setting (i.e., consider in those with left main disease, 3-vessel disease with LVEF less than 50%, high-risk unstable angina, non-ST-elevation MI, etc.). Routine prophylactic preoperative revascularization should never be performed for patients with stable coronary artery disease who do not meet these criteria.

Coronary Artery Bypass Surgery

There exist few clinical data regarding the utility of CABG prior to noncardiac surgery. Observational studies have demonstrated a low perioperative rate of death or MI in patients with prior CABG undergoing noncardiac surgery. This seems particularly true in those undergoing major vascular surgery. This finding, however, merits cautious interpretation as CABG prior to noncardiac surgery is not necessarily in the best interest of even high-risk patients. The combined physiologic stress of coronary artery bypass surgery plus subsequent noncardiac surgery may outweigh any benefits derived from this intervention. In other words, these studies evaluated CABG survivors who then underwent non-cardiac surgery, rather than the results of CABG plus non cardiac surgery versus noncardiac surgery alone.

In the Coronary Artery Surgery Study, Eagle et al. reported death and MI rates among patients revascularized via coronary bypass grafting who subsequently underwent noncardiac surgery. Patients with coronary artery disease and a history of CABG had perioperative death and MI rates that were half those of patients with coronary artery disease who did not undergo prior CABG. In a subgroup-analysis specifically evaluating those patients who underwent subsequent vascular surgery, death and MI rates among coronary artery disease patients with a history of CABG were approximately one-third of those among similar patients treated without CABG.

However, in the only prospective randomized controlled study to evaluate the effect of prophylactic revascularization prior to noncardiac surgery (Coronary Artery Prophylaxis Study, CARP), McFalls et al. showed that there was no benefit from coronary bypass grafting with respect to either immediate or long-term outcomes among 620 high-risk patients undergoing vascular surgery compared to medical therapy alone. Subsequent studies of CARP showed that the observed benefit may have been due to the enrichment of the CABG cohort by patients with poor left ventricular ejection fraction, peripheral arterial disease, and 3-vessel CAD, all of whom stood to benefit from revascularization. Further, the CARP study analysis in CABG was post-hoc and did not consider the cumulative risk of cardiac and subsequent non-cardiac surgery. Even in patients deemed at high risk for cardiac events (wall motion abnormalities on dobutamine stress-echocardiography), recent data shows no benefit from preoperative revascularization over optimal medical treatment.

In summary, it is prudent to pursue revascularization for those patients in whom it would provide long-term benefit. Such patients are well identified by current guidelines for PCI and CABG. Revascularization prior to noncardiac surgery in patients with stable CAD simply for the sake of perioperative cardiac-event prophylaxis is, quite simply, a formula for harm.

AHA/ACC PREOPERATIVE GUIDELINES

The 2009 AHA/ACCF perioperative guidelines summarize the available data and synthesize them into a meaningful clinical paradigm (Fleishmann et al., 2009). The guidelines feature an algorithmic approach to guide preoperative evaluation and perioperative treatment of patients facing noncardiac surgery (Fig. 28.1). Patients with PVD obviously fall into a high-risk category by definition. These guidelines provide a useful algorithm in even these high-risk patients for clinical evaluation and selective testing prior to noncardiac surgery.

Like most consensus guidelines, the ACCF/AHA guidelines are based on a synthesis of the available literature as well as expert panel opinion. Several studies have attempted to evaluate the impact of guideline implementation. Licker et al. evaluated the effect of implementation of these

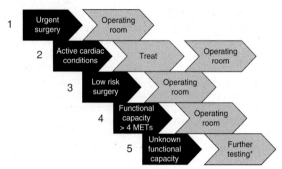

FIGURE 28-1. ACC/AHA guideline for perioperative cardiovascular evaluation for noncardiac surgery. (Adapted from Fleischmann KE, Beckman JA, Buller CE, et al. 2009 ACCF/AHA Focused Update on perioperative beta-blockade. *J Am Coll Cardiol* 2009;54:2102–2128.)

guidelines on patients undergoing aortic surgery at a single institution in Switzerland. The authors compared rates of noninvasive testing, cardiac catheterization, and revascularization, as well as rates of cardiac complications in 468 consecutive patients undergoing aortic surgery. Data were compared between those patients whose surgery occurred after implementation of the 1996 guidelines versus those who underwent surgery before. Prior to implementation of the guidelines, only 35% of patients facing elective aortic surgery underwent noninvasive cardiac testing prior to surgery and only 8% received beta-blocker therapy peri-operatively. After implementation of the guidelines, these investigators showed that 64% of patients facing major aortic surgery underwent appropriate noninvasive testing and 58% received perioperative beta-blockade. These practice changes were associated with a dramatic reduction in rates of perioperative cardiac events.

In another study from the University of Michigan in the United States, perioperative evaluation of 95 consecutive patients undergoing aortic surgery was compared to historical controls. The historical controls in this study underwent preoperative noninvasive testing in 88% of cases. After guideline implementation, testing was reduced to 47% with no negative effect on perioperative death or MI rates. These studies demonstrate a change in perioperative practice patterns that was brought about by implementation of the current guidelines. Using the current guidelines, institutions can reduce utilization of precious resources such as stress testing and/or revascularization and simultaneously preserve (if not improve) operative outcomes.

CONCLUSIONS

Proper preoperative evaluation and reduction of perioperative risk for patients with PVD should follow the same tenets of clinical evaluation and care as for any other medical condition. Clinical assessment alone, based on an informed history and physical examination, can capture risk prior to noncardiac surgery in the majority of patients. PVD may limit this clinical assessment, as functional status may be curtailed by claudication. Selective testing may identify patients at increased risk or those that would benefit long-term from coronary revascularization. This process should utilize stress testing only selectively where test results are likely to change management. Beta-blockers appear to lower risk in those considered very high-risk patients for perioperative cardiac events. However, perioperative beta blockade has a dark side, requiring controlled, strategic implementation only in those where the absolute benefit of such therapy is apparent. The recently updated ACCF/AHA 2009 Guidelines for Perioperative Cardiovascular Evaluation for Non-Cardiac Surgery provide a useful synthesis of the existing literature to guide perioperative therapies.

PRACTICAL POINTS

■ The goal of perioperative evaluation is not to clear patients for surgery but to accurately assess and minimize risk.

■ Patients with favorable invasive/noninvasive testing in the past 2 years need no further cardiac workup if asymptomatic since the test and functionally very active.

■ Patients with changing symptoms/signs of ischemia should be considered for further evaluation only if such testing is likely to alter management.

■ Poor functional capacity or a combination of high-risk surgery and moderate functional capacity in a patient with intermediate clinical predictors of cardiac risk (especially if there are two or more) often requires further noninvasive cardiac testing.

RECOMMENDED READING

Boersma E, Poldermans D, Bax JJ, et al. Predictors of cardiac events after major vascular surgery: role of clinical characteristics, dobutamine echocardiography, and beta-blocker therapy. *JAMA* 2001;285(14):1865–1873.

Cohn SL, Goldman L. Preoperative risk evaluation and perioperative management of patients with coronary artery disease. *Med Clin North Am* 2003;87(1):111–136.

Durazzo AE, Machado FS, Ikeoka DT, et al. Reduction in cardiovascular events after vascular surgery with atorvastatin: a randomized trial. *J Vasc Surg* 2004;39:967–975.

Eagle KA, Coley CM, Newell JB, et al. Combining clinical and thallium data optimizes preoperative assessment of cardiac risk before major vascular surgery. *Ann Intern Med* 1989;110(11):859–866.

Fleischmann KE, Beckman JA, Buller CE, et al. ACCF/AHA Focused Update on perioperative beta-blockade. *J Am Coll Cardiol* 2009;54:2102–2128.

Froehlich JB, Karavite D, Russman PL, et al. American College of Cardiology/American Heart Association preoperative assessment guidelines reduce resource utilization before aortic surgery. *J Vasc Surg* 2002;36(4):758–763.

Goldman L, Caldera DL, Nussbaum SR, et al. Multifactorial index of cardiac risk in noncardiac surgical procedures. *N Engl J Med* 1977;297(16):845–850.

Lee TH, Marcantonio ER, Manqione CM, et al. Derivation and prospective validation of a simple index for prediction of cardiac risk of major noncardiac surgery. *Circulation* 1999;100(10):1043–1049.

Licker M, Khatchatourian G, Schweizer A, et al. The impact of a cardioprotective protocol on the incidence of cardiac complications after aortic abdominal surgery. *Anesth Analg* 2002;95(6):1525–1533.

L'Italien GJ, Paul SD, Hendel RC, et al. Development and validation of a Bayesian model for perioperative cardiac risk assessment in a cohort of 1,081 vascular surgical candidates. *J Am Coll Cardiol* 1996;27(4):779–786.

Mangano DT, Layug EL, Wallace A, et al. Effect of atenolol on mortality and cardiovascular morbidity after noncardiac surgery. Multicenter Study of Perioperative Ischemia Research Group. *N Engl J Med* 1996;335(23):1713–1720.

McDermott MM, McCarthy W. Intermittent claudication. The natural history. *Surg Clin North Am* 1995;75(4):581–591.

McFalls EO, Ward HB, Moritz TE, et al. Coronary-artery revascularization Prophylaxis (CARP trial) before elective vascular surgery. *N Engl J Med* 2004;351:2795–2804.

Mukherjee D, Eagle KA. Perioperative cardiac assessment for non-cardiac surgery: eight steps to the best possible outcome. *Circulation* 2003;107:2771–2774.

Poldermans D, Bax JJ, Boersma E, et al. Guidelines for pre-operative cardiac risk assessment and perioperative cardiac management in noncardiac surgery. *Eur Heart J* 2009;30:2769–2812.

Poldermans D, Boersma E, Bax JJ, et al. The effect of bisoprolol on perioperative mortality and myocardial infarction in high-risk patients undergoing vascular surgery. Dutch Echocardiographic Cardiac Risk Evaluation Applying Stress Echocardiography Study Group. *N Engl J Med* 1999;341(24):1789–1794.

Schouten O, Boersma E, Hoeks SE, et al. Fluvastatin and perioperative events in patients undergoing vascular surgery. *N Engl J Med* 2009;361:980–989.

Vicenzi MN, Meislitzer T, Heitzinger B, et al. Coronary artery stenting and non-cardiac surgery-a prospective outcome study. *Br J Anaesth* 2006;96:686–693.

Ward RP, Leeper NJ, Kirkpatrick JN, et al. The effect of preoperative statin therapy on cardiovascular outcomes in patients undergoing infrainguinal vascular surgery. *Int J Cardiol* 2005;104:264–268.

Wijeysundera DN, Naik JS, Beattie WS. Alpha-2 adrenergic agonists to prevent perioperative cardiovascular complications: a meta-analysis [comment]. *Am J Med* 2003;114(9):742–752.

Williams TM, Harken AH. Statins for surgical patients. *Ann Surg* 2008;247:30–37.

CHAPTER 29 ■ Bypass Grafts: Surgical Aspects and Complications

Siddharth Bhende and Patrick S. Vaccaro

VASCULAR CONDUITS

Modern vascular surgical bypass grafts are credited to work done by Carrel in the early 1900s where he described the use of autogenous vein bypass grafts in dogs. Since then there have been long-standing attempts to identify the best conduit for arterial reconstruction. The success of vascular bypasses depends on certain host characteristics including the quality of inflow, quality of outflow, and the characteristics of the bypass graft. These graft characteristics vary depending on whether it is a biologic or manufactured graft.

The ideal graft would be readily available in a variety of sizes, be antithrombogenic, and provide long-term durability and patency. It should be easy to handle and elastic to account for the normal pulsatility of the artery. The graft should be biocompatible, as antigenicity can promote an intense inflammatory response and promote thrombosis. Currently, the ideal vascular graft does not exist and so we must make do with a variety of natural and prosthetic conduits, which will be discussed in more detail below (Table 29.1).

Vein Grafts

Vein grafts can be obtained from a variety of locations, but the most common site is the greater saphenous vein (GSV) (Fig. 29.1). The length and diameter of the GSV make it suitable for a variety of different bypasses. However, the saphenous vein may not be usable in 10 to 20% of cases for a variety of reasons, including previous saphenectomy for coronary or lower extremity revascularization, history of superficial phlebitis, poor caliber, or congenital absence. Contralateral GSV is an excellent choice for lower extremity revascularization if the ipsilateral vein is not available. In patients with peripheral artery disease, one must be cautious that the patient will be able to heal the vein harvest site from the contralateral leg. The lesser saphenous vein is another source for autogenous vein conduit. It generally extends from the lateral border of the Achille's tendon to the popliteal fossa where it drains into the popliteal vein. During its harvest, the surgeon must be careful to avoid injuring the sural nerve. Upper extremity veins (basilic and cephalic) can also be used as autogenous vein alternatives. However, there is much variability in the size and duplication of these veins. Futhermore, in patients who have undergone repeated venipuncture these veins may be quite sclerotic.

There are a number of factors that can affect the patency of vein bypass grafts. These include the pressure at which the vein is distended at the time

TABLE 29.1

TYPES OF VASCULAR BYPASS CONDUITS

- Autologous vein grafts
- Arterial autografts
- Biologic grafts
  - Umbilical vein grafts
  - Cryopreserved grafts
- Prosthetic grafts
- Composite grafts
- Endovascular grafts

of harvest, the use of vasoactive substances to dilate the vein, and the temperature at which the vein is stored after harvest and prior to implantation. Overdistension of a venous conduit has a negative effect on the biologic responsiveness of the graft. If the distending pressure exceeds 200 mm Hg, significant endothelial cell dysfunction is observed. The use of vasoactive substances, such as papaverine, helps to preserve endothelial morphology. Cold storage of a vein graft is deleterious, but storage at body temperature is ideal for preserving endothelial cell function and prostacyclin production.

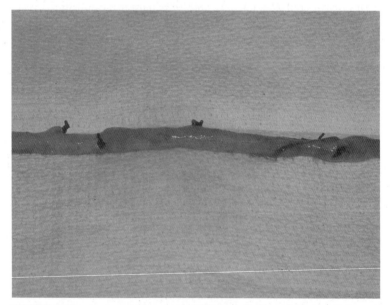

FIGURE 29-1.   A segment of harvested GSV. Note the ligated side branches—care was taken not to impinge on the lumen of the graft while ligating the side branches. The vein is gently dilated with a warm papaverine solution.

Care must be taken in harvesting vein grafts to prevent undue traction or pressure on the vein as well as to minimize handling. The vein can be removed through continuous or skip incisions. The use of skip incisions has been advocated when harvesting GSV to decrease the incidence of wound complications. Side branches are mobilized and ligated with silk sutures and hemoclips. Care must be taken to prevent crimping of the vein lumen during ligation of the side branches. Vein graft size is also important when determining whether a segment of vein is suitable for use as a bypass conduit. In general, veins less than 3 mm in diameter have lower patency rates. Vein sizes can be assessed preoperatively with the use of duplex ultrasonography (DUS). Smaller veins can be used if no other suitable conduit is available, but it requires meticulous dissection and the use of pharmacologic agents to prevent vasospasm. If a single segment of vein is not of adequate length for a bypass, particularly in lower extremity revascularization, multiple segments of veins can be spliced together. The patency rate of these spliced veins is less than that of a single piece of vein of adequate length.

Once implanted all vein grafts undergo morphologic changes in response to the hemodynamic forces of the arterial circulation. This process is termed arterialization and is a normal adaptive response. In some cases, however, the vein graft can deteriorate over time. Deterioration occurs in the first 30 days and is generally due to technical errors, patient selection, and the initial quality of the conduit. Between 30 days and 2 years of time, vein grafts can develop neointimal hyperplasia at anastomotic and valvulolysis sites. This occurs in approximately 10 to 30% of patients with the majority occurring within the first 12 months. After 24 months, changes that occur are generally due to progression of atherosclerosis. Aneurysmal degeneration of vein grafts can occur with time and is discussed later in more detail.

Arterial Grafts

Arterial bypass grafts are widely accepted as the best bypass conduit currently available. Many of their innate properties allow them to function with superiority. Arterial grafts are able to maintain their viability, do not degenerate with time, are resistant to infection, and demonstrate proportional growth when used in children. Arterial conduits are harvested from three main sites within the normal vascular tree: the internal iliac artery, the external iliac artery, and the superficial femoral artery. Most often, these donor sites can then be reconstructed using prosthetic conduits which are better tolerated in these locations than the original site of bypass. In children and young adults, the internal iliac artery has been harvested with no postoperative morbidity and no long-term morbidity. Even the thrombosed superficial femoral artery can be harvested to use as a bypass conduit. Patency is restored by performing an eversion endarterectomy of the resected portion. Most arterial bypass grafts are used in the abdomen for visceral vessel reconstruction or in the groin region. Due to size and availability, arterial conduits are rarely used in the aortic location or for lower extremity arterial bypass.

Biologic Grafts

When venous and arterial bypass grafts are not suitable, the surgeon must find another source for an adequate conduit. A variety of different conduits have been studied over the years and a few of the grafts that are still in clinical use are described here.

Umbilical Vein Grafts

The human umbilical cord provides approximately 50 cm of vein that can be dilated up to 7 mm in diameter. Initial experience involved the use of unmodified heterografts. Problems with immunologic rejection generally occurred several weeks after implantation. Rejection can lead to thrombosis or graft degeneration. This led to the use of glutaraldehyde-tanned umbilical veins. These grafts retain their basic architectural structure and the tanning process leads to protein cross-linking that increases the tensile strength of the grafts and masks its antigenicity. There are still instances of umbilical vein graft aneurysmal degeneration and therefore the graft is often wrapped in a polyester mesh.

Cryopreserved Grafts

Harvested vein and arterial segments from cadavers can be frozen for later use. Initial results with cryopreserved allografts resulted in high rates of immunologically derived biologic degradation and subsequent aneurysmal degeneration, calcification, rupture, and occlusion. Current cryopreservation techniques involve the use of cryoprotectants such as dimethylsulfoxide, atraumatic harvest of the vessel, and ultra-low-temperature freezing with liquid nitrogen. It has been reported that cryopreserved grafts can be stored up to a few years. Cryopreservation has been shown to preserve endothelium and reduce thrombogenicity. Degeneration of these grafts that is not attributable to immunologic rejection has been reported, including intimal disruption, luminal fibrin deposition, and cellular infiltrates in the media. Degenerative changes in the allograft are the major drawback of this technique. It has been suggested that a low dose of immunosuppression may prevent aneurysm formation, but many hesitate to use these drugs because of their serious potential adverse effects.

Prosthetic Grafts

Autogenous grafts are not always available or may be of inadequate length or caliber. The development of prosthetic vascular grafts arose to provide a substitute conduit in the absence of adequate autogenous material. Grafts are constructed in a variety of ways that affect their porosity, thrombogenicity, and compliance in order to help them mimic autogenous grafts. There are criteria that a prosthetic graft must meet in order to become an adequate conduit. First, the material must be biocompatible and free of toxic, allergic, and carcinogenic side effects. There is some reaction of the host to the foreign material, but this tissue reactivity is often a desirable response leading to incorporation of the graft. Second, the graft must be durable and resist degradation and deterioration with time. Third, the graft should be readily available in a variety of lengths and diameters and should have adequate flexibility, yet be resistant to kinking.

Porosity of prosthetic grafts is an important structural characteristic. The material obviously needs to be impervious to blood, but a porous framework has many potential advantages. Initial investigations suggested that a greater degree of porosity would promote fibrous encapsulation of the graft. Autogenous tissue ingrowth through the pores would initiate and provide adherence for a stable intimal lining. It has been hypothesized that unhindered ingrowth of tissue through large pores correlated with improved patency. This hypothesis has never been proven. In fact ,it is more likely the innate thrombogenicity of the luminal graft surface plays a larger role in determining graft patency.

A variety of graft characteristics influence a prosthetic graft's thrombogenicity. Upon exposure to blood, the graft is immediately coated with serum proteins, in particular fibrinogen. The ability of these proteins to interact with the graft is dependent upon the chemical and physical properties of the graft material. Platelets then adhere to the graft surface proteins to become activated, recruit more platelets, and activate local hemostatic reactions. The graft surface becomes lined with proteinaceous material and compacted fibrin to produce a pseudointima. Continuation of this process may lead to graft thrombosis. Much research has been devoted in attempts to "seed" prosthetic grafts with endothelial cells with the hopes of causing a complete endothelial lining, decreasing pseudointima formation and improving patency rates.

Graft compliance is an important mechanical property of grafts that affects their performance. Compliance is the ability of the graft to expand radially in response to increased pressure. In autogenous grafts this is related to the proportion of elastin and collagen within the vessel wall. Prosthetic grafts tend to be less compliant than autogenous grafts. Compliance has been shown to be directly related to the rate of thrombogenicity, but it is difficult to discern this factor from the many others that can affect graft thrombosis. External support can also be applied to prosthetic grafts that will minimize such events as kinking and mechanical compression.

A variety of materials have been investigated as possible materials from which to fabricate grafts. Two materials that have proven durable over time include Dacron (polyethylene terephthalate) and PTFE (polytetrafluoroethylene) (Fig. 29.2). Dacron is constructed into bypass graft material by a process that involves weaving, knitting, or braiding of the polymer yarns. Dacron grafts provide the advantage of decreased bleeding and better long-term integrity with lower chance of aneurysmal degeneration. The disadvantage of the Dacron graft is that it has a tendency to fray at cut edges decreasing compliance. The PTFE graft (Fig. 29.3) is an expanded polymer manufactured by a heating and mechanical stretching process and extruded through a die, producing a porous material that has solid nodes interconnected by fine fibrils. The material is chemically inert, electronegative, and hydrophobic. A thin layer of outer reinforcement is

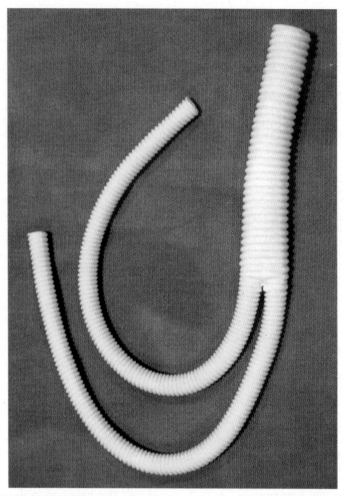

FIGURE 29-2. A Dacron prosthetic, bifurcated graft. Note the crimping along the length of the graft. The main body would be anastomosed to the aorta, while the smaller, bifurcated ends would be anastomosed to the iliac or femoral arteries.

added to prevent aneurysmal degeneration. PTFE grafts are generally more porous than Dacron grafts which promotes bleeding. Despite its increased porosity, minimal tissue ingrowth occurs, although the graft does become incorporated into the surrounding connective tissue. PTFE grafts are often supported with rings or coils, which may prevent external compression or kinking. The main disadvantage is the lower compliance, even when compared with Dacron grafts.

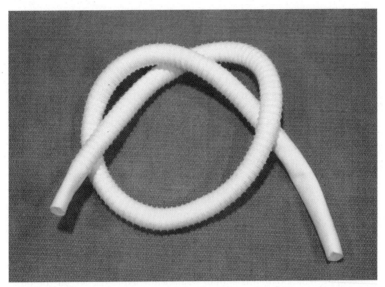

FIGURE 29-3. An ePTFE graft. Note the flexibility and resistance to kinking. The graft is externally supported with rings that help to protect against compression.

Composite Grafts

When an autogenous vein graft is available for bypass, but its length is not sufficient, as is seen in up to one third of lower extremity arterial reconstructions, a composite graft can be considered. Longer prosthetic grafts have a greater incidence of thrombosis compared with vein grafts, due to the increased thrombogenicity of the prosthetic graft's surface and lower flow rates occurring through these long grafts to smaller outflow vessels. Composite graft is a hybrid graft where the proximal portion of the graft is prosthetic and the distal portion is autogenous vein graft. The advantage of the composite graft is use of the more compliant and flexible vein graft to traverse the knee joint. The vein graft also facilitates anastomosis to the smaller diseased distal vessel, which may reduce the incidence of anastomotic narrowing.

GRAFT SELECTION

When selecting a graft for a particular arterial reconstructive procedure, the surgeon must weigh the advantages and disadvantages of the graft such as graft patency, convenience of use, and absence of complications. There is obviously controversy that arises in many situations as to which graft is most appropriate for particular situations.

In aortic reconstruction, size and length requirements nearly preclude the use of autogenous vein and arterial grafts. For these reasons, a prosthetic graft is generally required. In the location of the thoracic and abdominal aorta, bleeding is often of main concern and tightly woven Dacron grafts tend to be preferred; they also have excellent dimensional integrity and prolonged patency rates.

The preferred conduit for lower extremity bypass graft is the use of GSV. This can be placed in an in situ, reversed or nonreversed fashion. The valves need to be lysed if the vein is used in an in situ or nonreversed fashion. It can also be placed in a reversed fashion, but this may cause a significant size mismatch at the sites of anastomosis. The use of autogenous vein graft is highly preferable for all lower extremity bypasses. When it is unavailable, the alternatives are not as attractive given their lower patency rates. In addition, whenever a graft is being placed in an infected field, regardless of the location, preference is given to vein grafts as they have an increased resistance to infection compared with other biologic or prosthetic grafts.

Most extra-anatomic bypasses (i.e., femoral-femoral bypass, axillo-femoral bypass) are performed with PTFE. This is due to the lower incidence of hematoma formation from graft leakage and its resistance to kinking. This graft is also particularly amenable to graft thrombectomy, an important characteristic to consider in these types of bypasses.

SURGICAL CONSIDERATIONS

In deciding which conduits should be used for bypasses, one of the most important considerations is obtaining the appropriate size match between the native artery and conduit. Often an appropriate autograft can be obtained from a source within the same operative field. When this is not found, sources should be sought from other locations, provided it does not add significantly to the morbidity of the operation. If none is available, alternate sources of bypass conduit are needed.

Aortic Grafts

Aortic grafts are placed for treatment of aortoiliac occlusive disease as well as in the presence of aneurysmal disease. For aortoiliac occlusive disease the aorta may be approached through a midline or retroperitoneal incision. The retroperitoneal incision is advantageous in patients who have had multiple previous abdominal operations. The prosthetic graft is anastomosed to the aorta in either an end-to-end or an end-to-side technique. After completion of the proximal anastomosis, the graft is tunneled along the anatomic path of the iliac arteries. Care must be taken to pass the graft posterior to the ureter and to avoid juxtaposition with the bowel. The graft limbs are then anastomosed distally to the common femoral arteries. If there is significant disease at the orifice of the superficial femoral artery, the graft toe is extended onto the deep femoral artery. Aortofemoral bypass grafts have excellent long-term outcomes. Graft patency for standard repairs approach 85 to 90% at 5 years and 70 to 75% at 10 years. Thoraco-femoral bypass grafts have similar patency rates. These procedures are generally performed with few complications and have 30-day mortality rates of 2 to 3% in most large centers.

The repair of abdominal aortic aneurysm (AAA) is performed in a similar fashion. The aorta can be approached through a midline or retroperitoneal incision. The proximal anastomosis is performed in an end-to-end fashion. The distal anastomosis can often be performed to the terminal aorta, if it is not aneurysmal, or a bifurcated graft is used and anastomosed to the common iliac artery. In patients who can physiologically tolerate aortic surgery, the long-term durability is excellent with mortality rates less than 5% at most centers. In order to provide an improved approach to treatment of AAA, endovascular stent graft technology has been developed. This approach allows for the placement of a graft from within the arteries through the common femoral artery.

Extra-anatomic Grafts

Axillo-femoral and femoral–femoral bypass grafts are generally used in patients in whom multiple comorbidities exist, preventing direct aortoiliac reconstruction. Axillo-femoral grafts are constructed by providing inflow from the axillary artery exposed through an infraclavicular incision. Appropriate preoperative evaluation must be made to ensure the absence of more proximal brachiocephalic occlusive disease. The graft is generally constructed of externally supported PTFE. The graft is tunneled along the anterior axillary line and the distal anastomosis is performed to the common femoral artery. Patency rates for axillo-femoral bypass grafts have been significantly lower than for aorto-femoral bypass grafts. Five-year patency rates have been reported to range from 30 to 70%.

Femoral-femoral artery bypass graft is generally reserved for patients with unilateral iliac artery occlusive disease. The graft is anastomosed to the donor femoral artery, passed in a suprapubic subcutaneous tunnel, and anastomosed to the recipient femoral artery. Vein grafts have not been shown to provide better patency rates and are therefore reserved for use in infected fields. Five-year patency rates have ranged from 50 to 80%. Given an adequately patent profunda femoris artery, superficial femoral artery occlusion does not adversely affect long-term patency rates.

Lower Extremity Grafts

In lower extremity bypass grafts, vein grafts can be used in a reversed fashion, a nonreversed fashion or left in situ. The nonreversed and in situ grafts require disruption of the vein valves prior to their use. There are a variety of arguments made with regard to which method of bypass is most appropriate. The nonreversed and in situ grafts often provide a better size match for the proximal and distal vessels, particularly when the distal anastomosis is performed to an infrageniculate vessel. However these grafts do require intraluminal instrumentation to disrupt the valves, which injures the endothelium. The valves, despite being disrupted, may later prove a problem if an intact cusp becomes sclerotic. Reverse vein grafts can lead to a significant size mismatch between the native artery and vein graft. Currently there is no literature demonstrating statistically significant patency rates for reversed versus nonreversed versus in situ saphenous vein grafts. In general, patients who have surgery for limb-threatening ischemia have less desirable outcomes than do those who are operated on for disabling claudication. Femoral to above-the-knee bypass grafts with saphenous vein grafts have 5-year patency rates that approach 80%, whereas in infrageniculate bypasses this rate decreases to 60%.

Glutaraldehyde-stabilized human umbilical vein graft can be used for revascularization of the lower extremity in patients with peripheral vascular occlusive disease when adequate autologous vein is not available. During implantation several important technical points must be observed. These grafts must be handled gently as intimal fracture and extensive mural dissection of blood can occur if the graft is handled in a rough manner or if standard clamps are applied. It is suggested that the toe and the heel of the graft be anastomosed with interrupted sutures, which is not generally performed in saphenous vein grafts. The glutaraldehyde-treated human umbilical vein grafts must be tunneled through a rigid tunnel device in order to prevent damage to the polyester mesh. Outcomes for umbilical vein grafts in lower extremity reconstruction have reported primary patency rates of 61 and 39% for femoral to popliteal artery and tibial artery bypasses, respectively. Secondary patency rates are improved to 67 and 51% with limb salvage rates of 80 and 68% at 5 years, respectively. Despite better control of biodegradation in recent versions, there are still reported rates of aneurysmal degeneration in 36% of the umbilical vein grafts, and a 21% incidence of dilation after 5 years of implantation. Umbilical vein grafts have been used in locations such as aorto-renal bypasses and extraanatomic bypasses (axillo-femoral and femoral-femoral bypasses), but they have been shown to offer no clear advantage over other conduits, including prosthetics, in these regions.

The external iliac artery and the superficial femoral artery provide excellent conduits for bypasses of the common femoral artery, deep femoral artery, and popliteal artery. The lengths of diseased segments in these lesions are generally short and there are good diameter matches between the arterial homografts and the sites for bypass. The arterial homograft, given its ability to grow and resist infection, is the ideal conduit for reconstruction after oncologic surgery, particularly in children and young adults.

Prosthetic bypass grafts are used in lower extremity bypass grafting when no other conduit is available. They provide the benefit of allowing for shorter operative times and fewer incisions. However, the patency rates for prosthetic grafts are inferior to saphenous vein graft. Femoral to above-the-knee popliteal artery bypass grafts have 5-year primary patency rates of approximately 50%, with secondary patency rates of 60 to 70%. Infrageniculate and distal bypasses performed with prosthetic grafts have poor patency rates reported from 25 to 60% at 2 to 4 years. If some adequate vein is available, but is not of adequate length, a composite graft can be constructed. Patency rates for these bypass constructions have approached 40 to 50% at 4 years.

COMPLICATIONS

Graft Thrombosis

Bypass graft failure secondary to thrombosis does not occur infrequently. Determining the etiology of the thrombosis is crucial to formulating a treatment plan. It is imperative to assess the quality of inflow, quality of outflow, and the conduit for all bypass graft thrombosis. Patients presenting with acute graft thrombosis and evidence of acute limb ischemia should undergo immediate anticoagulation and surgical intervention. This would entail balloon catheter thrombectomy followed by an angiogram and subsequent revision of the graft. Patients with less severe symptoms may undergo thrombolysis of the graft, which would uncover the etiology of the graft thrombosis, and help prepare for the definitive intervention. No single approach is appropriate for all patients and thus the intervention performed must be tailored to the individual situation.

Graft Infection

The diagnosis and management of aortoiliac graft infections is quite difficult. Patients can present with a variety of symptoms ranging from nonspecific symptoms of fever and malaise to purulent discharge from a wound. Most patients undergo evaluation with computed tomography (CT) or magnetic resonance imaging (MRI) as well as angiography. Treatment involves the complete removal of all infected graft material and reconstruction which is challenging. Often patients undergo a staged procedure. In stage I an axillo-femoral or axillo-popliteal artery bypass (bilaterally if the infection involves both limbs) is performed. In stage II the entire graft is excised and the aortic stump is ligated. Others have advocated a one-stage approach if the patient is able to withstand the surgery. Other options include using reconstruction with superficial femoral-popliteal veins. In this technique the superficial femoral-popliteal vein is harvested and anastomosed to create a new aortic graft. In addition, experience is growing with the use of cryopreserved aortic allografts for reconstruction after removal of infected aortic grafts.

Treatment of lower extremity graft infection involves the control of systemic infection with antibiotics, excision of all infected tissue and graft material and preservation of blood flow. The most common infective organisms include *Staphylococcus epidermidis*, *S. aureus*, and *Escherichia coli*. Graft infections in the lower extremity often present as a draining sinus or mass. There is no specific test to diagnose graft infections, but most patients undergo one of the following: US, CT, MRI, or radioisotope-tagged white blood cell scan. Almost all patients undergoing treatment for an infected lower extremity graft infection should have preoperative arteriography. Patients should have the infected graft and surrounding infected tissue excised. Anastomotic sites can be closed primarily or with a vein patch. If the limb is not acutely threatened, revascularization should be delayed until the infection has cleared. If immediate reconstruction is necessary, vein grafts are the preferred bypass conduits. Attempts should be made to keep the path of the new bypass in an anatomic field that is separate for the previous graft. Another option in reconstructing the circulation after removal of an infected graft is using a prosthetic conduit to perform an extra-anatomic bypass. The glutaraldehyde-treated human umbilical vein graft, although not immune to infection, is imparted with some degree of infection resistance due to the tanning process. The incidence of infection in umbilical vein grafts is consistent with the rates seen for saphenous vein grafts (less than 3%).

Graft Pseudoaneurysm

Pseudoaneurysm formation occurs in prosthetic grafts at the site of proximal or distal anastomosis. Numerous factors have been implicated in the development of the anastomotic pseudoaneurysm including suture failure, graft infection, graft dilation, end-to-side anastomosis, and arterial degeneration. Most anastomotic aneurysms are asymptomatic and identified incidentally either on physical examination or during another diagnostic test. Pseudoaneurysms can develop at any time following graft placement. Early development generally signifies technical error or graft infection, while late development implies arterial wall degeneration. Repair involves resecting the pseudoaneurysm and replacing it with an interposition graft.

Aneurysmal degeneration of saphenous vein grafts can also occur and are primarily seen in children. This is due to the fact that in children the vein is dependent on an extensive network of vaso vasorum for continued vein wall nourishment which is disrupted during vein harvest. Aneurysmal degeneration of umbilical vein grafts is unusual because the superior tanning technology and use of a polyester mesh have contributed to preservation of the intrinsic anatomy and greater resistance to biodegradation.

Lymph Leak

The exact incidence of groin lymphatic complications is not known, but these are estimated to occur in 1 to 2% of patients. Careful dissection with ligation of all divided lymphatic vessels helps to prevent the development of lymph leak. However, factors that increase the risk of developing lymph leak include advanced age, repeated groin dissection, and extensive deep femoral artery dissection. Patients with a groin lymphocele present with a nontender, nonerythematous swelling in the groin. An ultrasound interrogation reveals a hypoechogenic mass. Aspiration reveals clear fluid with no white blood cells or bacteria and a protein content of 0.5 to 2 g/dL. Treatment by aspiration has limited success and risks the introduction of bacteria into a field with prosthetic material. Most surgeons will attempt aspiration for a lymphocele only once before proceeding with operative intervention. Although lymphocutaneous fistulas have previously been treated conservatively as well, most surgeons currently proceed to early surgical intervention. Surgery involves re-exploration of the groin with ligation of all leaking lymphatics. This can be assisted by subcutaneous injection of vital blue dye in the first web space between the first and second toe. The dye will be carried in the lymphatic system and can be seen pooling in the wound at the site of lymphatic leak.

Lymphatic disruption can also occur within the abdomen after aortic dissection resulting in chyloperitoneum. This is a rare complication and most patients present several weeks after surgery, once they have resumed a normal diet, and the chyle has had a chance to accumulate in the abdomen to a degree that causes symptoms. Patients often present with abdominal distention, nausea, vomiting, and early satiety. Paracentesis offers the definitive diagnosis. Initial management is conservative with the institution of a high-protein, low-fat diet supplemented with medium-chain triglycerides. If this is not successful, the patient's oral intake is restricted and is started on parenteral nutrition. Rarely is the placement of a peritoneal venous shunt required.

SPECIAL ISSUES

The most common cause of vein graft failure in the first 24 months after infrainguinal revascularization is the development of neointimal hyperplasia. This develops in 10 to 30% of bypass grafts, with the majority occurring within the first 12 months. These lesions are often detected on routine vein graft surveillance DUS, which is used to monitor grafts in the postoperative period with the intent of identifying potential areas of graft stenosis and compromise and intervening prior to graft thrombosis. Once identified, these lesions can be treated by a variety of techniques including open surgical patch angioplasty, bypass, or percutaneous balloon angioplasty.

CONCLUSION

There are a variety of options for bypass conduits, but none are ideal. Prosthetic grafts are an excellent option when aortic reconstruction is performed. Lower extremity revascularization should primarily be performed with GSV grafts. When these are not available, alternate sources must be utilized but result in significantly lower patency rates. The type of conduit used depends on multiple factors including patient's anatomy, availability of the graft and should be tailored specifically to each patient.

PRACTICAL POINTS

■ There are no ideal vascular conduits currently available.

■ GSV is the bypass conduit of choice for lower extremity reconstruction.

■ Alternate sources of conduit, such as prosthetic grafts and other biologic grafts, can be used for lower extremity revascularization, but have lower patency rates.

■ Aortic reconstruction can be performed with high patency rates with the use of large-diameter prosthetic grafts.

■ Extraanatomic grafts should be preferentially performed with prosthetic grafts as they have low porosity and are highly resistant to kinking. Vein grafts have shown no improved patency and are thus reserved for infected fields.

■ Multiple complications can occur with arterial reconstruction, but these can be limited by meticulous surgical techniques.

RECOMMENDED READING

Abbott WM, Purcell PN. Vascular grafts: characteristics and routine selection of prostheses. In: Moore WS, ed. *Vascular surgery: a comprehensive review*, 5th ed. Philadelphia: W. B. Saunders, 1998:399–414.

Angle N, Dorafsher AH, Farooq MM, et al. The evolution of the axillofemoral bypass over two decades. *Ann Vasc Surg* 2002;16:742–745.

Bandyk DF. Postoperative surveillance of infrainguinal bypass. *Surg Clin North Am* 1990;70(1):71–85.

Brewster DC. Prosthetic grafts. In: Rutherford RB, ed. *Vascular surgery*, 5th ed. Philadelphia: W. B. Saunders, 2000:559–584.

Criado E, Farber MA. Femorofemoral bypass: appropriate application based on factors affecting outcome. *Semin Vasc Surg* 1997;10:34–41.

Dardik G, Wengerter K. Biologic grafts for lower limb revascularization. In: Rutherford RB, ed. *Vascular surgery*, 5th ed. Philadelphia: W. B. Saunders, 2000:549–558.

Faruqi RM, Stoney RJ. The arterial autograft. In: Rutherford RB, ed. *Vascular surgery*, 5th ed. Philadelphia: W. B. Saunders, 2000:532–539.

Green RM, Abbott WM, Matsumoto T, et al. Prosthetic above-knee femoropopliteal bypass grafting five-year results of a randomized trial. *J Vasc Surg* 2000;31:417–425.

Hertzer NR, Mascha EJ, Karafa MT, et al. Open infrarenal abdominal aortic aneurysm repair: the Cleveland Clinic experience from 1989 to 1998. *J Vasc Surg* 2002;1145–1154.

Johnson WC, Lee KK. A comparative evaluation of polytetrafluorethylene, umbilical vein, and saphenous vein bypass grafts for femoral-popliteal above-knee revascularization: a prospective randomized Department of Veterans Affairs cooperative study. *J Vasc Surg* 2000;32:268–277.

Kempczinski RF. Vascular conduits: an overview. In: Rutherford RB, ed. *Vascular surgery*, 5th ed. Philadelphia: W. B. Saunders, 2000:527–532.

Leseche G, Castier Y, Petie M-D, et al. Long-term results of cryopreserved arterial allograft reconstruction in infected prosthetic grafts and mycotic aneurysms of the abdominal aorta. *J Vasc Surg* 2001;34:616–622.

McCarthy WJ, Mesh CL, McMillan WD, et al. Descending thoracic aorta-to-femoral artery bypass: ten years' experience with a durable procedure. *J Vasc Surg* 1993;17:336–348.

McCarthy WJ, Pearce WH, Flinn WR, et al. Long-term evaluation of composite sequential bypass for limb threatening ischemia. *J Vasc Surg* 1992;15:761–770.

Mii S, Mori A, Sakata H, et al. Para-anastomotic aneurysms: incidence, risk factors, treatment and prognosis. *J Cardiovasc Surg* 1998;39:259–266.

Ouriel K. Endovascular repair of abdominal aortic aneurysms: the Cleveland Clinic experience with five different devices. *Semin Vasc Surg* 2003;16:8894.

Ouriel K, Greenberg RK, Clair DG. Endovascular treatment of aortic aneurysms. *Curr Prob Surg* 2002;39:233–348.

Pabst TS, McIntyre KE, Schilling JD, et al. Management of chyloperitoneum after abdominal aortic surgery. *Am J Surg* 1993;166:194–198.

Sanchez LA, Suggs WD, Marin ML, et al. Is percutaneous balloon angioplasty appropriate in the treatment of graft and anastomotic lesions responsible for failing vein bypasses? *Am J Surg* 1994;168:97–101.

Schwartz MA, Schanzer H, Skladany M, et al. A comparison of conservative therapy and early selective ligation in the treatment of lymphatic complications following vascular procedures. *Am J Surg* 1995;170:206–208.

Seidel SA, Modrall G, Jackson MR, et al. The superficial femoral-popliteal vein graft: a reliable conduit for large-caliber arterial and venous reconstructions. *Perspect Vasc Surg Endovasc Ther* 2001;14:57–80.

Shah DM, Darling RC, Chang BB, et al. Long-term results of in situ saphenous vein bypass. Analysis of 2058 cases. *Ann Surg* 1995;222:438–446.

STILE Investigators. Results of a prospective randomized trial evaluating surgery versus thrombolysis for ischemia of the lower extremity. *Ann Surg* 1994;220:251–268.

Szilagyi DE, Elliott JR, Smith RF, et al. A 30-year survey of the reconstructive surgical treatment of aortoiliac occlusive disease. *J Vasc Surg* 1986;3:421–436.

Towne JB. The autogenous vein. In: Rutherford RB, ed. *Vascular surgery*, 5th ed. Philadelphia: W. B. Saunders, 2000:539–549.

QUESTIONS

1. A 67-year-old male presents with severe tearing back pain that started 1 hour ago. On examination his blood pressure is 198/112 and pulse is 110. A CT of the chest reveals Type A aortic dissection. The best initial drug for his hypertension is:
A. Nitroprusside
B. Nitroglycerin
C. Beta-blocker
D. Hydralazine

2. Which of the following statements regarding the application of CTA in the assessment of acute abdominal aorta syndrome is incorrect?
A. CTA in addition to assessing the vasculature can also provide information on soft tissue structures including complications such as hemorrhage.
B. A noncontrast study may illustrate acute hemorrhage within an aortic dissection plane, perio-arotic, or retroperitoneal structures.
C. A precontrast study allows for comparison of subtle changes in thrombus opacification post contrast suggesting a slow bleed.
D. Delayed acquisitions 1 to 2 minutes post contrast can help identify slow hemorrhage
E. All of the above are correct

3. A 71-year-old female has been admitted to the hospital with recurrent, unexplained congestive heart failure and sudden, unexplained pulmonary edema. An abdominal CTA performed for vague abdominal pain during one of her hospitalizations had revealed severe left renal artery stenosis. The best course of action would be:
A. Confirm renal artery stenosis with ultrasound
B. Coronary angiography
C. High dose diuretic therapy
D. Revascularization

4. Optimal angiographic angle to assess origin of the mesenteric vessels is:
A. Anteroposterior
B. LAO 30 angulation
C. RAO 30 angulation
D. Lateral projection
E. Cranial 30 angulation

5. Which of these scenarios often require further cardiac testing?
A. A patient with poor functional capacity
B. Patient with high-risk surgery and moderate functional capacity
C. Patient with intermediate clinical predicators of cardiac risk
D. All of the above

6. The stent of preference for an ostial subclavian artery stenosis is:
A. Balloon expandable stent
B. Self expanding stainless steel stent
C. Self expanding nitinol stent
D. Balloon angioplasty alone is best

7. What is the best treatment for lower extremity prosthetic bypass graft infections?
A. Intravenous antibiotics
B. Complete graft excision with extraanatomic bypass
C. Complete graft excision without extraanatomic bypass
D. Local wound debridement

8. A 63-year-old former college basketball player is seen in your clinic with a complaint of lower extremity cramping and pain with walking. These symptoms are relieved with rest. He also notes hypertension and erectile dysfunction on review of systems. In addition to treatment for peripheral arterial disease, this patient should next undergo:
A. Noninvasive cardiac testing
B. Coronary angiogram
C. Trial of phosphodiesterase inhibitor Type 5 treatment
D. Penile Doppler ultrasound testing

9. A 40-year-old woman presents to the Emergency Department with pain and swelling of the left upper extremity after a day of moving heavy boxes into a new home. An upper extremity Duplex study shows occlusive thrombus in the left subclavian and axillary veins. What is the best therapeutic approach at this time?
A. Intravenous heparin and close observation for resolution of symptoms
B. Catheter directed thrombolysis
C. Systemic thrombolysis
D. Surgical thrombectomy

10. A 45-year-old male has been using a left IJ vein tunneled catheter for hemodialysis for the last 6 months. A left forearm radiocephalic AV fistula was placed about 3 weeks ago which seems to be developing well with good bruit and thrill. He is noted to have progressive swelling of his left forearm and hand. There is no pain or fever. Which one of the following is the best approach to this patient?
A. The fistula should be ligated immediately as it is causing steal syndrome.
B. The patient should be hospitalized for intravenous antibiotics for presumed infection.
C. A fistulogram should be done to detect and treat central vein stenosis.
D. An ultrasound evaluation of the forearm should be done to rule out a hematoma or abscess formation.
E. The progress of the fistula must be observed for 6 more weeks to let it mature prior to planning any further action.

11. A 63-year-old male presents with hypertension to your clinic. On exam his blood pressure is 159/93, and pulse is 78. He also shows you a copy of an abdominal ultrasound report which showed severe right renal artery stenosis and a small 3.2 cm abdominal aortic aneurysm. The antihypertensive of choice in this patient is:

A. Minoxidil
B. Prazosin
C. Hydralazine + nitrates
D. Lisinopril

12. A 77-year-old man is scheduled for aortic valve replacement due to aortic stenosis and a 48-mm supracoronary thoracic aortic aneurysm was noted on echocardiography. Which of the following should be done in addition to aortic valve replacement?

A. Yearly imaging of the aneurysm with CT angiography
B. Repeat echocardiogram 6 months after surgery to assess aortic size
C. Surgical repair of the aneurysm at the time of valve replacement
D. Genetic testing for fibrillin gene

13. Patients treated with phosphodiesterase inhibitors for vasculogenic erectile dysfunction have _____ likelihood of myocardial infarction relative to moderate exercise and should be avoided in patients on _____ therapy.

A. Increased; nitrate
B. Decreased; selective serotonin reuptake inhibitor
C. Increased; selective serotonin reuptake inhibitor
D. Equivalent; nitrate

14. A 60-year-old woman with a history of an idiopathic deep vein thrombosis 5 years ago presents with leg swelling for the past 2 weeks. She denies any pain or increased warmth of the leg. She recently returned from an 8-day trip to Germany. What is the best test to evaluate her current complaints?

A. Air plethysmography
B. Computed tomography (CT) venography
C. Descending venography
D. Duplex ultrasound

15. A 65-year-old female has advanced chronic kidney disease stage IV secondary to diabetes mellitus. During her recent hospitalization for foot infection her serum creatinine was noted to be 4 mg/dL. An AV fistula (AVF) is being planned. Regarding the role of vein mapping prior to the AV fistula placement, which of the following statements is true?

A. It reduces early AVF thrombosis.
B. It improves primary patency of AVF.
C. It reduces infection rate in permanent access.
D. It increases the number of potential AVF that can be created.
E. It improves maturation of AVF.

16. The following treatment approaches may be considered in the treatment of Buerger's disease except

A. ASA
B. Prednisone
C. IV Iloprost
D. Lumbar sympathectomy

17. A 54-year-old female presents with painful raised reddish lesions in the toes bilaterally (Fig. 30-1). The lesion began abruptly following several days of cold weather. They are pruritic. She denies smoking. There is no history of vascular disease in her family. Arterial pulses were normal bilaterally. The most likely diagnosis is:

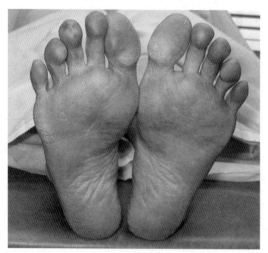

FIGURE 30-1.   (See color insert.)

A. Raynaud's disease
B. Pernio
C. Acrocyanosis
D. Buerger's disease

18. Patients with intermittent claudication (IC) can progress to limb threatening ischemia. All of the following statements regarding progression in IC patients is true except:
A. Progression of symptoms occurs in 25% of cases over a 5-year period.
B. The deterioration is most often during the first year after identification of cases.
C. Major amputation occurs in 10% of cases at 5 years.
D. A changing ABI is the best individual predictor of need for arterial surgery or major amputation.

19. All of the following constitute features of splenic artery aneurysm except:
A. Splenic artery aneurysms are commonly located in the hilum of the spleen.
B. Fibromuscular dysplasia is a common cause.
C. Rupture risk is heightened in pregnancy.
D. Splenic artery aneurysms are the commonest form of visceral artery aneurysms.

20. What is the treatment of choice for a patient with symptomatic significant large varicosities extending off the great saphenous vein and evidence

of superficial and deep reflux without relief with the use of grated compression stockings?
A. Venography and possible iliac stenting
B. Varicose vein excision only
C. Vein ablation and varicose vein excision
D. Deep system reconstruction

21. The signal used to create MRI images is most commonly obtained from:
A. Hydrogen nuclei
B. Oxygen nuclei
C. Carbon 13-nuclei
D. Nitrogen 14-nuclei

22. Carotid stenting is currently approved for the following indication:
A. Asymptomatic stenosis greater than 50%
B. Symptomatic stenosis greater than 50%
C. Asymptomatic stenosis greater than 70% at high risk for CEA
D. Symptomatic stenosis greater than 70% at high risk for CEA

23. The following conditions can predispose a patient to nephrogenic systemic fibrosis (NSF) with the administration of gadolinium contrast agents except?
A. GFR < 30 mL/min
B. Acute inflammatory state (e.g., sepsis)
C. High total dose of gadolinium
D. All the above can predispose patient to NSF

24. A 57-year-old woman presents with bilateral buttock numbness with walking 50 yards. These symptoms have been noticeable for the past 3 years, and have progressively worsened over the past 6 months. When the patient stops and stands, the numbness resolves within 5 minutes. She does not experience similar symptoms at rest, or with standing. Her right arm blood pressure is 170 mm Hg; left arm blood pressure is 200 mm Hg. The pressures via hand-held continuous wave Doppler are: right dorsalis pedis artery: 140 mm Hg; posterior tibial artery: 130 mm Hg; left dorsalis pedis artery: 110 mm Hg; posterior tibial artery: 90 mm Hg. Which of the following is true?
A. Based on the history and Doppler pressures, the symptoms are clearly nonvascular in nature.
B. The right leg ankle-brachial index is 0.65.
C. The left leg ankle-brachial index is 0.65.
D. The patient has right subclavian artery disease.
E. The right leg ankle-brachial index is 0.82.

25. A 67-year-old with chronic kidney disease is admitted to the hospital with acute pneumonitis complicated by new onset atrial fibrillation and is treated with intravenous unfractionated heparin. Admission labs: BUN 52 mg/dL, creatinine 3.8 mg/dL, WBCs 9 × 103/mm³; PLT 196 × 103/ mm. On hospital day 6, the patient develops acute right calf pain/ swelling. A venous duplex ultrasound displays an acute right femoropopliteal deep venous thrombosis. The PLT count is now 55 × 103/mm³. Heparin induced thrombocytopenia and thrombosis is suspected and serologic confirmation is pending. Which of the following is the most appropriate therapy for presumed HITT in this patient?

A. Enoxaparin
B. Argatroban
C. Warfarin
D. Lepirudin

26. The patency rates for surgical revascularization for aorto-iliac disease using an aorto-bifemoral bypass graft at 5 years in intermittent claudication is:

A. 75 to 80%
B. 90 to 95%
C. 65 to 70%
D. 80 to 85%

27. Which of the following ulcerations can be associated with pathergy?

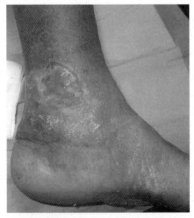

FIGURE 30-2A.   (See color insert.)

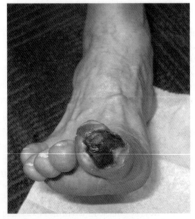

FIGURE 30-2B.   (See color insert.)

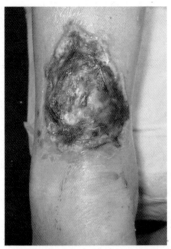

FIGURE 30-2C. (See color insert.)

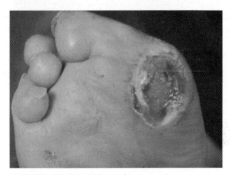

FIGURE 30-2D. (See color insert.)

28. A patient in perioperative assessment has a history of cardiac events and is of low functional capacity. You estimate that it is unclear whether or not this patient would benefit from beta-blockers. Would the use of beta-blockers be an acceptable treatment prior to intervention?
A. Yes—Patient is clearly high-risk.
B. Yes—Patient has a history of cardiac events and use of beta-blockers will lower risk.
C. No—Absolute benefit is unknown and may complicate condition.
D. No—Beta-blockers are unsafe for patients undergoing perioperative assessment.

29. According to the ESCHAR trial, what is the advantage of greater saphenous vein ablation in a patient with stage C6 disease?
A. Increased number of healed ulcers
B. Decreased ulcer recurrence
C. Increased rate of ulcer healing
D. Decreased rate of varicosity formation

30. A 58-year-old man presents to your office with a chief complaint of a swollen, painful left leg. A venous duplex ultrasound reveals an occlusive thrombus within the left superficial femoral vein. What is the most appropriate initial therapy for this patient?
A. Nonsteroidal anti-inflammatory medication with heat and elevation
B. Aspirin 325 mg daily
C. Enoxaparin 1 mg/kg twice daily with concurrent warfarin
D. Repeat venous duplex ultrasound in 5 to 7 days to assess for thrombotic propagation.

31. A 76-year-old man presents with a nonhealing ulcer of the right great toe. He is not a candidate for surgical or endovascular revascularization. Which of the following therapies is most likely to lead to improved wound healing?
A. Low-molecular-weight heparin
B. Intravenous naftidrofuryl
C. Debridement and a dry dressing
D. Intermittent pneumatic compression

32. All of the following are diagnostic criteria for Takayasu's arteritis except:
A. Onset of illness by age 40 years
B. Upper-extremity claudication
C. Association with smoking
D. Greater than 10 mm Hg difference between systolic blood pressure in the arms
E. Narrowing of the aorta or a major branch

33. Which of the following changes at the scanner console will help reduce the radiation dose delivered to the patient?
A. Decreasing tube voltage.
B. Increasing tube current.
C. Decreasing the pitch (from 1.0 to 0.5).
D. Increasing the thickness of the reconstructed slices.

34. Which of the following may improve symptoms in patients with erythermalgia?
A. Cilostazol
B. Nifedipine
C. Topical Lidocaine patches
D. Warfarin

35. The most important diagnostic criterion suggestive of a greater than 70% carotid stenosis on duplex ultrasonography is:
A. End-diastolic velocity 55 cm/s
B. Peak systolic velocity 350 cm/s
C. ICA/CCA systolic velocity ratio 3.2
D. Spectral broadening

36. Which of the following MRA techniques would be the best for assessment of vasculitis involving the thoracic aorta?
A. Contrast enhanced MRA
B. Time of flight imaging
C. Dark blood imaging—HASTE or SPACE
D. Phase contrast imaging

37. Endovenous ablation of the Great Saphenous vein with radiofrequency or laser is often performed in conjunction with all of the following procedures except:

A. Ligation of saphenofemoral junction

B. Stab avulsion phlebectomy

C. Ligation of the femoral vein

D. Sclerotherapy

38. Intermittent claudication (IC) is a symptom of PAD. The following is an accurate statement regarding IC in PAD:

A. 30% have classic claudication, 50% have atypical leg pain, and the remaining 20% did are asymptomatic.

B. 10% have classic claudication, 50% have atypical leg pain, and the remaining 40% did not have exercise induced leg pain.

C. 50% have classic claudication, 40% have atypical leg pain, and the remaining 10% did not have exercise induced leg pain.

D. 20% have classic claudication, 30% have atypical leg pain, and the remaining 50% did not have exercise induced leg pain.

39. Repair of TAA is indicated in asymptomatic patients with degenerative thoracic aneurysm, chronic aortic dissection, intramural hematoma, penetrating atherosclerotic ulcer, mycotic aneurysm, or pseudoaneurysm, and for whom the ascending aorta or aortic sinus diameter is:

A. 6.0 cm or greater

B. 5.5 cm or greater

C. 6.5 cm or greater

D. 5.0 cm or greater

40. A 65-year-old male is being evaluated for the management of an asymptomatic 2.0 cm aneurysm of the common hepatic artery. All of the following statements regarding this visceral aneurysm are true with the exception of:

A. The rupture rate of hepatic aneurysms is high at 20% of cases.

B. The appropriate management of the patient involves removal of the aneurysm by surgery or endovascular approaches.

C. Repair should be initiated only if the aneurysm exceeds 3.0 cm.

D. Etiologies include atherosclerosis, polyarteritis nodosa and cystic medial necrosis.

41. A 60-year-old male underwent EVAR for a 6 cm AAA 1 month ago. The patient underwent a follow-up CT scan that demonstrated an endoleak associated with a lumbar artery. The aneurysm diameter has not changed in size since the time of the procedure. What type of endoleak does this patient have, and what management/intervention is appropriate for this patient?

A. Type I, open surgical repair of the aneurysm.

B. Type II, CT surveillance every 6 months to evaluate for late-onset expansion.

C. Type III, selective catheterization of the lumbar artery with coil embolization.

D. Type III, laparoscopically clip the lumbar artery.

42. A 19-year-old woman presents with unilateral right lower limb enlargement that has been progressively getting worse over the last 12 months. The skin overlying the limb displays a bluish discoloration. There was no bruit over the limb. Stemer sign was negative. Branhams sign was negative. MR angiography/venography revealed numerous large venous channels with absence of a clearly differentiated venous system. The most likely diagnosis is:
A. Klippel Trenaunay syndrome
B. Parke-Weber form of Klippel Trenaunay syndrome
C. Sturge Weber syndrome
D. Klippel Feil syndrome

43. A 42-year-old patient presents with severe rest pain in his lower extremity and gives a history of smoking. Angiographic evaluation reveals classic distal involvement with absence of proximal involvement and cork-screw collaterals. Which one of the following additional factors may play a role in the pathogenesis of Buerger's disease?
A. Antiphospholipid antibodies.
B. Antibasement membrane antibodies
C. Matrix metalloproteinases
D. Anti-TGF antibodies

44. The recommended minimal anticoagulation treatment for upper extremity deep venous thrombosis is?
A. One month
B. Two months
C. Three months
D. Six months

45. A 60-year-old female presents to your clinic with the lower extremities shown in Figure 30-3.

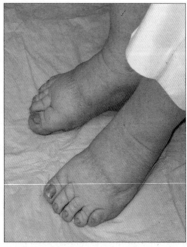

FIGURE 30-3.   (See color insert.)

A CT scan of her chest will most likely reveal a:
A. Pulmonary arteriovenous malformation
B. Pleural effusion
C. Pulmonary emboli
D. Pulmonary alveolar hemorrhage

46. What is the most common type of primary lymphedema?
A. Lymphedema tarda
B. Filariasis
C. Lymphedema praecox
D. Post mastectomy lymphedema

47. A 65-year-old male, status post EVAR for AAA 1 year ago, presents with 24 hours of worsening left flank pain. He is slightly tachycardic and normotensive. On examination, his abdomen is slightly distended, and he has a tender pulsatile mass in his left lower quadrant. CT scan demonstrates a large amount of retroperitoneal blood. What is the status of this patient's AAA, and what treatment option is appropriate for this patient?
A. Ruptured AAA
B. Perforated diverticulitis.
C. Nephrolithiasis with perforated calyx.
D. May-Thurner syndrome

48. The following features are suspicious for Livedo Racemosa:
A. Generalized distribution
B. Irregular "broken" rings
C. Asymmetric distribution
D. All of the above

49. Possible options for antiplatelet therapy for stroke prevention includes all of the following except:
A. Aspirin alone
B. Clopidogrel alone
C. Aspirin with clopidogrel
D. Aspirin with extended-release dipyridamole

50. All of the agents listed below are generally effective for sclerotherapy of varicose veins except:
A. Tetradecyl sulfate
B. Hypertonic saline
C. Polidocanol
D. Normal saline

51. Which of the following setting is needed to image the ascending thoracic aorta and coronary arteries simultaneously when there is a suspicion of thoracic aortic dissection?
A. Gated acquisition should be performed.
B. Field of view should extend from the thoracic inlet to the aortic bifurcation.
C. Minimal detector collimation should be used.
D. Pre and post contrast studies may be performed for the assessment of hemorrhage, intramural hematoma, and slow leaks.
E. All of the above are necessary.

52. An arteriogram is obtained on a 25-year-old left-handed man with exertional arm pain. What is the most likely cause of the abnormality illustrated in this arteriogram (Fig. 30-4)?

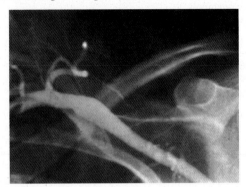

FIGURE 30-4.   (Courtesy of Dr. Thom Rooke, Mayo Clinic Foundation.)

A. Thoracic outlet syndrome
B. Takayasu's arteritis
C. Premature atherosclerosis
D. Ehlers-Danlos syndrome

53. A 47-year-old physician presents concerned about the appearance of her legs and varicose veins. On examination she has reticular veins and venous telangectasias over both extremities. She has 1+ late day edema without changes of lipodermatosclerosis or hemosiderin staining. She is an interventional cardiologist and spends several days a week standing in the imaging laboratory. What advice should you give her regarding her condition?
A. Recommend descending venography with plans for endovenous ablation.
B. Schedule her for duplex ultrasound of the great saphenous vein followed by radiofrequency ablation.
C. Recommend the use of compression stockings and elevation.
D. Prescribe diuretics and reassure her no additional therapy is warranted.

54. You are asked to provide anticoagulation recommendations on a 66-year-old patient with an acute left lower extremity proximal DVT in the setting of underlying Stage III ovarian carcinoma. According to current guidelines, which of the following anticoagulation regimens should you suggest?
A. Unfractionated or low-molecular-weight heparin for greater than 5 days followed by a Vitamin K antagonist for 6 to 12 months
B. Unfractionated or low-molecular-weight heparin for greater than 5 days followed by a Vitamin K antagonist for 6 to 12 months plus Inferior Vena Cava filter insertion
C. Unfractionated or low-molecular-weight heparin for greater than 5 days followed by a Vitamin K antagonist indefinitely
D. Low-molecular-weight heparin for at least the first 3 months of therapy.

55. Cilostazol is a Type III phosphodiesterase inhibitor that has been shown to be of modest efficacy in patients with intermittent claudication. The following are correct statements regarding its effects except:
A. Inhibition of vascular smooth muscle proliferation
B. Improvements in serum lipoproteins (10% decrease in triglycerides and 4% increase in HDL)
C. It is contraindicated in patients with advanced CHF with an LVEF of less than 35%.
D. Interference with the effects of clopidogrel contributing to clopidogrel resistance

56. A patient is referred for assessment of abdominal aortic aneurysm and has a GFR of 28 mL/min. Which of the following tests is appropriate?
A. CTA of the abdominal aorta with contrast.
B. Contrast enhanced MRA of the abdominal aorta.
C. Invasive angiogram.
D. Dark blood MRA imaging of the abdominal aorta.

57. Digital plethysmography is performed on a 51-year-old right-handed laborer with ischemic fingers (Fig. 30-5). What is the most likely diagnosis?

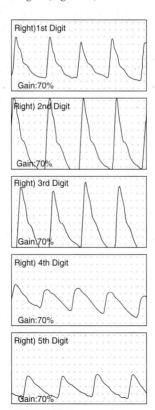

FIGURE 30-5.

A. C5-C6 cervical radiculopathy.
B. Hypothenar hammer syndrome
C. Vibration white finger
D. Carpal tunnel syndrome

58. What is the best conduit for bypasses in children?
A. Lesser saphenous vein
B. Internal iliac artery
C. Cryopreserved vein
D. Internal jugular vein

59. All of the following are thought to inhibit enlargement of thoracic aortic aneurysm except?
A. Doxycycline
B. Beta-blocker
C. Diuretics
D. Smoking cessation

60. Which of the following statements is most correct?
A. Patients without preexisting peripheral vascular disease with acute embolization typically have class I or IIa ischemia.
B. Thrombolysis is best for most cases of in situ thrombosis of native axial vessels or bypass grafts, provided that the limb is not immediately threatened.
C. Pharmacomechanical thrombolysis has been proven to be more effective than standard catheter directed thrombolysis in randomized trials.
D. Patients with preexisting peripheral vascular disease who develop in situ thrombosis typically have class IIb or III ischemia.

61. Which of the following sequences can be used to identify the hemodynamic consequence of an identified vascular stenosis?
A. CE-MRA
B. HASTE
C. Phase contrast imaging
D. SPACE

62. Which of the following is characteristic of patients with acrocyanosis?
A. Pain
B. Pallor
C. Episodic presentation
D. Bluish discoloration of skin

63. Bypass versus Angioplasty in Severe Ischemia of the Leg (BASIL), has compared outcome of a surgery-first with an angioplasty-first strategy in patients with severe limb ischemia due to infrainguinal disease in patients with CLI. Which of the following statements about the BASIL trial is incorrect?
A. The primary outcome measure of amputation free survival was no different between the two groups at 2 years.
B. Re-intervention was required in 50% of the surgical arm.

C. The use of evidence based pharmacotherapy for prevention of cardiovascular events was poor (statins, ASA, and ACE inhibitors) in the trial.

D. Short-term (30-day) events were higher in the surgical group compared to the endovascular group.

64. All of the features are consistent with symptoms of intermittent claudication except:

A. Pain in the buttocks and hips on exertion that extends to the calves on walking

B. Pain in the buttocks and hips on exertion that relieves immediately on resting/sitting down

C. Pain in the buttocks and hips on exertion that relieves on resting for less than 5 minutes

D. Pain in feet with exertion in a patient who smokes

65. A patient with a history of recently worsening claudication presents with a pale, cool foot. He has absent sensation, weakness of ankle plantar flexion, and is unable to dorsiflex his ankle. There is no arterial Doppler signal but he does have a venous Doppler signal. What is the most appropriate treatment for this patient?

A. Catheter directed thrombolysis

B. Admission, heparinization, and plan for angiography the next morning

C. Immediate transport to the OR/hybrid angiography suite for on table angiography and immediate revascularization

D. Pharmacomechanical thrombolysis

66. Median arcuate ligament syndrome is a cause of mesenteric ischemia. Features of the syndrome include all of the following except:

A. May be associated with a bruit

B. Occurs primarily in older males

C. Entrapment of celiac trunk by the median ligament of the diaphragm

D. Is often seen in asymptomatic individuals undergoing noninvasive vascular testing such as CTA or MRA

67. All of the following are forms of vasculitis that are most likely to lead to the loss of a pulse except:

A. Henoch-Schönlein purpura

B. Giant cell arteritis

C. Buerger's disease

D. Takayasu's arteritis

68. All of the following are reasonable to prevent contrast nephropathy except:

A. Staging procedures as appropriate

B. Sodium bicarbonate, 3 mL/kg·h, for 1 hour before and 1 mL/kg·h for 6 hours after contrast administration

C. Intravenous normal saline 150 to 250 mL prior to the procedure followed by 75 to 100 mL/h for 6 to 12 hours after contrast administration

D. Minimizing the total volume of the contrast given

E. Administer IV furosemide 80 mg prior to the procedure

69. The CE-MRA technique should be avoided in patients with a GFR of?
   A. GFR > 60 mL/min
   B. GFR > 30 mL/min
   C. GFR < 60 mL/min
   D. GFR < 30 mL/min

70. An ankle-brachial index greater than 1.30 is consistent with:
   A. Stiff, noncompliant arteries
   B. Normal arterial circulation
   C. A diagnosis of diabetes mellitus
   D. Hypertension

71. A 65-year-old Caucasian male patient presents with an apparent pulmonary-renal syndrome, and purpura. He claims no problems with the respiratory tract. Further testing reveals ANCA. What is the most reasonable diagnosis?
   A. Hypersensitivity vasculitis
   B. Microscopic polyangiitis
   C. Giant cell arteritis
   D. Kawasaki disease

ANSWERS

1. C. In this tachycardic patient with hypertension IV betablockers are the best initial therapy. If systolic blood pressures remain greater than 120 mm Hg after adequate heart rate control has been obtained, then angiotensin-converting enzyme inhibitors and/or other vasodilators should be administered intravenously to further reduce blood pressure that maintains adequate end-organ perfusion. (see Chapter 14).

2. E. A noncontrast CT can help in determining the presence of hematoma and hemorrhage in the adjacent structure. Delayed imaging can help in picking up slow bleeds (see Chapter 5).

3. D. Percutaneous revascularization is indicated for patients with hemodynamically significant RAS and recurrent, unexplained congestive heart failure and sudden, unexplained pulmonary edema as a class I indication (see Chapter 10).

4. D. Lateral projection accurately shows the origin of the mesenteric arteries, that is, celiac artery (CA), superior mesenteric artery (SMA), and inferior mesenteric arteries (IMA) (see Chapter 3).

5. D. Poor functional capacity or a combination of high-risk surgery and moderate functional capacity in a patient with intermediate clinical predictors of cardiac risk (especially if there are two or more) often requires further noninvasive cardiac testing (see Chapter 28).

6. A. Balloon expandable stents have more radial strength and are best suited for aorto-ostial stenosis. Self expanding stents and plain balloon angioplasty do not perform as well at these sites. Furthermore, accurate placement is more likely with balloon expandable stents with a mm or so of the stent sticking out in the aorta to completely cover the ostial lesion (see Chapter 17).

7. B. Prosthetic bypass infection is best treated by removal of the focus of infection and keeping the path of the new bypass in an anatomic field that is separate for the previous graft (see Chapter 29).

8. A. This patient has evidence placing him at intermediate risk based on the Second Princeton Consensus and therefore the recommendation is for noninvasive testing to attempt to place the patient in a low or high risk category based on the findings. Even patients at low risk are suggested to undergo noninvasive testing. A trial of phosphodiesterase treatment would be indicated once ensuring the patient is not at high risk and needing further testing. A penile Doppler ultrasound has little role until after a failed phosphodiesterase trial (see Chapter 24).

9. B. A pulse-wave catheter, centered in the obstructing thrombosis, delivering rTPA over 15 minutes, may be utilized (see Chapter 23).

10. C. Venography is required prior to the intervention to localize the stenosis. Access is achieved by inserting a needle antegrade into the fistula or graft and inserting a sheath. Once access is achieved and a fistulogram defines the lesion, angioplasty can be performed (see Chapter 27).

11. D. Angiotensin-converting enzyme inhibitors are effective medications for treatment of hypertension associated with unilateral RAS and recommended in the ACC/AHA guidelines (see Chapter 10).

12. C. The 2010 ACC/AHA guidelines for aortic disease recommend for patients undergoing aortic valve repair or replacement and who have an ascending aorta or aortic root of greater than 4.5 cm should be considered for concomitant repair of the aortic root or replacement of the ascending aorta (Level I, evidence C) (see Chapter 13).

13. D. Patients on treatment have shown in several studies to have no increase in myocardial infarction likelihood assuming they can tolerate moderate exercise. Nitrate therapy is a contraindication for the use of phosphodiesterase inhibitor therapy (see Chapter 24).

14. D. Given her history, the current complaint must be evaluated for acute DVT. Duplex ultrasound is the best option for this. In addition she may have symptoms of postthrombotic syndrome exacerbated by the flight. Duplex ultrasound is useful to evaluate for reflux or other chronic changes within the vein that may be contributing (see Chapter 19).

15. D. Use of vessel mapping has been shown to be associated with a higher rate of AVF placement, although this does not translate into a higher maturity rate of AVF (see Chapter 27).

16. B. Though the use of corticosteroids has never been shown to be of therapeutic benefit except in care reports, recent data have shown a role for immunosuppression with cyclophosphamide (see Chapter 9).

17. B. Pernio, a common condition in women. The photograph shows a clear case of pernio (see Chapter 18).

18. C. The vast majority of patients with IC (≈70%) do not alter their symptoms. Major amputation is relatively rare in IC, with 1 to 3% needing major amputation over a 5-year period (see Chapter 6).

19. A. Splenic artery aneurysms are the most common form of visceral aneurysms and are most commonly located in the distal third of the splenic artery. FMD is likely the most important etiology in the majority of cases. Rupture risk increases in pregnancy (see Chapter 15).

20. C. Patients without symptomatic relief are recommended to undergo varicose vein excision (VVE). Those patients found to have superficial reflux should undergo great saphenous ablation (VA) at the same time as VVE (see Chapter 22).

21. A. Hydrogen nuclei is the most commonly used nuclei for MRI applications (see Chapter 4).

22. D. Carotid stenting is currently approved for patients at high risk for CEA who have symptomatic carotid artery stenosis greater than 70%, as long as stenting is performed using FDA-approved systems with embolic-protection devices (see Chapter 11).

23. D. All the above described conditions can predispose patients to NSF (see Chapter 4).

24. D. Using the classic calculations of the ABI, the right ABI is 140/200 = 0.7. The left ABI is 110/200 = 0.55. Therefore, choices B, C, and E are incorrect. The history and Doppler pressures are, in fact, suggestive of a vascular etiology. Therefore, choice "A" is incorrect. Note the discrepancy in arm blood pressures, with the right arm pressure 30 mm Hg lower than the left, suggesting right subclavian artery disease (see Chapter 2).

25. B. Low-molecular-weight heparins such as enoxaparin are contraindicated in the setting of HITT. Warfarin use is also contraindicated in the setting of acute HIT and should never be initiated until the platelet count has recovered. The direct thrombin inhibitors argatroban and lepirudin are approved medications for treating HITT in the United States. However, lepirudin is renally excreted and thus the half life would be expected to unpredictably rise when used in a patient with significant azotemia (such as the patient presented above). Since argatroban is eliminated in the hepatobiliary system, it is the most logical agent to use in the setting of HITT and azotemia. Thus, the correct answer is B (see Chapter 21).

26. B. Most contemporary analysis estimates the long-term patency at greater than 90% (see Chapter 6).

27. C. "Pathergy" or hyperreactivity of the skin, is a process whereby minimal dermal trauma can provoke pustules and/or ulcerations in susceptible patients. Pyoderma gangrenosum ulcerations often evolve from a pathergic type response. Image "C" is a classic illustration of a pyoderma gangrenosum ulceration with a well-defined, edematous, violaceous border combined with a fibropurulent and partially necrotic base. Venous stasis (A), ischemic (B), and neuropathic (D) ulcerations do not exhibit the pathergic response (see Chapter 18).

28. C. Beta-blockers appear to lower risk in those considered very high-risk patients for perioperative cardiac events. However, perioperative beta blockade has a dark side, requiring controlled, strategic implementation only in those where the absolute benefit of such therapy is apparent (see Chapter 28).

29. B. Even if conservative measures are successful, these patients may benefit from a decreased risk of ulcer recurrence with treatment of superficial reflux though VVE and VA (see Chapter 22).

30. C. Although the term "superficial femoral vein" may suggest the diagnosis of superficial thrombophlebitis to some, this vein is a component of the deep system. Consequently, typical therapy for deep venous thrombosis is required when the superficial femoral vein is thrombosed. Since "superficial" femoral vein is somewhat of a misnomer, "femoral vein" is now the preferred anatomic nomenclature. Thus, the correct answer is C (see Chapter 21).

Reference:
Hammond I. The superficial femoral vein. *Radiology* 2003;229(2):604; discussion 604–606.

31. D. Intermittent pneumatic compression which has been shown in controlled studies to improve wound healing (see Chapter 8).

Reference:
Kavros SJ Delis KT, Turner NS, et al. Improving limb salvage in critical limb ischemia with intermittent pneumatic compression: a controlled study with 18-month follow-up. *J Vasc Surg* 2008;47:543–549.

32. C. The diagnostic criteria for Takayasu's arteritis includes onset of disease by 40 years of age, upper extremity claudication, greater than 10 mm systolic blood pressure difference in the arms and narrowing of the great vessels. Takayasu's arteritis is not associated with smoking (see Chapter 17).

33. A. Decreasing tube voltage and current and increasing the pitch will decrease the total dose of radiation delivered to the patient (see Chapter 5).

34. C. Topical Lidocaine may be effective in erythermalgia owing to the effects of Lidocaine in blocking sodium channels. A role for the neuronal voltage-gated sodium channel (Nav1.7) has been demonstrated in erythermalgia (see Chapter 18).

35. B. The most important criterion for the diagnosis of an internal carotid artery stenosis via duplex ultrasonography is the peak systolic velocity. Choice "A" is incorrect, as an end-diastolic velocity; a secondary criterion of 55 cm/s is normal and would not suggest greater than 70% stenosis. The ICA/CCA ratio of 3.2 does not correlate with greater than 70% stenosis. Spectral broadening is demonstrative of mild stenosis (greater than 20%) (see Chapter 2).

36. C. Dark blood imaging generally is best in assessment vessel wall pathology. HASTE is a 2D technique while SPACE is a 3D technique (see Chapter 4).

37. C. Answers A, B, and D can also be performed concomitantly if necessary with endovenous ablation with a laser of radio frequency. Ligation of the femoral vein is not an option for treatment of varicose veins and can lead to significant complications including deep venous thrombosis (see Chapter 20).

38. B. 10% have classic claudication, 50% have atypical leg pain, and the remaining 40% did not have exercise-induced leg pain (see Chapter 6).

Reference:
McDermott MM, Greenland P, Liu K, et al. Leg symptoms in peripheral arterial disease. *JAMA* 2001;286(13):1599–1606.

39. B. In general, the American Heart Association recommends that patients with infrarenal or juxtarenal AAAs measuring 5.5 cm or larger should undergo repair to eliminate the risk of rupture (see Chapter 14).

40. C. Repair is advocated regardless of size in majority of hepatic artery aneurysms. Intrahepatic aneurysm may be treated with catheter-based embolization while extrahepatic aneurysms may be excised or excluded (see Chapter 15).

41. B. The diameter has not changed, so there is no need to repair AAA, and surveillance for 6 months is suggested due to possible expansion at a later time. This is a classic type II endoleak (see Chapter 12).

42. A. Klippel-Trenaunay typically presents with discoloration or port wine stain involving an extremity with associated venous varicosities and absent deep venous system; Parke-Weber syndrome is a subset of Klippel-Trenaunay with direct arteriovenous malformations/communication with a tendency for high-output congestive heart failure. The lack of direct arterial venous communication excludes Parke-Weber syndrome. Sturge Weber syndrome presents with port-wine stain in the trigeminal nerve distribution characterized by the congenital fusion of any two of the seven cervical vertebra (see Chapter 1).

43. A. Antiphospholipid antibody syndrome or APS is an autoimmune disorder that has been associated with Buerger's disease. APS is the result of the production of antibodies in defense against the certain normal components of blood and/or cell membranes as foreign substances (see Chapter 9).

44. C. Either unfractionated or low-molecular-weight heparin is given initially and followed by warfarin or other anti-vitamin K agents for a minimum of 3 months with a goal international normalized ratio (INR) of 2.0 to 3.0 (see Chapter 23).

45. B. The photograph depicts two components of the triad of the "yellow nail syndrome," specifically, lymphedema and yellow nails. A pleural effusion is the remaining element of the classic YNS triad. The remaining detractors are not typical pulmonary conditions found in this disorder (see Chapter 26).

46. C. Lymphedema praecox is the most common subtype of primary lymphedema accounting for 77 to 94% of all primary forms. Lymphedema tarda is responsible for approximately 10% of primary lymphedema cases. Both filariasis and post mastectomy lymphedema are secondary causes of lymphedema (see Chapter 26).

47. A. The pathway of fluid flow from the retroperitoneal space into the pelvic extraperitoneal space on CT is often the result of AAA rupture. Given a history of AAA EVAR, suspect rupture with immediate worsening left flank pain (see Chapter 12).

48. D. In livedo reticularis, the discoloration is exemplified by symmetric, regular, "unbroken" rings whereas livedo racemosa is marked by irregular "broken" rings. Livedo reticularis symmetrically affects the extremities whereas livedo racemosa often involves the limbs in an asymmetric fashion. Livedo racemosa tends to be more generalized often involving the buttocks, trunk, and even the feet and hands (see Chapter 18).

49. C. Aspirin (50 to 325 mg/d) monotherapy, the combination of aspirin and extended-release dipyridamole, and clopidogrel monotherapy are all acceptable options for initial therapy for stroke prevention. The combination of aspirin with clopidogrel was associated with increased intracranial bleeds in the MATCH study and is not recommended (see Chapter 11).

50. D. Answers A, B, and C are all options for sclerosing varicose, reticular and spider veins. However, normal saline does not have a sclerosant effect (see Chapter 20).

51. E. All of the elements are required to avoid (a) artifact, (b) extent, (c) missing subtle aortic wall hematoma (c) complications (see Chapter 5).

52. A. The arteriogram illustrates a small subclavian artery aneurysm that arose from post stenotic dilatation secondary to compression in association with an elongated cervical rib. Thus, thoracic outlet syndrome is the most likely diagnosis. There is no arteriographic evidence of arteritis or atherosclerosis. Although Ehlers-Danlos syndrome is associated with aneurysms, it is not the most likely diagnosis in the presence of a prominent cervical rib (see Chapter 16).

53. C. Given her history and relatively asymptomatic venous disease compression and elevation are likely to provide the most relief. In the absence of more significant clinical findings it is unlikely that she has significant reflux that needs evaluation and intervention. Diuretics are of little use in this setting (see Chapter 19).

54. D. According to the eighth ACCP Consensus guidelines on antithrombotic therapy, "we recommend at least 3 months of treatment of LMWH for patients with VTE and cancer (Grade IA), followed by treatment with LMWH or VKA as long as the cancer is active (Grade IC)." In Lee's study, dalteparin was compared with VKA therapy for the long-term treatment of cancer patients with acute venous thromboembolic disease (proximal DVT and/or PE). At 6-month follow up, the long-term use of dalteparin was associated with a recurrent VTE disease RRR of ~50% when compared to a VKA ($p = 0.002$). Consequently, answer "D" is correct (see Chapter 21).

References:
Lee AY, Levine MN, Baker RI, et al. LMWH vs a coumarin for the prevention of recurrent venous thromboembolism in patients with cancer. *N Engl J Med* 2003;349:146–153.
Kearon C, Kahn SR, Agnelli G, et al. Antithrombotic therapy for venous thromboembolic disease. *American College of Chest Physicians Evidence-Based Clinical Practice Guidelines*, 8th ed. *Chest* 2008;133:454S–545S.

55. D. Cilostazol has been shown to inhibit platelet function. It does not interfere with the effects of clopidogrel (see Chapter 6).

56. D. All the other techniques are not appropriate in the context of such low GFR. Dark blood imaging is a noncontrast MRA technique which can provide high resolution assessment of the abdominal aorta (see Chapter 5).

57. B. A C5-C6 radiculopathy can be associated with vasospastic fingers; yet the thumb and index finger would be involved, but not the fourth and fifth digits.

Hypothenar hammer syndrome would be the most likely diagnosis since this condition commonly affects the digits supplied by the ulnar artery, specifically the fourth and fifth fingers. The plethysmographic waveforms from the right fourth and fifth digits display a diminished amplitude and loss of the dicrotic notch suggestive of ischemia.

Vibration white finger typically provokes diffuse vasospasm and therefore localized involvement of the fourth and fifth fingers would be less plausible.

Carpal tunnel syndrome can provoke digital vasospasm yet the thumb, index, and third fingers would be affected (see Chapter 16).

58. B. The arterial homograft, given its ability to grow and resistance to infection, is the ideal conduit for reconstruction after oncologic surgery, particularly in children and young adults (see Chapter 29).

59. C. There is no evidence that treatment with diuretics reduces aneurysmal size or mortality in patients with thoracic aortic aneurysm (see Chapter 13).

60. B. This is based on the TOPAS and STILE trials with intravenous thrombolysis that demonstrated a benefit in patients with Class I or II ischemia. A majority of patients in both of these trials had class I and IIa ischemia, with less than 25% having class IIb or III limb ischemia (see Chapter 7).

61. C. Stenosis can be identified using sequences 1, 2, or 4. However, to identify the hemodynamic consequence a flow based sequence called phase contrast imaging is used. This can be done in an in-plane view to visually assess the stenosis and in a through plane view to quantify the flow velocities at the site of stenosis (see Chapter 4).

62. D. Acrocyanosis is painless and is persistent (see Chapter 18).

63. B. In the BASIL trial re-intervention was far more frequent in the angioplasty arm (see Chapter 8).

Reference:
Adam DJ, Cleveland T Beard JD, et al. Bypass versus angioplasty in severe ischaemia of the leg (BASIL): multicentre, randomised controlled trial. *Lancet* 2005;366:1925–1934.

64. B. Pain in the buttocks and hips on exertion that relieves immediately on resting/sitting down is consistent with a diagnosis of spinal claudication (see Chapter 1).

65. C. This patient has both motor and sensory deficits and presents with class IIb ischemia. Thrombolytics or diagnostic angiography may require too much time and immediate revascularization is indicated. These patients should be taken immediately to surgery (see Chapter 7).

66. B. Median arcuate ligament syndrome is typically described in middle aged females. It is most commonly an incidental finding on imaging and may sometimes be associated with a bruit (see Chapter 15).

67. A. The three forms of vasculitis most likely to lead to loss of a pulse are TA, GCA, and Buerger's disease (see Practical Points in Chapter 25).

68. E. Staging procedures, administering hydration either with bicarbonate or normal saline, minimizing contrast volume have all been shown to reduce the incidence of contrast nephropathy. Administering a diuretic will increase the risk of contrast nephropathy (see Chapter 3).

69. D. Although GFR < 30 is not an absolute contraindication for gadolinium contrast based imaging, there must be a strong clinical indication where the benefits clearly outweigh the risks in order for gadolinium to be used. The risk of NSF is much higher with GFR < 30 (see Chapter 4).

70. A. A normal ABI is defined as 0.91 to 1.00. A high ankle brachial index suggests that the ankle arteries are stiff and noncompliant. Although this is commonly seen in patients with diabetes mellitus, there are other potential etiologies, including the elderly, those with chronic corticosteroid use, and those requiring hemodialysis (see Chapter 2).

71. B. Necrotizing glomerulonephritis is very common and pulmonary capillaritis is not an infrequent complication. Patients may thus present with a pulmonary-renal syndrome which must be distinguished from antiglomerular basement membrane disease. MPA has many similarities to WG, but prominent involvement of the upper respiratory tract is uncommon (see Chapter 25.)

Note: Page numbers followed by "f" indicate figures, and page numbers followed by "t" indicate tables.